Apoptosis Signals

Cytoplasm

TRANCE
RANK
ATAR
TACI
TNF
TNFR2
TNF
TNFR2
TNF
TNFR1
FasL
Fas
TRAIL
DR5
TRAIL
DR4
TRAIL
DCR2
TRAIL
DCR1
DR3

Jun/Fos
Granzyme B
Perforin

Growth Factor

Ceramide

Mitochondria

Radiation

Serum Starvation

Jun
Jun
Death

Nuclear Collapse
DNA fragmentation

Nucleus

Cell Activation

TCF ELK1
NF-κB
NF-AT
Atf2

Pathway Functions

↑ The path of cell death
↑ Neutral or bifunctional
↑ Cell activation
↑ Proteolytic activity
↑ Blocking or inhibition
↑ Opposes death

Functional Families

Bcl-2
A1 (homologous)
Bcl-2
BHRF1 (ebv)
vbcl-2 (hsv)
E1B 19K (adenov)
Mcl1

Bak
Bax
Bad
Bid
Bik/Nbk

Apoptosis Inhibitors
BHRF1
crmA (cowpox virus)
DEVD-CHO
E8
FLICE/FLAME, cFLIP
IETD-CHO
MC159
p35 (baculovirus)
XIAP (h-il-2, ilpA)
YVAD-CHO

Related Proteins
APAF-1 (ced4)
APAF-2 (cytochrome c)

Death Receptors
Fas (Apo1, Cd95)
DR3 (Apo3, Wsl1, TRAMP, LARD)
DR4 (Apo2, TRAILr1)
DR5 (Killer, TRAILr2, TRICK2)
DCR1 (TRAILr3, TRID)
DCR2 (TRAILr4, TRUNDD)
TNFR1

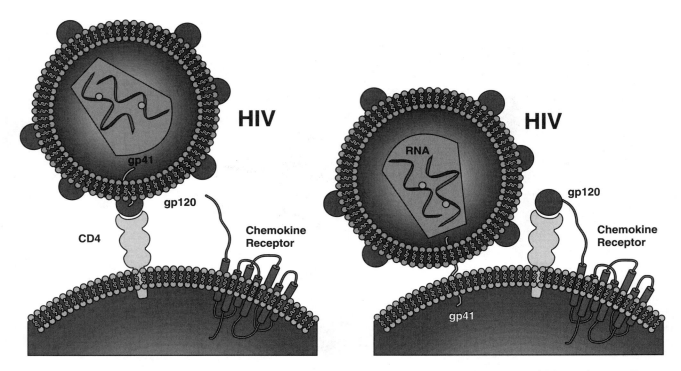

Proposed scheme for interaction of HIV with CD4 and CXCR4 (above). (Courtesy of PharMingen; *Science* 274: 602-5, 1996)

Apoptosis signaling (overleaf). (Courtesy of PharMingen)

ATLAS OF IMMUNOLOGY

JULIUS M. CRUSE
B.A., B.S., D.Med.Sc., M.D., PH.D., F.A.A.M., F.R.S.H.

Professor of Pathology
Director of Immunopathology and Transplantation Immunology
Director of Graduate Studies in Pathology
Department of Pathology
Associate Professor of Medicine and Associate Professor of Microbiology
University of Mississippi Medical Center
Investigator of the Wilson Research Foundation
Mississippi Methodist Rehabilitation Center
Jackson, MS

ROBERT E. LEWIS
B.S., M.S., Ph.D., F.R.S.H.

Professor of Pathology
Co-Director of Immunopathology and Transplantation Immunology
Department of Pathology
University of Mississippi Medical Center
Investigator of the Wilson Research Foundation
Mississippi Methodist Rehabilitation Center
Jackson, MS

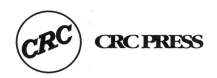 CRC PRESS

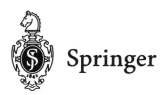 Springer

Library of Congress Cataloging-in-Publication Data

Catalog record is available from the Library of Congress.

Co-published by
CRC Press LLC
2000 Corporate Blvd., N.W.
Boca Raton, FL 33431, U.S.A.
(Orders from the U.S.A. and Canada (only) to CRC Press LLC)

and by
Springer-Verlag GmbH & Co. KG
Tiergartenstraße 17
D-69121 Heidelberg
Germany
(Orders from outside the U.S.A. and Canada to Springer-Verlag)
ISBN 3-540-64807-0 (alk. paper)

Dedicated to

Earl R. Wilson

Martha Lyles Wilson

Hyman F. McCarty, Jr.

Mary Ann McCarty

… truly persons of vision whose philanthropy and unselfish dedication to their fellow human beings in establishing the Mississippi Methodist Rehabilitation Center, the Wilson Research Foundation, and advancing medical education at the University of Mississippi Medical Center have inspired all of us who are beneficiaries of their generosity to create a better community, state and nation through medical research and improved patient care.

Editorial Staff for the Authors

CRC Press Editorial Staff

Authors

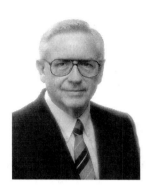

Julius M. Cruse, B.A., B.S., D.Med.Sc., M.D., Ph.D., is Professor of Pathology, Director of Immunopathology and Transplantation Immunology and Director of Graduate Studies in Medicine and Associate Professor of Microbiology. Formerly, Dr. Cruse was Professor of Immunology and of Biology in the University of Mississippi Graduate School.

Dr. Cruse graduated in 1958 with his B.A. and B.S. degrees in Chemistry from the University of Mississippi. He was a Fulbright Fellow at the University of Graz (Austria) Medical Faculty, where he wrote a thesis on *Russian Tickborne Encephalitis Virus* and received the D.Med.Sc. degree *summa cum laude* in 1960. On his return to the United States, he entered the M.D., Ph.D. program at the University of Tennessee College of Medicine, Memphis, completing the M.D. degree in 1964 and the Ph.D. in Pathology (immunopathology) in 1966. Dr. Cruse also trained in Pathology at the University of Tennessee Center for the Health Sciences, Memphis.

Dr. Cruse is a member of numerous professional societies which include the American Association of Immunologists (Historian), the American Society for Investigative Pathology, the American Society for Histocompatibility and Immunogenetics (Member of Council, formerly Chairman [1987-1995], Publications Committee 1987-1995), the Societe Francaise d'Immunologie, the Transplantation Society, the Society for Experimental Biology and Medicine, among many others. He is a Fellow of the American Academy of Microbiology and a Fellow of the Royal Society of Health (U.K.).

Dr. Cruse's research has centered on transplantation and tumor immunology, autoimmunity, MHC genetics in the pathogenesis of AIDS, and neuroendocrine immune interactions. He has received many research grants during his career and is presently funded by the Wilson Research Foundation for neuroendocrine-immune system interactions in spinal cord injury and stroke patients. He is the author of more than 250 publications in scholarly journals and 35 books, and has directed dissertation and thesis research for more than 40 graduate students during his career. He is the founding editor of the journals *Immunologic Research, Pathobiology and Transgenics.*

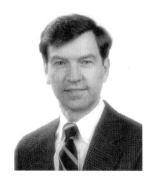

Robert E. Lewis, B.A., M.S., Ph.D., is Professor of Pathology and Co-Director of Immunopathology and Transplantation Immunology in the Department of Pathology at the University of Mississippi Center in Jackson.

Dr. Lewis received B.A. and M.S. in Microbiology degrees from the University of Mississippi and earned his Ph.D. in Pathology (Immunopathology) degree from the University of Mississippi Medical Center. Following specialty post-doctoral training at several medical institutions, Dr. Lewis has risen through the academic rank from Instructor to Professor at the University of Mississippi Medical Center.

Dr. Lewis is a member of numerous professional societies which include the American Immunologists, the American Society for Investigative Pathology, the Society for Experimental Biology and Medicine, the American Society for Microbiology, the Canadian Society for Immunology, the American Society for Histocompatibility and Immunogenetics (Vice Chairman, Publications Committee), among numerous other scientific organizations. He is a Fellow of the Royal Society of Health of Great Britain. Dr. Lewis has been the recipient of a number of research grants in his career and is currently funded by the Wilson Research Foundation for his research on neuroendocrine–immune system interaction in spinal cord injury and stroke patients.

Dr. Lewis has authored or co-authored more than 100 papers and 125 abstracts and has made numerous scientific presentations at both the national and international levels. In addition to neuroendocrine-immune interactions, his current research also includes immunogenetic aspects of AIDS progression. Dr. Lewis is a founder and editor of *Immunologic Research, Pathobiology* and *Transgenics.*

Preface

The *Atlas of Immunology* is designed to provide a pictorial reference and serve as a primary resource for the most up-to-date and thorough illustrated treatise available in the complex science of immunology. The book contains more than 1,000 illustrations and depicts essentially every concept of importance in understanding the subject matter of immunology. It is addressed to immunologists and nonimmunologists alike, including students, researchers, practitioners, and basic biomedical scientists. Use of the book does not require prior expertise. Some of the diagrams illustrate basic concepts, whereas others are designed for the specialist interested in a more detailed treatment of the subject matter of immunology. The group of illustrations is relatively complete and eliminates the need to refer to another source. The subject matter ranges from photographs of historical figures to molecular structures of recently characterized cytokines, the major histocompatibility complex molecules, immunoglobulins, and molecules of related interest to immunologists.

The subject matter is divided into chapters that follow an outline that correlates with a standard immunology textbook. This provides for a logical and sequential presentation and gives the reader ready access to each part of the subject matter as it relates to the other parts of the publication. These descriptive illustrations give the reader a concise and thorough understanding of basic immunological concepts that often intersect the purview of other basic and clinical scientific disciplines. A host of new illustrations, such as cellular adhesions molecules, is presented in a manner that facilitates better understanding of their role in intercellular and immune reactions. Figures that are pertinent to all of the immunological subspecialties, such as transplantation, autoimmunity, immunophysiology, immunopathology, antigen presentation, the T-cell receptor, to name a few, may be found in this publication. Those individuals with a need for ready access to a visual image of immunological information will want this book to be readily available in their bookshelf. No other publication provides the breadth or detail of illustrated immunological concepts as may be found in the *Atlas of Immunology*.

Acknowledgments

Although many individuals have offered help or suggestions in the preparation of this book, several deserve special mention. We are very grateful to Dr. Sherman Bloom, Chairman, and to Dr. Michael Hughson, Vice Chairman, Department of Pathology, University of Mississippi Medical Center, Jackson, for their genuine interest and generous support of our academic endeavors at this institution. Dr. Fredrick H. Shipkey, Professor of Pathology and Chief of Surgical Pathology, at the University of Mississippi Medical Center provided valuable assistance in selecting and photographing appropriate surgical pathology specimens to illustrate immunological lesions. We express genuine appreciation to Dr. Edwin and Dr. Marsha Eigenbrodt for many photomicrographs. We thank Prof. Albert Wahba for offering constructive criticism related to a number of the chemical structures and express genuine appreciation to Dr. Virginia Lockard for providing the electron micrographs that appear in the book. We also thank Dr. Robert Peace for a case of Job's syndrome, Dr. Ray Shenefelt for the photomicrograph of cytomegalovirus, Dr. Jonathan Fratkin for photomicrographs of eye and muscle pathology, Dr. C. J. Chen for VKH photos, Dr. Howard Shulman for GVH photos, Dr. David DeBauche for providing an illustration of the Philadelphia chromosome, Dorothy Whitcomb for the history photos, and Mr. Jerry Berndt for the photo of Dr. Thomas and Dr. Murray. We thank Dr. G. Reid Bishop of Emory University for his generous contribution of molecular models of cytokines and other configurations critical to immunology.

We express genuine appreciation to Mary Blaine, Dana Roe, Smaroula Dilioglou, and Jean Henderson for their dedicated efforts in helping us to complete this publication in a timely manner and making valuable editorial contributions. We also appreciate the constructive criticisms of Patsy Foley, B.S., M.T., C.H.T., Paula Hymel, B.S., M.T., C.H.T., Elisa Rodabough, B.S., M.T., C.H.T., Maxine Crawford, B.S., Kathy VanLandingham, B.S., M.T., C.H.T., and Susan Touchstone, B.S., M.T., S.B.B., C.H.T., C.H.S. We thank doctoral candidates Martha Brackin and Andrew Achord for constructive criticisms and William Buhner for scanning selected figures. We are most grateful to Joanna Arentz, of R&D Corp. for providing the artwork for the cover illustration and sharing with us a number of schematic diagrams of immunological molecules and concepts owned by R&D. We would also like to commend the individuals at CRC Press — Liz Covello, Acquiring Editor, Gerry Jaffe, Production Manager, Life Sciences and Forensics, Becky McEldowney, former Marketing Manager, Gary Bennett, Prepress Manager, and all members of their staff for their professionalism and unstinting efforts to bring this book to publication. To these individuals, we offer our grateful appreciation.

The authors' cellular immunology research is funded through the generous support of the Wilson Research Foundation, Mississippi Methodist Rehabilitation Center, Jackson, MS 39216.

Special thanks are expressed to Dr. A. Wallace Conerly, Dean of Medicine and Vice Chancellor for Health Affairs, University of Mississippi Medical Center, and to Mr. Mark Adams, CEO of Mississippi Methodist Rehabilitation Center, for their unstinting support of our research endeavors.

Illustration Credits

Figure 11-4 redrawn from Arlaud, G. J., Colomb, M. G., and Gagnon J. "A functional model of the human C1 complex." *Immunology Today* 8:107-109, 1987.

Figure 9-2 reprinted from *Atlas of Tumor Pathology*, 2d Series, Fascicle 13. Armed Forces Institute of Pathology.

Figures 9-3 and **9-8** reprinted from *Atlas of Tumor Pathology*, 3d Series, Fascicle 21. Armed Forces Institute of Pathology.

Figures 2-16, 2-39, 2-78, 2-85, 2-87, 4-18, 4-19, 9-22, 9-23, 9-28, 9-29, 9-38 and **9-39** redrawn from Barclay, A. N., Birkeland, M. L., Brown, M. H., Beyers, A. D., Davis, S. J., Somoza, C., and Williams, A. F. *The Leucocyte Antigen Facts Book*. Academic Press, Orlando, FL, 1993.

Figures 3-2, 6-19, 20-20, and **21-5** redrawn from Bellanti, J. A. *Immunology II*. W.B. Saunders Co., Philadelphia, PA, 1978.

Figure 1-55 reprinted with permission of Jerry Berndt.

Figure 4-22 reprinted with permission from *Nature*. Bjorkman, P. J., Saper, M. A., Samraoui, B., Bennet, W. S., Strominger, J. L., and Wiley, D. C. "Structure of the human class I histocompatibility antigen, HLA-A2." 329:506-512. ©1987 Macmillan Magazines Ltd.

Figure 7-11 reprinted by permission from *Nature*. Brambell, F. W. R., Hemmings, W. A., and Morris, I. G. "A theoretical model of gamma globulin catabolism." 203:1352-1355. ©1964 Macmillan Magazines Ltd.

Figure 7-12 reprinted from Brambell, F. W. R. "The transmission of immunity from mother to young and the catabolism of immunoglobulins." *The Lancet* 1966; ii:1087-1093.

Figure 6-55 redrawn from Capra, J. D. and Edmundson, A. B. "The antibody combining site." *Scientific American* 236:50-54, 1977. ©George V. Kelvin/*Scientific American*.

Figure 6-63 courtesy of Dr. Leon Carayannopoulos, Department of Microbiology, University of Texas, Southwestern Medical School, Dallas, TX.

Figure 7-28 redrawn from Conrad, D. H., Keegan, A. D., Kalli, K. R., Van Dusen, R., Rao, M., and Levine, A. D. "Superinduction of low affinity IgE receptors on murine B lymphocytes by LPS and interleukin-4." *Journal of Immunology*. 141:1091-7, 1988.

Figures 16-8 and **16-69** redrawn from Cotran, R. S., Kumar, V., and Robbins, S.L. *Robbins Pathologic Basis of Disease*. W. B. Saunders Co., Philadelphia, PA, 1989.

Figures 15-12, 15-24, and **15-26** reprinted from Daniels, G. *Human Blood Groups*. Blackwell Science Ltd, Oxford, UK, 1995. pp. 13, 271, 432

Figures 9-33 and **16-90** redrawn from Davis, M. M. "T cell receptor gene diversity and selection." *Annual Review of Biochemistry*. 59:477, 1990.

Figure 2-33 reprinted from Deutsch, M. and Weinreb, A. "Apparatus for high-precision repetitive sequential optical measurement of lifting cells." *Cytometry* 16:214-226. 1994. Adapted by permission of Wiley-Liss, Inc., a subsidiary of John Wiley & Sons, Inc.; and Marder, O. et al. "Effect of interleukin-1α, interleukin-1β, and tumor necrosis factor-α on the intercellular fluorescein fluorescence polarization of human lung fibroblasts." *Pathobiology*. 64(3): 123-130.

Figure 16-112 redrawn from Dieppe, P. A., Bacon, P. A., Bamji, A. N., and Watt, I. *Atlas of Clinical Rheumatology*. Lea & Febiger, Philadelphia, PA, 1986.

Figure 10-28 redrawn from Ealick, S. E., Cook, W. J., and Vijay-Kumar, S. "Three-dimensional structure of recombinant human interferon-γ." *Science* 252: 698-702. ©1991 American Association for the Advancement of Science.

Figures 16-27 and **16-28** adapted from Edmundson, A. B., Ely, K. R., Abola, E. E., Schiffer, M., and Panagotopoulos, N. "Rotational allomerism and divergent evolution of domains in immunoglobulin light chains." *Biochemistry* 14:3953-3961. ©1975 American Chemical Society.

Figures 2-30, 2-31, 2-41, 2-50, 2-68, 2-69, 2-71, 2-75, 2-76, 2-84, 2-85, 2-90, 2-94, 2-95, 2-98, 2-99, 2-103, 9-7, 20-33, 20-34, 20-35, 20-36, 20-37, 20-38, 20-39, 20-40, 20-41, 20-42, 20-43, 20-44, 20-45, 20-46, and **20-47** compliments of Marsha L. Eigenbrodt, M.D., M.P.H., Assistant Professor, Department of Medicine, and Edwin H. Eigenbrodt, M.D., Professor of Pathology, University of Mississippi Medical Center.

Figures 8-9, 8-37, 8-39, and **8-42** redrawn from Eisen, H. *Immunology*. Lippincott-Raven Publishers, New York, 1974, p.p 371, 373, 385–386.

Figure 23-19 redrawn from Elek, S. D. *Staphylococcus Pyogenes and its Relation to Disease*. E. & S. Livingstone Ltd., Edinburgh and London, 1959.

Figure 3-26 ©1997 by Facts and Comparisons. Adapted with permission from *Immunofacts: Vaccines and Immunologic Drugs*. Facts and Comparisons, St. Louis, MO, a Wolters Kluwer Company, 1996

Figure 7-18 adapted from Haber, E., Quertermous, T., Matsueda, G. R., and Runge, M. S. "Innovative approaches to plasminogen activator therapy." *Science* 243:52-56. ©1989 American Association for the Advancement of Science.

Figure 6-32 reprinted with permission from *Nature*. Harris, L. J., Larson, S. E., Hasel, K. W., Day, J., Greenwood, A., and McPherson, A. "The three-dimensional structure of an intact monoclonal antibody for canine lymphoma." 360(6402):369-372. ©1992 Macmillan Magazines Ltd.

Figure 1-8 courtesy of the Cruse collection; adapted from Hemmelweit, F. *Collected Papers of Paul Ehrlich*. Pergamon Press, Inc., Tarrytown, NY, 1956–1960.

Figure 22-36 courtesy of S. Farr-Jones, University of California at San Francisco.

Figures 23-3 and **23-4** redrawn from Hudson, L. and Hay, F. C. *Practical Immunology*. Blackwell Scientific Publications, Cambridge, MA, 1989.

Figure 6-21 redrawn from Hunkapiller, T. and Hood, L. "Diversity of the immunoglobulin gene superfamily." *Advances in Immunology* 44:1-63, 1989.

Figure 6-31 courtesy of Mike Clark, Ph.D., Division of Immunology, Cambridge University.

Figure 4-15 reprinted from Janeway, C. A., Jr., and Travers, P. *Immunobiology: The immune system in health and disease*. 3rd Edition, pp. 4–5, 1997.

Figures 8-43 and **8-44** reprinted from Kabat, E. A. *Structural concepts in immunology and immunochemistry*. 1968.

Figure 6-68 adapted from Kang, C. and Kohler, H. *Immunoregulation and Autoimmunity*, Vol. 3. J. M. Cruse and R. E. Lewis, Eds., 226. S. Karger, Basel, Switzerland, 1986.

Figure 11-19 redrawn from Kinoshita, T. *Complement Today*. Cruse, J. M. and Lewis, R. E., Eds., 48. S. Karger, Basel, Switzerland, 1993.

Figures 2-4, 7-29, and **11-18** redrawn from Lachmann, P. J. *Clinical Aspects of Immunology*. Blackwell Scientific Publications, Inc., Cambridge, MA, 1993. Reprinted by permission of Blackwell Science, Inc.

Figure 9-13 reprinted from Lo, D., Reilly, C. R., DeKoning, J., Laufer, T. M., and Glimcher, L. H. "Thymic stromal cell specialization and the T cell receptor repertoire." *Immunologic Research*. 16(1):3-14. 1997.

Figure 23-10 redrawn from Miller, L. E. *Manual of Laboratory Immunology*. Lea & Febiger, Malvern, PA, 1991.

Figures 9-4, 9-5, and **9-6** reprinted from Muller-Hermelink, H. K., Marino, M., and Palestra, G. "Pathology of thymic epithelial tumors." In *The Human Thymus. Current Topics in Pathology*. Muller-Hermelink HK, Ed. 1986; 75:207-68.

Figures 2-79, 6-43, 6-45, 6-48, 12-2, 12-18, 12-22, 12-28 , and **14-9** redrawn from Murray, P. R. *Medical Microbiology*. Mosby-Year Book, Inc., St. Louis, MO, 1994.

Figures 1-1, 1-5, 1-8, 1-11, 1-12, 1-14, 1-15, 1-18, 1-19, 1-20, 1-21, 1-40, 1-41, 1-42, 1-46, and **1-49** reprinted from U.S. National Library of Medicine.

Figures 6-40, 6-42, 6-43, 6-44, 6-45, 6-48, 6-49, 6-50, and **6-52** for imunoglobulins redrawn from Oppenheim, J., Rosenstreich, D. L., and Peter, M. *Cellular Function Immunity and Inflammation*. Elsevier Science Publishing Co. Inc., New York, NY, 1984.

Figures 6-6, 6-9, and **23-50** redrawn from Paul, W. E. *Fundamental Immunology* 3rd edRaven Press, Ltd., . New York, NY, 1993.

Figure 20-17 adapted from *Splits, Associated Antigens and Inclusions*, PEL-FREEZE Clinical Systems, Brown Deer, WI, 1992.

Figures 11-9 and **11-11** redrawn from Podack, E. R. "Molecular mechanisms of cytolysis by complement and cytolytic lymphocytes." *Journal of Cellular Biochemistry* 30:133-170, 1986.

Figures 2-5, 2-6, 2-9, 2-19, 2-52, 4-4, 4-17, 4-20, 7-24, 7-27, 9-24, 9-25, 9-26, 9-29, 9-30, 9-37, 10-4, 10-5, 10-6, 10-10, 10-19, 10-24, 10-26, 10-30, 10-35 10-37, 10-39, 10-40, 18-8, 18-9, 18-10, 19-16, 19-19, 19-22, 20-4, 20-5, 20-6, 21-8, 21-25, 22-25, 22-29, 22-40, and **22-41** reprinted from Protein Data Bank. Abola. E. E., Bernstein, F. C., Bryant, S. H., Koetzle, T. F., and Weng, J. Protein Data Bank, in *Crystallographic Databases-Information Content, Software Systems, Scientific Applications*. F. H. Allen, G. Bergerhoff, and R. Wievers, Eds. Data Commission of the International Union of Crystallography, Bonn/Cambridge/Chester, 1987, pp. 107–132. Bernstein, F. C., Koetzle, T. F., Williams, G. J. B., Meyer, E. F., Jr., Brice, M. D., Rodgers, J. R., Kennard, O., Shimanouchi, T., and Tasumi M. "The Protein Data Bank: a Computer-based Archival File for Macromolecular Structures." *J. Mol. Biol.* 112, 535–542, 1977. These images are part of the Swiss-3D Image Collection. Manuel C. Peitsch, Geneva Biomedical Research Institute, Glaxo Wellcome R & D, Geneva, Switzerland.

Figure 7-10 reprinted with permission from Raghavan M. et al. "Analysis of the pH dependence of the neonatal Fc receptor/immunoglobulin G interaction usint antibody and receptor variants." *Biochemistry* 34:14,649-14,657. ©1995 American Chemical Society; and from Junghans, R. P. Finally, the Brambell Receptor (FcRB). *Immunologic Research* 16:29-57.

Figure 2-44 redrawn from Ravetch, J. V. and Kinet, J. P. "Fc receptors." *Annual Review of Immunology* 9:462, 1991.

Figure 11-12 redrawn from Rooney, I. A., Oglesby, T. J., and Atkinson, J. P. "Complement in human reproduction: activation and control." *Immunologic Research* 12(3):276-294, 1993.

Figures 22-31 and **22-32** reprinted from Seifer, M. and Standring, D. N. "Assembly and antigenicity of hepatitis B virus core particles." *Intervirology*. 38:47-62. 1995.

Figures 21-1, 21-2, and **21-3** reprinted from Monoclonal Antiadhesion Molecules. Nov. 8, 1994. Seikagaku Corp.

Figures 20-48, 20-49, 20-50, 20-51, 20-52, 20-53, 20-54, 20-55, 20-56, 20-57, 20-58, 20-59, 20-60, 20-61, and **20-62** compliments of Dr. Howard M. Shulman, Professor of Pathology, University of Washington, Member Fred Hutchinson Cancer Research Center.

Figure 12-26 reprinted from Shwartzman, G. *Phenomenon of local tissue reactivity and its immunological, pathological, and clinical significance*. Lippincott-Raven Publishers, New York, 1937, p. 275.

Figure 16-46 redrawn from Stites, D. P. *Basic and Clinical Immunology*. Appleton & Lange, East Norwalk, CT, 1991.

Figure 2-86 redrawn from Tedder, T. F. "Structure of the gene encoding the human B lymphocyte differentiation antigen CD20 (B1). *Journal of Immunology*. 142 (7): 2567, 1989.

Figure 22-17 reproduced from the *Journal of Cell Biology*. Tilney, L. G. and Portnoy, D. A. "Actin filaments and the growth, movement, and spread of the intracellular bacterial parasite," *Listeria monocytogenes*. 1989, 109:1597-1608, by ©permission of the Rockefeller University Press.

Figure 9-10 reprinted from van Wijngaert, F. P., Kendall, M. D., Schuurman, H. J., Rademakers, L. H., Kater, L. "Heterogeneity of epithelial cells in the human thymus. An ultrastructural study." *Cell and Tissue Research*. 1984; 227-37.

Figure 16-23 and **16-87** reprinted from *Immunoflourescent Patterns in Skin Diseases* by Valenzuela, R., Bergfeld, W. F., and Deodhar, S. D. American Society of Clinical Pathologists Press, Chicago, IL, 1984. With permission of the ASCP Press.

Figures 15-5 and **15-22** adapted from Vengelen-Tyler, V., Ed. *Technical Manual*, 12th edition. American Association of Blood Banks, Bethesda, MD, 1996:231, 282.

Figure 15-33 (for major platelet membrane glycoproteins) and **15-11** (Rh polypeptides) adapted from Walker, R. H., Ed. *Technical Manual*, 11th edition. American Association of Blood Banks, Bethesda, MD, 1993: 242, 281.

Figures 1-2, 1-3, 1-4, 1-6, 1-9, 1-10, 1-13, 1-16, 1-17, 1-22, 1-23, 1-24, 1-25, 1-26, 1-27, 1-28, 1-29, 1-30, 1-32, 1-33, 1-34, 1-35, 1-36, 1-37, 1-38, 1-39, 1-43, 1-44, 1-45, 1-47, 1-48, 1-50, 1-51, 1-52, 1-53, and **1-54** reprinted from Whitcomb, D. *Immunology to 1980*. University of Wisconsin, Center of Health Sciences Library, Madison, WI, 1985.

Figure 1-56 compliments of Professor Dr. Rolf Zinkernagel, Institute of Pathology, University of Zurich.

Contents

1
History of Immunology

The metamorphosis of immunology from a curiosity of medicine associated with vaccination to a modern science focused at the center of basic research in molecular medicine is chronicled here. The people and events that led to this development are no less fascinating than the subject itself. A very great number of researchers in many diverse areas of medicine and science contributed to building the body of knowledge we now possess. It will be possible to name only a few but we owe a debt to them all. We are standing on the shoulders of giants, and in remembering their achievements we come to understand better the richness of our inheritance.

Resistance against infectious disease agents was the principal concern of bacteriologists and pathologists to establish the basis of classical immunology in the latter half of the nineteenth and early twentieth centuries. Variolation was practiced for many years prior to Edward Jenner's famous studies proving that inoculation with the cowpox could protect against subsequent exposure to smallpox. This established him as the founder of immunology. He contributed the first reliable method of conferring lasting immunity to a major contagious disease. Following the investigations by Louis Pasteur on immunization against anthrax, chicken cholera and rabies, and Robert Koch's studies on hypersensitivity in tuberculosis, their disciples continued research on immunity against infectious disease agents. Emil von Behring and Paul Ehrlich developed antitoxin against diphtheria while Elie Metchnikoff studied phagocytosis and cellular reactions in immunity. Hans Buchner described a principle in the blood later identified by Jules Bordet as alexine or complement. Bordet and Octave Gengou went on to develop the complement fixation test that was useful to assay antigen-antibody reactions. Karl Landsteiner described the ABO blood groups of man in 1900 followed by his elegant studies establishing the immunochemical basis of antigenic specificity.

Charles Robert Richet and Paul Jules Portier, in the early 1900s, attempted to immunize dogs against toxins in the tentacles of sea anemones but inadvertently induced a state of hypersusceptibility which they termed anaphylaxis. Since that time, many other hypersensitivity and allergic phenomena that are closely related to immune reactions have been described. Four types of hypersensitivity reactions are now recognized as contributory mechanisms in the production of immunological diseases. From the early 1900s until the

1940s, immunochemistry was a predominant force maintaining that antibody was formed through a template mechanism. With the discovery of immunological tolerance by Peter Medawar in the 1940s, David Talmage's cell selection theory and Frank Burnet's clonal selection theory of acquired immunity, it became apparent that a selective theory based on genetics was more commensurate with the facts than was the earlier template theory of the immunochemists. With the elucidation of immunoglobulin structure by Rodney Robert Porter and Gerald Edelman, among others, in the late 1950s and 1960s, modern immunology emerged at the frontier of medical research. Jean Baptiste Dausset described human histocompatibility antigens and transplantation immunology develop into a major science making possible the successful transplantation of organs. Bone marrow transplants became an effective treatment for severe combined immunodeficiency and related disorders. The year 1960 marked the beginning of a renaissance in cellular immunology, and the modern era dates from that time. Many subspecialties of immunology are now recognized and include such diverse topics as molecular immunology (immunochemistry), immunobiology, immunogenetics, immunopathology, tumor immunology, transplantation, comparative immunology, immunotoxicology, immunopharmacology, among others. Thus, it is apparent that immunology is only at the end of the beginning and has bright prospects for the future as evidenced by the exponential increase in immunologic literature in recent years.

In 1948, Astrid Elsa Fagraeus established the role of the plasma cell in antibody formation. The fluorescence antibody technique developed by Albert Coons was a major breakthrough for the identification of antigen in tissues and subsequently demonstrated antibody synthesis by individual cells. While attempting to immunize chickens in which the bursa of Fabricius had been removed, Bruce Glick et al. noted that antibody production did not take place. This was the first evidence of bursa-dependent antibody formation. Robert A. Good immediately realized the significance of this finding for immunodeficiencies of childhood. He and his associates in Minneapolis and J.F.A.P. Miller in England went on to show the role of the thymus in the immune response, and various investigators began to search for bursa equivalence in man and other animals. Thus, the immune system of many species was found to have distinct bursa-dependent, antibody-synthesizing and thymus-dependent cell-mediated limbs. In 1959, James Gowans proved that lymphocytes actually recirculate. In 1966, Tzvee Nicholas Harris et al. demonstrated clearly that lymphocytes could form antibodies. In 1966 and 1967, Claman et al., Davis et al. and Mitchison et al. showed that T and B lymphocytes cooperate with one another in the production of an immune response. Various phenomena such as the switch from forming one class of immunoglobulin to another by B cells were demonstrated to be dependent upon a signal from T cells activating B cells to change from IgM to IgG or IgA production. B cells stimulated by antigen in which no T cell signal was given continued to produce IgM antibody. Such antigens were referred to as thymus-independent antigens and others requiring T cell participation as thymus-dependent antigens. Mitchison et al. described a subset of T lymphocytes demonstrating helper activity, i.e., helper T cells. In 1971, Gershon and Condo described suppressor T cells. Suppressor T cells have been the subject of much investigation but have eluded confirmation by the techniques of molecular biology. Baruj Benacerraf et al. demonstrated the significant role played by gene products of the major histocompatibility complex in the specificity and regulation of T cell-dependent immune response. Jerne described the network theory of immunity in which antibodies formed against idiotypic specificities of antibody molecules followed by the formation of anti-idiotypic antibodies constitutes a significant additional immunoregulatory process for immune system function. This postulate has been proven valid by numerous investigators. Tonegawa et al. and Leder et al. identified and cloned the genes that code for variable and constant regions of immunoglobulin molecules leading to increased understanding of the origin of diversity in antibody-combining sites. In 1975, George Kohler and Cesar Milstein successfully produced monoclonal antiodies by hybridizing mutant myeloma cells with antibody producing B cells (hybridoma technique). The B cells conferred the antibody-producing capacity while the myeloma cells provided the capability for endless reproduction. Monoclonal antibodies are the valuable homogeneous products of hybridomas that have widespread application in diagnostic laboratory medicine.

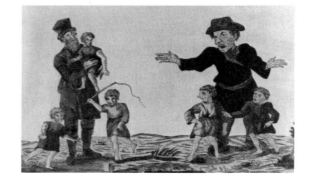

Smallpox cartoon, artist unknown   From the Clement C. Fry Collection. Yale Medical Library, contributed by Jason S. Zielonka, published in *J. Hist. Med.* 27-447-7, 1972. Legend translated: Smallpox disfigured father says, "How shameful that your pretty little children should call my children stupid and should run away, refusing to play with them as friends…" Meanwhile, the children lament: "Father dear, it appears to be your fault that they're avoiding us. To tell the truth, it looks as though you should have inoculated us against smallpox."

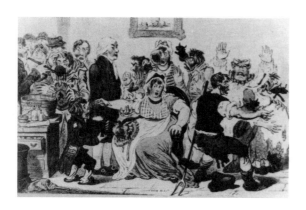

L. Gillray Cowpox Cartoon   The Cowpox or the wonderful effects of the new inoculation 1802. Courtesy of the National Library of Medicine.

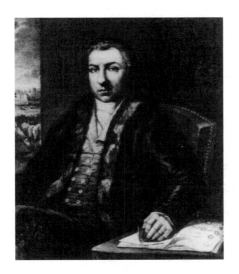

Lady Mary Wortley Montagu (1689–1762)   Often credited as the first to introduce inoculation as a means of preventing smallpox in England in 1722. After observing the practice in Turkey where her husband was posted as Ambassador to the Turkish court, she had both her young son and daughter inoculated and interested the Prince and Princess of Wales in the practice. Accounts of inoculation against small pox are found in her *Letters*, 1777. Robert Halsband authored a biography *The Life of Lady Mary Wortley Montagu*. Clarendon, Oxford, 1956.

Edward Jenner (1749–1822)   Often is termed the founder of immunology for his contribution of the first reliable method of conferring lasting immunity to a major contagious disease. He studied medicine under John Hunter and for most of his career was a country doctor in Berkeley in Southern England. Although it was common knowledge in the country that an eruptive skin disease of cattle, cowpox, and a similar disease in horses called grease conferred immunity to smallpox on those who cared for the animals and caught the infection from them, Jenner carefully observed and recorded 23 cases. The results of his experiments were published, establishing his claim of credit for initiating the technique of vaccination. He vaccinated an 8-year-old boy, James Phipps with matter taken from the arm of the milkmaid, Sara Nelmes, who was suffering from cowpox. After the infection subsided, he inoculated the child with smallpox and found that the inoculation had no effect. His results led to widespread adoption of vaccination in England and elsewhere in the world leading ultimately to eradication of smallpox.

Louis Pasteur (1822–1895)   French. Father of Immunology. One of the most productive scientists of modern times, Pasteur's contributions included the crystallization of L- and O-tartaric acid, disproving the theory of spontaneous generation, studies of diseases in wine, beer and silkworms, and the use of attenuated bacteria and viruses for vaccination. He used attenuated vaccines to protect against anthrax, fowl cholera and rabies. He successfully immunized sheep and cattle against anthrax, terming the technique vaccination in honor of Jenner. He produced a vaccine for rabies by drying the spinal cord of rabbits and using the material to prepare a series of 14 injections of increasing virulence. A child's (Joseph Meister's) life was saved by this treatment. *Les Maladies des Vers a Soie*, 1865; *Etudes sur le Vin*, 1866; *Etudes sur la Biere*, 1876; *Oeuvres*, 1922–1939.

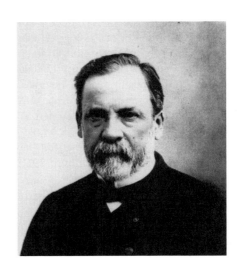

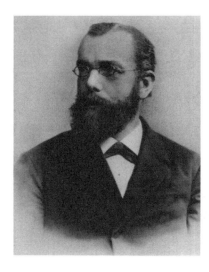

Robert Koch (1843–1910)   German Bacteriologist awarded the Nobel Prize in 1905 for his work on tuberculosis. Koch made many contributions to the field of bacteriology. Along with his postulates for proof of etiology, Koch instituted strict isolation in culture methods in bacteriology. He studied the life cycle of anthrax and discovered both the cholera vibrio and the tubercle bacillus. The Koch phenomenon and Koch-Weeks bacillus both bear his name.

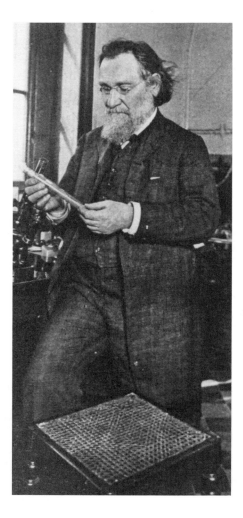

Elie (Ilya) Metchnikoff (1845–1916)   Born at Ivanovska, Ukraine, where he was a student of zoology with a very special interest in comparative embryology. He received a Ph.D. degree at the University of Odessa where he also served as Professor of Zoology. He studied phagocytic cells of starfish larvae in 1884 in a marine laboratory in Italy. This served as the basis for his cellular phagocytic theory of immunity. On leaving Russia for political reasons, Pasteur offered him a position at the Institute Pasteur in Paris where he extended his work on the defensive role of phagocytes and championed his cellular theory of immunity. He also made numerous contributions to immunology and bacteriology. He shared the 1908 Nobel Prize for medicine or physiology with Paul Ehrlich "In recognition for their work on immunity." *Lecons sur le Pathologie de l'Inflammation*, 1892; *L'Immunite dans les Maladies Infectieuses*, 1901; *Etudes sur la Nature Humaine*, 1903.

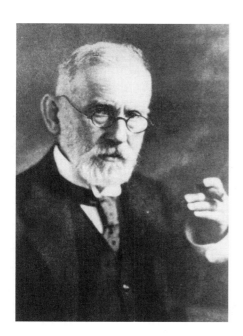

Paul Ehrlich (1854–1915)   Born in Silesia, Germany, and graduated Doctor of Medicine from the University of Leipzig. His scientific work included three areas of investigation. He first became interested in stains for tissues and cells and perfected some of the best ones to demonstrate the tubercle bacillus and for leukocytes in blood. His first immunological studies were begun in 1890 when he was an assistant at the Institute for Infectious Diseases under Robert Koch. After first studying the antibody response to the plant toxins abrin and ricin, Ehrlich published the first practical technique to standardize diphtheria toxin and antitoxin preparations in 1897. He proposed the first selective theory of antibody formation known as the "side chain theory" which stimulated much research by his colleagues in an attempt to disprove it. He served as Director of his own institute in Frankfurt am Main where he published papers with a number of gifted colleagues including Dr. Julius Morgenroth on immune hemolysis and other immunological subjects. He also conducted a number of studies on cancer and devoted the final phase of his career to the development of chemotherapeutic agents for the treatment of disease. He shared the 1908 Nobel prize with Metchnikoff for their studies on immunity. Fruits of these labors led to treatments for trypanosomiasis and syphilis (Salvarsan) — "The magic bullet". *Collected Studies on Immunity, 1906; Collected Papers of Paul Ehrlich*, Vol 3, 1957.

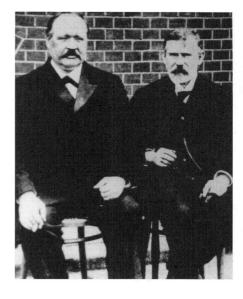

Svante Arrhenius (1859–1927)   Photographed with Paul Ehrlich, 1903. Coined the term "immunochemistry" and hypothesized that antigen-antibody complexes are reversible. He was awarded the Nobel Prize for chemistry, 1903. Book: *Immunochemistry*. MacMillan Publishers, New York, 1907.

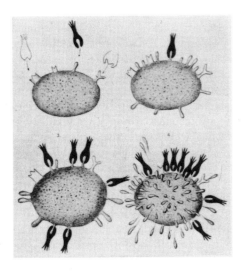

DIAGRAMMATIC REPRESENTATION OF THE SIDE-CHAIN THEORY
(PLATES I AND II)

Fig. 1   "The groups [the haptophore group of the side-chain of the cell and that of the food-stuff or the toxin] must be adapted to one another, *e.g.,* as male and female screw (PASTEUR), or as lock and key (E. FISCHER)."

Fig. 2   ". . . the first stage in the toxic action must be regarded as being the union of the toxin by means of its haptophore group to a special side-chain of the cell protoplasm."

Fig. 3   "The side-chain involved, so long as the union lasts, cannot exercise its normal, physiological, nutritive function . . ."

Fig. 4   "We are therefore now concerned with a defect which, according to the principles so ably worked out by . . . Weigert, is . . . [overcorrected] by regeneration."

Side-Chain Theory

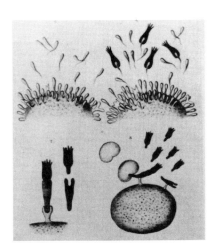

DIAGRAMMATIC REPRESENTATION OF THE SIDE-CHAIN THEORY
(*cont.*)

Fig. 5   ". . . the antitoxins represent nothing more than the side-chains reproduced in excess during regeneration and therefore pushed off from the protoplasm—thus coming to exist in a free state."

Fig. 6   [The free side-chains (circulating antitoxins) unite with the toxins and thus protect the cell.]

Fig. 7   ". . . two haptophore groups must be ascribed to the 'immune-body [haemolytic amboceptor], one having a strong affinity for a corresponding haptophore group of the red blood corpuscles, . . . and another . . . which . . . becomes united with the 'complement' . . ."

Fig. 8   "If a cell . . . has, with the assistance of an appropriate side-chain, fixed to itself a giant [protein] molecule . . . there is provided [only] one of the conditions essential for the cell nourishment. Such . . . molecules . . are not available until . . . they have been split into smaller fragments This will be . . . attained if . . . the 'tentacle' . . . possesses . . . second haptophore group adapted to take to itself ferment-like materia . . ."

Side-Chain Theory

Ehrlich side chain theory   The first selective theory of antibody synthesis developed by Paul Ehrlich in 1900. Although elaborate in detail, the essential feature of the theory was that cells of the immune system possess the genetic capability to react to all known antigens and that each cell on the surface bears receptors with surface haptophore side chains. On combination with antigen, the side chains would be cast off into the circulation and new receptors would replace the old ones. These cast-off receptors represented antibody molecules in the circulation. Although far more complex than this explanation, the importance of the theory was in the amount of research stimulated to try to disprove it. Nevertheless, it was the first effort to account for the importance of genetics in immune responsiveness at a time when Mendel's basic studies had not even yet been "rediscovered" by De Vries.

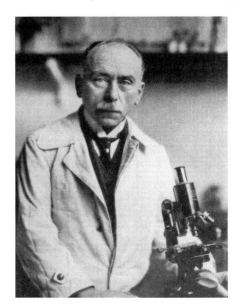

Jules Bordet (1870–1961)   Belgian. Physician who graduated Doctor of Medicine from the University of Brussels. He was preparateur in Metchnikoff's laboratory at the Institut Pasteur from 1894–1901 where he discovered immune hemolysis and elucidated the mechanisms of complement-mediated bacterial lysis. He and Gengou described complement fixation and pointed to its use in the diagnosis of infectious diseases. Their technique was subsequently used by von Wassermann to develop a complement fixation test for syphilis which enjoyed worldwide popularity. His debates with Paul Ehrlich on the nature of antigen-antibody-complement interactions stimulated much useful research. He was awarded the Nobel Prize in Medicine or Physiology for his studies on immunity, 1919. Book: *Traite de l'Immunite dans les Maladies Infectieuses*, 1920.

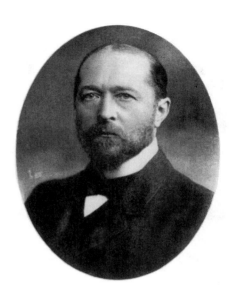

Emil Adolph von Behring (1854–1917) German bacteriologist who worked at the Institute for Infectious Diseases in Berlin with Kitasato and Wernicke in 1890–1892 and demonstrated that circulating antitoxins against diphtheria and tetanus toxins conferred immunity. He demonstrated that the passive administration of antitoxin-serum containing antitoxin could facilitate recovery. This represented the beginning of serum therapy, especially for diphtheria. Books: *Die Blutserumtherapie*, 1902; *Gesammelte Abhandlungen*, 1914; *Behring, Gestalt und Werk*, 1940; *Emil von Behring zum Gedächtnis*, 1942.

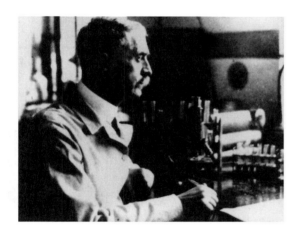

Karl Landsteiner (1868–1943) Viennese pathologist and immunologist who later worked at the Rockefeller Institute for Medical Research in New York. Recieved the Nobel Prize in 1930 "for his discovery of the human blood groups." He was the first to infect monkeys with poliomyelitis and syphilis to allow controlled studies of those diseases. He established the immunochemical specificity of synthetic antigens and haptens. Landsteiner felt his most important contribution was in the area of antibody-hapten interactions. Books: *Die Spezifizität der serologiochen Reactionen*, 1933; *The Specificity of Serological Reactions*, 1945.

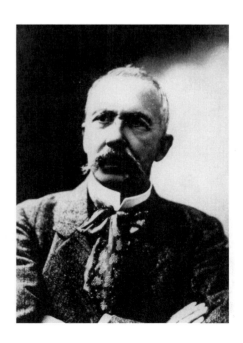

Charles Robert Richet (1850–1935) Parisian physician who became professor of physiology in the University of Paris. He was interested in the physiology of toxins and with Portier discovered anaphylaxis for which he was awarded the Nobel Prize in Physiology or Medicine in 1913. He and Portier discovered anaphylaxis in dogs exposed to the toxins of murine invertebrates to which they had been previously sensitized. Thus, an immune type reaction that was harmful rather than protective was demonstrated. Experimental anaphylaxis was later shown to be similar to certain types of hypersensitivity which lent clinical as well as theoretical significance to the discovery. Book: *L'anaphylaxie*, 1911.

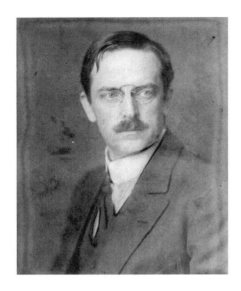

Clemens Freiherr von Pirquet (1874–1929)   Viennese physician who coined the term "allergy" and described serum sickness and its pathogenesis. He also developed a skin test for tuberculosis. He held academic appointments at Vienna, Johns Hopkins, Breslau and returned to Vienna in 1911 as Director of the University Children's Clinic. Books: *Die Serumkrankheit* (with Schick), 1905; *Klinische Studien uber vakzination und Vakzinale Allergie*, 1907; Allergy, 1911.

Almroth Edward Wright (1861–1947)   British pathologist and immunologist who graduated with a Doctor of Medicine degree from Trinity College Dublin in 1889. He became Professor of Pathology at the Army Medical School in Netley in 1892. He later became associated with the Institute of Pathology at St. Mary's Hospital Medical School, London, in 1902. Together with Douglas, he formulated a theory of opsonins and perfected an antitoxoid inoculation system. He studied immunology in Frankfurt-am-Main under Paul Ehrlich and made important contributions to the immunology of infectious diseases and immunization. He played a significant role in the founding of the American Association of Immunologists. His published works include: *Pathology and Treatment of War Wounds*, 1942; *Researches in Clinical Physiology*, 1943; *Studies in Immunology*, 2 vols., 1944.

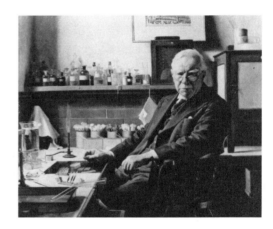

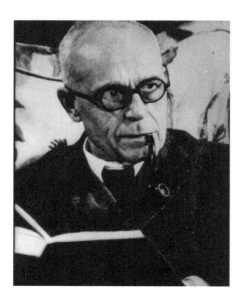

Carl Prausnitz-Giles (1876–1963)   German physician from Breslau who conducted extensive research on allergies. He and Küstner successfully transferred food allergy with serum. This became the basis for the Prausnitz-Küstner test. He worked at the State Institute for Hygiene in Breslau and spent time at the Royal Institute for Public Health in London earlier in the century. In 1933, he left Germany and practiced medicine on the Isle of Wight.

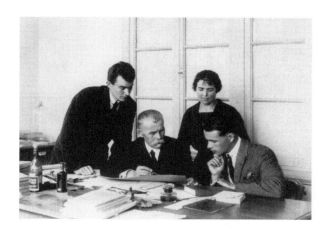

Nicolas Maurice Arthus (1862–1945)   Paris physician. He studied venoms and their physiological effects; first to describe local anaphylaxis or the Arthus reaction 1903. Arthus investigated the local necrotic lesion resulting from a local antigen antibody reaction in an immunized animal. *De l'Anaphylaxie a l'Immunite*, 1921.

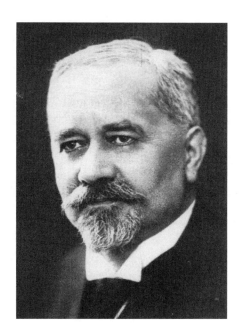

Albert Calmette (1863–1933)   French physician who was subdirector of the Institut Pasteur in Paris. In a popular book published in 1920, *Bacillary Infection and Tuberculosis*, he emphasized the necessity of separating tuberculin reactivity from anaphylaxis. Together with Guerin, he perfected BCG vaccine and also investigated snake venom and plague serum.

Michael Heidelberger (1888–1991)   American. A founder of immunochemistry. He began his career as an organic chemist. His contributions to immunology include the perfection of quantitative immunochemical methods and the immunochemical characterization of pneumococcal polysaccharides. His contributions to immunologic research are legion. During his career, he received the Lasker Award, the National Medal of Science, the Behring Award, the Pasteur Medal and the French Legion of Honor. Book: *Lectures on Immunochemistry*, 1956.

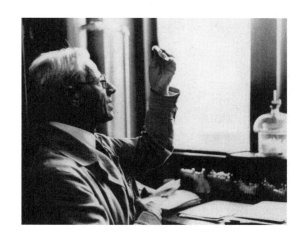

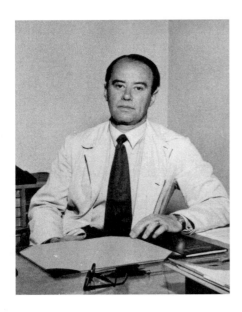

Arne W. K Tiselius (1902–1971). Swedish chemist who was educated at the University of Uppsala where he also worked in research. In 1934, he was at the Institute for Advanced Study in Princeton, worked for the Swedish National Research Council in 1946 and became President of the Nobel Foundation in 1960. Awarded the Nobel Prize in chemistry in 1948, he perfected the electrophoresis technique and classified antibodies as γ globulins together with Elvin A. Kabat. He also developed synthetic blood plasmas.

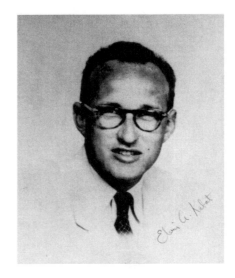

Elvin Abraham Kabat (1914–)   American immunochemist. With Tiselius he was the first to separate immunoglobulins electrophoretically. He also demonstrated that globulins can be distinguished as 7S or 19S. Other contributions include research on antibodies to carbohydrates, the antibody combining site, and the discovery of immunoglobulin chain variable regions. He received the National Medal of Science. Books: *Experimental Immunochemistry* (with Mayer), 1948; *Blood Group Substances: Their Chemistry and Immunochemistry, Structural Concepts in Immunology and Immunochemistry*, 1956, 1968.

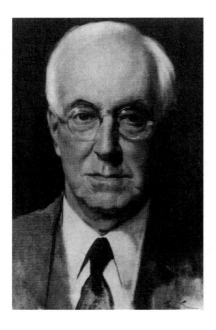

Henry Hallett Dale (1875–1968). British investigator who made a wide range of scientific contributions including work on the chemistry of nerve impulse transmission, the discovery of histamine and the development of the Schultz-Dale test for anaphylaxis. He received a Nobel Prize in 1935.

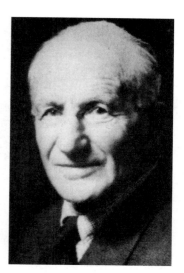

John Richardson Marrack (1899–1976)   British physician who served as Professor of Chemical Pathology at Cambridge and at the London Hospital. He hypothesized that antibodies are bivalent, labeled antibodies with colored dyes and proposed a lattice theory of antigen-antibody complex formation in fundamental physico-chemical studies.

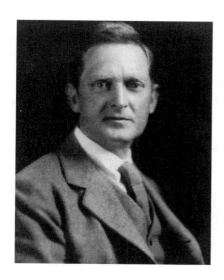

Hans Zinsser (1878–1940)   A leading American bacteriologist and immunologist who was a Columbia, Stanford and Harvard educator whose work in immunology included hypersensitivity research, plague immunology, formulation of the unitarian theory of antibodies and demonstration of differences between tuberculin and anaphylactic hypersensitivity. His famous text, *Microbiology* (with Hiss), 1911, has been through two dozen editions since its first appearance.

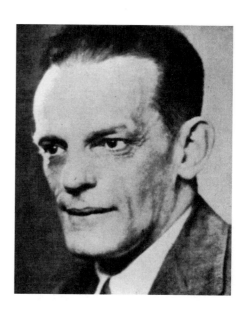

Max Theiler (1899–1972)   South African virologist who received the Nobel Prize in 1951 "for his development of vaccines against yellow fever."

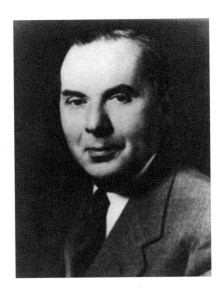

Gregory Shwartzman (1896–1965). Russian-American microbiologist who described systemic and local reactions that follow the injection of bacterial endotoxins. The systemic Shwartzman reaction, a nonimmunologic phenomenon, is related to disseminated intravascular coagulation. The local Schwartzman reaction in skin resembles the immunologically based Arthus reaction in appearance. Book: *Phenomenon of Local Tissue Reactivity and Its Immunological and Clinical Significance*, 1937.

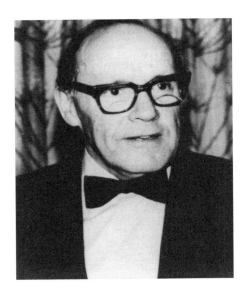

Robin R. A. Coombs (1921–)   British pathologist and immunologist who is best known for the Coombs' test as a means for detecting immunoglobulin on the surface of a patient's red blood cells. The test was developed in the 1940s to demonstrate autoantibodies on the surface of red blood cells that failed to cause agglutination of these erythrocytes. It is a test for autoimmune hemolytic anemia. He also contributed much to serology, immunohematology and immunopathology. Books: *The Serology of Conglutination and Its Relation to Disease*, 1961; *Clinical Aspects of Immunology* (with Gell), 1963.

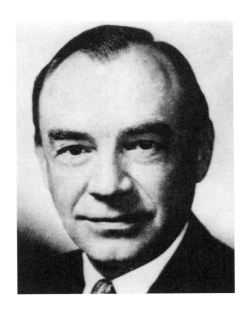

Albert Hewett Coons (1912–1978)   American immunologist and bacteriologist who was an early leader in immunohistochemistry with the development of fluorescent antibodies. Coons, a Professor at Harvard, received the Lasker medal in 1959, the Ehrlich Prize in 1961 and the Behring Prize in 1966.

Ernest Witebsky (1901–1969)   German-American immunologist and bacteriologist who made significant contributions to transfusion medicine and to concepts of autoimmune diseases. He was a direct descendent of the Ehrlich school of immunology, having worked at Heidelberg with Hans Sachs, Ehrlich's principal assistant, in 1929. He came to Mt. Sinai Hospital in New York in 1934 and became Professor at the University of Buffalo in 1936, where he remained until his death. A major portion of his work on autoimmunity was the demonstration with Noel R. Rose of experimental autoimmune thyroiditis.

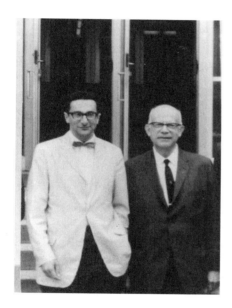

Noel Richard Rose (1927–)   American immunologist and authority on autoimmune diseases, who first discovered with Witebsky, experimental autoimmune thyroiditis. His subsequent contributions to immunology are legion. He has authored numerous books and edited leading journals in the field.

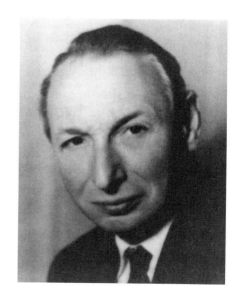

Peter Alfred Gorer (1907–1961)   British pathologist who was professor at Guy's Hospital Medical School, London, where he made major discoveries in transplantation genetics. With Snell, he discovered the H-2 murine histocompatibility complex. Most of his work was in transplantation genetics. He identified antigen II and described its association with tumor rejection. *The Gorer Symposium*, Blackwell, Oxford, 1985.

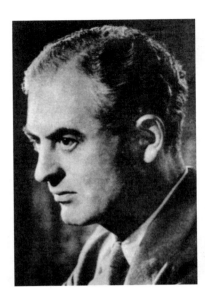

Peter Brian Medawar (1915–1987)   British transplantation biologist who received his Ph.D. at Oxford, 1935, where he served as lecturer in zoology. He was subsequently a Professor of Zoology at Birmingham (1947) and at University College, London, 1951. He became Director of the Medical Research Council, 1962 and of the Clinical Research Center at Northwick Park, 1971. Together with Billingham and Brent, he made seminal discoveries in transplantation and immunobiology and described immunological tolerance and its importance for tissue transplantation. He shared the 1960 Nobel Prize in Medicine or Physiology with Sir MacFarlane Burnet.

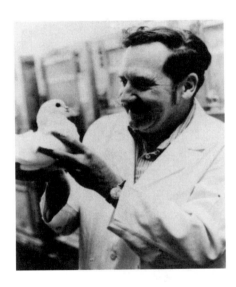

Ray David Owen (1915–)   American geneticist who described erythrocyte mosaicism in dizygotic cattle twins. This discovery of reciprocal erythrocyte tolerance contributed to the concept of immunological tolerance. This observation that cattle twins, which shared a common fetal circulation, were chimeras and could not reject transplants of each other's tissues later in life provided the groundwork for Burnet's ideas about tolerance and Medawar's work in transplantation.

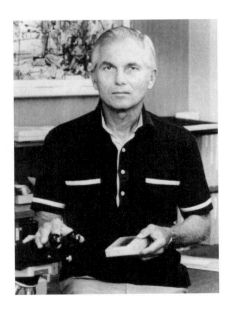

Frank James Dixon (1920–)   American physician and researcher noted for his fundamental contributions to immunopathology that include the role of immune complexes in the production of disease. He is also known for his work on antibody formation. Dixon was the founding Director of the Research Institute of Scripps Clinic, La Jolla, CA.

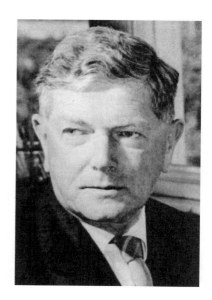

Niels Kaj Jerne (1911–) Immunologist, born in London and educated at Leiden and Copenhagen, who shared the Nobel Prize in 1984 with Kohler and Milstein for his contribution to immune system theory. These include his selective theory of antibody formation, the functional network of interacting antibodies and lymphocytes and distinction of self from nonself by T lymphocytes. He studied antibody synthesis and avidity, perfected the hemolytic plaque assay, developed the natural selection theory of antibody formation and formulated the idiotypic network theory. He was Director of the Paul Ehrlich Institute in Frankfurt-am-Main, 1966 and Director of the Basel Institute for Immunology, 1969.

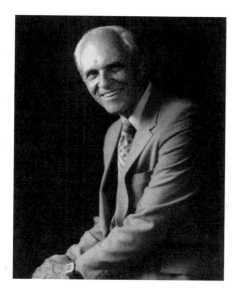

David Wilson Talmage (1919–) American physician and investigator who in 1956 developed the cell selection theory of antibody formation. His work was a foundation for Burnet's subsequent clonal selection theory. After training in immunology with Taliaferro in Chicago where he became a Professor in 1952, Talmage subsequently became Chairman of Microbiology, 1963; Dean of Medicine, 1968; and Director of the Webb-Waring Institute in Denver, 1973. In addition to his investigations of antibody formation, he also studied heart transplantation tolerance. Book: *The Chemistry of Immunity in Health and Disease* (with Cann), 1961.

Frank MacFarlane Burnet (1899–1985) Australian virologist and immunologist who shared the Nobel Prize in medicine or physiology with Peter B. Medawar in 1960 for the discovery of acquired immunological tolerance. Burnet was a theoretician who made major contributions to the developing theories of self tolerance and clonal selection in antibody formation. Burnet and Fenner's suggested explanation of immunologic tolerance was tested by Medawar et al. who confirmed the hypothesis in 1953 using inbred strains of mice. Books: *Production of Antibodies (with Fenner), 1949; Natural History of Infectious Diseases*, 1953; *Clonal Selection Theory of Antibody Formation, 1959; Autoimmune Diseases* (with Mackay), 1962; *Cellular Immunology*, 1969; *Changing Patterns* (autobiography), 1969.

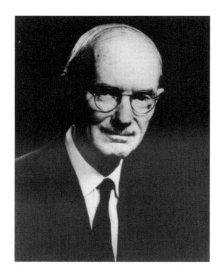

George Davis Snell (1903–1996)   American geneticist who shared the 1980 Nobel Prize in Medicine or Physiology with Jean Dausset and Baruj Benacerraf "For their work on genetically determined structures of the cell surface that regulate immunologic reactions." Snell's major contributions were in the field of mouse genetics, including discovery of the H-2 locus (together with Gorer) and the development of congenic mice. He made many seminal contributions to transplantation genetics and received the Gairdner Award in 1976. Book: *Histocompatibility* (with Dausset and Nathenson), 1976.

Jean Baptiste Gabriel Dausset (1916–)   French physician and investigator. He pioneered research on the HLA system and the immunogenetics of histocompatibility. For this work, he shared a Nobel Prize with Benacerraf and Snell in 1980. He made numerous discoveries in immunogenetics and transplantation biology. Books: *Immunohematologie Biologique et Clinique*, 1956; *HLA and Disease* (with Svejaard), 1977.

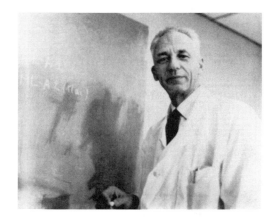

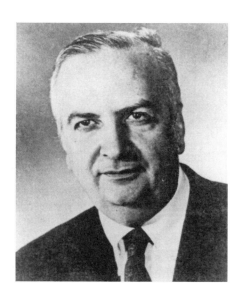

Baruj Benacerraf (1920–)   American immunologist born in Caracas, Venezuela. His multiple contributions include the carrier effect in delayed hypersensitivity, lymphocyte subsets, MHC and Ir immunogenetics, for which he shared the Nobel Prize in 1980 with Jean Dausset and George Snell. Benacerraf et al. showed that many of the genes within the MHC control the immune response to various immunogens. Using synthetic polypeptides as antigens, Benacerraf, McDevitt et al. demonstrated that immune response Ir genes control an animal's response to a given antigen. These genes were localized in the I region of the MHC. Book: *Textbook of Immunology* (with Unanue). Williams & Wilkins, Baltimore, MD, 1979.

Henry George Kunkel (1916–1983)   American physician and immunologist. The primary focus of his work was immunoglobulins. He characterized myeloma proteins as immunoglobulins and rheumatoid factor as an autoantibody. He also discovered IgA and idiotypy and contributed to immunoglobulin structure and genetics. Kunkel received the Lasker award and the Gairdner Award. A graduate of Johns Hopkins Medical School, he served as Professor of Medicine at the Rockefeller Institute for Medical Research.

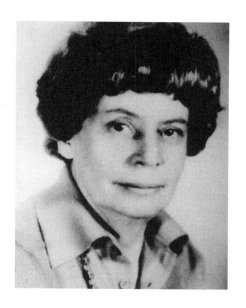

Astrid Elsa Fagraeus-Wallbom (1913–)   Swedish investigator noted for her doctoral thesis which provided the first clear evidence that immunoglobulins are made in plasma cells. In 1962, she became Chief of the Virus Department of the National Bacteriological Laboratory and in 1965, Professor of Immunology at the Karolinska Institute in Stockholm. She also investigated cell membrane antigens and contributed to the field of clinical immunology. Book: *Antibody Production in Relation to the Development of Plasma Cells*, Stockholm, 1948.

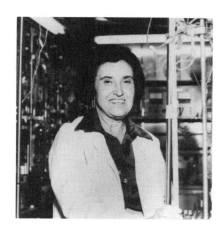

Rosalyn Sussman Yalow (1921–)   American investigator who shared the 1977 Nobel Prize with Guillemin and Schally for her endocrinology research and perfection of the radioimmunoassay technique. With Berson, Yalow made an important discovery of the role antibodies play in insulin resistant diabetes. Her technique provided a test to estimate nanogram or picogram quantities of various types of hormones and biologically active molecules, thereby advancing basic and clinical research.

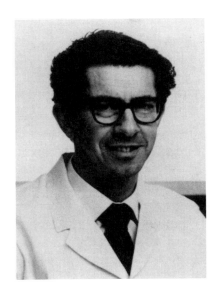

J. F. A. P. Miller (1931–)   Proved the role of the thymus in immunity while investigating Gross Leukemia in Neonatal Mice.

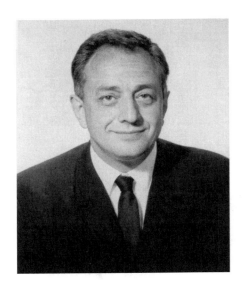

Robert Alan Good (1922–)   American immunologist and pediatrician who has made major contributions to studies on the ontogeny and phylogeny of the immune response. Much of his work focused on immunodeficiency diseases and the role of the thymus and the bursa of Fabricius in immunity. He and his colleagues demonstrated the role of the thymus in the education of lymphocytes. Books: *The Thymus in Immunobiology*, 1964; *Phylogeny of Immunity*, 1966.

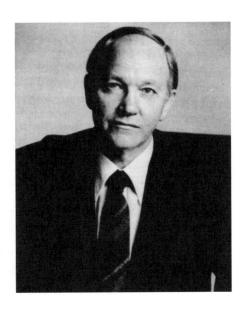

James Gowans (1924–)   British physician and investigator whose principal contribution to immunology was the demonstration that lymphocytes recirculate via the thoracic duct, which radically changed understanding of the role lymphocytes play in immune reactions. He also investigated lymphocyte function. He served as Director of the MRC Cellular Immunobiology Unit, Oxford, 1963.

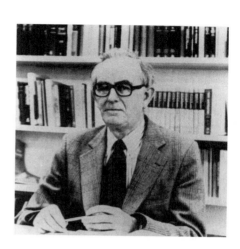

Rodney Robert Porter (1917–1985)   British biochemist who received the Nobel Prize in 1972, with Gerald Edelman, for their studies of antibodies and their chemical structure. Porter cleaved antibody molecules with the enzyme papain to yield Fab and Fc fragments. He suggested that antibodies have a four-chain structure. Fab fragments were shown to have the antigen-binding sites whereas the Fc fragment conferred the antibody's biological properties. He also investigated the sequence of complement genes in the MHC. Book: *Defense and Recognition*, 1973.

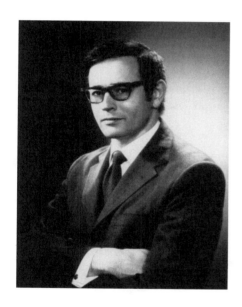

Gerald Maurice Edelman (1929–)   American investigator who was professor at the Rockefeller University and shared the Nobel Prize in 1972 with Porter for their work on antibody structure. Edelman was the first to demonstrate that immunoglobulins are composed of light and heavy polypeptide chains. He also did pioneering work with Bence-Jones protein, cell adhesion molecules, immunoglobulin amino acid sequence and neurobiology.

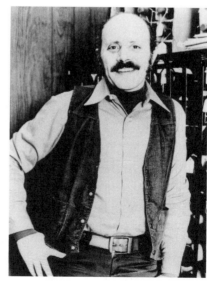

Richard K. Gershon (1932–1983)   One of the first to demonstrate the suppressor role of the T cell. The suppressor T cell was described as a subpopulation of lymphocytes that diminish or suppress antibody formation by B cells or down regulate the ability of T lymphocytes to mount a cellular immune response. The inability to confirm the presence of receptor molecules on their surface has cast a cloud over the suppressor cell; however, functional suppressor cell effects are indisputable.

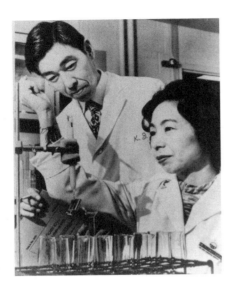

Kimishige Ishizaka (1925–) and **Terako Ishizaka**   Discovered IgE and have contributed to elucidation of its function.

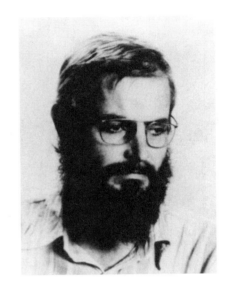

Georges J. F. Köhler (1946–)   German immunologist who shared the Nobel Prize in 1984 with Cesar Milstein for their work on the production of monoclonal antibodies by hybridizing mutant myeloma cells with antibody producing B cells (hybridoma technique). Monoclonal antibodies have broad applications in both basic and clinical research as well as in diagnostic assays.

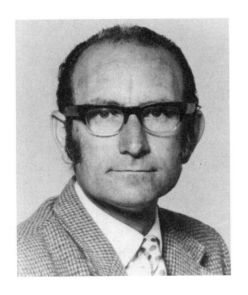

Cesar Milstein (1927–)   Immunologist born in Argentina who worked in the United Kingdom. He shared the 1984 Nobel Prize with G. F. Kohler for their production of monoclonal antibodies by hybridizing mutant myeloma cells with antibody-producing B cells (hybridoma technique). The production of monoclonal antibodies by hybridoma technology revolutionized immunological research.

Susumu Tonegawa (1939–)   Japanese born immunologist working in the United States. He received the Nobel Prize in 1987 for his research on immunoglobulin genes and antibody diversity. Tonegawa and many colleagues were responsible for the discovery of immunoglobulin gene C, V, J and D regions and their rearrangement.

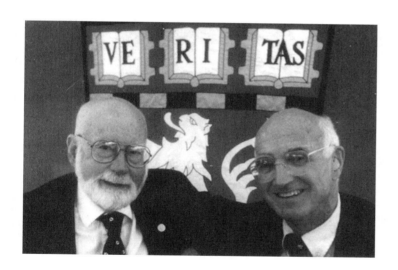

E. Donnall Thomas (1920–) and **Joseph E. Murray** (1919–)   Recipients of the 1990 Nobel Prize for physiology or medicine for their work during the 1950s and 1960s on reducing the risk of organ rejection by the body's immune system. Murray performed the first successful organ transplant in the world, which was a kidney from one identical twin to another, at the Peter Bent Brigham Hospital in 1954. Two years later, Thomas was the first to perform a successful transplant of bone marrow, which he achieved by administering a drug that prevented rejection. The two doctors have made significant discoveries that "have enabled the development of organ and cell transplantation into a method for the treatment of human disease," said the Nobel Assembly in its citation for the prize.

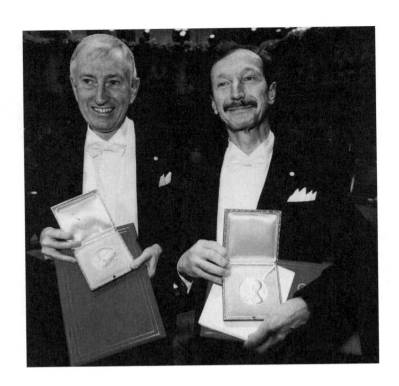

Rolf Zinkernagel (1944–) and *Peter Doherty* (1940–) Recipients of the 1996 Nobel Prize for physiology or medicine for their demonstration of MHC restriction. In an investigation of how T lymphocytes protect mice against lymphocytic choriomeningitis virus (LCMV) infection, they found that T cells from mice infected by the virus killed only infected target cells expressing the same major histocompatibility complex (MHC) class I antigens but not those expressing a different MHC allele. In their study, murine cytotoxic T cells (CTL) would only lyse virus-infected target cells if the effector and target cells were H-2 compatible. This significant finding had broad implications, demonstrating that T cells did not recognize the virus directly but only in conjunction with MHC molecules.

2

Molecules, Cells, and Tissue of the Immune Response

The generation of an immune response of either the innate or acquired variety requires the interaction of specific molecules, cells and tissues. The present chapter provides an overview of these structures with brief descriptions enhanced by schematic representations, light and electron micrographs of those elements whose interactions yield a highly tailored immune response that is critical to survival of the species. Many of the molecules of immunity are described in subsequent chapters. Adhesion molecules that are important in bringing cells together in the generation of immune responses or of directing cellular traffic through vessels or interaction of cells with matrix are presented here.

All lymphocytes in the body are derived from stem cells in the bone marrow. Those cells destined to become T cells migrate to the thymus where they undergo maturation and education prior to their residence in the peripheral lymphoid tissues. B cells undergo maturation in the bone marrow following their release. Both B and T cells occupy specific areas in the peripheral lymphoid tissues. Depictions of the thymus, lymph nodes, spleen and other lymphoid organs are presented to give the reader a visual concept of immune system structure and development. The various cells involved in antigen presentation and development of an immune response are followed by a description of cells involved in effector immune functions. Understanding the molecules, cells and tissues described in the pages that follow prepares the reader to appreciate the novel and fascinating interactions of these molecules and cells in the body tissues and organs that permit the generation of a highly specific immune response. Immunity may perform many vital functions such as the elimination of invading microbes, the activation of amplification mechanisms such as the complement pathway or the development of protective antibodies or cytotoxic T cells that prevent the development of potentially fatal infectious diseases. By contrast, the immune system may generate responses that lead to hypersensitivity or tissue injury and disease. In either case, the process is fascinating and commands the attention and respect of the reader for Nature's incomparable versatility.

CAM (cell adhesion molecules) are cell-selective proteins that promote adhesion of cells to one another and are calcium independent. They are believed to help direct migration of cells during embryogenesis.

Adhesion molecules are extracellular matrix proteins that attract leukocytes from the circulation. For example, T and B lymphocytes possess lymph node homing receptors on their membranes which facilitate passage through high endothelial venules. Neutrophils migrate to areas of inflammation in response to endothelial leukocyte adhesion molecule-1 (ELAM-1) stimulated by TNF and IL-1 on the endothelium of vessels. B and T lymphocytes that pass through high endothelial venules have lymph node homing receptors.

Adhesion receptors (Figure 1) are proteins in cell membranes that facilitate the interaction of cells with matrix. They play a significant role in adherence and chemoattraction in cell migration. They are divided into three groups that include the immunoglobulin superfamily which contains the T cell receptor/CD3, CD4, CD8, MHC class I, MHC class II, sCD2/LFA-2, LFA-3/CD58, ICAM-1, ICAM-2 and VCAM-2. The second group of adhesion receptors is made up of the integrin family which contains LFA-1, Mac-1, p150,95, VLA-5, VLA-4/LPAM-1, LPAM-2 and LPAM-3. The third family of adhesion receptors consists of selectin molecules that include Mel-14/LAM-1, ELAM-1 and CD62.

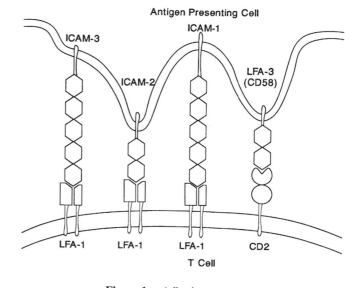

Figure 1. Adhesion receptors.

Integrins are a family of cell membrane glycoproteins that are heterodimers comprised of α and β chain subunits. They serve as extracellular matrix glycoprotein receptors. They identify the RGD sequence of the β subunit which consists of the arginine-glycine-aspartic acid tripeptide that occasionally also includes serine. The RGD sequence serves as a receptor recognition signal. Extracellular matrix glycoproteins for which integrins serve as receptors include fibronectin, C3, lymphocyte function associated antigen-1 (LFA-1) among other proteins. Differences in the β chain serve as the basis for division of integrins into three categories. Each category has distinctive α chains. The β chain provides specificity. The same 95kD β chain is found in one category of integrins that includes lymphocyte function associated antigen-1 (LFA-1) p150,95 and complement receptor 3 (CR3). The same 130kD β chain is shared among VLA-1, VLA-2, VLA-3, VLA-4, VLA-5, VLA-6 and integrins found in chickens. A 110kD β chain is shared in common by another category that includes the vitronectin receptor and platelet glycoprotein IIb/IIIa. There are four repeats of 40 amino acid residues in the β chain extracellular domains. There are 45 amino acid residues in the β chain intracellular domains. The principal function of integrins is to link the cytoskeleton to extracellular ligands. They also participate in wound healing, cell migration, killing of target cells and in phagocytosis. Leukocyte adhesion deficiency syndrome occurs when the β subunit of LFA-1 and Mac-1 are missing. VLA proteins facilitate binding of cells to collagen (VLA-1, -2, -3), laminin (VLA-1, -2, -6) and fibronectin (VLA-3, -4, -5).

Lymphocyte function-associated antigen-1 (LFA-1) (Figure 2) is a glycoprotein comprised of a 180-kD α chain and a 95-kD β chain expressed on lymphocyte and phagocytic cell membranes. LFA-1's ligand is the intercellular adhesion molecule-1 (ICAM-1). It facilitates natural killer cell and cytotoxic T cell interaction with target cells. Complement receptor 3 and p150,95 share the same specificity of the 769-amino acid residue β chain found in LFA-1. A gene on chromosome 16 encodes the α chain whereas a gene on chromosome 21 encodes the β chain.

Lymphocyte function associated antigen-3 (LFA-3) (Figures 3 and 4) is a 60kD polypeptide chain expressed on the surfaces of B cells, T cells, monocytes, granulocytes, platelets, fibroblasts and endothelial cells of vessels. LFA-3 is the ligand for CD2 (Figures 5–7) and is encoded by genes on chromosome 1 in man.

Intercellular adhesion molecule-1 (ICAM-1) (Figure 8) is a 90kD cellular membrane glycoprotein that occurs in multiple cell types including dendritic cells and endothelial cells. It is the lymphocyte function associated antigen-1 (LFA-1) ligand. The LFA-1 molecules on cytotoxic T lymphocytes (CTL) interact with ICAM-1 molecules found on CTL target cells. Interferon γ, tumor necrosis factor and IL-1 can elevate ICAM-1 expression.

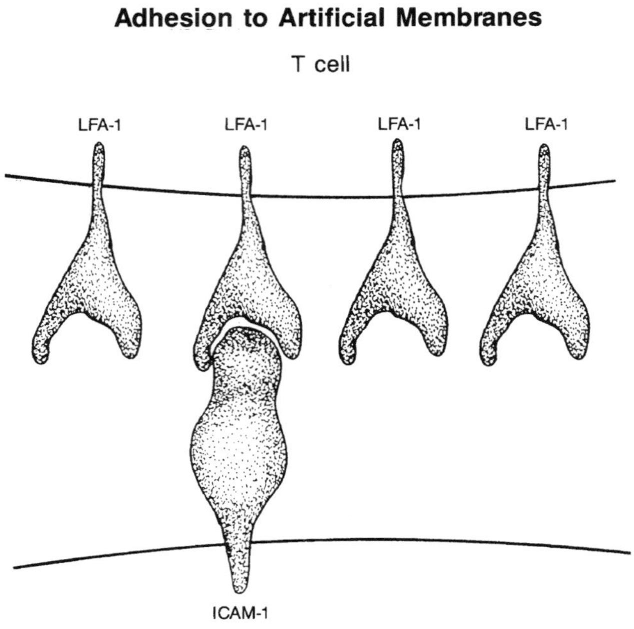

Adhesion to Artificial Membranes

T cell

Figure 2.   Lymphocyte function associated antigen-1.

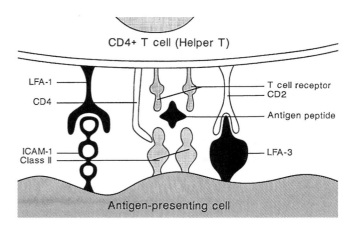

Figure 3.   Lymphocyte function associated antigen-3.

Intercellular adhesion molecule-2 (Figure 9) is a protein that is a member of the immunoglobulin superfamily that is important in cellular interactions. It is a cell surface molecule that serves as a ligand for leukocyte integrins. ICAM-2 facilitates lymphocyte binding to antigen-presenting cells or to endothelial cells. ICAM-2 binds to LFA-1, a T lymphocyte integrin.

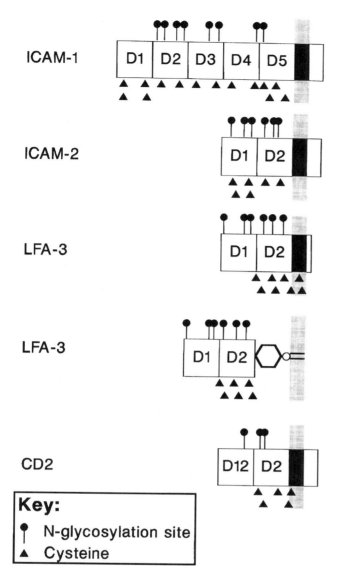

Key:
- N-glycosylation site
- Cysteine

Figure 4. Immunoglobulin superfamily adhesion receptors.

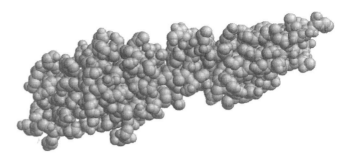

Figure 6. CD2. Space fill. Resolution. 2.0 angstroms.

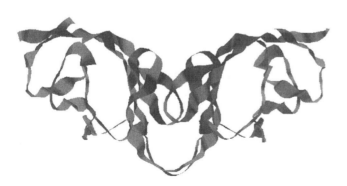

Figure 5. CD2. Ribbon diagram. Resolution. 2.0 angstroms.

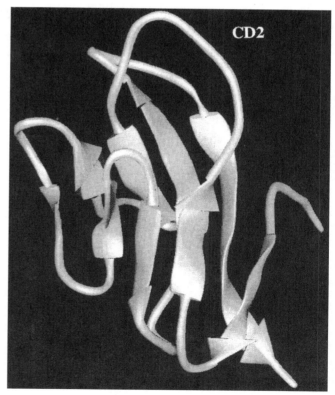

Figure 7. CD2. Ribbon structure.

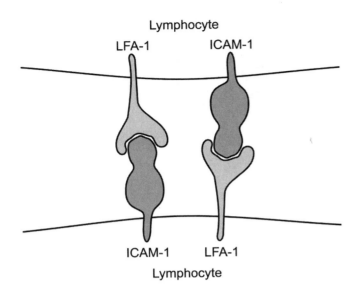

Figure 8.   ICAM-1.

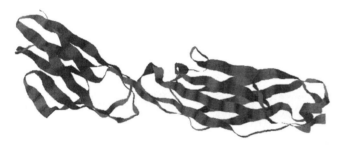

Figure 9.   ICAM-2. Ribbon diagram. Resolution. 2.2 angstroms.

Intercellular adhesion molecule-3 (ICAM-3) is a leukocyte cell surface molecule that plays a critical role in the interaction of T lymphocytes with antigen presenting cells. The interaction of the T lymphocyte with an antigen presenting cell through union of ICAM-1, ICAM-2 and ICAM-3 with LFA-1 molecules is also facilitated by the interaction of the T cell surface molecule CD2 with LFA-3 present on antigen-presenting cells.

Very late activation antigens (VLA molecules) are β-1 integrins that all have the CD19 β chain in common. They were originally described on T lymphocytes grown in long-term culture, but were subsequently found on additional types of leukocytes and on cells other than blood cells. VLA proteins facilitate leukocyte adherence to vascular endothelium and extracellular matrix. Resting T lymphocytes express VLA-4, VLA-5, and VLA-6. VLA-4 is expressed on multiple cells that include thymocytes, lymphocytes in blood, B and T cell lines, monocytes, NK cells, and eosinophils. The extracellular matrix ligand for VLA-4 and VLA-5 is fibronectin, and for VLA-6 it is laminin. The

binding of these molecules to their ligands gives T lymphocytes costimulator signals. VLA-5 is present on monocytes, memory T lymphocytes, platelets, and fibroblasts. It facilitates B and T cell binding to fibronectin. VLA-6, which is found on platelets, T cells, thymocytes, and monocytes, mediates platelet adhesion to laminin. VLA-3 is a laminin receptor, binds collagen, and identifies fibronectin. It is present on B cells, the thyroid, and the renal glomerulus. Platelet VLA-2 binds to collagen only, whereas endothelial cell VLA-2 combines with collagen and laminin. Lymphocytes bind through VLA-4 to high endothelial venules and to endothelial cell surface proteins (VCAM-1) in areas of inflammation. VLA-1, which is present on activated T cells, monocytes, melanoma cells, and smooth muscle cells, binds collagen and laminin.

Vascular Cell Adhesion Molecule-1 (VCAM-1) (Figures 10 and 11) is a molecule that binds lymphocytes and monocytes. It is found on activated endothelial cells, dendritic cells, tissue macrophages, bone marrow fibroblasts, and myoblasts. VCAM-1 belongs to the immunoglobulin gene superfamily and is a ligand for VLA-4 (integrin α4/β1) and integrin α4/β7. It plays an important role in leukocyte recruitment to inflammatory sites and facilitates lymphocyte, eosinophil, and monocyte adhesion to activated endothelium. It participates in lymphocyte-dendritic cell interaction in the immune response.

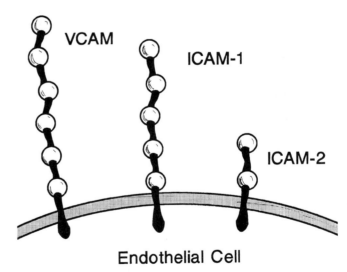

Figure 10.   VCAM-1 bound to an endothelial cell.

Platelet Endothelial Cell Adhesion Molecule-1 (PECAM-1) (CD31) is an antigen that is a single chain membrane glycoprotein, with a MW of 140kD. It is found on granulocytes, monocytes, macrophages, B cells, platelets, and endothelial cells. Although it is termed gpIIa′, it is different from the CD29 antigen. At present the function of CD31 is unknown. It may be an adhesion molecule.

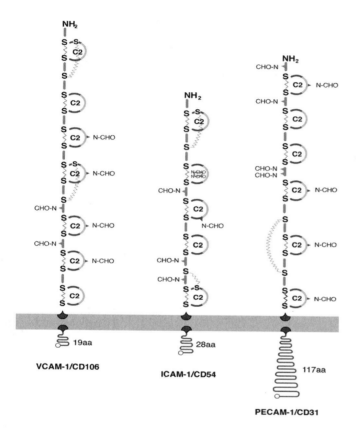

Figure 11. Schematic representation of VCAM-1.

Endothelial leukocyte adhesion molecule-1 (ELAM-1) facilitates focal adhesion of leukocyte to blood vessel walls. It is induced by endotoxins and cytokines and belongs to the adhesion molecule family. It is considered to play a significant role in the pathogenesis of atherosclerosis, infectious and autoimmune diseases. Neutrophil and monocyte adherance to endothelial cells occurs during inflammation *in vivo* where there is leukocyte margination and migration to areas of inflammation. Endothelial cells activated by IL-1 and TNF synthesize ELAM-1, at least in culture. A 115kD chain and a 100kD chain comprise the ELAM-1 molecule.

Fibronectin is an adhesion-promoting dimeric glycoprotein found abundantly in the connective tissue and basement membrane. The tetrapeptide, Arg-Gly-Asp-Ser, facilitates cell adhesion to fibrin, Clq, collagens, heparin and type I-, II-, III-, V-, and VI-sulfated proteoglycans. Fibronectin is also present in plasma and on normal cell surfaces. Approx-

imately 20 separate fibronectin chains are known. They are produced from the fibronectin gene by alternative splicing of the RNA transcript. Fibronectin is comprised of two 250kD subunits joined near their carboxy-terminal ends by disulfide bonds. The amino acid residues in the subunits vary in number from 2145 to 2445. Fibronectin is important in contact inhibition, cell movement in embryos, cell-substrate adhesion, inflammation and wound healing. It may also serve as an opsonin.

Vitronectin (Figure 12) is a cell adhesion molecule that is a 65kD glycoprotein. It is found in the serum at a concentration of 20 mg/l. It combines with coagulation and fibrinolytic proteins and with C5b67 complex to block its insertion into lipid membranes. Vitronectin appears in the basement membrane, together with fibronectin in proliferative viteroretinopathy. It decreases nonselective lysis of autologous cells by insertion of soluble C5b67 complexes from other cell surfaces. Vitronectin also is called epibolin and protein S.

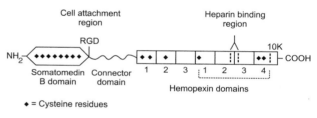

Figure 12. Vitronectin.

Collagen (Figure 13) is a 285kD extracellular matrix protein that contains proline hydroxyproline, lysine, hydroxylysine and glycine 30%. The structure consists of a triple helix of 95kD polypeptides forming a tropocollagen molecule that is resistance to proteases. Collagen types other than IV form fibrils with quarter stagger overlap between molecules that provide a fibrillar structure that resists tension. Several types of collagen have been described and most of them can be cross-linked through lysine side-chain.

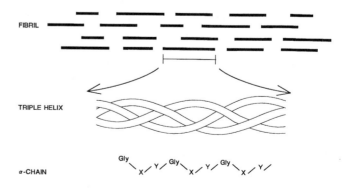

Figure 13. Collagen.

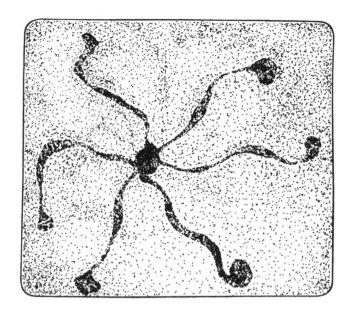

Figure 14.   Tenascin.

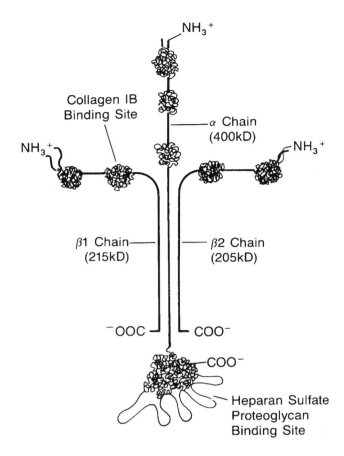

Figure 15.   Laminin.

Tenascin (Figure 14) is a matrix protein produced by embryonic mesenchymal cells. It facilitates epithelial tissue differentiation and consists of six 210kD proteins that are all alike.

Laminin (Figure 15) is a relatively large (820kD) basement membrane glycoprotein comprised of three polypeptide subunits. It belongs to the integrin receptor family which includes a 400kD α heavy chain and two 200kD light chains designated β1 and β2. By electron microscopy the molecule is arranged in the form of a cross. The domain structures of the α and β chains resemble one another. There are six primary domains. I and II have repeat sequences forming α helices. III and V are comprised of cysteine-rich repeating sequences. The globular regions are comprised of domains IV and VI. There is an additional short cysteine-rich α domain between the I and II domains in the β1 chain. There is a relatively large globular segment linked to the C-terminal of domain I, designated the "foot" in the α chain. Five "toes" on the foot contain repeat sequences. Laminins have biological functions and characteristics that include facilitation of cellular adhesion and linkage to other basement membrane constituents such as collagen type IV, heparan and glycosaminoglycans. Laminins also facilitate neurite regeneration, an activity associated with the foot of the molecule. There is more than one form of laminin, each representing different gene products, even though they possess a high degree of homology. S laminin describes a form found only in synaptic and non-muscle basal lamina. This is a single 190kD polypeptide (in the reduced form) and is greater than 1000kD in the nonreduced form. It is associated with the development or stabilization of synapses. It is homologous to the β1 chain of laminin. Laminin facilitates cell attachment and migration. It plays a role in differentiation and

metastasis and is produced by macrophages. Macrophages, endothelial cells, epithelial cells and Schwann cells produce it.

The **laminin receptor** is a membrane protein comprised of two disulfide bond-linked subunits, one relatively large and one relatively small. Its function appears to be for attachment of cells and for the outgrowth of neurites. It may share structural similarities with fibronectin and vitronectin, both of which are also integrins.

Mac-1 (Figure 16) is found on mononuclear phagocytes, neutrophils, NK cells and mast cells. It is an integrin molecule comprised of an alpha chain (CD11b) linked noncovalently to a beta chain (CD18) that is the same as the beta chains of leukocyte function-associated antigen-1 (LFA-1) and of p150,95. It facilitates phagocytosis of microbes that are coded with iC3b. It also facilitates neutrophil and monocyte adherence to the endothelium.

LFA-2 is a T cell antigen that is the receptor molecule for sheep red cells and is also referred to as the T11 antigen, the leukocyte function associated antigen-2 (LFA-2). The molecule has a mol wt of 50 kD. The antigen also seems to

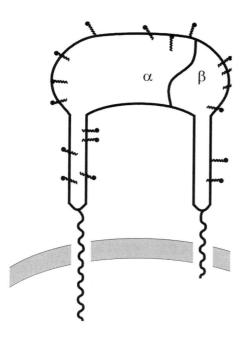

Figure 16.   Mac-1.

be involved in cell adhedrence, probably binding LFA-3 as its ligand.

A **human T lymphocyte** encircled by a ring of sheep red blood cells is referred to as an E rosette. This was used previously as a method to enumerate T lymphocytes (Figure 17).

Selectins (Figure 18) are a group of cell adhesion molecules (CAMs) that are glycoproteins and play an important role in the relationship of circulating cells to the endothelium. The members of this surface molecule family have three separate structural motifs. They have a single N-terminal (extracellular) lectin motif preceeding a single epidermal growth factor repeat and various short consensus repeat homology units. They are involved in lymphocyte migration, selective IgA, and IgG deficiency. This disease, which affects both males and females, is either X-linked, autosomal recessive, or can be acquired later in life. There may be a genetic defect in the switch mechanism for immunoglobulin producing cells to change from IgM to IgG or IgA synthesis. Respiratory infections with pyogenic microorganisms or autoimmune states that include hemolytic anemia, thrombocytopenia, and neutropenia may occur. Numerous IgM-synthesizing plasma cells are demonstrable in both lymph nodes and spleen of affected individuals.

L-selectin (CD62L) is a molecule found on lymphocytes that is responsible for the homing of lymphocytes to lymph node high endothelial venules. L-selectin is also found on neutrophils where it acts to bind the cells to activated endothelium early in the inflammatory process.

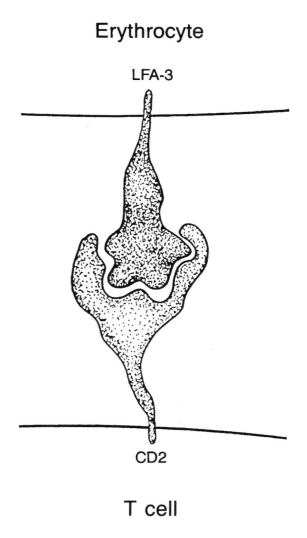

Figure 17.   E rosette.

LAM-1 (leukocyte adhesion molecule-1) is a homing protein found on membranes that combines with target cell specific glycoconjugates. It helps to regulate migration of leukocytes through lymphocyte-binding to high endothelial venules and to regulate neutrophil adherence to endothelium at inflammatory sites.

CD44 is a transmembrane molecule with a mol wt of 80 to 90 kD. It is found on some white and red cells. It is weakly expressed on platelets. It functions probably as a homing receptor. CD44 is a receptor on cells for hyaluronic acid. It binds to hyaluronate. CD44 mediates leukocyte adhesion.

E-selectin (CD62E) is a molecule found on activated endothelial cells that recognizes sialylated Lewis X and related glycans. Its expression is associated with acute cytokine mediated inflammation.

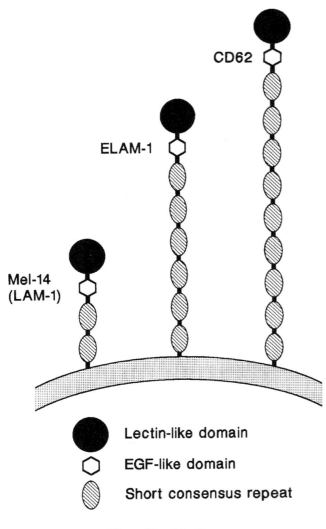

CD62

ELAM-1

Mel-14
(LAM-1)

⬤ Lectin-like domain

⬡ EGF-like domain

▱ Short consensus repeat

Figure 18. Selectins.

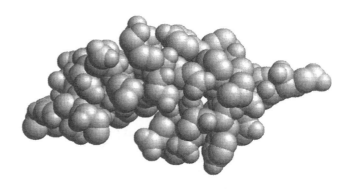

Figure 19. P-selectin. NMR.

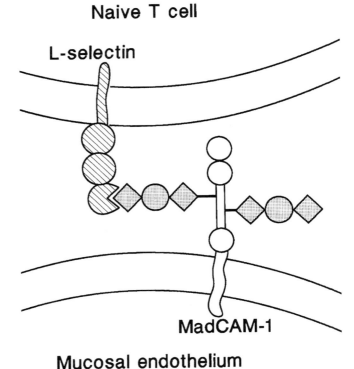

Naive T cell

L-selectin

MadCAM-1

Mucosal endothelium

Figure 20. MadCAM-1.

P-selectin (CD62P) (Figure 19) is a molecule found in the storage granules of platelets and the Weible-Palade bodies of endothelial cells. Ligands are sialylated Lewis X and related glycans. P-selectins are involved in the binding of leukocytes to endothelium and platelets to monocytes in areas of inflammation.

Addressin is a molecule such as a peptide or protein that serves as a homing device to direct a molecule to a specific location (an example is ELAM-1). Lymphocytes from Peyer's patches home to mucosal endothelial cells bearing ligands for the lymphocyte homing receptor.

MadCAM-1 (Figure 20) facilitates access of lymphocytes to the mucosal lymphoid tissue, as in the gastrointestinal tract.

Cadherins are one of the four specific families of cell adhesion molecules that enable cells to interact with their environment. Cadherins help cells to communicate with other

cells, in immune surveillance, extravasation, trafficking, tumor metastasis, wound healing and tissue localization. Cadherins are calcium-dependent. The five different cadherins include N-cadherin, P-cadherin, T-cadherin, V-cadherin and E-cadherin. Cytoplasmic domains of cadherins may interact with proteins of the cytoskeleton. They may bind to other receptors based on homophilic specificity but still depend on intracellular interactions linked to the cytoskeleton.

Chemotaxis (Figure 21) is the process whereby chemical substances direct cell movement and orientation. The orientation

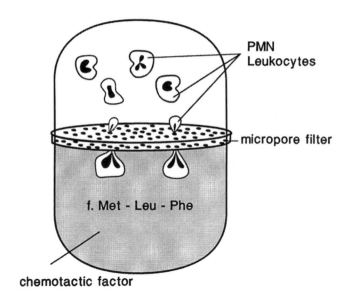

Figure 21.   Chemotaxis.

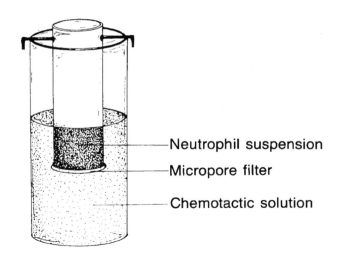

Figure 22.   Boyden chamber.

and movement of cells in the direction of a chemical's concentration gradient is positive chemotaxis, whereas movement away from the concentration gradient is termed negative chemotaxis. Substances that induce chemotaxis are referred to as chemotaxins and are often small molecules, such as C5a, formyl peptides, lymphokines, bacterial products, leukotriene B_4, etc., that induce positive chemotaxis of polymorphonuclear neutrophils, eosinophils, and monocytes. These cells move into inflammatory agents by chemotaxis. A dual chamber device called a Boyden chamber is used to measure chemotaxis in which phagocytic cells in culture are separated from a chemotactic substance by a membrane. The number of cells on the filter separating the cell chamber from the chemotaxis chamber reflect the chemotactic influence of the chemical substance for the cells.

A **Boyden chamber** (Figure 22) is a two compartment structure used in the laboratory to assay chemotaxis. The two chambers in the apparatus are separated by a micropore filter. The cells to be tested are placed in the upper chamber and a chemotactic agent such as F-met-leu-phe is placed in the lower chamber. As cells in the upper chamber settle to the filter surface, they migrate through the pores if the agent below chemoattracts them. On staining of the filter, cell migration can be evaluated.

Chemotactic factors include substances of both endogenous and exogenous origin. Among them are bacterial extracts, products of tissue injury, chemical substances, various proteins, and secretory products of cells. The most important among them are those generated from complement and described as anaphylatoxins. This name is related to their concurrent ability of stimulating the release of mediators from mast cells. Some chemotactic factors act specifically in directing migration of certain cell types. Others

have a broader spectrum of activity. Many of them have additional activities besides acting as chemotactic factors. Such effects of aggregation and adhesion of cells, discharge of lysosomal enzymes, and phagocytosis by phagocytic cells may be concurrently stimulated. Participation in various immunologic phenomena such as cell triggering of cell-cell interactions is known for certain chemotactic factors. The structure of chemotactic factors and even the active region in their molecules have been determined in many instances. However, advances in the clarification of their mechanism of action have been facilitated by the use of synthetic oligopeptides with chemotactic activities. The specificity of such compounds depends both on the nature of the amino acid sequence and the position of amino acids in the peptide chain. Methionine at the NH_2 terminal is essential for chemotactic activity. Formylation of Met leads to a 3,000–30,000-fold increase in activity. The second position from the NH_2-terminal is also essential and Leu, Phe, and Met in this position are essentially equivalent. Positively charged His and negatively charged Glu in this position are significantly less active, substantiating the role of a neutral amino acid in the second position at the N-terminal.

Chemotactic receptors are specific for chemotactic factors. In bacteria such receptors are designated sensors and signalers and are associated with various transport mechanisms. The cellular receptors for chemotactic factors have not been isolated and characterized. In leukocytes, the chemotactic receptor appears to activate a serine proesterase enzyme, which sets in motion the sequence of events related to cell locomotion. The receptors appear specific for the chemotactic factors under consideration and apparently the same receptors mediate all types of cellular responses inducible by a given chemotactic factor. However, these responses can be dissociated from each other suggesting that binding to the putative receptor initiates a series of parallel, interdependent and coordinated biochemical events leading to one or another type of response. Using a synthetic peptide, N-formyl-methionyl-leucyl-phenylalanine, about 2,000 binding sites have been demonstrated per PMN leukocyte. The binding sites are specific, have high affinity for the ligand, and are saturable. Competition for the binding sites is shown only by the parent or related compounds; the potency of the latter varies. Positional isomers may inhibit binding. Full occupancy of the receptors is not required for a maximal response and occupancy of only 10–20% of them is sufficient. The presence of spare receptors may enhance the sensitivity in the presence of small concentrations of chemotactic factors and may contribute to the detection of a gradient. There also remains the possibility that some substances with chemotactic activity do not require specific binding sites on cell membranes.

The **fluid mosaic model** (Figure 23) is a fluid bilayer of lipid molecules in the plasma membrane and organelle membranes of cells. This structure permits membrane proteins and glycoproteins to float. The lipid molecules are situated in a manner that arranges the polar heads toward outer surfaces and their hydrophobic side chains projecting into the interior. There can be lateral movement of molecules in the bilayer plane or they may rotate on their long axes. This is the Singer-Nicholson "fluid mosaic." The bilayer consists of phospholipids and glycolipids. Amphipathic lipids and globular proteins are spaced throughout the membrane. The fluid consistency permits movement of the proteins, glycoprotein and receptors laterally.

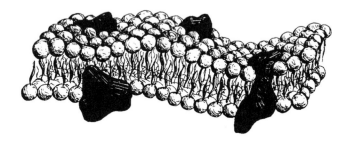

Figure 23. Fluid mosaic model.

The **endoplasmic reticulum** (Figure 24) is a structure in the cytoplasm comprised of parallel membranes that are connected to the nuclear membranes. Lipids and selected proteins are synthesized in this organelle. The membrane is continuous and convoluted. Electron microscopy reveals rough endoplasmic reticulum which contains ribosomes on the side exposed to the cytoplasm and smooth endoplasmic reticulum without ribosomes. Fatty acids and phospholipids are synthesized and metabolized in smooth endoplasmic reticulum. Selected membrane and organelle proteins as well

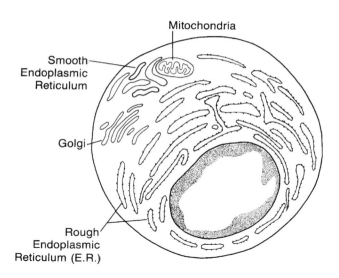

Figure 24. Eukaryotic cell.

as secreted proteins are synthesized in the rough endoplasmic reticulum. Cells such as plasma cells that produce antibodies or other specialized secretory proteins have abundant rough endoplasmic reticulum in the cytoplasm. Following formation, proteins move from the rough endoplasmic reticulum to the Golgi complex. They may be transported in vesicles that form from the endoplasmic reticulum and fuse with Golgi complex membranes. Once secreted protein reaches the endoplasmic reticulum lumen, it does not have to cross any further barriers prior to exit from the cell.

The **Golgi apparatus** consist of a stack of vesicles enclosed by membranes found within a cell and serve as a site of glycosylation and packaging of secreted proteins. It is a part of the GERL complex.

A **lysosome** (Figure 25) is an organelle in the cytoplasm enclosed by a membrane that contains various hydrolytic enzymes that may escape into either a phagosome or to the outside. Lysosomal enzymes may autolyze a dead cell.

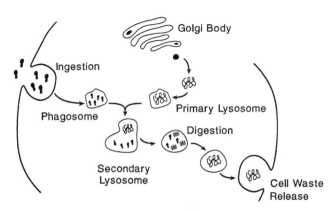

Figure 25. Lysosome

The **mitochondria** are cytoplasmic organelles that are sites of metabolism in cells.

Stem cells (Figure 26) are relatively large cells with a cytoplasmic rim that stains with methyl green pyronin and a nucleus that has thin chromatin strands and contains nucleoli that are pyroninophilic. They are found in hematopoietic tissues such as the bone marrow. These stem cells are a part of the colony forming unit (CFU) pool which indicates that individual cells are able to differentiate and proliferate under favorable conditions. The stem cells, CFU-S which are pluripotent, are capable of differentiating into committed precursor cells of the granulocyte and monocyte lineage (CFU-C) of erythropoietic lineage (CFU-E and BFU-E), and of megakaryocyte lineage (CFU-Mg). Lymphocytes, like other hematopoietic cells are generated in the bone marrow. The stem cell compartment is composed of a continuum of cells that include the most primitive with the greatest capacity for self renewal and the least evidence of cell cycle activity, to the most committed with a lesser capacity for self renewal and the most evidence of cell cycle activity. Stem cells are precursor cells that are multipotential with the capacity to yield differentiated cell types with different functions and phenotypes. The proliferative capacity of stem cells is, however, limited.

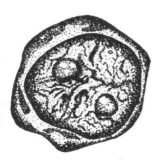

Figure 26. Stem cell.

Leukocytes are white blood cells. The principal types of leukocytes in the peripheral blood of man include polymorphonuclear neutrophils, eosinophils and basophils (granulocytes), lymphocytes and monocytes.

Mononuclear cells are leukocytes with single round nuclei such as lymphocytes and macrophages, in contrast to polymorphonuclear leukocytes. Thus, the term refers to the mononuclear phagocytic system or to lymphocytes.

A **lymphoblast** (Figure 27) is a relatively large cell of the lymphocyte lineage that bears a nucleus with fine chromatin and basophilic nucleoli. They frequently form following antigenic or mitogenic challenge of lymphoid cells, which leads to enlargement and division to produce effector lymphocytes

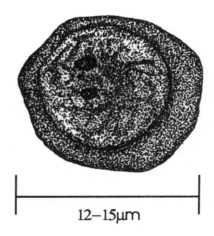

12–15μm

Figure 27. Lymphoblast.

that are active in immune reactions. The Epstein-Barr virus is commonly used to transform B cells into B lymphoblasts in tissue culture to establish B lymphoblast cell lines.

A **lymphocyte** (Figures 28–33) is a round cell that measures 7 to 12 μ and contains a round to ovoid nucleus that may be indented. The chromatin is densely packed and stains dark blue with Romanowsky stains. Small lymphocytes contain a thin rim of robin's egg blue cytoplasm, and a few azurophilic granules may be present. Large lymphocytes have more cytoplasm and a similar nucleus. Electron microscopy reveals villi that cover most of the cell surface. Lymphocytes are divided into two principal groups termed B and T lymphocytes. They are distinguished not on morphology but on the expression of distinctive surface molecules that have precise roles in immune reaction. In addition, natural killer cells, which are large granular lymphocytes, comprise a small percentage of the lymphocyte population.

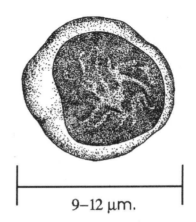

9–12 μm.

Figure 28. Lymphocyte.

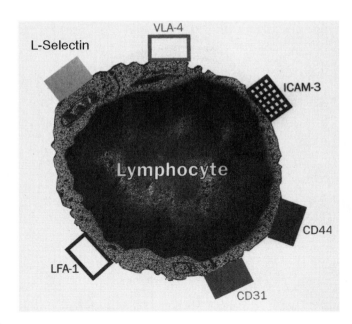

Figure 29.   Lymphocyte.

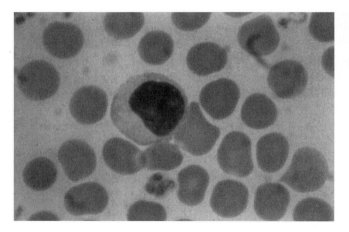

Figure 30.   Lymphocyte in peripheral blood.

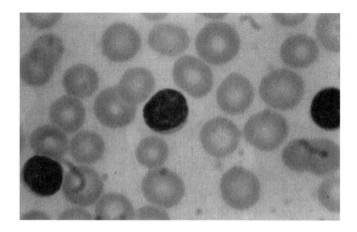

Figure 31.   Small lymphocyte in peripheral blood.

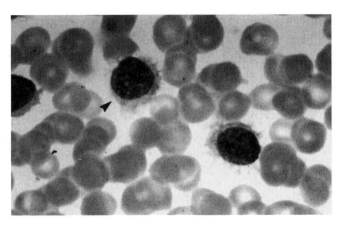

Figure 32.   Lymphocytes in peripheral blood.

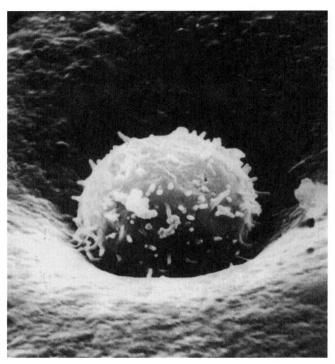

Figure 33.   Lymphocyte scanning electron micrograph.

Circulating lymphocytes are the lymphocytes present in the systemic circulation represent a mixture of cells derived from different sources: (1) B and T cells exiting from bone marrow and thymus on their way to seed the peripheral lymphoid organs, (2) lymphocytes exiting the lymph nodes via lymphatics, collected by the thoracic duct and discharged into the superior vena cava, and (3) lymphocytes derived from direct discharge into the vascular sinuses of the spleen. About 70% of cells in the circulating pool are recirculating; that is, they undergo a cycle during which they exit the systemic circulation to return back to lymphoid follicles, lymph nodes and spleen and start the cycle again. The cells in this recirculating pool are mostly long lived mature T

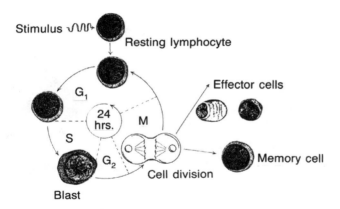

Figure 34. Lymphocyte activation.

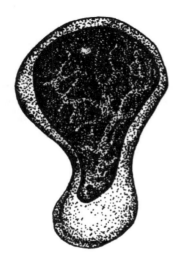

Figure 35. Uropod.

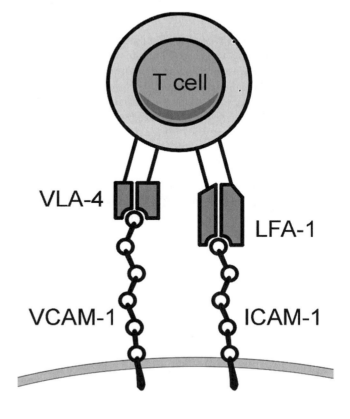

Figure 36. T cell.

cells. About 30% of the lymphocytes of the intravascular pool do not recirculate. They comprise mostly short-lived immature T cells which either live their life span intravascularly or are activated and exit the intravascular space. The exit of lymphocytes into the spleen occurs by direct discharge from the blood vessels. In lymph nodes and lymphoid follicles, the exit of lymphocytes occurs through specialized structures, the postcapillary venules. These differ from other venules in that they have a tall endothelial covering. The exiting lymphocytes percolate through the endothelial cells, a mechanism whose real significance is not known. A number of agents such as cortisone or the bacterium Bordetella pertussis increase the extravascular exit of lymphocytes and prevent their return to circulation. The lymphocytes travel back and forth between the blood and lymph. They attach to and pass through the high endothelial cells of the postcapillary venules of lymph nodes or the spleen's marginal sinuses. Within 24–48 hours they return via the lymphatics to the thoracic duct where they then reenter the blood.

Lymphocyte activation (Figure 34) follows stimulation of lymphocytes *in vitro* by antigen or mitogen which renders them metabolically active. Activated lymphocytes may undergo transformation or blastogenesis.

Uropod (Figure 35) describes lymphocyte cytoplasm extending as an elongated tail or pseudopod in locomotion. The uropod may resemble the handle of a hand mirror. The plasma membrane covers the uropod cytoplasm.

T cells (Figure 36) are derived from hematopoietic precursors that migrate to the thymus where they undergo differentiation which continues thereafter to completion in the various lymphoid tissues throughout the body or during their circulation to and from these sites. T cells primarily are involved in the control of immune responses by providing specific cells capable of helping or suppressing these responses. They also have a number of other functions related to cell-mediated immune phenomena.

Veto cells (Figures 37 and 38) comprise a proposed population of cells suggested to facilitate maintenance of self tolerance through veto of autoimmune responses by T cells. A "veto cell" would neutralize the function of an autoreactive T lymphocyte. A T cell identifies itself as an autoreactive lymphocyte by recognizing surface antigen on the "veto cell." No special receptors with specificity for the autoreactive T lymphocyte are required for the "veto cell" to render the T lymphocyte nonfunctional.

B cells are B lymphocytes that derive from the fetal liver in the early embryonal stages of development and from the bone marrow thereafter. In birds, maturation takes place in the bursa of Fabricius, a lymphoid structure derived from an outpouching of the hindgut near the cloaca. In mammals, maturation is in the bone marrow. Plasma cells that synthesize antibody develop from precursor B cells.

CD22 (Figure 39) is a molecule, with a MW of α130 and β140kD, that is expressed in the cytoplasm of B cells of the pro-B and pre-B cell stage, and on the cell surface of mature B cells with surface Ig. The antigen is lost shortly before

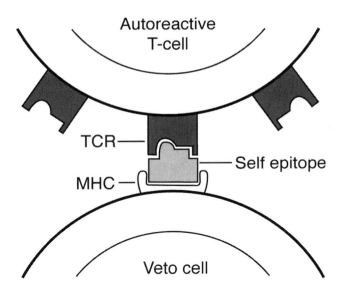

Figure 37.   Veto Effect.

the terminal plasma cell phase. The molecule has five extracellular immunoglobulin-domains and shows homology with myelin adhesion glycoprotein and with N-CAM (CD56). It participates in B cell adhesion to monocytes and T cells. It also is called BL-CAM.

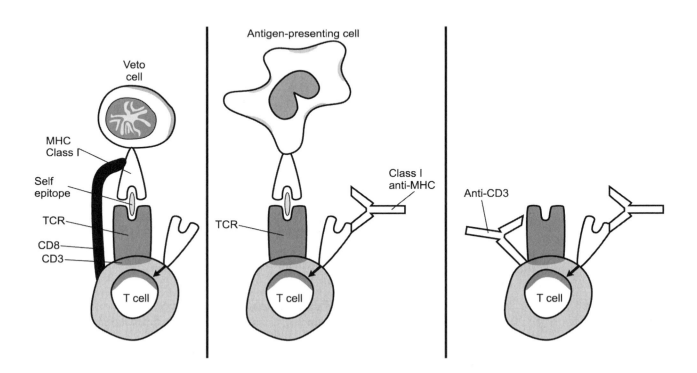

The Three Mechanisms of the Veto Effect

Figure 38.   Veto Effect.

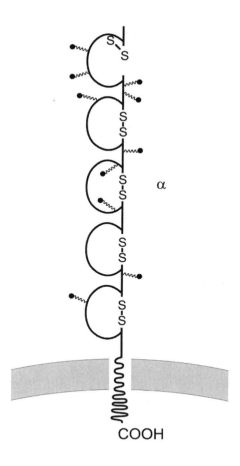

Figure 39.   CD22.

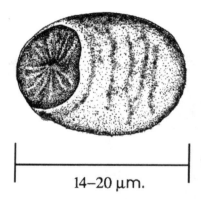

14–20 μm.

Figure 40.   Plasma cell.

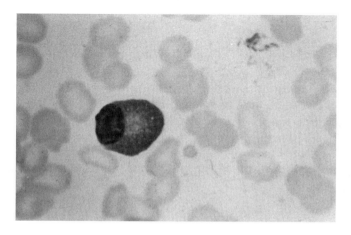

Figure 41.   Plasma cell in peripheral blood.

Plasma cells (Figures 40 and 41) are antibody producing cells. Immunoglobulins are present in their cytoplasm and secretion of immunoglobulin by plasma cells has been directly demonstrated *in vitro*. Increased levels of immunoglobulins in some pathologic conditions are associated with increased numbers of plasma cells and conversely, their number at antibody producing sites increases following immunization. Plasma cells develop from B cells and are large, spherical or ellipsoidal cells, 10–20 μ in size. Mature plasma cells have abundant cytoplasm, staining deep blue with Wright's stain, and have an eccentrically located, round or oval nucleus, usually surrounded by a well defined perinuclear clear zone. The nucleus contains coarse and clumped masses of chromatin, often arranged in a cartwheel fashion. The nuclei of normal, mature plasma cells, have no nucleoli but those of neoplastic plasma cells such as those seen in multiple myeloma, have conspicuous nucleoli. The cytoplasm of normal plasma cells has conspicuous Golgi complex and rough endoplasmic reticulum and frequently contains vacuoles. The nuclear to cytoplasmic ratio is 1:2. By electron microscopy, plasma cells show very abundant endoplasmic reticulum, indicating extensive and active protein synthesis. Plasma cells do not express surface immunoglobulin or complement receptors which distinguishes them from B lymphocytes.

Hof (Figure 42) is a German word for courtyard which refers to the perinuclear clear zone adjacent to the nucleus in plasma cells. Lymphoblasts and Reed-Sternberg cells may also exhibit a hof.

A **null cell** is a lymphocyte that does not manifest any markers of T or B cells including cluster of differentiation (CD) antigens or surface immunoglobulins. Approximately 20% of peripheral lymphocytes are null cells. They play a role in antibody-dependent cell-mediated cytotoxicity (ADCC). They may be the principal cell in certain malignancies such as acute lymphocytic leukemia of children. The three types of null cells include: (1) undifferentiated stem cells that may mature into T or B lymphocytes, (2) cells with labile IgG and high-affinity Fc receptors that are resistant to trypsin and (3) large granular lymphocytes that constitute NK and K cells. The null cell compartment comprises 37% of the bone marrow. Null cells may differentiate into either B or T cells upon appropriate induction, the mechanism of

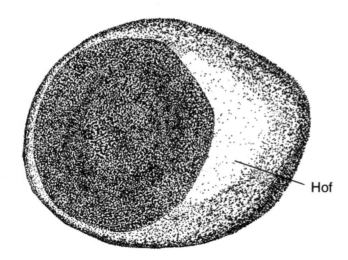

Figure 42.   Hof.

which is unknown. Some null cells differentiate into killer (K) cells by developing Fc and complement receptors. The NK cells are also present in this cell population. Null cells, K and NK cells, like committed lymphocytes, also migrate to the peripheral lymphoid organs such as spleen and lymph nodes or to the thymus but represent only a very small fraction of the total cells present there. At all locations, the null cells are part of the rapidly renewed pool of immature cells with a short life span (five–six days). The null cells which have been committed to the T cell lineage migrate to the thymus to continue their differentiation.

Natural killer (NK) cells (Figure 43) are cells that attack and destroy certain virus-infected cells. They constitute an important part of the natural immune system, do not require prior contact with antigen, and are not MHC restricted by the major histocompatibility complex (MHC) antigens. NK cells are lymphoid cells of the natural immune system that express cytotoxicity against various nucleated cells including tumor cells and virus-infected cells. NK cells, killer (K) cells or antibody-dependent cell-mediated cytotoxicity (ADCC) cells induce lysis through the action of antibody. Immunologic memory is not involved as previous contact with antigen is not necessary for NK cell activity. The NK cell is approximately 15 μm in diameter and has a kidney shaped nucleus with several, often three, large cytoplasmic granules. The cells are also called large granular lymphocytes (LGL). In addition to the ability to kill selected tumor cells and some virus-infected cells, they also participate in antibody-dependent cell-mediated cytotoxicity (ADCC) by anchoring antibody to the cell surface through an Fc γ receptor. Thus, they are able to destroy antibody coated nucleated cells. NK cells are believed to represent a significant part of the natural immune defense against spontaneously developing neoplastic cells and against infection by viruses. NK cell activity is measured by a ^{51}Cr release

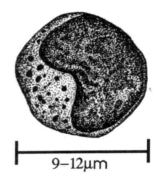

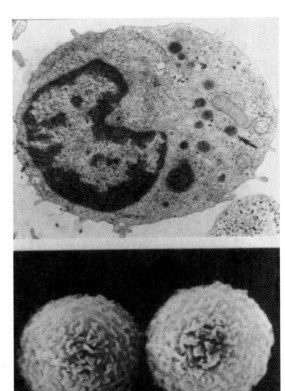

Figure 43.   NK (Natural killer) cell schematic representation, transmission, and scanning E.M. of human large granular lymphocyte.

assay employing the K562 erythroleukemia cell line as a target.

CD16 (Figure 44) is an antigen that is also known as the low affinity Fc receptor for complexed IgG-FcγRIII. It is expressed on NK cells, granulocytes (neutrophils), and macrophages. Structural differences in the CD16 antigen from granulocytes and NK cells have been reported. This apparent polymorphism suggests two different genes for the FcγRIII molecule in polymorphonuclear leukocytes (PMN) and in NK cells. The CD16 molecule in NK cells has a transmembrane form, whereas it is phosphatidylinositol (PI)-linked in

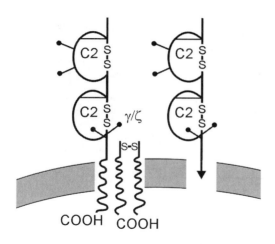

Figure 44. CD16.

granulocytes. CD16 mediates phagocytosis. It is the functional receptor structure for performing antibody dependent-cell-mediated cytotoxicity (ADCC). CD16 is also termed FcγRIII.

CD56 (Figure 45) is a 220/135 kD molecule that is an isoform of the neural adhesion molecule (N-CAM). It is used as a marker of NK cells, but it is also present on neuroectodermal cells.

K562 cells (Figures 46 and 47) are a chronic myelogenous leukemia cell line that serves as a target cell in a chromium-51 release assay of natural killer (NK) cells. Following incubation of NK cells with ^{51}Cr-labeled target K562 cells, the amount of chromium released into the supernatant is measured and the cytotoxicity determined by use of a formula.

K (killer) cells (Figure 48), also called null cells, have lymphocyte-like morphology but functional characteristics different from those of B and T cells. They are involved in a particular form of immune response, the antibody-dependent cellular cytotoxicity (ADCC), killing target cells coated with IgG antibodies. A K cell is an Fc-bearing killer cell that has an effector function in mediating antibody-dependent cell-mediated cytotoxicity. An IgG antibody molecule binds through its Fc region to the K cell's Fc receptor. Following contact with a target cell bearing antigenic determinants on its surface for which the Fab regions of the antibody molecule attached to the K cell are specific, the lymphocyte-like K cell releases lymphokines that destroy the target. This represents a type of immune effector function in which cells and antibody participate. Besides K cells, other cells that mediate antibody-dependent cell-mediated cytotoxicity include natural killer (NK) cells, cytotoxic T cells, neutrophils and macrophages.

Macrophages (Figures 49 and 50) are mononuclear phagocytic cells derived from monocytes in the blood that were

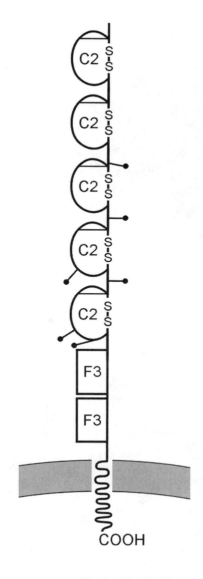

Figure 45. CD56.

produced from stem cells in the bone marrow. These cells have a powerful, although nonspecific role in immune defense. These intensely phagocytic cells contain lysosomes and exert microbicidal action against microbes which they ingest. They also have effective tumoricidal activity. They may take up and degrade both protein and polysaccharide antigens and present them to T lymphocytes in the context of major histocompatibility complex class II molecules. They interact with both T and B lymphocytes in immune reactions. They are frequently found in areas of epithelium, mesothelium and blood vessels. Macrophages have been referred to as adherent cells since they readily adhere to glass and plastic and may spread on these surfaces and manifest chemotaxis. They have receptors for Fc and C3b on their surfaces, stain positively for non-specific esterase and peroxidase, and are Ia antigen positive when acting as accessory

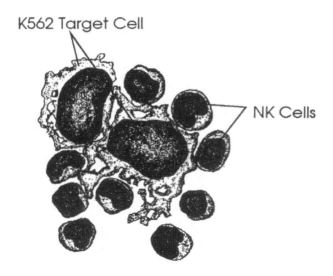

Figure 46. Schematic representation of a K562 target cell bound to NK cells.

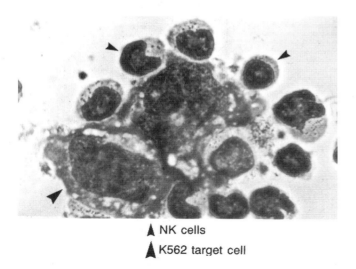

Figure 47. K562 target cells (large arrow) bound to NK cells (small arrows).

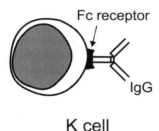

Figure 48. Schematic representation of a K cell.

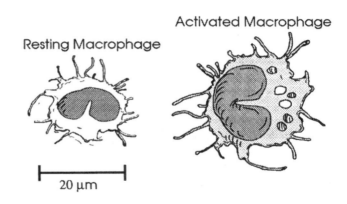

Figure 49. Schematic representation of a resting macrophage vs. an activated macrophage.

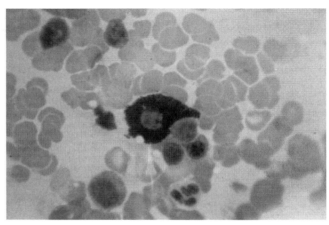

Figure 50. Macrophage-histiocyte in bone marrow.

cells that present antigen to CD4$^+$ lymphocytes in the generation of an immune response. Monocytes, which may differentiate into macrophages when they migrate into the tissues, make up 3–5% of leukocytes in the peripheral blood. Macrophages that are tissue-bound may be found in the lung alveoli, as microglial cells in the central nervous system, as Kupffer cells in the liver, as Langerhans cells in the skin, as histiocytes in connective tissues, as well as macrophages in lymph nodes and peritoneum. Multiple substances are secreted by macrophages including complement components C1 through C5, factors B and D, properdin, C3b inactivators and β-1H. They also produce monokines such as interleukin 1, acid hydrolase, proteases, lipases and numerous other substances.

Multiple processes are involved in **macrophage activation**. These include an increase in size and number of cytoplasmic granules and spreading membrane ruffling. Functional alterations include elevated metabolism and transport of amino acids and glucose, increased enzymatic activity, and an elevation in prostaglandins, cGMP, plasminogen activator, intracellular calcium ions, phagocytosis, pinocytosis and the ability to lyse bacteria and tumor cells.

CD9 is a single chain protein, with a MW of 24 kD, that is present on pre-B cells, monocytes, granulocytes, and platelets. Antibodies against the molecule can cause platelet aggregation. The CD9 antigen has protein kinase activity. It may be significant in aggregation and activation of platelets.

CD13 is an antigen that is a single chain membrane glycoprotein with a MW of 130 kD. It is present on monocytes, granulocytes, some macrophages, and connective tissue. CD13 has recently been shown to be aminopeptidase-N. It functions as a zinc metalloproteinase.

CD33 is an antigen that is a single chain transmembrane glycoprotein, with a MW of 67 kD. It is restricted to myeloid cells and is found on early progenitor cells, monocytes, myeloid leukemias, and weakly on some granulocytes.

An **accessory cell** (Figure 51) is a cell such as a monocyte, macrophage, dendritic cell or Langerhans cell that facilitates the generation of an immune response through antigen presentation to helper T cells. B cells may also act as antigen presenting cells, thereby serving an accessory cell function.

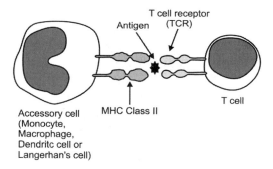

Figure 51.   Accessory cell.

Macrophage activating factor (MAF) is a lymphokine such as gamma interferon that accentuates the ability of macrophages to kill microbes and tumor cells. A lymphokine that enhances a macrophage's phagocytic activity, bactericidal and tumoricidal properties.

Macrophage chemotactic factor (MCF) refers to cytokines that act together with macrophages to induce facilitating migration. Among these substances are interleukins and interferons.

Macrophage chemotactic and activating factor (MCAF) is a chemoattractant and activator of macrophages produced by fibroblasts, monocytes, and endothelial cells as a result of exogenous stimuli and endogenous cytokines such as TNF, IL-1 and PDGF. It also has a role in activating monocytes to release an enzyme that is cytostatic for some tumor cells. MCAF also has a role in ELAM-1 and CD11a&b

surface expression in monocytes and is a potent degranulator of basophils.

Macrophage inflammatory protein-1-α (MIP-1) (Figure 52) is an endogeneous fever-inducing substance that binds heparin and is resistant to cyclo-oxygenase inhibition. Macrophages stimulated by endotoxin may secrete this protein, termed MIP-1, which differs from tumor necrosis factor (TNF) and IL-1, as well as other endogenous pyrogens because its action is not associated with prostaglandin synthesis. It appears indistinguishable from hematopoietic stem cell inhibitor and may function in growth regulation of hematopoietic cells.

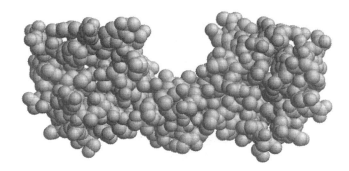

Figure 52.   MIP-1α. NMR.

Macrophage inflammatory peptide-2 (MIP-2) is a IL-8 type II receptor competitor and chemoattractant that is also involved in hemopoietic colony formation as a costimulator. It also degranulates murine neutrophils. The inflammatory activities of MIP-2 are very similar to IL-8.

Macrophage cytophilic antibody (Figure 53) is an antibody that becomes anchored to the Fc receptors on macrophage surfaces. This cytophilic antibody can be demonstrated by the immunocytoadherence test.

Macrophage functional assays are tests of macrophage function that include (1) chemotaxis: macrophages are placed in one end of a Boyden chamber and a chemoattractant is added to the other end. Macrophage migration toward the chemoattractant is assayed. (2) Lysis: macrophages acting against radiolabeled tumor cells or bacterial cells in suspension can be measured after suitable incubation by measuring the radioactivy of the supernatant. (3) Phagocytosis: radioactivity of macrophages that have ingested a radiolabed target can be assayed.

Alveolar macrophages (Figure 54) in the lung alveoli that may remove inhaled particulate matter.

A **veiled cell** (Figure 55) is a mononuclear phagocytic cell that serves as an antigen-presenting cell. It is found in the afferent lymphatics and in the marginal sinus. It may manifest IL-2 receptors in the presence of GM-CSF.

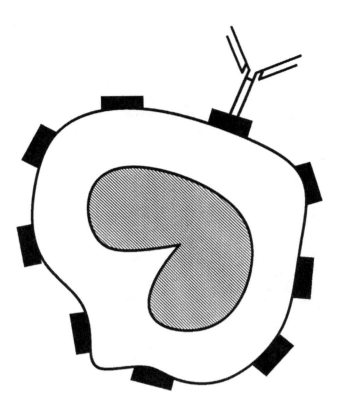

Figure 53. Macrophage cytophilic antibody.

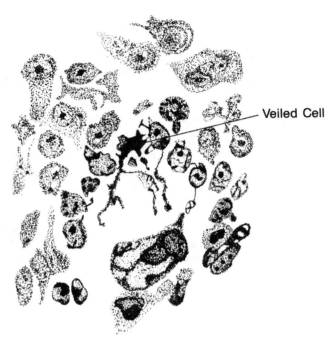

Figure 55. Veiled cell.

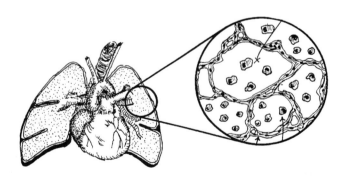

Figure 54. Alveolar macrophages

Dendritic cells are mononuclear phagocytic cells found in the skin as Langerhans cells, in the lymph nodes as interdigitating cells, in the paracortex as veiled cells in the marginal sinus of afferent lymphatics and as mononuclear phagocytes in the spleen where they present antigen to T lymphocytes. Dendritic reticular cells may have non-specific esterase, Birbeck granules, endogenous peroxidase, possibly CD1, complement receptors CR1 and CR3 and Fc receptors.

Langerhans cells (Figure 56) are dendritic-appearing accessory cells interspersed between cells of the upper layer of the epidermis. They can be visualized by gold chloride

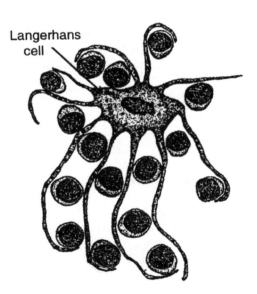

Figure 56. Langerhans cell.

impregnation of unfixed sections and show dendritic processes but no intercellular bridges. By electron microscopy, they lack tonofibrils or desmosomes, have indented nuclei and contain tennis racket-shaped Birbeck granules, which are relatively small vacuoles, round to rectangular and measuring 10 nm. Following their formation from stem cells in the bone marrow, Langerhans cells migrate to the epidermis and then to the lymph nodes, where they are described as dendritic cells based upon their thin cytoplasmic processes that

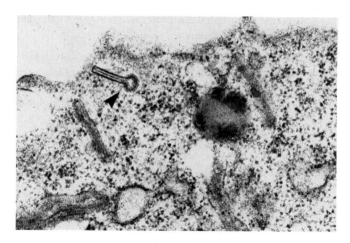

Figure 57.   Birbeck granules.

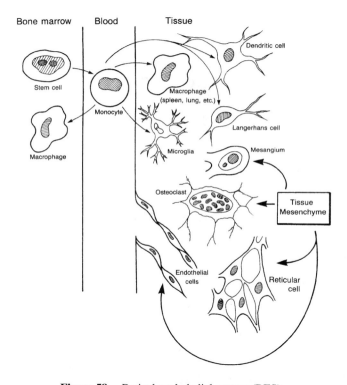

Figure 58.   Reticuloendothelial system (RES).

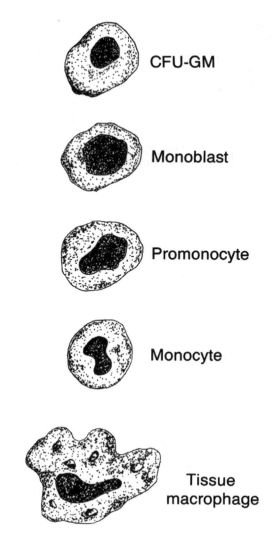

Figure 59.   Mononuclear phagocyte system.

course between adjacent cells. Langerhans cells express both class I and class II histocompatibility antigens, as well as C3b receptors and IgG Fc receptors on their surfaces. They function as antigen-presenting cells. Epidermal Langerhans cells express complement receptors 1 and 3, Fc γ receptors and fluctuating quantities of CD1. Dendritic cells do not express Fc γ receptors or CD1. Langerhans cells in the lymph nodes are found in the deep cortex. Epidermal Langerhans cells are important in the development of delayed-type hypersensitivity through the uptake of antigen in the skin and transport of it to the lymph nodes. Veiled cells in the lymph are indistinguishable from Langerhans cells.

Birbeck granules (Figure 57) are 10–30nm diameter round cytoplasmic vesicles present in the cytoplasm of Langerhans cells in the epidermis.

The **Reticuloendothelial system (RES)** (Figure 58) is a former term for the mononuclear phagocyte system that includes Kupffer cells lining the sinusoids of the liver as well as macrophages of the spleen and lymph nodes. Aschoff introduced the term to describe cells that could take up and retain vital dyes and particles that had been injected into the body. In addition to macrophages, less active phagocytic cells such as fibroblasts and endothelial cells were also included in the original definition. The principal function of the mononuclear phagocyte system is to remove unwelcome particles from the blood. RES activity can be measured by the elimination rate of radiolabeled molecules or cells, such as albumin or erythrocytes coated with antibody.

The **mononuclear phagocyte system** (Figure 59) consists of mononuclear cells with pronounced phagocytic ability that are distributed extensively in lymphoid and other organs. "Mononuclear phagocyte system" should be used in place of the previously popular "reticulo-endothelial system" to describe this group of cells. Mononuclear phagocytes originate from stem cells in the bone marrow that first differentiate into monocytes that appear in the blood for approximately 24 or more hours with final differentiation into macrophages in the tissues. Macrophages usually occupy perivascular areas. Liver macrophages are termed Kupffer cells, whereas those in the lung are alveolar macrophages. The microglia represent macrophages of the central nervous system, whereas histiocytes represent macrophages of connective tissue. Tissue stem cells are monocytes that have wandered from the blood into the tissues and may differentiate into macrophages. Mononuclear phagocytes have a variety of surface receptors that enable them to bind carbohydrates or such protein molecules as C3 via complement receptor 1 and complement receptor 3, and IgG and IgE through Fcγ and Fcε receptors. The surface expression of MHC class II molecules enables both monocytes and macrophages to serve as antigen presenting cells to CD4+ T lymphocytes. Mononuclear phagocytes secrete a rich array of molecular substances with various functions. A few of these include interleukin 1; tumor necrosis factor α; interleukin 6; C2, C3, C4 and factor B complement proteins; prostaglandins; leukotrienes and other substances.

Polymorphonuclear leukocytes (PMNs) (Figures 60 and 61) are white blood cells with lobulated nuclei that are often tri-lobed. These cells are of the myeloid cell lineage and in the mature form can be differentiated into neutrophils, eosinophils

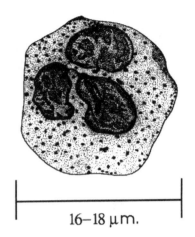

16–18 μm.

Figure 60.   Schematic representation of a PMN cell.

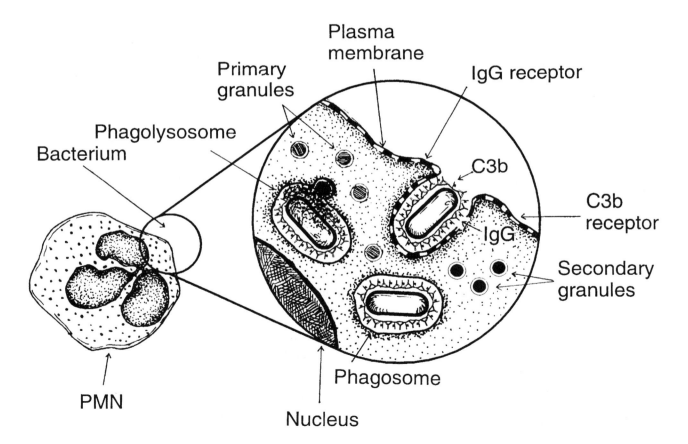

Figure 61.   Polymorphonuclear leukocyte (PMN).

and basophils. This distinction is based on the staining characteristics of their cytoplasmic specific or secondary granules. These cells, which measure approximately 13 μ in diameter, are active in acute inflammatory responses.

A **neutrophil leukocyte** (Figure 62) is a peripheral blood polymorphonuclear leukocyte derived from the myeloid lineage. Neutrophils comprise 40–75% of the total white blood count numbering 2,500–7,500 cells/cu mm. They are phagocytic cells and have a multilobed nucleus and azurophilic and specific granules that appear lilac following staining with Wright's or Giemsa stains. They may be attracted to a local site by such chemotactic factors as C5a. They are the principal cells of acute inflammation and actively phagocytize invading microorganisms. Besides serving as the first line of cellular defense in infection, they participate in such reactions as the uptake of antigen-antibody complexes in the Arthus reaction.

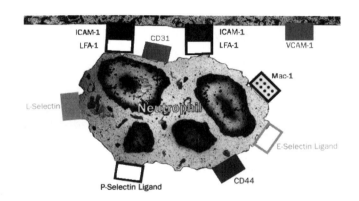

Figure 62. Neutrophil leukocyte.

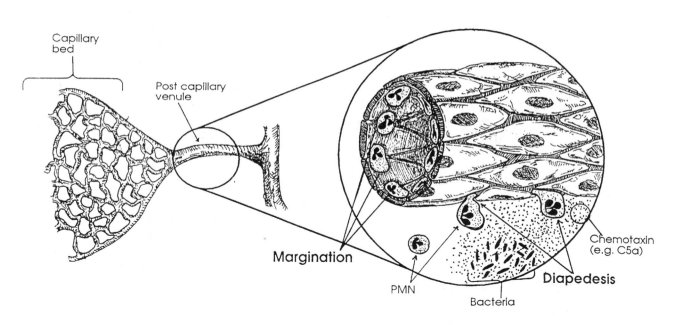

Figure 63. Diapedesis and margination.

Diapedesis (Figures 63 and 64) refers to cell migration from the interior of small vessels into tissue spaces as a consequence of constriction of endothelial cells in the wall.

Margination refers to the adherence of leukocytes in the peripheral blood to the endothelium of vessel walls. Approximately 50% of polymorphonuclear neutrophils marginate at one time. During inflammation, there is margination of leukocytes followed by their migration out of the vessels.

Phagocytes (Figures 65 and 66) are cells such as mononuclear phagocytes and polymorphonuclear neutrophils that ingest, and frequently digest particles such as bacteria, blood

cells, and carbon particles among many other particulate substances.

A **phagolysosome** is a cytoplasmic vesicle with a limiting membrane produced by the fusion of a phagosome with a lysosome. Substances within a phagolysosome are digested by hydrolysis.

Eosinophils (Figure 67 and 68) are polymorphonuclear leukocytes identified in Wright or Giemsa stained preparations by staining of secondary granules in the leukocyte cytoplasm as brilliant reddish-orange refractile granules. Cationic peptides are released from these secondary granules when an

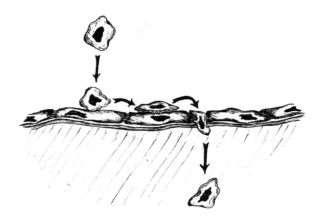

Figure 64.   Diapedesis.

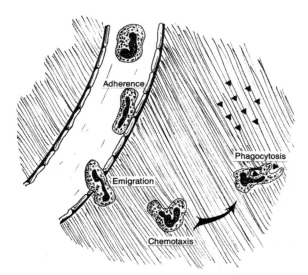

Figure 65.   Phagocytosis.

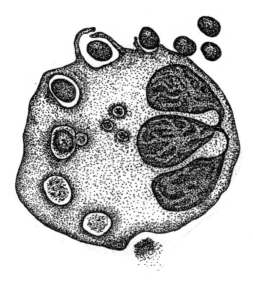

Figure 66.   Schematic representation of phagocytosis.

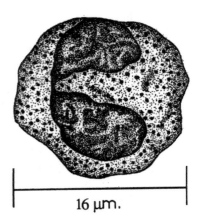

Figure 67.   Eosinophil with segmented nucleus.

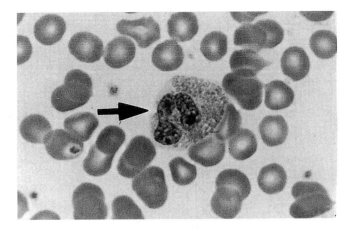

Figure 68.   Eosinophil in peripheral blood.

eosinophil interacts with a target cell and may lead to death of the target. Eosinophils make up 2–5% of the total white blood cells in man. After a brief residence in the circulation, eosinophils migrate into tissues by passing between the lining endothelial cells. It is believed that they do not return to the circulation. The distribution corresponds mainly to areas exposed to external environment such as skin, mucosa of the bronchi and gastro-intestinal tract. Eosinophils are elevated during allergic reactions, especially type I immediate hypersensitivity responses and are also elevated in individuals with parasitic infestations.

Basophils (Figure 69) are polymorphonuclear leukocytes of the myeloid lineage with distinctive basophilic secondary granules in the cytoplasm that frequently overlie the nucleus. These granules are storage depots for heparin, histamine, platelet activating factor and other pharmacological mediators of immediate hypersensitivity. Degranulation of the cells with release of these pharmacological mediators takes place following cross-linking by allergen or antigen of Fab regions of IgE receptor molecules bound through Fc receptors to the cell surface. They comprise less than 0.5% of peripheral blood leukocytes. Following cross-linking of surface bound

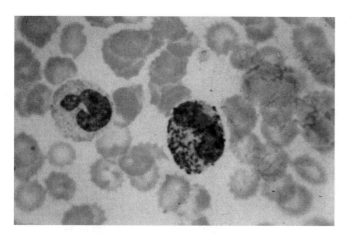

Figure 69. Basophil and neutrophil in peripheral blood.

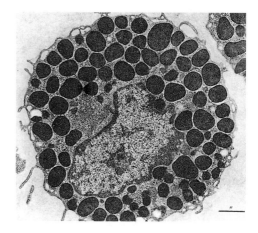

Figure 71. Mast cell in peripheral blood.

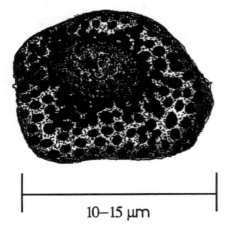

Figure 70. Mast cell.

IgE molecules by specific allergen or antigen, granules are released by exocytosis. Substances liberated from the granules are pharmacological mediators of immediate (Type I) anaphylactic hypersensitivity.

Mast cells (Figures 70 and 71) are normal components of the connective tissue that play an important role in immediate (type I) hypersensitivity and inflammatory rections by secreting a large variety of chemical mediators from storage sites in their granules upon stimulation. Their anatomical location at mucosal and cutaneous surfaces and about venules in deeper tissues is related to this role. They can be identified easily by their characteristic granules which stain metachromatically. The size and shape of mast cells vary, i.e., 10–30 μm in diameter. In adventitia of large vessels, they are elongated; in loose connective tissue they are round or oval; and the shape in fibrous connective tissue may be angular. On their surfaces, they have Fc receptors for IgE. Cross-linking by either antigen for which the IgE Fab regions are specific or by anti-IgE or anti-receptor antibody, leads to degranulation with the release of pharmacological mediators of immediate hypersensitivity from their storage

sites in the mast cell granules. Leukotrienes, prostaglandins and platelet-activating factor are also produced and released following Fcε receptor cross-linking. Mast cell granules are approximately 0.5 μ in diameter and are electron-dense. They contain many biologically active compounds, of which the most important are heparin, histamine, serotonin and a variety of enzymes. Histamine is stored in the granule as a complex with heparin or serotonin. Mast cells also contain proteolytic enzymes such as plasmin, and also hydroxylase, β glucuronidase, phosphatase and a high uronidase inhibitor, to mention only the most important. Zinc, iron and calcium are also found. Some substances released from mast cells are not stored in a preformed state but are synthesized following mast cell activation. These represent secondary mediators as opposed to the first, primary mediators. Mast cell degranulation involves adenylate cyclase activation with rapid synthesis of cyclic AMP, protein kinase activation, phospholipid methylation and serine esterase activation. Mast cells of the gastrointestinal and respiratory tracts that contain chondroitin sulfate produce leukotriene C_4, whereas connective tissue mast cells that contain heparin produce prostaglandin D_2.

Monocytes (Figures 72–76) are mononuclear phagocytic cells in the blood that are derived from promonocytes in the bone marrow. Following a relatively brief residence in the blood, they migrate into the tissues and are transformed into macrophages. They are less mature than are macrophages, as suggested by fewer surface receptors, cytoplasmic organelles and enzymes than the latter. Monocytes are larger than polymorphonuclear leukocytes, are actively phagocytic and constitute 2–10% of the total white blood cell count in humans. The monocyte in the blood circulation is 15–25 μm in diameter. It has grayish-blue cytoplasm that contains lysosomes with enzymes such as acid phosphatase, arginase cachetepsin, collagenase, deoxyribonuclease, lipase, glucosidase and plasminogen activator. The cell has a reniform nucleus with delicate lace-like chromatin. The monocyte has surface receptors such as the Fc receptor for IgG and a receptor for CR3. It is actively phagocytic and plays a significant role in antigen processing. Monocyte numbers are

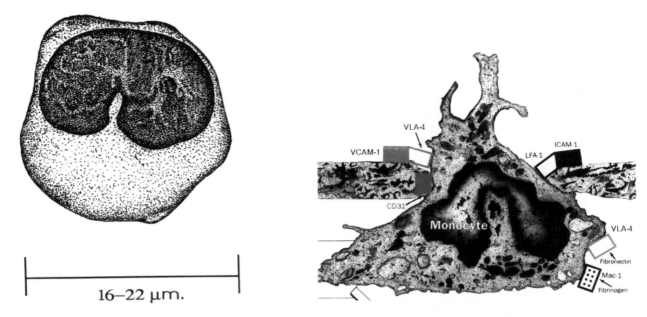

Figure 72.   Monocyte.

Figure 74.   Monocyte.

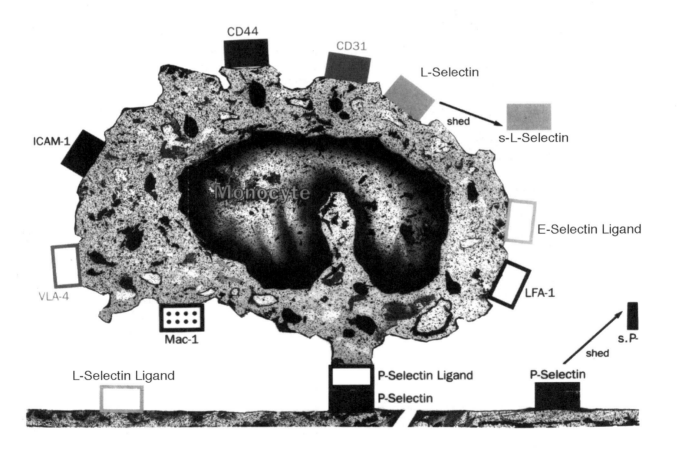

Figure 73.   Monocyte.

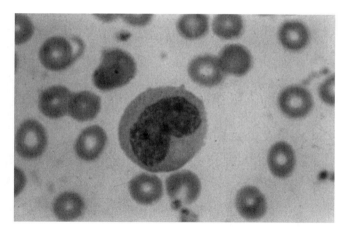

Figure 75.   Monocyte in peripheral blood.

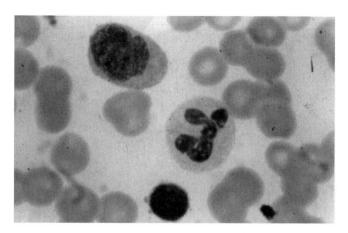

Figure 76.   Monocyte, lymphocyte, and polymorphonuclear neutrophil.

elevated in both benign and malignant conditions. Certain infections stimulate a reactive type of monocytosis such as in tuberculosis, brucellosis, HIV-1 infection and malaria.

Trophoblast consists of a layer of cells in the placenta that synthesizes immunosuppressive agents. These cells are in contact with the lining of the uterus.

A **blast cell** is a relatively large cell that is of greater than 8μm diameter with abundant RNA in the cytoplasm, a nucleus with loosely arranged chromatin and a prominent nucleolus. Blast cells are active in synthesizing DNA and contain numerous polyribosomes in the cytoplasm.

Megakaryocytes (Figure 77) are relatively large bone marrow giant cells that are multinuclear and from which blood platelets derived by the breaking up of membrane-bound cytoplasm to produce the thrombocytes.

CD42a is an antigen, equivalent to glycoprotein IX, that is a single chain membrane glycoprotein with a mol. wt. of 23 kD. It is found on megakaryocytes and platelets. CD42a forms a noncovalent complex with CD4b (gpIb) which acts

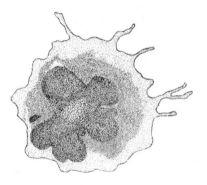

Figure 77.   Megakaryocyte.

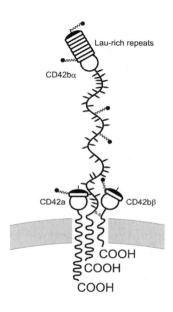

Figure 78.   CD42.

as a receptor for von Willebrand factor. It is absent or reduced in the Bernard–Soulier syndrome.

CD42b is an antigen, equivalent to glycoprotein Ib, that is a two-chain membrane glycoprotein with a mol. wt. of 170 kD. CD42b has an a-chain of 135 kD and b chain of 23 kD. It is found on platelets and megakaryocytes. CD42b forms a noncovalent complex with CD42a (gpIX) which acts as a receptor for von Willebrand factor. The antigen is absent or reduced in the Bernard-Soulier syndrome.

CD42c (Figure 78) is a 22 kD antigen found on platelets and megakaryocytes. It is also referred to as GPIB-β.

CD42d is a 85 kD antigen present mainly on platelets and megakaryocytes. It is also referred to as GPV.

Lymphoid tissues (Figure 79) are tissues that include the lymph nodes, spleen, thymus, Peyer's patches, tonsils, bursa of Fabricius in birds, and other lymphoid organs in which the predominant cell type is the lymphocyte.

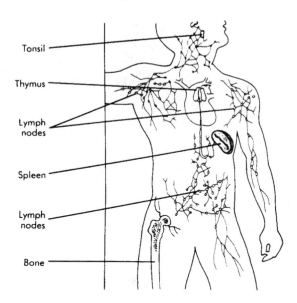

Figure 79.   Lymphoid tissue.

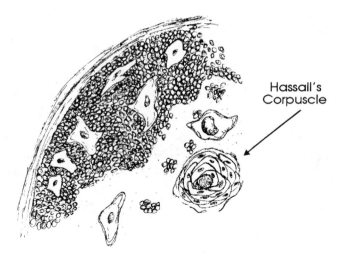

Figure 80.   Histology of the thymus.

The **thymus** (Figure 80) is a triangular bilobed structure enclosed in a thin fibrous capsule and located retrosternally. Each lobe is subdivided by prominent trabeculae into interconnecting lobules and each lobule comprises two histologically and functionally distinct areas, cortex and medulla. The cortex consists of a mesh of epithelial-reticular cells enclosing densely packed large lymphocytes. It has no germinal centers. The epithelial cell component is of endodermal origin; the lymphoid cells are of mesenchymal origin. The prothymocytes, which migrate from the bone marrow to the subcapsular regions of the cortex, are influenced by this microenvironment which directs their further development. The process of education is exerted by hormonal substances produced by the thymic epithelial cells. The cortical cells proliferate extensively. Part of these cells are short lived and die. The surviving cells acquire characteristics of thymocytes.

Peripheral lymphoid organs (Figure 81) are not required for ontogeny of the immune response. They include the lymph nodes, spleen, tonsils and Peyer's patches.

A **lymph node** (Figures 82–85) is a relatively small, i.e., 0.5 cm secondary lymphoid organ that is a major site of immune reactivity. It is surrounded by a capsule and contains lymphocytes, macrophages and dendritic cells in a loose reticulum environment. Lymph enters this organ from afferent lymphatics at the periphery, percolates through the node until it reaches the efferent lymphatics, where it exits at the hilus and circulates to central lymph nodes and finally to the thoracic duct. The lymph node is divided into a cortex and medulla. The superficial cortex contains B lymphocytes in

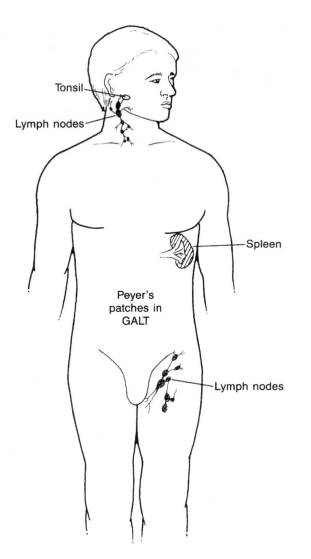

Figure 81.   Peripheral lymphoid organs.

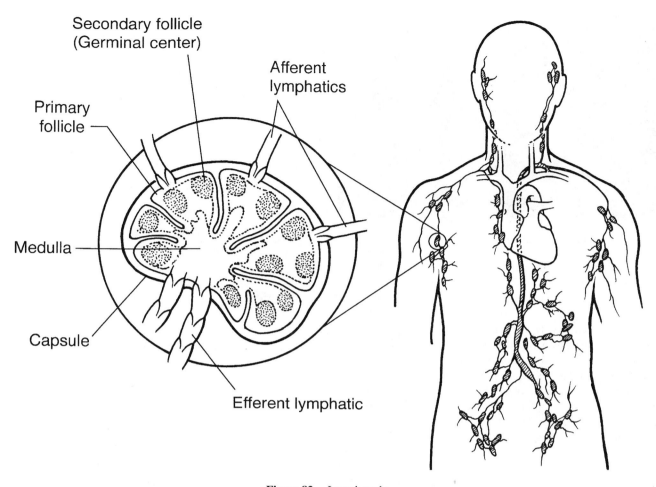

Secondary follicle
(Germinal center)

Afferent
lymphatics

Primary
follicle

Medulla

Capsule

Efferent lymphatic

Figure 82.   Lymph node.

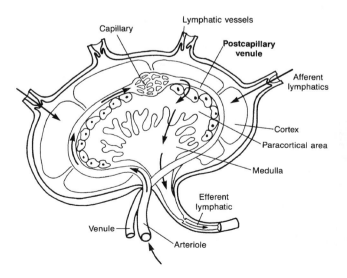

Capillary

Lymphatic vessels

**Postcapillary
venule**

Afferent
lymphatics

Cortex

Paracortical area

Medulla

Efferent
lymphatic

Venule

Arteriole

Figure 83.   Structure of a lymph node.

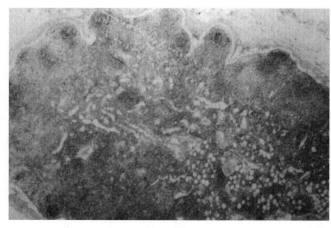

Figure 84.   Lymph node (low power).

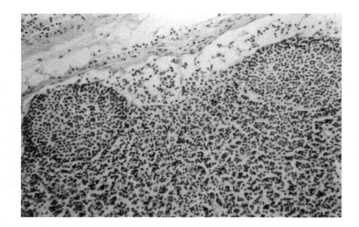

Figure 85.   Subcapsular sinus lymph node.

follicles, and the deep cortex is comprised of T lymphocytes. Differentiation of the specific cells continues in these areas and is driven by antigen and thymic hormones. Conversion of B cells into plasma cells occurs chiefly in the medullary region where enclosed lymphocytes are protected from undesirable influences by a macrophage sleeve. The post capillary venules from which lymphocytes exit the lymph node are also located in the medullary region. Macrophages and follicular dendritic cells interact with antigen molecules that are transported to the lymph node in the lymph. Reticulum cells form medullary cords and sinuses in the central region. T lymphocytes percolate through the lymph nodes. They enter from the blood at the post capillary venules of the deep cortex. They then enter the medullary sinuses and pass out of the node through the efferent lymphatics. T cells that interact with antigens are detained in the lymph node which may be a site of major immunologic reactivity. The lymph node is divided into B and T lymphocyte regions. Individuals with B cell or T cell immunodeficiencies may reveal an absence of one or the other lymphocyte types in the areas of the lymph node normally occupied by that cell population. The lymph node acts as a filter and may be an important site for phagocytosis and for the initiation of immune responses.

Follicular dendritic cells (Figure 86) are cells manifesting narrow cytoplasmic processes that interdigitate between densely populated areas of B lymphocytes in lymph node follicles and in spleen. Antigen-antibody complexes adhere to the surfaces of follicular dendritic cells and are not generally endocytosed but are associated with the formation of germinal centers. These cells are bereft of class II histocompatibility molecules although Fc receptors, complement receptor 1 and complement receptor 2 molecules are demonstrable on their surfaces.

CD21 (Figure 87) is an antigen, with a MW of 145 kD, that is expressed on B cells, and even more strongly, on follicular dendritic cells. It appears when surface Ig is expressed after the pre-B cell stage and is lost during early stages of terminal B cell differentiation to the final plasma cell stage. CD21 is

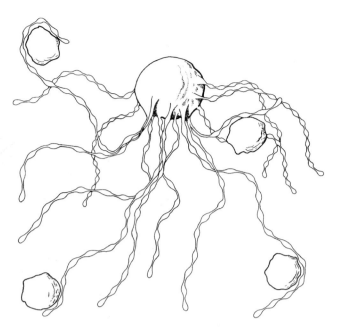

Figure 86.   Follicular dendritic cell.

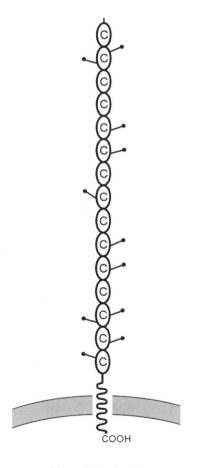

COOH

Figure 87.   CD21.

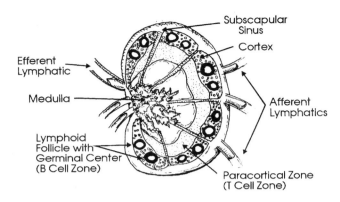

Figure 88. Germinal center.

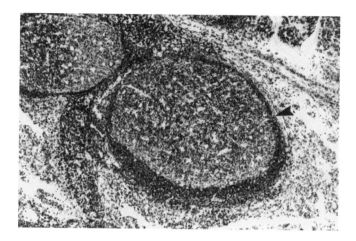

Figure 89. Germinal center.

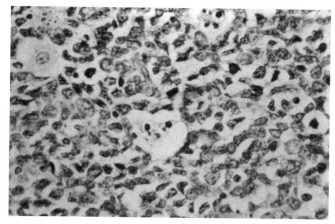

Figure 90. Tangible body macrophages in germinal center.

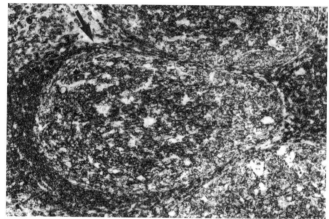

Figure 91. Mantle zone.

coded for by a gene found on chromosome 1 at band q32. The antigen functions as a receptor for the C3d complement component and also for Epstein-Barr virus. CD21, together with CD19 and CD81, constitutes the co-receptor for B cells. It is also termed CR2.

Germinal centers (Figures 88–90) develop in lymph nodes and lymphoid aggregates within primary follicles of lymphoid tissues following antigenic stimulation. The mixed cell population in the germinal center is comprised of B lymphoblasts (both cleaved and transformed lymphocytes), follicular dendritic cells and numerous tingible body-containing macrophages. Germinal centers seen in various pathologic states include "burned out" germinal centers comprised of accumulations of pale histiocytes and scattered immunoblasts; "progressively transformed" centers that show a "starry sky" pattern containing epithelioid histiocytes, dendritic reticulum cells, increased T lymphocytes and mantle zone lymphocytes; and "regressively transformed" germinal centers that are relatively small with few lymphocytes and reveal an onion-skin layering of dendritic reticulum cells, vascular endothelial cells and fibroblasts. The mantle zone (Figure 91) is a dense area of lymphocytes that encircles a germinal center.

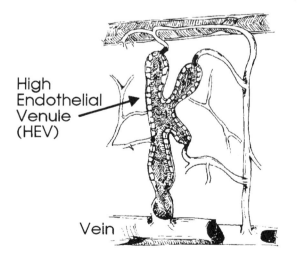

Figure 92. High endothelial venules (HEV).

High endothelial venules (HEV) (Figure 92) are post capillary venules of lymph node paracortical areas. They also

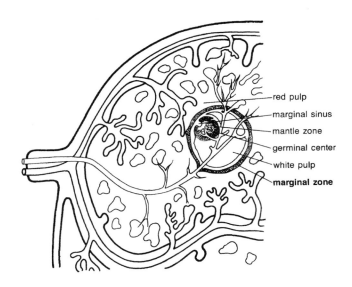

Figure 93.   Spleen.

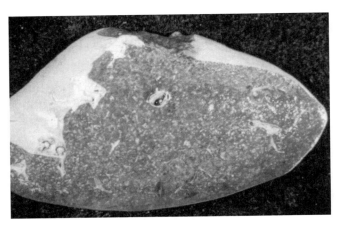

Figure 94.   Spleen gross specimen.

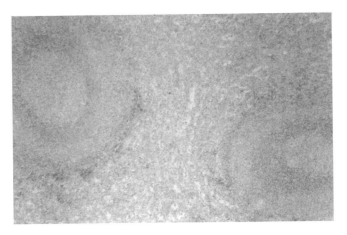

Figure 95.   Spleen follicle with central follicular artery.

occur in Peyer's patches which are part of the gut-associated lymphoid tissue (GALT). Their specialized columnar cells bear receptors for antigen-primed lymphocytes. They signal lymphocytes to leave the peripheral blood circulation. A homing receptor for circulating lymphocytes is found in lymph nodes.

High endothelial postcapillary venules are lymphoid organ vessels that are especially designed for circulating lymphocytes to gain access into the parenchyma of the organ. They contain cuboidal endothelium which permits lymphocytes to pass between the cells into the tissues. Lymphocyte recirculation from the blood to the lymph occurs through these vessel walls.

The **spleen** (Figures 93–95) is an encapsulated organ in the abdominal cavity which has important immunologic and nonimmunologic functions. Vessels and nerves enter the spleen at the hilum, as in lymph nodes, and travel part of their course within the fibrous trabeculae that emerge from the capsule. The splenic parenchyma has two regions that are functionally and histologically distinct. The white pulp consists of a thick layer of lymphocytes surrounding the arteries that have left the trabeculae. They form a periarterial sheath which contains mainly T cells. The sheaths then expand along their course to form well developed lymphoid nodules called Malpighian corpuscles. The red pulp consists of a mesh of reticular fibers, continuous with the collagen fibers of the trabeculae. These fibers enclose an open system of sinusoids that drain into small veins and are lined by endothelial cells with reticular properties. The endothelium is discontinuous leaving small slits that cells have to pass during transit. Within the sinusoidal mesh are red blood cells, macrophages, lymphocytes, and plasma cells. The red pulp between adjacent sinusoids forms the pulp cords sometimes called the cords of Billroth. The marginal zone consists of

a poorly defined area between the white and the red pulp where the periarterial sheath and the lymphoid nodules merge. The blood vessels branch and at the periphery of the marginal zone, the blood empties into the pulp. Lymphocytes of the marginal zone are mainly T cells. They surround the periphery of the lymphoid nodules that comprise B cells. In this marginal region, the T and B cells contact each other. Some B cells may convert into immunoblasts. Further maturation to plasma cells occurs in the red pulp. Active follicles contain germinal centers in which lymphoblasts may be generated. They are discharged into sinusoids and plasma cells may form. The spleen also contains dendritic cells which have long cytoplasmic extensions. Dendritic cells serve as antigen-presenting cells, interacting with lymphocytes. The spleen filters blood as the lymph nodes filter the lymph. The spleen is active in the formation of antibodies against intravenously administered particulate antigens. It has numerous additional functions including the sequestration and destruction of senescent red blood cells, platelets and lymphocytes.

Red pulp (Figure 96) describes areas of the spleen comprised of the cords of Billroth and sinusoids.

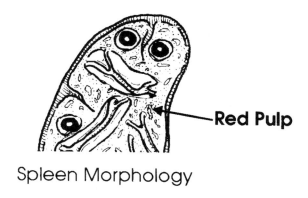

Spleen Morphology

Figure 96. Red pulp.

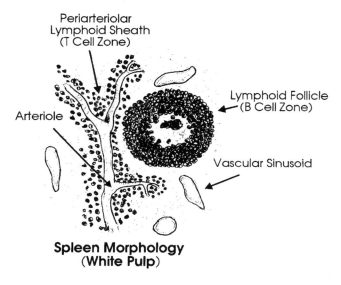

Figure 97. White pulp.

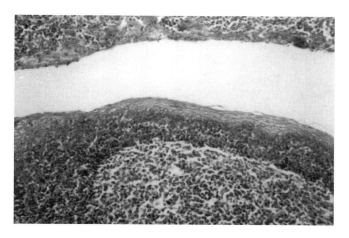

Figure 98. Mucosa of ileum with Peyer's patch.

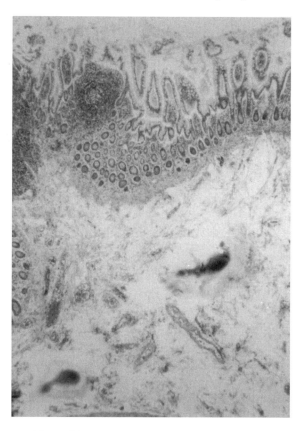

Figure 99. Peyer's patch (higher magnification).

White pulp (Figure 97) refers to the peri-arteriolar lymphatic sheaths encircled by small lymphocytes which are mainly T cells that surround germinal centers comprised of B lymphocytes and B lymphoblasts in normal splenic tissue. Following interaction of B cells in the germinal center with antigen in the blood, a primary immune response is generated within 24 hours revealing immunoblastic proliferation and enlargement of germinal centers.

The **marginal zone** is an exterior layer of lymphoid follicles of the spleen where T and B lymphocytes are loosely arranged encircling the periarterial lymphatic sheath. When antigens are injected intravenously, macrophages in this area actively phagocytize them.

Peyer's patches (Figure 98 and 99) are lymphoid tissues in the submucosa of the small intestine. They are comprised of lymphocytes, plasma cells, germinal centers, and thymus-dependent areas.

The **vermiform appendix** (Figure 100) is a lymphoid organ situated at the ileocecal junction of the gastrointestinal tract.

Waldeyer's ring (Figure 101) describes a circular arrangement of lymphoid tissue comprised of tonsils and adenoids encircling the pharynx-oral cavity junction.

Tonsils (Figures 102 and 103) are lymphoid tissue masses at the intersection of the oral cavity and the pharynx, i.e., in the oropharynx. Tonsils contain mostly B lymphocytes and are classified as secondary lymphoid organs. There are several types of tonsils designated as palatine, flanked by the palatoglossal and palatopharyngeal arches, the pharyngeal,

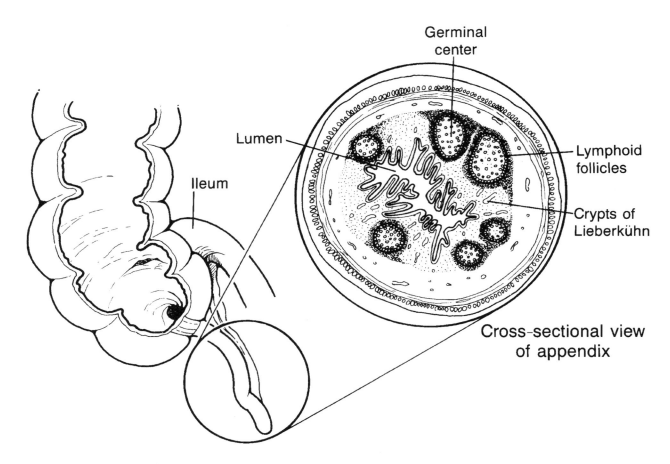

Figure 100. Appendix.

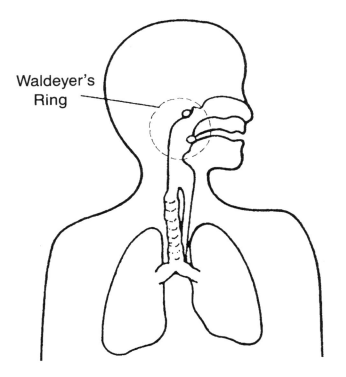

Figure 101. Waldeyer's ring.

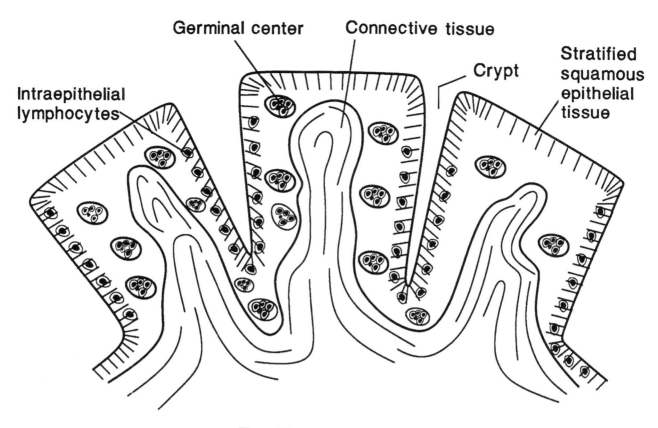

Figure 102. Histology of the tonsil

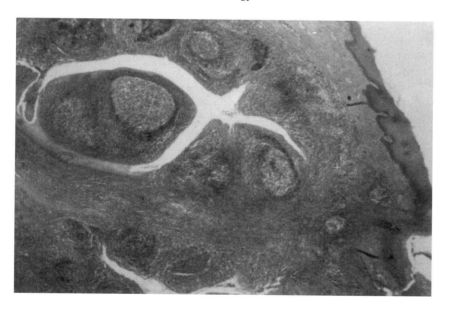

Figure 103. Tonsil.

which are adenoids in the posterior pharynx and the lingual, at the tongue's base.

Inflammation is a defense reaction of living tissue to injury. The literal meaning of the word is burning and originates from the cardinal symptoms of rubor, calor, tumor, and dolor, the Latin terms equivalent to redness, heat, swelling, and pain, respectively. It is beneficial for the host and essential for survival of the species, although in some cases the response is exaggerated and may be itself injurious.

Inflammation is the result of multiple interactions which have as a first objective localization of the process and removal of the irritant. This is followed by a period of repair.

Inflammation is not necessarily of immunologic nature, although immunologic reactions are among the immediate causes inducing inflammation, and the immunologic status of the host determines the intensity of the inflammatory response. Inflammation tends to be less intense in infants whose immune system is not fully mature.

The causes of inflammation are numerous and include living microorganisms such as pathogenic bacteria and animal parasites which act mainly by the chemical poisons they produce and less by mechanical irritation, viruses which become offenders after they have multiplied in the host and cause cell damage, and fungi which grow at the surface of the skin but produce little or no inflammation in the dermis; physical agents such as trauma, thermal and radiant energy; and chemical agents which represent a large group of exogenous or endogenous causes which include immunologic offenders. Refer to inflammatory response.

An **acute inflammatory response** represents an early defense mechanism to contain an infection and prevent its spread from the initial focus. When microbes multiply in host tissues, two principal defense mechanisms mounted against them are antibodies and leukocytes. The three major events in acute inflammation are (1) dilation of capillaries to increase blood flow, (2) changes in the microvasculature structure leading to escape of plasma proteins and leukocytes from the circulation, and (3) leukocyte emigration from the capillaries and accumulation at the site of injury. Widening of interendothelial cell junctions of venules or injury of endothelial cells facilitates the escape of plasma proteins from the vessels. Neutrophils attached to the endothelium through adhesion molecules, escape the microvasculature and are attracted to sites of injury by chemotactic agents. This is followed by phagocytosis of microorganisms that may lead to their intracellular destruction. Activated leukocytes may produce toxic metabolites and proteases that injure endothelium and tissues when they are released. Activation of the third complement component (C3) is also a critical step in inflammation.

Multiple chemical mediators of inflammation derived from either plasma or cells have been described. Mediators and plasma proteins such as complement are present as precursors that require activation to become biologically active. Mediators derived from cells are present as precursors in intracellular granules, such as histamine and mast cells. Following activation, these substances are secreted. Other mediators such as prostaglandins may be synthesized following stimulation. These mediators are quickly activated by enzymes or other substances such as antioxidants. A chemical mediator may also cause a target cell to release a secondary mediator with a similar or opposing action.

Besides histamine, other preformed chemical mediators in cells include serotonin and lysosomal enzymes. Those that are newly synthesized include prostaglandins, leukotrienes, platelet activating factors, cytokines and nitric oxide. Chemical mediators in plasma include complement fragments C3a and C5a and the C5b-g sequence. Three plasma-derived factors including kinins, complement and clotting factors are involved in inflammation. Bradykinin is produced by activation of the kinin system. It induces arteriolar dilation and increased venule permeability through contraction of endothelial cells and extravascular smooth muscle. Activation of bradykinin precursors involves activated factor XII (Hageman factor) generated by its contact with injured tissues.

During clotting, fibrinopeptides produced during the conversion of fibrinogen to fibrin increase vascular permeability and are chemotactic for leukocytes. The fibrinolytic system participates in inflammation through the kinin system. Products produced during arachidonic acid metabolism also affect inflammation. These include prostaglandins and leukotrienes, which can mediate essentially every aspect of acute inflammation.

An **acute phase response** (APR) (Figure 104) is a nonspecific response by an individual stimulated by interleukin-1, interleukin-6, tumor necrosis factor and interferons. C reactive protein may show a striking rise within a few hours. Infection, inflammation, tissue injury and very infrequently neoplasm may be associated with APR. The liver produces acute phase proteins at an accelerated rate, the endocrine system is affected with elevated gluconeogenesis, impaired thyroid function and other changes. Immunologic and hematopoietic system changes include hypergammaglobulinemia and leukocytosis with a shift to the left. There is diminished formation of albumin, elevated ceruloplasmin and diminished zinc and iron.

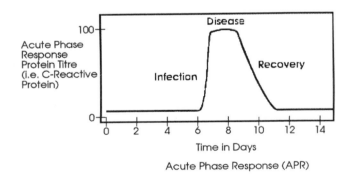

Figure 104. Acute phase response.

Acute phase reactants are serum proteins that increase during acute inflammation. These proteins, which migrate in the α-1 and α-2 electrophoretic regions include α-1-antitrypsin, α-1 glycoprotein, amyloid A&P, antithrombin III, C-reactive protein, C1-esterase inhibitor, C3 complement, ceruloplasmin, fibrinogen, haptoglobin, orosomucoid, plasminogen, and transferrin.

3

Antigens, Immunogens, Vaccines, and Immunization

An infectious agent, whether a bacterium, fungus, virus or parasite contains a plethora of substances capable of inducing an immune response. These are called immunogens or antigens. Specifically, an immunogen is a substance capable of stimulating B cell, T cell, or both limbs of the immune response. An antigen is a substance that reacts with the products of an immune response stimulated by a specific immunogen, including both antibodies and/or T lymphocyte receptors. The "traditional" definition of antigen more correctly refers to an immunogen. A complete antigen is one that both induces an immune response and reacts with the products of it, whereas an incomplete antigen or hapten is unable to induce an immune response alone but is able to react with the products of it, e.g., antibodies. Haptens could be rendered immunogenic by covalently linking them to a carrier molecule.

Following the administration of an antigen (immunogen) to a host animal, antibody synthesis and/or cell mediated immunity or immunologic tolerance may result. To be immunogenic, a substance usually needs to be foreign although some autoantigens represent an exception. They should usually have a molecular weight of at least 10,000 and be either proteins or polysaccharides. Nevertheless, immunogenicity depends upon the genetic capacity of the host to respond rather than merely upon the antigenic properties of an injected immunogen.

The specific parts of antigen molecules that elicit immune reactivity are known as antigenic determinants or epitopes. Even the earliest investigators in immunology recognized that small molecular weight substances such as simple chemicals could react with the products of an immune response but were not themselves immunogenic. These were termed haptens. Thus, a hapten is a relatively small molecule which by itself is unable to elicit an immune response when injected into an animal but is capable of reacting *in vitro* with an antibody specific for it. However, a hapten may be covalently linked to a carrier macromolecule such as a foreign protein that renders it immunogenic and can form new antigenic determinants. Haptens often have highly reactive chemical groupings which permit them to autocouple with a substance such as a tissue protein. This type of reaction

occurs in individuals who develop contact hypersensitivity to poison ivy or poison oak.

An **antigenic determinant (epitope)** (Figure 1) interacts with the specific antigen binding site in the variable region of an antibody molecule known as a paratope. The excellent fit between epitope and paratope is based upon their three dimensional interaction and non-covalent union. An antigenic determinant or epitope may also react with a T cell receptor for which it is specific. A single antigen molecule may have several different epitopes. Whereas an epitope interacts with the antigen binding region of an antibody molecule or with the T cell receptor, a separate region of the antigen that combines with class II MHC molecules is known as an agretope.

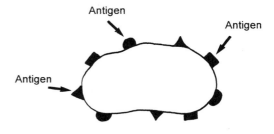

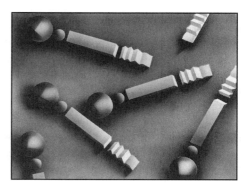

Figure 1. Schematic of antigenic determinants (epitopes).

Antigenic determinants may be either conformational or linear. A conformational determinant is produced by spatial juxtaposition during folding of amino acid residues from different segments of the linear amino acid sequence. Conformational determinants are usually associated with natural rather than denatured proteins. A linear determinant is one produced by adjacent amino acid residues in the covalently sequenced proteins. They are usually available for interaction with antibody only following denaturation of a protein and are not customarily in the native configuration. Antigenic determinants or epitopes are sometimes called immunodominant groups. In contrast to the natural antigens that constitute part of a microbe, one derived exclusively by laboratory synthesis and not obtained from living cells is termed a **synthetic antigen**.

An antigen molecule has two or more epitopes or (antigenic determinants) per molecule. Epitopes consist of approximately 6 amino acids or 6 monosaccharides. Epitopes that stimulate a greater antibody response than others are referred to as immunodominant epitopes.

The principal chemical features of antigens include their large size, complexity and ability to be degraded by enzymes within phagocytes. Most antigens are of 10,000 d or greater molecular weight. Exceptions include such substances as insulin with 5700 d. Antigenicity is usually more easily demonstrated with molecules of greater molecular weight. However, size alone does not make the molecule antigenic. It must have a certain amount of internal structural complexity. Linear polymers of polylysine comprised of a repeating simple structure are not antigenic. The majority of protein antigens contain 20 different amino acids in an assorted arrangement. Oligosaccharides comprised of both monosaccharides and complex sugars are antigenic. The antigen must also be degradable by phagocytes to be antigenic. Antigen processing includes enzymatic digestion to prepare soluble macromolecular antigen. Substances such as D-amino acid polypeptides that cannot be degraded in phagocytes are not antigenic even through they might otherwise possess the characteristics of antigens. Foreignness is another characteristic that is critical for antigenicity. We do not respond to our own self antigens because we are immunologically tolerant of them. During development, the body becomes tolerant to self antigens, as well as foreign antigens that may have been artificially introduced into the host prior to development of the immune system. The latter situation describes the induction of actively acquired immunologic tolerance which was discovered by Medawar, Billingham and Brent in the 1950s in studies on skin grafting. They inoculated fetal or newborn mice with cells of a different mouse strain prior to development of immunologic competence in the recipients. Once the recipient mice reached maturity, they were able to accept skin grafts from the donor strain without rejecting them. Since that time, many studies have been conducted defining the nature of T cell and B cell tolerance. In general, T cells are rendered tolerant with lower doses of antigen and for longer periods of time than are B cells. B cell tolerance is for relatively brief duration and requires much greater quantities of antigen than does T cell tolerance. Tolerance is a type of antigen-induced specific immunosup-

pression and antigen must remain in contact with immunocompetent cells for the tolerant state to be maintained. Tolerance induction is favored by the route of administration and the physical nature of the injected antigen. For example, the intravenous route of injection of solubilized antigen favors tolerance induction. By contrast, the injection of antigen in particulate form into the skin favors the development of immunity. An antigen that induces tolerance is often referred to as a tolerogen.

To mount an immune response to an antigen, a host must have appropriate immune response (Ir) genes. This has been proven in animal studies in which inbred strain 2 guinea pigs were shown to be responders whereas strain 13 were not. Lymphocyte proteins in man encoded by Ir genes include the class II MHC molecules designated DP, DQ, and DR that are found on human B cells and macrophages. This enables recognition among B cells, T cells and macrophages. Antigens may be classified as either T cell dependent or (TD) or T cell independent (TI). As shown in Table 1, TD antigens are much more complex than TI antigens, are usually proteins, stimulate a full complement of immunoglobulins with all five classes represented, elicit an anamnestic or memory response and are present in most pathogenic microorganisms. This ensures that an effective immune response can be generated in a host infected with these pathogens. By contrast, the simpler TI antigens are often polysaccharides or lipopolysaccharides, elicit an IgM response only and fail to stimulate an anamnestic response compared to T cell dependent antigens.

A **superantigen** is a substance such as a bacterial toxin capable of stimulating many CD4+ T lymphocytes. Selected bacterial toxins may stimulate all T lymphocytes in the body that contain a certain family of Vbeta T cell receptor genes. Superantigens assume significance through their capacity to stimulate multiple T lymphocytes leading to the release of relatively large quantities of cytokines that provoke pathophysiologic manifestations resembling endotoxin shock.

Superantigens are TD antigens that do not require phagocyte processing. Instead of fitting into the TCR internal grove where a typical processed peptide antigen fits, superantigens bind to the external region of the TCR and simultaneously link to DP, DQ or DR molecules on antigen presenting cells. Superantigens react with multiple TCR molecules whose peripheral structure is similar from one TCR to another. Thus, they stimulate multiple T cells that augment a protective T and B cell antibody response. This is especially important in responding to the toxins of such microorganisms as streptococci and staphylococci.

An **antigen** is a substance that reacts with the products of an immune response stimulated by a specific immunogen, including both antibodies and/or T lymphocyte receptors. It is one of many kinds of substances with which an antibody molecule or T cell receptor may bind. These include sugars, lipids, intermediary metabolites, autocoids, hormones, complex carbohydrates, phospholipids, nucleic acids and proteins. By contrast, the "traditional" definition of antigen is a substance that may stimulate B and/or T cell limbs of the immune response and react with the products of that response including immunoglobulin antibodies and/or specific receptors on T cells. See immunogen definition. The "traditional" definition of antigen more correctly refers to an immunogen. A complete antigen is one that both induces an immune response and reacts with the products of it, whereas an incomplete antigen or hapten is unable to induce an immune response alone but is able to react with the products of it, e.g., antibodies. Haptens could be rendered immunogenic by covalently linking them to a carrier molecule. Following the administration of an antigen (immunogen) to a host animal, antibody synthesis and/or cell mediated immunity or immunologic tolerance may result. To be immunogenic, a substance usually needs to be foreign although some autoantigens represent an exception. They should usually have a molecular weight of at least 1,000 and be either proteins or polysaccharides. Nevertheless, immunogenicity depends also upon the genetic capacity of the host to respond rather than merely upon the antigenic properties of an injected immunogen.

Whereas an **artificial antigen** is prepared by chemical modification of a natural antigen, a synthetic antigen (Figure 2) is derived exclusively by laboratory synthesis and not obtained from living cells. **Synthetic polypeptide antigens** have a backbone consisting of amino acids that usually include lysine. Side chains of different amino acids are attached directly to the backbone and then elongated with a homopolymer, or conversely, attached via the homopolymer. They have contributed much to our knowledge of epitope structure and function. They have well defined specificities determined by the particular arrangement, number

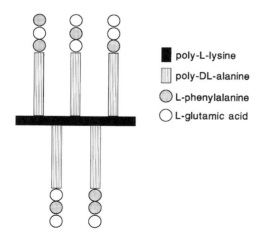

Figure 2.   Synthetic polypeptide antigen with multichain copolymer (Phe, G)-A-L.

and nature of the amino acid components of the molecule, and they may be made more complex by further coupling to haptens or derivatized with various compounds. The size of the molecule is less critical with synthetic antigens than with natural antigens. Thus, molecules as small as those of p-azobenzenearsonate coupled to three L-lysine residues (mol. wt. 750) or even of p-azobenzenearsonate-N-acetyl-L-tyrosine (mol. wt. 451) may be immunogenic. Specific antibodies are markedly stereospecific, and there is no cross-reaction between, e.g., poly-D-alanyl and poly-L-alanyl determinants. Studies employing synthetic antigens demonstrated the significance of aromatic, charged amino acid residues in proving the ability of synthetic polypeptides to induce an immune response.

An **immunogen** is a substance that is able to induce a humoral antibody and/or cell-mediated immune response rather than immunological tolerance. The term "immunogen" is sometimes used interchangeably with "antigen", yet the term signifies the ability to stimulate an immune response as well as reacting with the products of it, e.g., antibody. By contrast, "antigen" is reserved by some to mean a substance that reacts with antibody. The principal immunogens are proteins and polysaccharides, whereas lipids may serve as haptens.

Immunogenicity is the ability of an antigen serving as an immunogen to induce an immune response in a particular species of recipient. Immunogenicity depends upon a number of physical and chemical characteristics of the immunogen (antigen) as well as on the genetic capacity of the host response.

Immunogenic is an adjective that denotes the capacity to induce humoral antibody and/or cell-mediated immune responsiveness, but not immunological tolerance. Immunogenicity depends on characteristics of the immunogen and on the injected animal's genetic capacity to respond to the immunogen. To be immunogenic, a substance must be foreign to the recipient. An immunogen that is of significant molecular size and complexity, as well as host factors such as previous exposure to the immunogen and immunocompetence are all critical factors in immunogenicity.

Antigenicity is the property of a substance that renders it immunogenic or capable of stimulating an immune response. Antigenicity was more commonly used in the past to refer to what is now known as immunogenicity, although the two are still used interchangably by various investigators. An antigen is considered by many to be a substance that reacts with the products of immunogenic stimulation. It is a substance that combines specifically with antibodies formed or receptors of T cells stimulated during an immune response.

Antigenic refers to the ability of a substance to induce an immune response and to react with its products, which include antibodies and T lymphocyte receptors. The term "antigenic" has been largely replaced by "immunogenic".

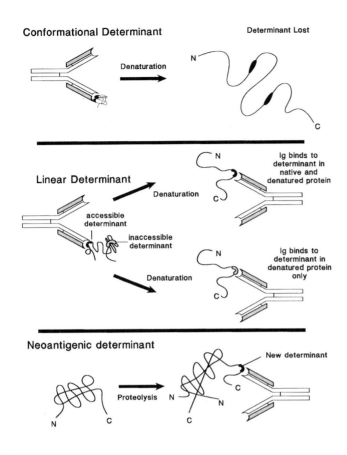

Figure 3. Antigenic determinants.

An **antigenic determinant** (Figure 3) is the site on an antigen molecule that is termed an epitope and interacts with the specific antigen-binding site in the variable region of an antibody molecule known as a paratope. The excellent fit between epitope and paratope is based on their three dimensional interaction and non-covalent union. An antigenic determinant or epitope may also react with a T cell receptor for which it is specific. A single antigen molecule may have several different epitopes available for reaction with antibody or T cell receptors.

A **conformational determinant** is an epitope composed of amino acid residues that are not contiguous and represent separated parts of the linear sequence of amino acids that are brought into proximity to one another by folding of the molecule. A conformational determinant is dependent on 3-dimensional structure. Conformational determinants are, therefore, usually associated with native rather than denatured proteins. Antibodies specific for linear determinants and others specific for conformational determinants may give clues as to whether a protein is denatured or native, respectively.

Linear determinants are antigenic determinants produced by adjacent amino acid residues in the covalent sequence in proteins. Linear determinants of 6 amino acids interact with specific antibody. Occasionally, linear determinants may be

on the surface of a native folded protein, but they are more commonly unavailable in the native configuration and only become available for interaction with antibody upon denaturation of the protein.

Determinant groups (or epitopes) are chemical mosaics found on macromolecular antigens that induce an immune response.

Primary structure (Figure 4) refers to a polypeptide or protein molecule's linear amino acid sequence. **Secondary structure** (Figure 5) is based on polypeptide chain or polynucleotide strand folding along the axis or backbone of a molecule. This is a consequence of the formation of intramolecular hydrogen bonds joining carbonyl oxygen and amide nitrogen atoms. Secondary structure is based on the local spatial organization of polypeptide chain segments or polynucleotide strands irrespective of the structure of side chains or of the relationship of the segments to one another. **Tertiary structure** (Figure 6) describes the folding of a polypeptide chain as a result of the interactions of its amino acid side chains which may be situated either near or distant along the chain. This three-dimensional folding occurs in globular proteins. Tertiary structure also refers to the spatial arrangement of protein atoms irrespective of their relationship to atoms in adjacent molecules. **Quaternary structure** (Figure 7) refers to four components that are associated with one another. Two or more folded polypeptide chains packed into a configuration such as a tetramer. Quaternary antigenic determinants may be difficult to demonstrate in such structures as hemoglobulin molecules.

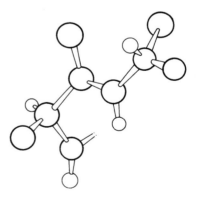

Figure 4. Primary structure.

2,4-dinitrophenyl (DNP) (Figures 8 and 8A) groups may serve as haptens after they are chemically linked to -NH$_2$ groups of proteins that interact with chlorodinitrobenzene, 2,4-dinitrobenzene sulphonic acid or dinitrofluorobenzene. These protein carrier-DNP hapten antigens are useful as experimental immunogens. Antibodies specific for the DNP hapten, which are generated through immunization with the carrier-hapten complex, interact with low molecular weight substances that contain the DNP groups.

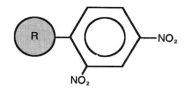

Figure 8.   2,4-dinitrophenyl (DNP).

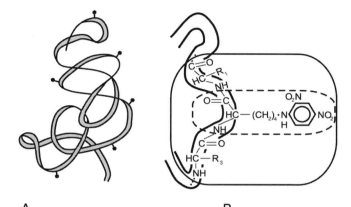

A   B
A. Conjugated protein with substituents
B. Broken line refers to the haptenic group and the
   solid line refers to the antigenic determinant

Figure 8A.

A **trinitrophenyl (picryl) group** (Figure 9) is a chemical grouping that may serve as a hapten when it is linked to a protein through -NH$_2$ groups by reaction with picryl chloride or trinitrobenzene sulfonic acid.

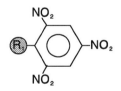

Figure 9.   Trinitrophenyl group.

Dinitrochlorobenzene (DNCB) (Figure 10) is a substance employed to test an individual's capacity to develop a cell-mediated immune reaction. A solution of DNCB is applied to the skin of an individual not previously sensitized against this chemical, where it acts as a hapten, interacting with proteins of the skin. Reexposure of this same individual to a second application of DNCB two weeks after the first challenge results in a T cell-mediated delayed-type hypersensitivity (contact dermatitis) reaction. Persons with impaired delayed-type hypersensitivity or cell-mediated immunity might reveal an impaired response. The 2,4-dinitro-1-chlorobenzene interacts with free "-amino-terminal groups in polypeptide chains

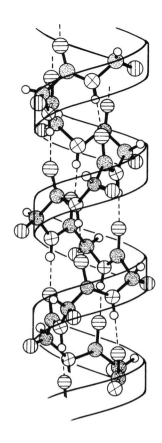

Figure 5.   Secondary structure.

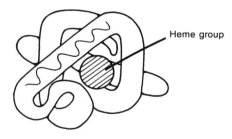

Heme group

Figure 6.   Tertiary structure.

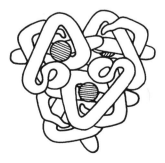

Figure 7.   Quaternary structure.

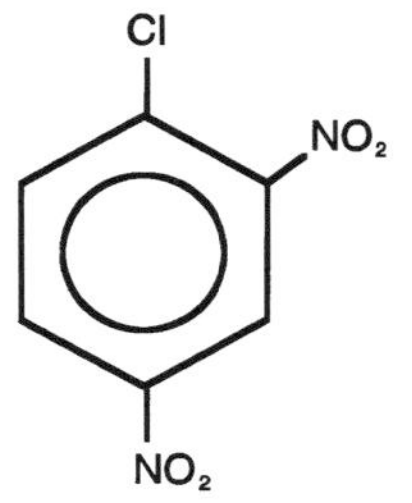

Figure 10.   Dinitrochlorobenzene.

as well as with side chains of lysine, tyrosine, histidine, cysteine or other amino acid residues."

An **epitope** is an antigenic determinant. It is the simplest form or smallest structural area on a complex antigen molecule that can combine with an antibody or T lymphocyte receptor. It must be at least 1 kD to elicit an antibody response. A smaller molecule, such as a hapten, may induce an immune response if combined with a carrier protein molecule. Multiple epitopes may be found on large non-polymeric molecules. Based on X-ray crystallography, epitopes consist of prominently exposed "hill and ridge" regions that manifest surface rigidity. Antigenicity is diminished in more flexible sites.

A **carrier** is an immunogenic macromolecular protein such as ovalbumin, to which an incomplete antigen termed a hapten may be conjugated either *in vitro* or in vivo. Whereas the hapten is not immunogenic by itself, conjugation to the carrier molecule renders it immunogenic.

Carrier specificity refers to an immune response, either humoral antibody or cell-mediated immunity, that is specific for the carrier portion of a hapten-carrier complex that has been used as an immunogen. The carrier-specific part of the immune response does not react with the hapten either by itself or conjugated to a different carrier.

Schlepper is the name used by Landsteiner to refer to large macromolecules that serve as carriers for simple chemical molecules serving as haptens. The immunization of rabbits or other animals with a hapten-carrier complex leads to the formation of antibodies specific for the hapten as well as the carrier. T cells were later shown to be carrier-specific and B cells hapten-specific. Carriers are conjugated to haptens through covalent linkages such as the diazo linkage.

A **hapten** is a relatively small molecule which by itself is unable to elicit an immune response when injected into an animal but is capable of reacting *in vitro* with an antibody specific for it. Only if complexed to a carrier molecule prior to administration can a hapten induce an immune response. Haptens usually bear only one epitope. Pneumococcal polysaccharide is an example of a larger molecule that may act as a hapten in rabbits but as a complete antigen in humans.

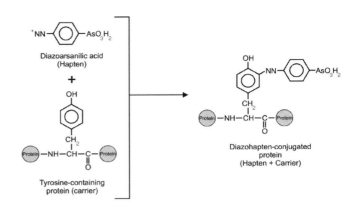

Figure 11.   Hapten Conjugates.

The response to **hapten conjugates** (Figure 11) requires two populations of lymphocytes, T and B cells. The cells producing the antibodies are derived from B cells. T cells act as helpers in this process. B cell preparations, depleted of T cells, cannot respond to hapten conjugates. The T cells are responsive to the carrier portion of the conjugate, although in some cases they also recognize the hapten. The influence of the carrier on the ensuing response is called carrier effect. The experimental design for demonstrating the carrier effect involves adoptive transfer of hapten sensitive B cells, and of T cells primed with one or another carrier. The primed cells are those which have already had a past opportunity to encounter the antigen.

The **hapten inhibition** test is an assay for serological characterization or elucidation of the molecular structure of an epitope by blocking the antigen binding site of an antibody specific for the epitope with a defined hapten.

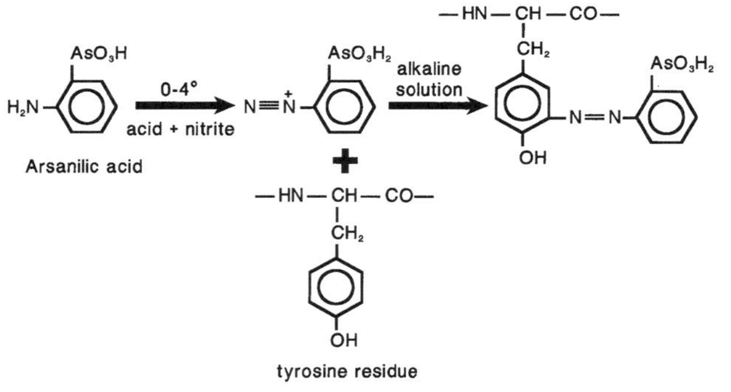

Figure 12.   Diazotization.

Diazotization (Figure 12) is a method to introduce the diazo group ($-N^+ \equiv N^-$) into a molecule. Landsteiner used this technique extensively in coupling low molecular weight chemicals acting as haptens to protein macromolecules serving as carriers. Aromatic amine derivatives can be coupled to side chains of selected amino acid residues to prepare protein-hapten conjugates, which, when used to immunize experimental animals such as rabbits, stimulate the synthesis of antibodies. Some of these antibodies are specific for the hapten, which by itself is unable to stimulate an immune response. First an aromatic amine reacts with nitrous acid generated through the combination of sodium nitrite with HCl. The diazonium salt is then combined with the protein at a pH that is slightly alkaline. The reaction products include monosubstituted tyrosine and histidine, and lysine residues that are disubstituted.

An **azoprotein** is produced by joining a substance to a protein through a diazo linkage $-N = N-$. Karl Landsteiner (in early 1900s) made extensive use of diazotization to prepare hapten-protein conjugates to define immunochemical specificity.

An **antigen-binding site** is the location on an antibody molecule where an antigenic determinant or epitope combines with it. The antigen-binding site is located in a cleft bordered by the N-terminal variable regions of heavy and light chain parts of the Fab region. Called also paratope.

Antigen clearance   The liver has important immunologic functions by virtue of its mass of Kupffer cells which represent the major part (90%) of the body's phagocytic capacity. Antigens escaping the intestinal barrier by passage through the liver are removed. The liver's anatomical position at the border between the splanchnic and systemic circulations substantiates its function as a filter for noxious substances, whether antigen or otherwise. The same removal mechanism is operative during liver passage, in situations in which antigen circulates in the blood.

A **superantigen** is a substance such as a bacterial toxin that is capable of stimulating multiple T lymphocytes, especially $CD4^+$ T cells, leading to the release of relatively large quantities of cytokines. Selected bacterial toxins may stimulate all T lymphocytes in the body that contain a certain family of V β T cell receptor genes. Superantigens may induce proliferation of 10% of $CD4^+$ T cells by combining with the T cell receptor V8 and to the MHC HLA-DR α−1 domain. Superantigens are thymus-dependent (TD) antigens that do not require phagocytic processing. Instead of fitting into the T cell receptor (TCR) internal groove where a typical processed peptide antigen fits, superantigens bind to the external region of the αβ TCR and simultaneously link to DP, DQ, or DR molecules on antigen-presenting cells. Superantigens react with multiple TCR molecules whose peripheral structure is similar. Thus, they stimulate multiple T cells that augment a protective T and B cell antibody response. This enhanced responsiveness to antigens such as toxins produced by staphylococci and streptococci is an important protective mechanism in the infected individual.

The simultaneous injection of two closely related antigens may lead to suppression or decrease of the immune response to one of them compared to the antigen's ability to elicit an immune response if injected alone. This is known as **antigenic competition**. Proteins that are thymus-dependent antigens are the ones with which antigenic competition occurs. The phenomenon has been claimed to be due in part to the competition by antigenic peptides for one binding site on class II MHC molecules. Antigenic competition was observed in the early days of vaccination when it was found that the immune response of a host to the individual components of a vaccine might be less than if they had been injected individually.

The immune response against a virus, such as a parental strain, to which an individual was previously exposed may be greater than it is against the immunizing agent, such as type A influenza virus variant. This concept is known as the **doctrine of original antigenic sin**.

Antigenic variation represents a mechanism whereby selected viruses, bacteria and animal parasites may evade the host immune response, thereby permitting antigenically altered etiologic agents of disease to produce a renewed infection. The variability among infectious disease agents is of critical significance in the development of effective vaccines. Antigenic variation affects the surface antigens of the viruses, bacteria, or animal parasite in which it occurs. By the time the host has developed a protective immune response against the antigens originally present, the latter have been replaced in a few surviving microorganisms by new antigens to which the host is not immune, thereby permitting survival of the microorganism or animal parasite and its evasion of the host immune response. Thus, from these few surviving viruses, bacteria or animal parasites, a new population of infectious agents is produced. This cycle may be repeated, thereby obfuscating the protective effects of the immune response.

Antigenic drift (Figure 13) refers to spontaneous variation, as in influenza virus, expressed as relatively minor differences exemplified by slow antigenic changes from one year to the next. Antigenic drift is believed to be due to mutation of the genes encoding the hemagglutinin or the neuraminidase components. Antigenic variants represent those viruses that have survived exposure to the host's neutralizing antibodies. Minor alterations in a viral genome might occur every few years, especially in influenza A subtypes that are made up of H1, H2 and H3 hemagglutinins and N1 and N2 neuraminidases. Antigenic shifts follow point mutations of DNA encoding these hemagglutinins and neuraminidases.

Antigenic shift (Figure 13) also describes a major antigenic change in which a strain with distinctive new antigens may appear, such as Asian or A2 influenza in 1957. Antigenic variants of type A influenza virus are known as subtypes. Influenza virus antigenic shift is attributable mainly to alterations in the hemagglutinin antigens with less frequent alterations in the neuraminidase antigens. The appearance of a new type A influenza virus signals the addition of a new

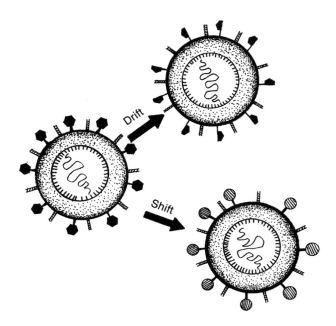

Figure 13.   Antigenic drift and shift.

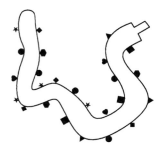

Figure 14.   Thymus dependent antigen.

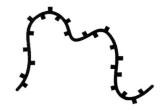

Figure 15.   Thymus independent antigen.

epitope even through several original antigenic determinants are still present.

In contrast to antigenic drift, antigenic shift involves a principal alteration in a genome attributable to gene rearrangement between two related microorganisms. Since antigenic shift involves the acquisition of totally new antigens against which the host population is not immune, this alteration may lead to an epidemic of significant proportions.

Antigenic mosaicism refers to antigenic variation first discovered in pathogenic *Neisseria*. It is the result of genetic transformation between gonococcal strains. This is also observed in penicillin resistance of several bacterial species where the resistant organism contains DNA from a host commensal organism.

A **thymus-dependent (TD) antigen** (Figure 14) is an immunogen that requires T lymphocyte cooperation for B cells to synthesize specific antibodies. Presentation of thymus-dependent antigen to T cells must be in the context of MHC class II molecules. Thymus-dependent antigens include proteins, polypeptides, hapten-carrier complexes, erythrocytes, and many other antigens that have diverse epitopes.

A **thymus-independent (TI) antigen** (Figure 15) is an immunogen that can stimulate B cells to synthesize antibodies without participation by T cells. These antigens are less complex than are thymus-dependent antigens. They are often polysaccharides that contain repeating epitopes or lipopolysaccharides derived from gram negative microorganisms. Thymus-independent antigens induce IgM synthesis by B lymphocytes without cooperation by T cells. They also do not stimulate immunological memory.

	T-cell dependent antigen	T-cell independent antigen
Structural properties	Complex	Simple
Chemistry	Proteins; protein-nucleoprotein conjugates; glycoproteins; lipoproteins	Polysaccharide of pneumococcus; dextran polyvinyl pyrolidone; bacterial lipo-polysaccharide
Antibody class induced	IgG, IgM, IgA (+IgD and IgE)	IgM
Immunological memory response	Yes	No
Present in most pathogenic microbes	Yes	No

Figure 16.   Comparison of T cell dependent with T cell independent antigens.

A **private antigen** (Figure 16) is 1) an antigen confined to one major histocompatibility complex (MHC) molecule; 2) an antigenic specificity restricted to a few individuals; 3) a tumor antigen restricted to a specific chemically induced tumor; or 4) a low frequency epitope present on red blood cells of fewer than 0.1% of the population, i.e., Pta, By, Bpa, etc; HLA antigen encoded by one allele such as HLA-B27.

A **public antigen (supratypic antigen)** (Figure 17) is an epitope which several distinct or private antigens have in common. A public antigen is one such as a blood group antigen that is present in greater than 99.9% of a population. It is detected by the indirect anti-globulin (Coombs' test). Examples include Ve, Ge, Jr, Gy[a], and Ok[a]. Antigens that

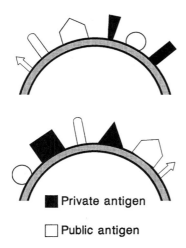

Figure 17.   Public and private antigen.

occur frequently but are not public antigens include MNs, Lewis, Duffy, P, etc. In blood banking, there is a problem finding a suitable unit of blood for a transfusion to recipients who have developed antibodies against public antigens.

Forssman antigen is a heterophile or heterogenetic glycolipid antigen that stimulates the synthesis of anti-sheep hemolysin in rabbits. Its broad phylogenetic distribution spans both animal and plant kingdoms. The antigen is present in guinea pig and horse organs but not in their red blood cells. In sheep, it is found exclusively in erythrocytes. Forssman antigen occurs in both red blood cells and organs in chickens. It is also present in goats, ostriches, mice, dogs, cats, spinach, *Bacillus anthracis* and on the gastrointestinal mucosa of a limited number of people. It is absent in rabbits, rats, cows, pigs, cuckoos, beans and Salmonella typhi. Forssman substance is ceramide tetrasaccharide. The Forssman antigen contains N-acylsphingo-sine (ceramide), galactose and N-acetylactosamine. As originally defined, it is present in guinea pig kidney, is heat stable and alcohol soluble. Forssman antigen-containing tissue is effective in absorbing the homologous antibody from serum. Antibodies to the Forssman antigen occur in the sera of patients recovering from infectious mononucleosis.

A **heterophile antigen (epitope)** is present in divergent animal species, plants and bacteria that manifest broad cross-reactivity with antibodies of the heterophile group. Heterophile antigens induce the formation of heterophile antibodies when introduced into a species where they are absent. Heterophile antigens are often carbohydrates.

An **immune response** is the reaction of an animal body to challenge by an immunogen. This is expressed as antibody production and/or cell-mediated immunity or immunologic tolerance. Immune response may follow stimulation by a wide variety of agents such as pathogenic microorganisms, tissue transplants or other antigenic substances deliberately introduced for one purpose or another. Infectious agents may also induce inflammatory reactions characterized by the production of chemical mediators at the site of injury.

A **primary immune response** refers to the animal body's response to first contact with antigen (Figure 18). It is characterized by a lag period of a few days following antigen administration before antibodies or specific T lymphocytes are detectable. The antibody produced consists mostly of IgM, is of relatively low titer and low affinity. This is in contrast to the secondary immune response in which the latent period is relatively brief and IgG is the predominant antibody. The most important event that occurs in the primary response is the activation of memory cells that recognize antigen immediately on second encounter with antigen leading to a secondary response. A similar pattern is followed in cell-mediated responses.

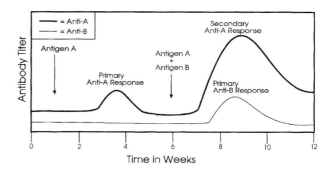

Figure 18.   Primary immune response.

The **secondary immune response** describes a heightened antibody response following second exposure to antigen in animals that have been primed by previous contact with the same antigen. The secondary immune response depends upon immunological memory learned from the first encounter with antigen. It is characterized by a steep and rapid rise in antibody titer, usually of the IgG class, accompanied by potent cell-mediated immunity. Protein and glycoprotein immunogens stimulate this type of response. The rapid rise in antibody synthesis is followed by a gradual exponential decline in titer. This is also known as the booster response as observed following administration of antigens subsequent to the secondary exposure.

An **anamnestic immune response** (Figure 19) is one that is accentuated and occurs following exposure of immunocompetent cells to an immunogen to which they have been exposed before. Commonly called the secondary or anamnestic response. It occurs rapidly, i.e., within hours following secondary immunogen inoculation and does not have the lag period observed with primary immunization. Immunologic memory is involved in the production of this response which generally consists of IgG antibodies of high titer and high affinity. There may also be heightened T cell (cell-mediated) immune reactivity. It also is called memory or booster response or secondary immune response.

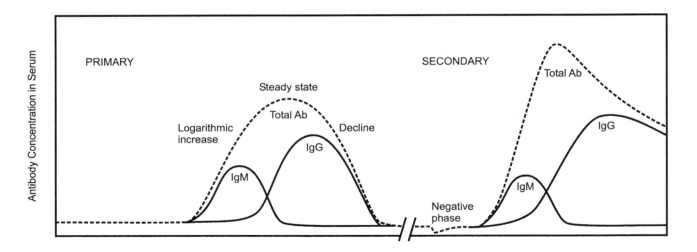

Schematic Representation of Humoral and Cellular Events
in the Primary and Secondary (Anamnestic) Antibody Responses

Figure 19.   Anamnestic immune response.

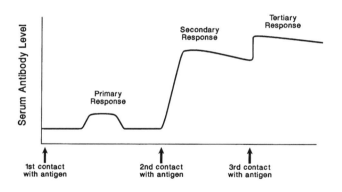

Figure 20.   Tertiary immune response.

A **tertiary immune response** (Figure 20) is one that is induced by a third (second booster) administration of antigen. It closely resembles the secondary (or booster) immune response.

An **adjuvant** (Figure 21) is a substance that facilitates or enhances the immune response to an antigen with which it is combined. Various types of adjuvants have been described, including Freund's complete and incomplete adjuvants, aluminum compounds and muramyl dipeptide. Some of these act by forming a depot in tissues from which antigen is slowly released. In addition, Freund's adjuvant attracts a large number of cells to the area of antigen deposition to provide increased immune responsiveness to it. Modern adjuvants include such agents as muramyl dipeptide. The ideal adjuvant is one that is biodegradable with elimination from the tissues once its immunoenhancing activity has been completed. An adjuvant nonspecifically facilitates an immune response to antigen. An adjuvant usually combines with the immunogen but is sometimes given prior to or following antigen administration. Adjuvants represent a heterogenous class of compounds capable of augmenting the humoral or cell-mediated immune response to a given antigen. They are widely used in experimental work and for therapeutic purposes in vaccines. Adjuvants comprise compounds of mineral nature, products of microbial origin and synthetic compounds. The primary effect of some adjuvants is postulated to be retention of antigen at the inoculation site so that the immunogenic stimulus persists for a longer period of time. However, the mechanism by which adjuvants augment the immune response is poorly understood. The macrophage may be the target and mediator of action of some adjuvants, whereas others may require T cells for their response augmenting effect. Adjuvants such as lipopolysaccharide (LPS) may act directly on B lymphocytes.

Freund's adjuvant is a water-in-oil emulsion that facilitates or enhances an immune response to antigen that has been incorporated into the adjuvant. There are two forms. Freund's complete adjuvant (CFA) consists of light-weight mineral oil that contains killed, dried mycobacteria. Antigen in an aqueous phase is incorporated into the oil phase containing mycobacteria with the aid of an emulsifying agent such as Arlacel A. This emulsion is then used as the immunogen. Freund's incomplete adjuvant (IFA) differs from the complete form only in that it does not contain mycobacteria. In both cases, the augmenting effect depends on and parallels the magnitude of the local inflammatory lesion, essentially a nonnecrotic monocytic reaction with fibrous encapsulation. Whereas the complete form facilitates stimulation of both T and B limbs of the immune response, the incomplete variety enhances antibody formation but does not stimulate cell-mediated immunity except for transient Jones-Mote

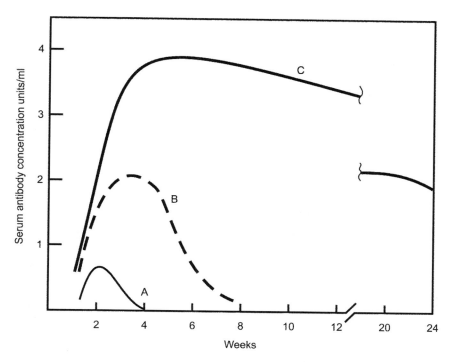

Figure 21. Effect of adjuvants. Schematic representation of the quantities of antibodies formed by rabbits following a single injection of a soluble protein antigen (arrow), such a bovine gammaglobulin in dilute physiologic saline solution (A), adsorbed on precipitated alum (B), or incorporated into Freund's complete adjuvant (C).

reactivity. The adjuvant principle in mycobacteria is the cell wall wax D fraction. CFA does not potentiate the immune response to the so-called thymus-independent antigens such as pneumococcal polysaccharide or polyvinylpyrrolidone. CFA may be combined with normal tissues and injected into animals of the type supplying the tissue to induce autoimmune diseases such as thyroiditis, allergic encephalomyelitis or adjuvant arthritis.

Muramyl dipeptide (MDP) (N-acetyl-muramyl-L-alanyl-D-isoglutamine) (Figure 22) is the active principle responsible for the immunlogic adjuvant properties of complete Freund's adjuvant. It is an extract of the peptidoglycan of the cell walls of mycobacteria in complete Freund's adjuvant that have the immunopotentiating property of inducing delayed-type hypersensitivity and boosting antibody responses. It induces fever and lyses blood platelets and may produce a temporary leukopenia. However, purified derivatives without adverse side effects have been prepared for use as immunologic adjuvants and may prove useful for use in human vaccines.

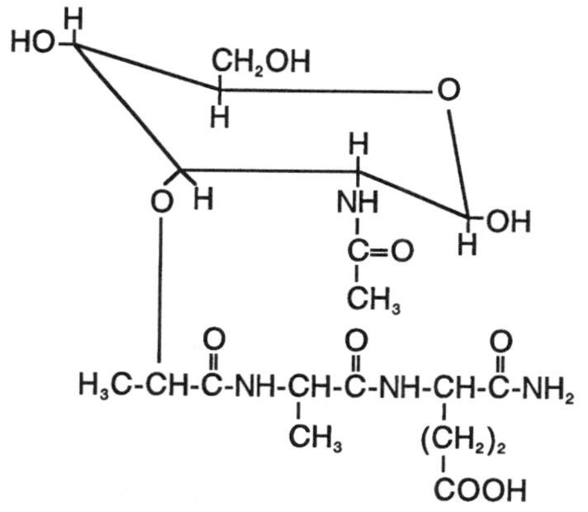

A **vaccine** may contain live attenuated or killed microorganisms or antigenic parts or products from them capable of stimulating a specific immune response conprised of protective antibodies and T cell immunity. A vaccine should stimulate a sufficient number of memory T and B lymphocytes to yield effector T cells from memory cells. Viral vaccine should also be able to stimulate high titers of neutralizing

N-acetylmuramyl-L-alanyl-D-isoglutamine

Figure 22. Muramyl dipeptide (MDP).

antibodies to protect against virus infection. Injection of a vaccine into a nonimmune subject induces active immunity against the modified pathogens.

A **heterologous vaccine** induces protective immunity against pathogenic microorganisms which the vaccine does not contain. Thus, the microorganisms that are present in the heterologous vaccine possess antigens that cross-react with those of the pathogenic agent absent from the vaccine. Measles vaccine can stimulate protection against canine distemper. Vaccinia virus was used in the past to induce immunity against smallpox because the agents of vaccinia and variola share antigens in common.

Historically the intracutaneous inoculation of pus from lesions of smallpox victims into healthy, non-immune subjects to render them immune to smallpox was known as **variolation**. In China lesional crusts were ground into a powder and inserted into the recipient's nostrils. These procedures protected some individuals but often led to life-threatening smallpox infection in others. Edward Jenner's introduction of vaccination with cowpox to protect against smallpox rendered variolation obsolete.

Vaccination is immunization against infectious disease through the administration of vaccines for the production of active (protective) immunity in man or other animals.

Cowpox (Figure 23) is a bovine virus disease that induces vesicular lesions on the teats. It is of great historical significance in immunology because Edward Jenner observed that milkmaids who had cowpox lesions on their hands failed to develop smallpox. He used this principle in vaccinating humans with the cowpox preparation to produce harmless vesicular lesions at the site of inoculation (vaccination). This stimulated protective immunity against smallpox (variola) because of shared antigens between vaccinia virus and variola virus.

Vaccinia refers to a virus termed *Poxvirus officinale* derived from cowpox and used to induce active immunity against smallpox through vaccination (Figure 24). It differs from both cowpox and smallpox viruses in minor antigens.

Tetanus antitoxin is an antibody raised by immunizing horses against *Clostridium tetani* exotoxin. It is a therapeutic agent to treat or prevent tetanus in individuals with contaminated lesions. Anaphylaxis or serum sickness (type III hypersensitivity) may occur in individuals receiving second injections because of sensitization to horse serum proteins following initial exposure to horse antitoxin. One solution to this has been the use of human antitetanus toxin of high titer. Treatment of the IgG fraction yields F(ab′)$_2$ fragments which retain all of the toxin neutralizing capacity but with diminished antigenicity of the antitoxin preparation.

A **toxoid** is formed by treating a microbial toxin with formaldehyde to inactivate toxicity but leave the immunogenicity (antigenicity) of the preparation intact. Toxoids are prepared from exotoxins produced in diphtheria and tetanus. These are used to induce protective immunization against adverse effects of the exotoxins in question.

Tetanus toxoid is prepared from formaldehyde-treated toxins of *Clostridium tetani*. It is an immunizing preparation to protect against tetanus. Individuals with increased likelihood of developing tetanus as a result of a deep penetrating wound with a rusty nail or other contaminated instrument are immunized by subcutaneous inoculation. The preparation is available in both fluid and adsorbed forms. It is included in a mixture with diphtheria toxoid and pertussis vaccine and is known as DTP or triple vaccine. It is employed to routinely immunize children less than 6 years old.

An **inactivated vaccine** is an immunizing preparation that contains microorganisms such as bacteria or viruses that have been killed to stop their replication while preserving their protection-inducing antigens. Formaldehyde, phenol and β-propiolactone have been used to inactivate viruses, whereas formaldehyde, acetone, phenol or heating have been methods used to kill bacteria to be used in vaccines.

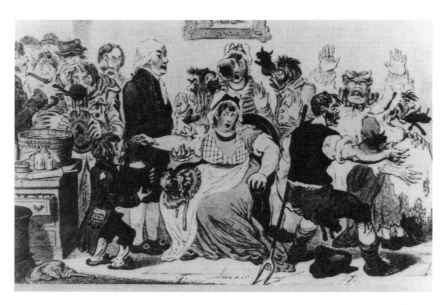

Figure 23.   James Gillray's cartoon of the cowpock.

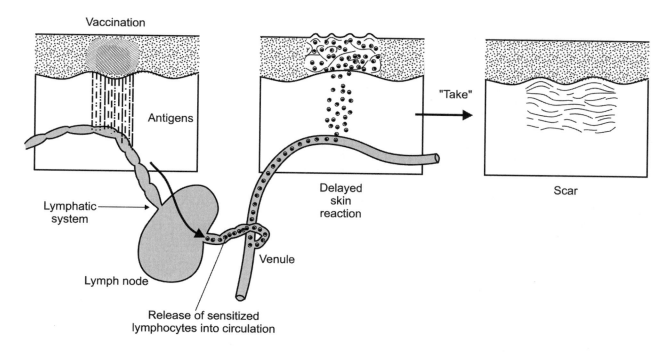

Figure 24.   Vaccination against smallpox.

A **polyvalent vaccine** is comprised of multiple antigens from more than one strain of a pathogenic microorganism or from a mixture of immunogens such as the diphtheria, pertussis, tetanus toxoid preparation.

An **autogenous vaccine** (Figure 25) is prepared by isolating and culturing of microorganisms from an infected subject. The microorganisms in culture are killed and used as an immunogen, i.e., a vaccine, to induce protective immunity in the same subject from which they were derived. In earlier years, this was a popular method to treat *Staphylococcus aureus*-induced skin infections.

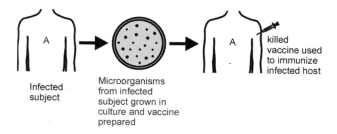

Figure 25.   Autogenous vaccine.

DTP vaccine (Figure 26) is a preparation used for protective immunization that is comprised of diphtheria and tetanus toxoids and pertussis vaccine. Children should receive DTP vaccine at the ages of 2, 4, 6 and 15 months with a booster given at 4 to 6 years of age. The tetanus and diphtheria toxoids should be repeated at 14 to 16 years of age. The vaccine is contraindicated in individuals who have shown prior allergic reactions to DTP or in subjects with acute or developing neurologic disease. DTP vaccine is effective in preventing most cases of the diseases it addresses. Because of the occasional production of neurologic complications by the pertussis part of the vaccine, a genetically altered mutant is being developed for use in the vaccine.

Pertussis vaccine (Figure 27) is a preparation used for prophylactic immunization against whooping cough in children. It consists of virulent *Bordetella pertussis* microorganisms that have been killed by treatment with formalin. It is administered in conjunction with diphtheria toxoid and tetanus toxoid as a so-called triple vaccine. In addition to stimulating protective immunity against pertussis, the killed *Bordetella pertussis* microorganisms act as an adjuvant and facilitate antibody production against the diphtheria and tetanus toxoid components in vaccine. Rarely, hypersensitivity reaction may occur.

Triple vaccine is an immunizing preparation comprised of three components and is used to protect infants against diphtheria, pertussis (whooping cough) and tetanus. It is made up of diphtheria toxoid, pertussis vaccine and tetanus toxoid. The first of four doses is administered between 3 and 6 months of age. The second dose is administered one month later and the third dose is given 6 months after the second. The child receives a booster injection when beginning school.

Pneumococcal polysaccharide vaccine contains a polysaccharide found in the *Streptococcus pneumoniae* capsule that is type specific antigen. It is a virulence factor. Serotypes of

	Diphtheria, tetanus toxoids, and whole cell pertussis vaccine	Diphtheria, tetanus toxoids and acellular pertussis vaccine	Diphtheria and tetanus toxoid (pediatric)	Tetanus and diphtheria toxoids (adult)	Diphtheria and tetanus toxoids and Hib conjugate and whole cell pertussis vaccines
Synonyms	DTP, DTwP	DTP, DTaP	DT	Td	DTwP-Hib
Manufacturers	several	Connaught, Lederle	several	several	Lederle
Concentration (per 0.5 ml) Diphtheria Tetanus Pertussis Hib	6.5-12.5 Lf u 5-5.5 Lf u 4 u none	6.7-7.5 Lf u 5 Lf u either 46.8 mcg or 300 HA u none	6.6-12.5 Lf u 5-7.6 Lf u none none	2 Lf u 2-5 Lf u none none	6.7 or 12.5 Lf u 5 Lf u 4 u 10 mcg
Packaging	5 or 7.5 ml vials	5 or 7.5 vials	5 ml vial, 0.5 ml syringe	5 or 30 ml vials, 0.5 ml syringe	5 ml vial
Appropriate age range	2 months to <7 years	18 months to <7 years	2 months to <7 years	7 years to adult	typically 2 to 15 months
Standard schedule	Five 0.5 ml doses: at 2, 4, 6, and 18 months and 4-6 years of age	For doses 4 and 5: at 18 months and at 4-6 years of age	Three 0.5 ml doses: at 2, 4 and 10-16 months of age	Three 0.5 ml doses: the second 4-8 weeks after the first and the third 6-12 months after the second	Four 0.5 ml doses: at 2, 4, 6, and 15 months of age
Routine additional doses	none	none	none	every 10 years	none
Route	IM	IM	IM	IM, jet	IM

Figure 26.   Diphtheria, tetanus, and pertussis — combination summary.

	Risk of occurrence after	
Problem	Vaccination	Disease
Seizures	1:1750	1:25-1:50
Encephalitis	1:100,000	1:1000-1:4000
Severe brain damage	1:310,000	1:2000-1:8000
Death	1:1,000,000	1:200-1:1000

Figure 27.   Pertussis vaccine.

this microorganism are based upon different specificities in the capsular polysaccharide which is comprised of oligosaccharide repeating units. Glucose and glucuronic acid are the repeating units in type III polysaccharide.

Rabies vaccine. In humans, significant levels of neutralizing antibody can be generated by immunization with a virus grown in tissue culture in diploid human embryo lung cells. A vaccine adapted to chick embryos, especially egg passage material, is used for prophylaxis in animals prior to exposure. The "historical" vaccine originally prepared by Pasteur made use of rabbit spinal cord preparations to which the virus had become adapted. However, they were discontinued because of the risk of inducing post-rabies vaccination encephalomyelitis.

TAB vaccine is an immunizing preparation used to protect against enteric fever. It is comprised of *Salmonella typhi* and *Salmonella paratyphi* A and B microorganisms that have been killed by heat and preserved with phenol. The bacteria used in the vaccine are in the smooth specific phase. They also contain both O antigens and Vi antigens. The vaccine is administered subcutaneously. Lipopolysaccharide from the gram negative bacteria may induce fever in vaccine recipients. If *Salmonella paratyphi* C is added, the vaccine is referred to as TABC. If tetanus toxoid is added, it is referred to as TABT.

Yellow fever vaccine is a lyophilized attenuated vaccine prepared from the 17D strain of live attenuated yellow fever virus grown in chick embryos. A single injection may confer immunity that persists for a decade.

Salk vaccine is an injectable poliomyelitis virus vaccine, killed by formalin, that was used for prophylactic immunization against poliomyelitis prior to development of the Sabin oral polio vaccine.

Sabin vaccine is an attenuated live poliomyelitis virus vaccine that is administered orally to induce local immunity in the gut, which is the virus's natural route of entry, thereby stimulating local as well as systemic immunity against the causative agent of the disease.

Influenza vaccine is a purified and inactivated immunizing preparation made from viruses grown in eggs. It cannot lead to infection. It contains (H1N1) and (H3N2) type A strains and one type B strain. These are the strains considered most likely to cause influenza in the United States. Whole virus and split virus preparations are available. Children tolerate the split virus preparation better than the whole virus vaccine.

BCG (bacille Calmette-Guerin) is a *Mycobacterium bovis* strain maintained for more than three quarters of a century on potato, bile glycerine agar which preserves the immunogenicity but dissipates the virulence of the microorganism. It has long been used in Europe as a vaccine against tuberculosis although it never gained popularity in the United

States. It also has been used in tumor immunotherapy to nonspecifically activate the immune response in selected tumor-bearing patients, such as those with melanoma. It has been suggested as a possible vector for genes that determine HIV proteins such as *gag, pol, env*, reverse transcriptase, gp20, gp40 and tetanus toxin.

Measles vaccine is an attenuated virus vaccine administered as a single injection to children either two years of age or between 1 and 10 years old. Contraindications include a history of allergy or convulsions. Puppies may be protected against canine distemper in the neonatal period by the administration of attenuated measles virus which represents a heterologous vaccine. Passive immunity from the mother precludes early immunization with live canine distemper vaccine.

Mumps vaccine is an attenuated virus vaccine prepared from virus generated in chick embryo cell cultures.

Rubella vaccine is an attenuated virus vaccine used to immunize girls 10–14 years of age. It is not to be used during pregnancy.

Hepatitis vaccines (Figure 29) is a vaccine used to actively immunize subjects against hepatitis B virus and contains purified hepatitis B surface antigen. Current practice uses an immunogen prepared by recombinant DNA technology referred to as Recombivax®. The antigen preparation is administered in three sequential intramuscular injections to individuals such as physicians, nurses and other medical personnel who are at risk. Temporary protection against hepatitis A is induced by the passive administration of pooled normal human serum immunoglobulin which protects against hepatitis A virus for a brief time. Antibody for passive protection against hepatitis must be derived from the blood sera of specifically immune individuals.

Vaccine	Birth	2 months	4 months	6 months	12 months	15 months	18 months	4-6 years	11-12 years	14-16 years
Hepatitis B	HB-1									
		HB-2		HB-3						
Diphtheria, Tetanus, Pertussis		DTP	DTP	DTP	DTP or DTaP at ≥15 months			DTP or DTaP	Td	
H. influenzae type b		Hib	Hib	Hib	Hib					
Measles, mumps, and rubella		OPV	OPV	OPV				OPV		
Measles, mumps, and rubella					MMR			MMR or MMR		

Figure 28. Childhood immunization schedule recommended by U.S. Public Health Service, January 1996.

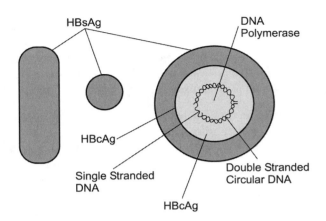

Figure 29. Hepatitis B virus and its antigens.

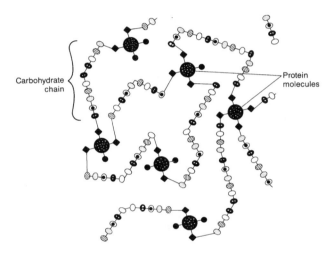

Figure 30. Conjugate vaccine.

Conjugate vaccine (Figure 30) is an immunogen comprised of polysaccharide bound covalently to proteins. The conjugation of weakly immunogenic, bacterial polysaccharide antigens with protein carrier molecules considerably enhances their immunogenicity. Conjugate vaccines have reduced morbidity and mortality for a number of bacterial diseases in vulnerable populations such as the very young or adults with immunodeficiencies. An example of a conjugate vaccine is *H. influenzae* 6 polysaccharide polyribosyl-ribitol-phosphate vaccine.

Hib (*Hemophilus influenzae type b*) is a microorganism that induces infection mostly in infants less than 5 years of age. Approximately 1,000 deaths out of 20,000 annual cases are recorded. A polysaccharide vaccine (Hib Vac) was of only marginal efficacy and poorly immunogenic. By contrast, anti-Hib vaccine which contains capsular polysaccharide of Hib bound covalently to a carrier protein such as polyribosylribitol-diphtheria toxoid or PRP-D induces a very high level of protection that reached 94% in one cohort of Finnish infants. PRP-tetanus toxoid has induced 75% protection. PRP-diphtheria toxoid vaccine has been claimed to be 88% effective.

Although there is no effective vaccine against **malaria** (Figure 31), several vaccine candidates are under investigation including an immunogenic but nonpathogenic *Plasmodium* sporozoite that has been attenuated by radiation. Circumsporoite proteins combined with sporozoite surface protein 2(SSP-2) are immunogenic. Murine studies have shown the development of transmission-blocking antibodies following immunization with vaccinia into which has been inserted the *Plasmodium falciparum* surface 25kD protein designated Pfs25. Attempts have been made to increase natural antibodies against circumsporozoite (CS) protein to prevent the pre-hepatoinvasive stage. The high mutability of *Plasmodium falciparum* makes prospects for an effective vaccine dim.

Hookworm vaccine (Figure 32) is a live vaccine to protect dogs against the hookworm, *Ancylostoma caninum*. The vaccine is comprised of X-irradiated larvae to halt their development to adult forms.

Several experimental **AIDS vaccines** (Figure 33) are under investigation. HIV-2 inoculation into cyomologus monkeys apparently prevented them from developing simian AIDS following injection of the SIV virus. Various problems relate

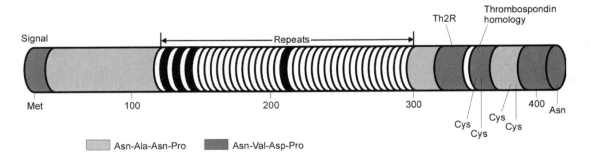

Figure 31. Circumsporate protein of malaria.

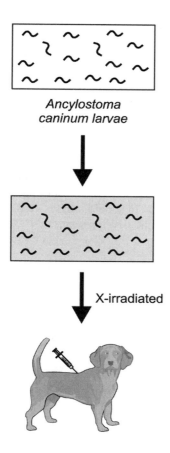

Figure 32. Hookworm vaccine.

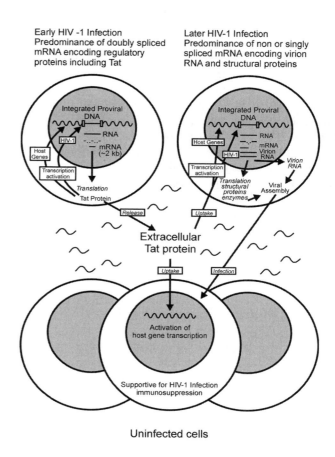

Figure 33. Possible AIDS vaccine.

DEVELOPMENT OF HUMAN VACCINES

Live Attenuated	Killed Whole Organism	Purified Protein or Polysaccharide	Genetically Engineered
Eighteenth Century Smallpox, 1798			
Nineteenth Century Rabies,1885	Typhoid, 1896 Cholera, 1896 Plague, 1897		

Early Twentieth Century
Bacille Calmette-Guerin,
  1927 (tuberculosis)
Yellow fever, 1935
	Pertussis, 1926
	  (whole cell)
	Influenza,1936
		Diphtheria, 1923
		Tetanus, 1927	

After World War II
  (Cell culture)
Polio (oral)
Measles
Mumps
Rubella
Adenovirus
Typhoid (Salmonella Ty21a)
Varicella
	Polio (injected)
	Rabies
	Japanese encephalitis
	Hepatitis A
		Pneumococcus
		Meningoccus
		Haemophilus influenzae PRP
		Hepatitis B (plasma derived)
		Tick-borne encephalitis
		H. influenzae PRP-protein
		  (conjugate)
		Acellular pertussis
			Hepatitis B recombinant

to the successful development of an HIV vaccine to protect against AIDS. There is no precise animal model that can be employed to evaluate a vaccine against HIV. Studies of vaccine efficacy in humans are also problematic. The simian immunodeficiency virus (SIV), a close relative of HIV that infects macaques, produces a disease that closely resembles AIDS in Asian macaques but not in the African variety. This variability of SIV points to the problem in attempting to extrapolate results of vaccine trials in macaques to trials in humans. The requirements to establish immunity against HIV infection are unknown. Unlike infections that induce long lasting protective immunity, HIV coexists with an intensive immune response. HIV infection leads to a progressive immunodeficiency even though there is variability among individuals in resistance to HIV which could be attributable either to their infection by a mutant HIV or to resistance to HIV infection mediated by their $CD8^+$ T cells. The type of immunity induced is also significant. A $CD8^+$ T cell or T_H1 cell immune response would probably be most desirable. AIDS patients usually produce T_H2 cell cytokines and their $CD4^+$ T cell response to HIV components is affected by T_H1 cytokines. Subunit vaccines have also been attempted but these induce immunity to only some proteins of the virus, and when tested in chimpanzees have induced immunity specific only for the exact virus strain used to make the vaccine. Such subunit vaccines fail to protect against natural infection. In addition, there are ethical issues involved in AIDS vaccine development.

4

Major Histocompatibility Complex

The first recognition of MHC genes was based on their ability to encode proteins that serve as identity markers on tissues and cells that have been transplanted into an incompatible recipient. Their recognition by the recipient's lymphocytes leads to prompt rejection. The preoccupation of investigators with the role of histocompatibility antigens in transplantation obscured their real purpose of serving as identity markers on cells interacting with T cells carrying out specific immune functions through their own T cell receptors. In fact, T lymphocytes recognize antigens only in the context of MHC molecules.

Histocompatibility means tissue compatibility as in the transplantation of tissues or organs from one member to another of the same species, i.e., an allograft, or from one species to another, a xenograft. The genes that encode antigens which should match if a tissue or organ graft is to survive in the recipient are located in the major histocompatibility complex (MHC) region. Genes that encode the major, as opposed to minor, histocompatibility antigens that are expressed on cell membranes. The MHC gene is located on the short arm of chromosome 6 in man and of chromosome 17 in the mouse (Figures 1 and 2). Class I (Figures 3 and 4) and class II MHC antigens are important in tissue transplantation. The greater the match between donor and recipient, the more likely the transplant is to survive. For example, a six-antigen match implies sharing of two HLA-A antigens, two HLA-B antigens, and two HLA-DR antigens between donor and recipient. Even though antigenically dissimilar grafts may survive when a powerful immunosuppressive drug such as cyclosporine is used, the longevity of the graft still is improved by having as many antigens match as possible.

Calnexin (Figure 5) is a 88 kD membrane molecule that combines with newly formed α chains that also interact with nascent β_2-microglobulin. Calnexin maintains partial folding of the MHC-class I molecule in the endoplasmic reticulum.

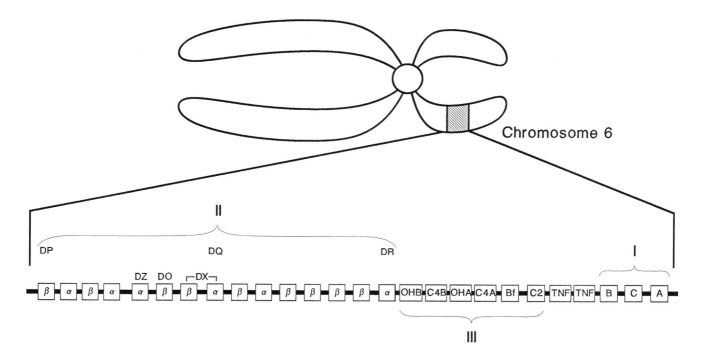

Figure 1. **HLA** is an abbreviation for human leukocyte antigen. The HLA locus in humans is found on the short arm of chromosome 6. The class I region consists of HLA-A, HLA-B, and HLA-C loci and the class II region consists of the D region which is subdivided into HLA-DR, HLA-DQ and HLA-DR subregions.

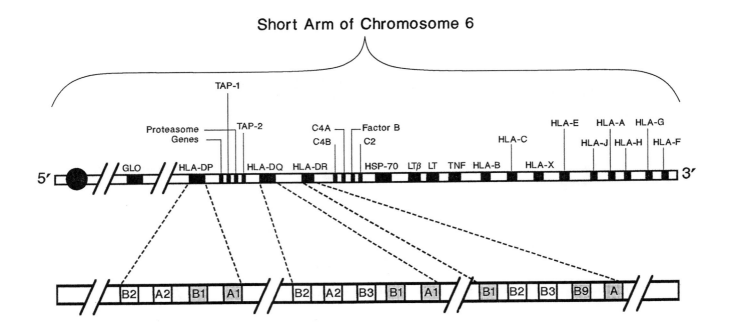

Figure 2. **MHC genes** (major histocompatibility complex genes) encode the major histocompatibility antigens that are expressed on cell membranes. MHC genes in the mouse are located at the H-2 locus on chromosome 17 whereas the MHC genes in man are located at the HLA locus on the short arm of chromosome 6.

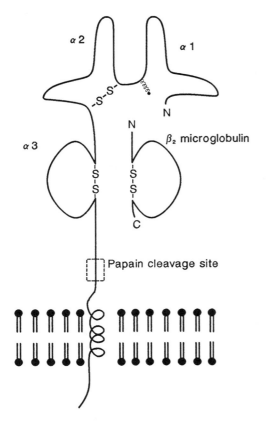

Figure 3. **Class I MHC** molecules are glycoproteins that play an important role in the interactions among cells of the immune system.

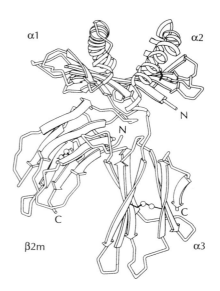

Figure 4. Schematic representation of the three-dimensional structure of the external domains of a human class I HLA molecule based on X-ray crystallographic analysis. The β strands are depicted as thick arrows and the α helices as spiral ribbons. Disulfide bonds are shown as two interconnected spheres. The α_1 and α_2 domains interact to form the peptide-binding cleft. Note the immunoglobulin-fold structure of the α_3 domain and β_2 microglobulin.

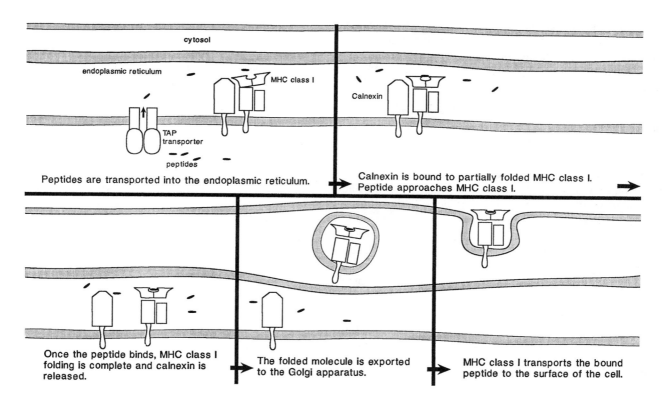

cytosol

endoplasmic reticulum

MHC class I

TAP transporter

peptides

Peptides are transported into the endoplasmic reticulum.

Calnexin

Calnexin is bound to partially folded MHC class I.
Peptide approaches MHC class I.

Once the peptide binds, MHC class I folding is complete and calnexin is released.

The folded molecule is exported to the Golgi apparatus.

MHC class I transports the bound peptide to the surface of the cell.

Figure 5. **Calnexin** is an 88 kD membrane molecule that combines with newly formed α chains that also interact with nascent β_2-microglobulin. Calnexin maintains partial folding of the MHC-class I molecule in the endoplasmic reticulum. It also interacts with MHC class II molecules, T cell receptors and immunoglobulins that are partially folded.

It also interacts with MHC class II molecules, T cell receptors and immunoglobulins that are partially folded. Class III MHC genes encode secreted proteins such as complement components, tumor necrosis factor and soluble stem proteins. The A, B and C regions encode class I MHC molecules in man, whereas DP, DQ and DR regions encode class II molecules in humans. The C4, CD2 and Bf regions encode class III molecules in humans. Class I and class II MHC antigens are important in tissue transplantation. The greater the match between donor and recipient, the more likely the transplant is to survive. For example, a 6 antigen match implies sharing of two HLA-A antigens, two HLA-B antigens, and two HLA-DR antigens between donor and recipient. Even though antigenically dissimilar grafts may survive when a powerful immunosuppressive drug such as cyclosporine is used, the longevity of the graft is still improved by having as many antigens to match as possible.

The **major histocompatibility complex (MHC)** is a locus on a chromosome comprised of multiple genes that encode histocompatibility antigens that are cell surface glycoproteins which play a significant role in interaction among immune cells. MHC genes encode both class I and class II MHC antigens. These antigens play critical roles in interactions among immune system cells, such as class II antigen participation in antigen presentation by macrophages to CD4+ lymphocytes; the participation of class I MHC antigens in cytotoxicity mediated by CD8+ T lymphocytes against target cells such as those infected by viruses, as well as various other immune reactions. MHC genes are very polymorphic and also encode a third category termed class III molecules that include complement proteins C2, C4 and factor B, P-450 cytochrome 21-hydroxylase, tumor necrosis factor and lymphotoxin. The MHC locus in man is designated HLA, in the mouse H2, in the chicken B, in the dog DLA, in the guinea pig GPLA and the rat RT1. The mouse and human MHC loci are the most widely studied. When organs are transplanted across major MHC locus differences between donor and recipient, graft rejection is prompt.

A **histocompatibility locus** is the specific site on a chromosome where the histocompatibility genes that encode histocompatibility antigens are located. There are major histocompatibility loci such as HLA in the human and H-2 in the mouse across which incompatible grafts are rejected within 1 to 2 weeks. There are also several minor histocompatibility loci, with more subtle antigenic differences, across which only slow, low level graft rejection reactions occur.

A **histocompatibility antigen** is one of a group of genetically encoded antigens present on tissue cells of an animal that provoke a rejection response if the tissue containing them is transplanted to a genetically dissimilar recipient.

These antigens are detected by typing lymphocytes on which they are expressed. These antigens are encoded in the human by genes at the HLA locus on the short arm of chromosome 6. In the mouse, they are encoded by genes at the H-2 locus on chromosome 17.

Coisogenic refers to inbred mouse strains that have an identical genotype except for a difference at one genetic locus. A point mutation in an inbred strain provides the opportunity to develop a coisogenic strain by inbreeding the mouse in which the mutation occurred. The line carrying the mutation is coisogenic with the line not expressing the mutation. Considering the problems associated with developing coisogenic lines, congenic mouse strains were developed as an alternative. Congenic strains of inbred mice (Figure 6) are believed to be genetically identical except for a difference at one genetic locus. Congenic strains are produced by crossing a donor strain and a background strain. Repeated backcrossing is made to the background strain and selecting in each generation for heterozygosity at a certain locus. Following 12–14 backcrosses, the progeny are inbred through brother-sister matings to yield a homozygous inbred strain. Mutation and genetic linkage may lead to random differences at a few other loci in the congenic strain. Designations for congenic strains consist of the symbol for the background strain followed by a period and then the symbol for the donor strain.

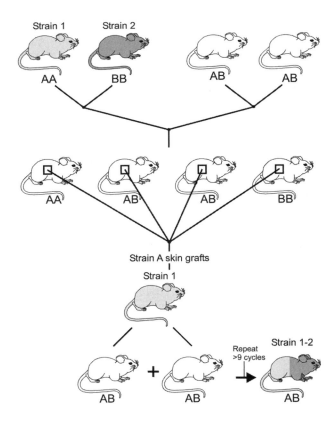

Figure 6. Congenic strains.

H-2 (Figure 7) designates the major histocompatibility complex in the mouse. H-2 genes are located on chromosome 17. They encode somatic cell surface antigens as well as the host immune response (*Ir*) genes. Each of these has a length of 600 base pairs. There are four regions in the H-2 complex designated K, I, S and D. K region genes encode class I histocompatibility molecules designated K. I region genes encode class II histocompatibility molecules designated I-A and I-E. S region genes encode class III molecules designated C2, C4, Factor B and P-450 cytochrome (21-hydroxylase). D region genes encode class I histocompatibility molecules designated D and L. Antigens that represent the H-2 type of a particular inbred strain of mice are encoded by H-2 alleles. Thus, differences in the antigenic structure between inbred mice of differing H-2 alleles is of critical importance in the acceptance or rejection of tissue grafts exchanged between them. K, D and L subregions of H-2 correspond to A, B, and C subregions of HLA in humans. The I-A and I-E regions are equivalent to the human HLA-D region. The **H-2D** and **H-2K** are murine H-2 loci whose gene products are class I antigens. Both H-2D and H-2K loci have multiple alleles.

The **Qa locus** is a subregion of the murine MHC located on the telomeric side of the H2 complex in a 1.5 centiMorgan stretch of DNA.

The **Qa region** is a part of the Tla complex which also contains Tla. The Qa region is comprised of 220 kilobases that encode for class I MHC α chains that associate noncovalently with β_2 microglobulin. The Qa region is comprised of 8 to 10 genes designated as Q1, Q2, Q3, etc.

Qa antigens are Class I histocompatibility antigens in mice designated Qa1, Qa2 and Qa10. They are encoded by genes in the QA region of the H-2 complex on the telomeric side. Lymphoid cells express Qa1 and Qa2 antigens whereas hepatic cells express Q10 antigens. The Qa represents one of two regions of the Tla complex with Tla representing the second region of this complex.

The **Tla complex** consists of genes that map to the MHC region telomeric to H2 loci on chromosome 17 in mice. These genes encode MHC class I proteins such as Qa and Tla that have no known immune function. Qa and Tla proteins that closely resemble H2 MHC class I proteins in sequence, associate noncovalently with β_2 microglobulin. Expression of Qa and Tla proteins, unlike expression of MHC H-2 class I proteins is limited to only selected mouse cells. For example, only hepatocytes express Q10 protein and only selected lymphocyte subpopulations, such as activated T lymphocytes, express Qa-2 proteins and T lymphocytes express Tla proteins. Thus, Qa and Tla class I molecules differ in structure and expression from the remaining MHC class I genes and proteins in the mouse. This could account for their failure to function in antigen presentation to T lymphocytes.

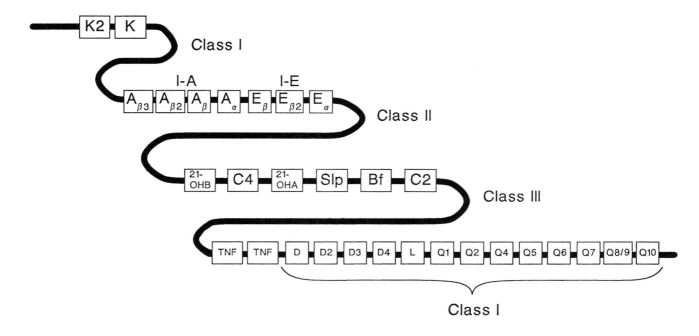

Figure 7.   H-2 histocompatibility system is the major histocompatibility complex in the mouse.

The **Tla antigen** is a murine MHC class I histocompatibility antigen encoded by genes that are situated near the Qa region on chromosome 17. Thymocytes may express products of up to 6 alleles. Leukemia cells may aberrantly express Tla antigens.

In the mouse, the **I region** (Figure 8) is the DNA segment of the major histocompatibility complex where the genes that encode MHC class II molecules are located. The 250 kilobase I region consists of I-A and I-E subregions. The genes designated pseudo $A_\beta 3$, $A_\beta 2$, $A_\beta 1$ and A_α are located in the 175 kilobase I-A subregion. The genes designated $E_\beta 2$ and E_α are located in the 75 kilobase I-E subregion. $E_\beta 1$ is located where the I-A and I-E subregions join. The S region contains the $E_\beta 3$ gene. **Ia antigens** (immune-associated antigens) are products of major histocompatibility complex (MHC) **I region** genes that encode murine cellular antigens. B lymphocytes, monocytes and activated T lymphocytes express Ia antigens.

HLA is the abbreviation for human leukocyte antigen. The HLA histocompatibility system in humans represents a complex of MHC class I molecules distributed on essentially all nucleated cells of the body and MHC class II molecules that are distributed on B lymphocytes, macrophages and a few other cell types. These are encoded by genes at the major histocompatibility complex. The HLA locus in humans is found on the short arm of chromosome 6. This has now been well defined and in addition to encoding surface isoantigens, genes at the HLA locus also encode immune response (*Ir*) genes. The class I region consists of HLA-A, HLA-B and HLA-C loci and the class II region consists of the D region which is subdivided

into HLA-DP, HLA-DQ and HLA-DR subregions. Class II molecules play an important role in the induction of an immune response since antigen presenting cells must complex an exogenous antigen with class II molecules to present it in the presence of interleukin-1 to CD4+ T lymphocytes. Class I molecules are important in presentation of intracellular endogenous antigen to CD8+ T lymphocytes as well as effector functions of target cells (Figures 9 and 10). Class III molecules encoded by genes located between those that encode class I and class II molecules include C2, BF, C4a, and C4b. Class I and class II molecules play an important role in the transplantation of organs and tissues. HLA-C molecules act as inhibitors of the lytic capacity of natural killer (NK) cells and non-MHC-restricted T cells. The microlymphocytotoxicity assay has been used for HLA-A, -B, -C, -DR and -DQ typing, but is gradually being replaced by molecular (DNA) typing. The primed lymphocyte test is used for DP typing.

Proteasome (Figure 11) is a 650-kD organelle in the cytoplasm termed the low molecular mass polypeptide complex. The proteasome is believed to generate peptides by degradation of proteins in the cytosol. It is a cylindrical structure comprised of as many as 24 protein subunits. The proteasome participates in degradation of proteins in the cytosol that are covalently linked ubiquinated prior to presentation to MHC class 1-restricted T lymphocytes. Proteasomes that include MHC gene encoded subunits are especially adept at forming peptides that bind MHC class I molecules.

The **transporter in antigen processing (TAP) 1 and 2 genes** (Figure 12) are in the MHC class II region that must be expressed for MHC class I molecules to be assembled

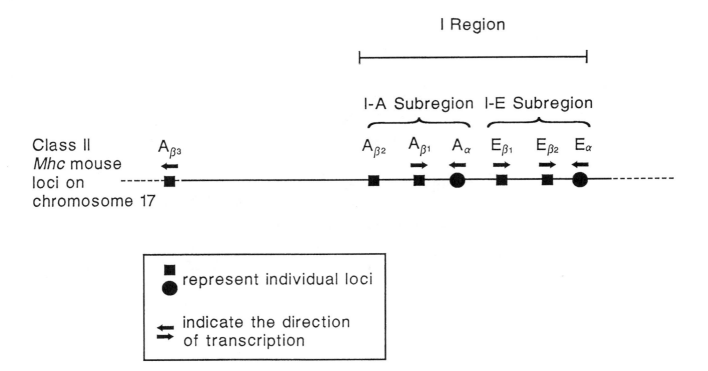

Figure 8.   In the mouse, the I region is the DNA segment of the major histocompatibility complex where the genes that encode MHC class II molecules are located.

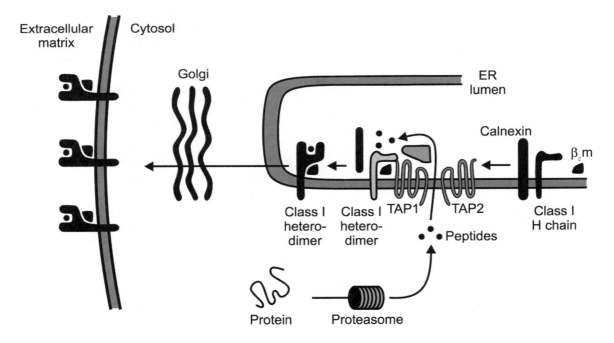

Figure 9.   Class I MHC assembly.

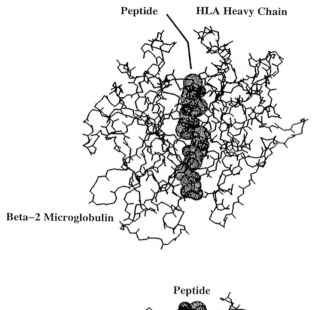

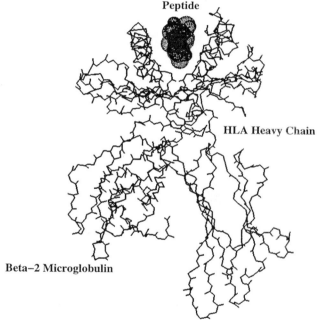

Figure 10. A schematic backbone structure of human class I histocompatibility antigen (HLA-A 0201) complexed with a decameric peptide from hepatitis B nucleocapsid protein (residues 18-27). Determined by X-ray crystallography.

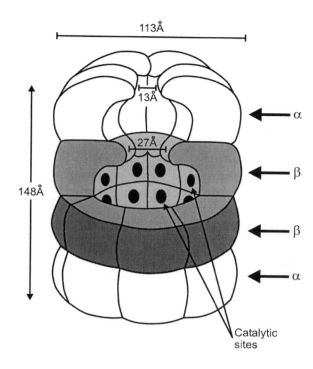

Figure 11. Longitudinal and transverse section through the 20S proteasome. The 20S proteasome is composed of two outer and two inner rings. The two outer rings each comprise seven copies of the 25.9 kDa α subunit.

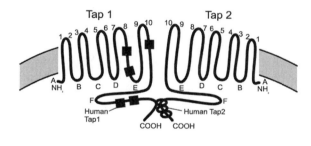

Figure 12. Topology of Tap 1 and Tap 2 proteins.

efficiently. TAP 1 and 2 are postulated to encode components of a heterodimeric protein pump that conveys cytosolic peptides to the endoplasmic reticulum. Here they associate with MHC class I heavy chains.

The human **MHC class II region** (Figure 13), HLA-D, is comprised of three subregions designated DR, DQ and DP. Multiple genetic loci are present in each of these. DN (previously DZ) and DO subregions are each comprised of one genetic locus. Each class II HLA molecule is comprised of one α and one β chain that constitute a heterodimer

(Figures 14 and 15). Genes within each subregion encode a particular class II molecule's α and β chains. Class II genes that encode α chains are designated A whereas class II genes that encode β chains are designated B. A number is used following A or B if a particular subregion contains two or more A or B genes.

The **HLA-DP subregion** is a site of two sets of genes designated HLA-DPA1 and HLA-DPB1 and the pseudogenes HLA-DPA2 and HLA-DPB2. DPα and DPβ chains encoded by the corresponding genes DPA1 and DPB1 unite to produce the DPab molecule. DP antigen or type is determined principally by the very polymorphic DPβ chain in contrast to the much less polymorphic DPα chain. DP molecules carry DPw1-DPw6 antigens.

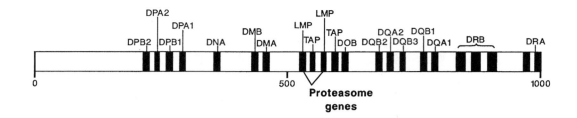

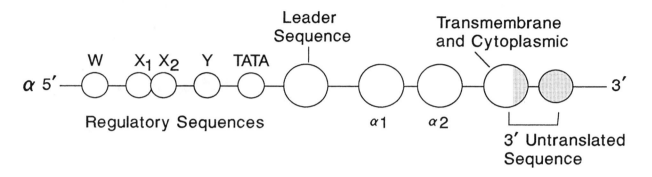

Figure 13.   MHC Class II.

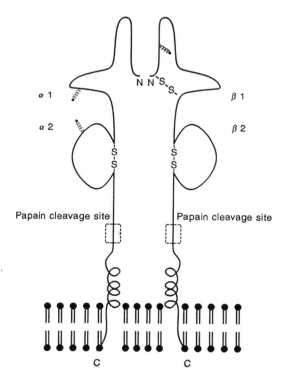

Figure 14.   Class II MHC molecules are glycoprotein histocompatibility antigens that play a critical role in immune system cellular interactions. Each class II MHC molecule is comprised of a 32-34kD α chain and a 29-32kD β chain, each of which possesses N-linked oligosaccharide groups, amino termini that are extracellular and carboxyl termini that are intracellular. Approximately 70% of both α and β chains are extracellular.

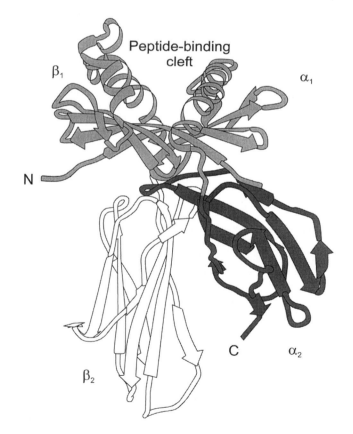

Figure 15.   MHC Class II Molecular Structure.

The **HLA-DQ subregion** contains two sets of genes designated DQA1 and DQB1 and DQA2 and DQB2. DQA2 and DRB2 are pseudogenes. DQα and DQβ chains, encoded by DQA1 and DQB1 genes, unite to produce the DQαβ molecule. Although both DQα and DQβ chains are polymorphic, the DQβ chain is the principal factor in determining the DQ antigen or type. DQαβ molecules carry DQw1-DQw9 specificities.

The **HLA-DR subregion** is the site of one HLA-DRA gene. Although DRB gene number varies with DR type, there are usually three DRB genes, termed DRB1, DRB2, and DRB3 (or DRB4). The DRB2 pseudogene is not expressed. The DR α chain, encoded by the DRA gene, can unite with products of DRB1 and DRB3 (or DRB4) genes which are the DRβ1 and DRβ3 (or DRβ4) chains. This yields two separate DR molecules, DRαβ1 and DRαβ3 (or DRαβ4). The DRβ chain determines the DR antigen (DR type) since it is very polymorphic, whereas the DRα chain is not. DRαβ1 molecules carry DR specificities DR1-DRw18. Yet DRαβ3 molecules carry the DRw52 and the DRαβ4 molecules carry the DRw53 specificity.

HLA-DR antigenic specificities reflect the epitopes on DR gene products. Selected specificities have been mapped to defined loci. HLA serologic typing requires the identification of a prescribed antigenic determinant on a particular HLA molecular product. One typing specificity can be present on many different molecules. Different alleles at the same locus may encode these various HLA molecules. Monoclonal antibodies are now used to recognize certain antigenic determinants shared by various molecules bearing the same HLA typing specificity. Monoclonal antibodies have been employed to recognize specific class II alleles with disease associations.

HLA-DM (Figure 16) facilitates the loading of antigenic peptides onto MHC class II molecules. As a result of the proteolysis of the invariant chain a small fragment called the class II-associated invariant chain peptide, or CLIP, remains bound to the MHC class II molecule. CLIP peptide is replaced by antigenic peptides but in the absence of HLA-DM, this does not occur. The HLA-DM molecule must therefore play some part in removal of the CLIP peptide and in the loading of antigenic peptides.

HLA nonclassical class I genes include genes located within the MHC class I region that encode products that can associate with β_2 microglobulin. However, their function and tissue distribution are different from those of HLA-A,B,C molecules. Examples include HLA-E, F and G. HLA-E,-F and -G. Of these only HLAG is expressed on the cell surface. It is uncertain whether or not these HLA molecules are involved in peptide binding and presentation like classical class I molecules.

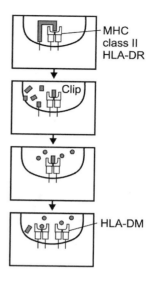

Figure 16. HLA-DM.

HLA-G is a nonclassical class I HLA antigen which exhibits a certain amount of polymorphism with the most extensive variability in the α-2 domain. It is found on trophoblast, i.e., that is placenta cells and trophoblastic neoplasms. HLA-G is expressed only on cells such as placental extravillous cytotrophoblasts and choriocarcinoma that fail to express HLA-A, B and C antigens. HLA-G expression is most pronounced during the first trimester of pregnancy. Trophoblast cells expressing HLA-G at the maternal-fetal junction may protect the semiallogeneic fetus from "rejection". Prominent HLA-G expression suggests maternal immune tolerance.

The **C2** and **B genes** are situated within the MHC locus on the short arm of chromosome 6. They are termed MHC class III genes. *TNF-α* and *TNF-β* genes are situated between the *C2* and *HLA-B* genes. Another gene designated *FD* lies between the *Bf* and *C4a* genes. C2 and B complete primary structures have been deduced from cDNA and protein sequences. C2 is comprised of 732 residues and is an 81kD molecule, whereas B contains 739 residues and is an 83kD molecule. Both proteins have a three-domain globular structure.

Certain HLA alleles occur in a higher frequency in individuals with particular diseases than in the general population. This type of data permits estimation of the "relative risk" of developing a disease with every known HLA allele. For example, there is a strong association between ankylosing spondylitis, which is an autoimmune disorder involving the vertebral joints, and the class I MHC allele, HLA-B27. There is a strong association between products of the polymorphic class II alleles HLA-DR and DQ and certain autoimmune diseases, since class II MHC molecules are of great importance in the selection and activation of CD4+ T lymphocytes which regulates immune responses against protein antigens. For example, 95% of Caucasians with insulin-dependent (type I) diabetes mellitus have HLA-DR3 or HLA-DR4 or

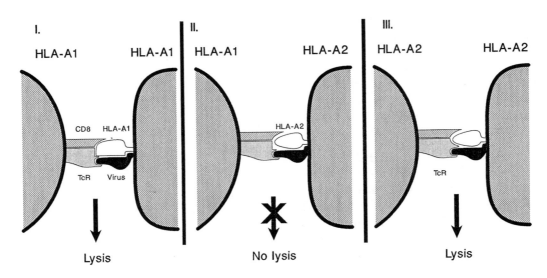

Figure 17.   MHC restriction.

both. There is also a strong association of HLA-DR4 with rheumatoid arthritis. Numerous other examples exist and are the targets of current investigations, especially in extended studies employing DNA probes. Calculation of the relative risk (RR) and absolute risk (AR) can be found elsewhere in this dictionary under definitions for those terms.

Genomic analysis has identified specific individual **allelic variants** to explain HLA associations with rheumatoid arthritis, type I diabetes mellitus, multiple sclerosis and celiac disease. There is a minimum of 6 α and 8 β genes in distinct clusters, termed HLA-DR, DQ, and DP within the HLA class II genes. DO and DN class II genes are related but map outside DR, DQ, and DP regions. There are two types of dimers along the HLA cell-surface HLA-DR class II molecules. The dimers are made up of either DRα-polypeptide associated with DRβ_1-polypeptide or DR with DRβ_2-polypeptide. Structural variation in class II gene products is linked to functional features of immune recognition leading to individual variations in histocompatibility, immune recognition and susceptibility to disease. There are two types of structural variations which include variation among DP, DQ, and DR products in primary amino acid sequence by as much as 35% and individual variation attributable to different allelic forms of class II genes. The class II polypeptide chain possesses domains which are specific structural subunits containing variable sequences that distinguish among class II α genes or class II β genes. These allelic variation sites have been suggested to form epitopes which represent individual structural differences in immune recognition.

MHC restriction (Figure 17) is the recognition of antigen in the context of either class I or class II molecules by the T cell receptor for antigen. In the afferent limb of the immune response, when antigen is being presented at the surface of a macrophage or other antigen presenting cell to CD4$^+$ T lymphocytes, this presentation must be in the context of MHC class II molecules for the CD4$^+$ lymphocyte to recognize the antigen and proliferate in response to it. By contrast, cytotoxic (CD8$^+$) T lymphocytes recognize foreign antigen, such as viral antigens on infected target cells, only in the context of class I MHC molecules. Once this recognition system is in place, the cytotoxic T cell can fatally injure the target cell through release of perforin molecules that penetrate the target cell surface.

CD4 (Figure 18) is a single chain glycoprotein, also referred to as the T4 antigen, that has a MW of 56 kD and is present on approximately two thirds of circulating human T cells, including most T cells of helper/inducer type. The antigen is also found on human monocytes and macrophages. The molecule is a receptor for gp120 of HIV-1 and HIV-2 (AIDS viruses). This antigen binds to class II MHC molecules on antigen-presenting cells (APC), and may stabilize antigen presenting cell and T cell interactions. It is physically associated with the intracellular tyrosine protein kinase, known as p56^{lck}, which phosphorylates nearby proteins. This antigen is thereby relaying a signal to the cells. Cross-linking of CD4 may induce activation of this enzyme and phosphorylation of CD3.

CD8 (Figures 19 and 20) is an antigen, also referred to as the T8 antigen, that has a MW of 32–34 kD. The CD8 antigen consists of two polypeptide chains, α and β, which may exist in the combination α/α homodimer or α/β heterodimer. Most antibodies are against the α-chain. This antigen binds to class I MHC molecules on antigen presenting cells (APC), and may stabilize APC/class I cell interactions.

The **CD4 molecule** exists as a monomer and contains four immunoglobulin-like domains. The first domains of CD4 form a rigid rod-like structure that is linked to the two carboxyl-terminal domains by a flexible link. The binding site for MHC class II molecules is thought to involve the D$_1$ and D$_2$ domains of CD4.

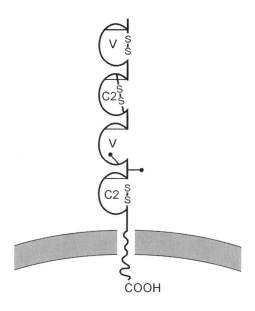

Figure 18.   CD4.

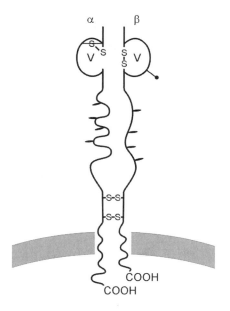

Figure 19.   CD8.

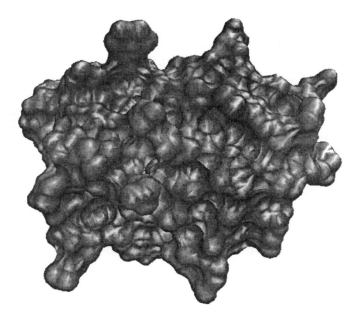

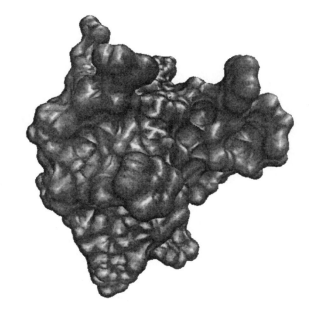

Figure 20.   This structure consists of the N-terminal 114 residues of CD8. These residues make up a single immunoglobulin axis which coincides with a crystallographic two-fold axis.

The **CD8 molecule** is a heterodimer of an α and β chain that are covalently associated by a disulfide bond. The two chains of the dimer have similar structures, each having a single domain resembling an immunoglobulin variable domain and a stretch of peptide believed to be in a relatively extended confirmation (Figure 21)

Antigen presentation (Figures 22 and 23) is the expression of antigen molecules on the surface of a macrophage or other antigen presenting cell in association with MHC class II molecules when the antigen is being presented to a CD4+ T helper lymphocyte or in association with cell surface MHC class I molecules when presentation is to CD8+ cytotoxic T

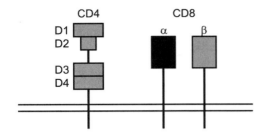

Figure 21. The outline structure of the CD4 and CD8 co-receptor molecules.

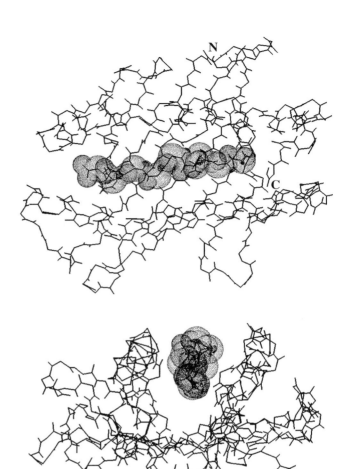

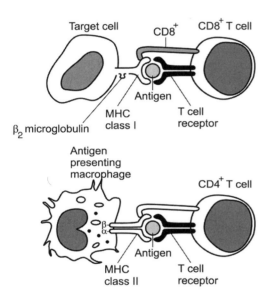

Figure 22. Antigen presentation.

Figure 23. Presentation of MHC histocompatibility antigen HLA-B 270S complexed with nonapetide ARG-ARG-ILE-LYS-ALA-ILE-THR-LEU-LYS. The C-terminal amino acid of the antigen binding domain is protected by a N-methyl group. Three water molecules bridge the binding of the peptide to the histocompatibility protein

lymphocytes. Antigen presenting cells, known also as accessory cells, include macrophages, dendritic cells and Langerhan cells of the skin as well as B lymphocytes.

Each set of alleles is referred to as a **haplotype** (Figure 24). An individual inherits one haplotype from the mother and one haplotype from the father. In an outbred population, the offspring are generally heterozygous at many loci and will express both maternal and paternal MHC alleles. The alleles are therefore codominantly expressed, that is both maternal and paternal gene products are expressed in the same cells. In inbred mice, however, each H-2 locus is homozygous because the maternal and paternal haplotypes are identical, and all offspring express identical haplotypes.

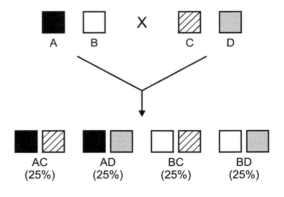

Figure 24. Each set of alleles is referred to as a haplotype.

Name	Previous equivalents	Molecular characteristics
HLA-A	-	Class I α-chain
HLA-B	-	Class I α-chain
HLA-C	-	Class I α-chain
HLA-E	E,"6.2"	associated with class I 6.2-kB Hind III fragment
HLA-F	F, "5.4"	associated with class I 5.4-kB Hind III fragment
HLA-G	G,"6.0"	associated with class 6.0 Hind III fragment
HLA-H	H, AR, "12.4"	Class I pseudogene associated with 5.4-kB Hind III fragment
HLA-J	cda 12	Class I pseudogene associated with 5.9-kB Hind III fragment
HLA-K	HLA-70	Class I pseudogene associated with 7.0-kB Hind III fragment
HLA-L	HLA-92	Class I pseudogene associated with 9.2-kB Hind III fragment
HLA-DRA	DRα	DR α chain
HLA-DRB1	DRβI,DR1B	DR β1 chain determining specificities DR1, DR2, DR3, DR4, DR5, etc.
HLA-DRB2	DRβII	pseudogene with DR β-like sequences
HLA-DRB3	DRβIII, DR3B	DR β3 chain determining DR52 and Dw24, Dw25, Dw26 specificities
HLA-DRB4	DRβIV, DR4B	DR β4 chain determining DR53
HLA-DRB5	DRβIII	DR β5 chain determining DR51
HLA-DRB6	DRBX, DRBσ	DRB pseudogene found on DR1, DR2, and DR10 haplotypes
HLA-DRB7	DRBψ1	DRB pseudogene found on DR4, DR7 and DR9 haplotypes
HLA-DRB8	DRBψ2	DRB pseudogene found on DR4, DR7 and DR9 haplotypes
HLA-DRB9	M4.2 β exon	DRB pseudogene, isolated fragment
HLA-DQA1	DQα1, DQ1A	DQ α chain as expressed
HLA-DQB1	DQβ1, DQ1B	DQ β chain as expressed
HLA-DQA2	DXα, DQ2A	DQ α-chain-related sequence, not known to be expressed
HLA-DQB2	DXβ, DQ2B	DQ β-chain-related sequence, not known to be expressed
HLA-DQB3	DVβ,DQB3	DQ β-chain-related sequence, not known to be expressed
HLA-DOB	DOβ	DO β chain
HLA-DMA	RING6	DM α chain
HLA-DMB	RING7	DM β chain
HLA-DNA	DZα, DOα	DN α chain
HLA-DPA1	DPα1, DP1A	DP α chain as expressed
HLA-DPB1	DPβ2, DP2B	DP β chain as expressed
HLA-DPA2	DPα2, DP2A	DP α-chain-related pseudogene
HLA-DPB2	DPβ2, DP2B	DP β-chain-related pseudogene
TAP-1	RING4, Y3, PSF1	ABC (ATP binding cassette) transporter
TAP-2	RING11, Y1, PSF2	ABC (ATP binding cassette) transporter
LMP2	RING12	Proteasome-related sequence
LMP7	RING10	Proteasome-related sequence

Figure 25.   Names for genes in the HLA region.

5

Antigen Presentation

T lymphocytes recognize antigens only in the context of self-MHC molecules on the surface of accessory cells. During processing, intact protein antigens are degraded into peptide fragments. Most epitopes that T cells recognize are peptide chain fragments. B cells and T cells often recognize different epitopes of an antigen leading to both antibody and cell-mediated immune responses. Before antigen can bind to MHC molecules, it must be processed into peptides in the intracellular organelles. CD4+ helper T lymphocytes recognize antigens in the context of class II MHC molecules, a process known as class II MHC-restriction. By contrast, CD8+ cytotoxic T lymphocytes recognize antigens in the context of class I molecules, which is known as class I MHC-restriction. Following the generation of peptides by proteolytic degradation in antigen-presenting cells, peptide-MHC complexes are presented on the surface of antigen-presenting cells where they may be recognized by T lymphocytes. Antigens derived from either intracellular or extracellular proteins may be processed to produce peptides from either self or foreign proteins that are presented by surface MHC molecules to T cells. In the class II MHC processing pathway, professional antigen-presenting cells, such as macrophages, dendritic cells or B lymphocytes incorporate extracellular proteins into endosomes where they are processed (Figures 1 and 2). Enzymes within the vesicles of the endosomal pathway cleave proteins in the acidic environment.

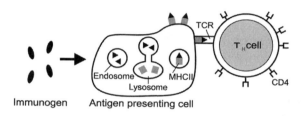

Figure 1. Capture, processing and presentation of antigen by an antigen-presenting cell.

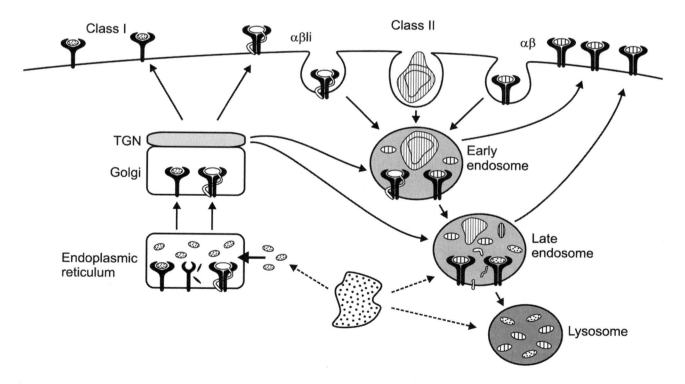

Figure 2. Processing pathways for class II-restricted antigen presentation.

Class II MHC heterodimeric molecules unite with invariant chain and are shifted to endosomal vesicles from the endoplasmic reticulum. Following cleavage of the invariant chain, DM molecules remove a tiny piece of invariant chain from the MHC molecules peptide binding groove. Following complexing of extracellular derived peptide with the class II MHC molecule, the MHC-peptide complex is transported to the cell surface where presentation to CD4+ T cells occurs. Proteins in the cytosol, such as those derived from viruses may be processed through the class I MHC route of antigen presentation. The multiprotein complex in the cytoplasm known as the proteasome effects involve proteolytic degradation of proteins in the cytoplasm to yield many of the peptides that are presented by class I MHC molecules. TAP molecules transport peptides from the cytoplasm to the endoplasmic reticulum where they interact and bind to class I MHC dimeric molecules. Once the class I MHC molecules have become stabilized through peptide binding, the complex leaves the endoplasmic reticulum entering the Golgi apparatus enroute to the surface of the cell. Thus, mechanisms are provided through MHC-restricted antigen presentation to guarantee that peptides derived from extracellular microbial proteins can be presented by class II MHC molecules to CD4+ helper T cells and that peptides derived from intracellular microbes can be presented by class I MHC molecules to CD8+ cytotoxic T lymphocytes. The generation of microbial peptides produced through antigen processing to combine with self MHC molecules is critical to the development of an appropriate immune response.

Antigen presentation is the expression of antigen molecules on the surface of a macrophage or other antigen-presenting cell in association with MHC class II molecules when the antigen is being presented to a CD4+ T helper lymphocyte or in association with cell surface MHC class I molecules when presentation is to CD8+ cytotoxic T lymphocytes (Figure 3). Antigen-presenting cells, known also as accessory cells, include macrophages, dendritic cells and Langerhans cells of the skin as well as B lymphocytes. Target cells such as fibroblasts present antigen to CD8+ cytotoxic T lymphocytes. Mononuclear phagocytes ingest proteins and split them into peptides in endosomes. These eight to ten amino acid residue peptides link to cell surface MHC class II molecules. For appropriate presentation, it is essential that peptides bind securely to the MHC class II molecules since those that do not bind or are bound only weakly are not presented and fail to elicit an immune response. Following interaction of the presented antigen and MHC class II molecules with the CD4+ helper T cell receptor, the CD4+ lymphocyte is activated, interleukin-2 is released and IL-2 receptors are expressed on the CD4+ lymphocyte surface. The IL-2 produced by the activated cell stimulates its own receptors as well as those of mononuclear phagocytes increasing their microbicidal activity. IL-2 also stimulates B cells to synthesize antibodies. Whereas B cells may recognize a protein antigen in its native state, T lymphocytes recognize the peptides that result from antigen processing.

An **antigen-presenting cell (APC)** is a cell that can process a protein antigen, breaking it into peptides and presenting it in conjunction with class II major histocompatibility molecules on the cell surface where it may interact with appropriate T cell receptors (Figure 4). Macrophages, Langerhans cells, B cells and dendritic reticulum cells process and present antigens to immunoreactive lymphocytes such as CD4+ helper/inducer T cells (Figure 5). A MHC transporter gene-encoded peptide supply factor may mediate peptide antigen presentation. Other antigen-presenting cells that serve mainly as passive antigen transporters include B cells, endothelial cells, keratinocytes, and Kupffer cells. APC include cells that present exogenous antigen processed in

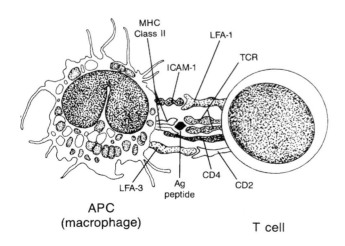

Figure 3.   Antigen presentation.

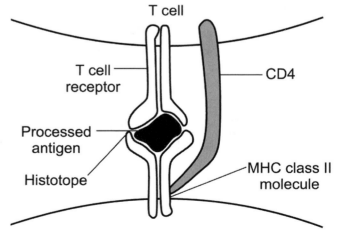

Figure 4.   Antigen-presenting cell.

Cell type	Class II	Costimulators	Principle functions
Dendritic cells (langerhan's cells, lymphoid dendritic cells)	Constitutive	Constitutive	Inflamation of CD4 T cell response; allograft rejection
Macrophages	Inducible by IFN	Inducible by LPS	Development of CD4 effector T cells
B lymphocytes	Constitutive	Constitutive	Stimulation by CD4 helper T cells in humoral immune responses
Vascular endothelial cells	Inducible by IFN	Constitutive	Recruitment of antigen-specific T cells to site of antigen exposure or inflammation

Figure 5. Properties and functions of antigen-presenting cells.

their endosomal compartment and presented together with MHC class II molecules. Other APCs present antigens that have been endogeneously produced by the body's own cells with processing in an intracellular compartment and presentation together with class I MHC molecules. A third group of APCs present exogenous antigens that are taken into the cell and processed followed by presentation together with MHC class I molecules.

MHC restriction is the recognition of an antigen in the context of either class I or class II molecules by the T cell receptor for antigen. In the afferent limb of the immune response, when the antigen is being presented at the surface of a macrophage or other antigen-presenting cell to CD4$^+$ T lymphocytes, this presentation must be in the context of MHC class II molecules for the CD4$^+$ lymphocyte to recognize the antigen and proliferate in response to it. By contrast, cytotoxic (CD8$^+$) T lymphocytes recognize foreign antigens, such as viral antigens on infected target cells, only in the context of class I MHC molecules. Once this recognition system is in place, the cytotoxic T cell can fatally injure the target cell through release of perforin molecules that penetrate the target cell surface.

CTLA-4 is a molecule that is homologous to CD28 and expressed on activated T cells (Figure 6). The genes for CD28 and CTLA-4 are closely linked on chromosome 2. The binding of CTLA-4 to its ligand B7 is an important costimulatory mechanism. **CTLA4-Ig** is a soluble protein composed of the CD28 homolog CTLA and the constant region of an IgG1 molecule. It is used experimentally to inhibit the immune response by blocking CD28-B7 interaction.

B7 is the ligand for CD28. B7 is expressed by accessory cells and is important in costimulatory mechanisms (Figure 7). Some APCs may upregulate expression of B7 following activation by various stimuli including IFN-α, endotoxin and MHC class II binding. B7 is also termed CD80. **B7.2** is a costimulatory molecule whose sequence resembles that of B7. Dendritic cells, monocytes, activated T cells, and activated B lymphocytes may express B7.2.

Activated T Cell

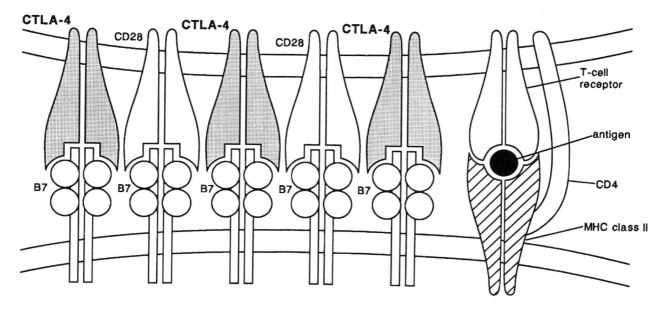

Figure 6. Participation of CTLA-4 molecules during an antigen presentation.

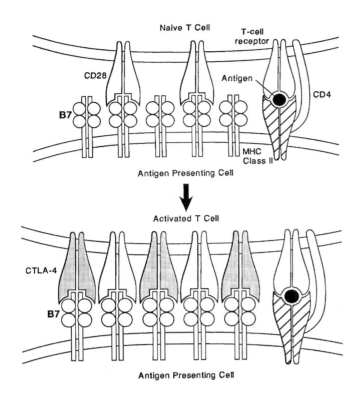

Figure 7. B7.

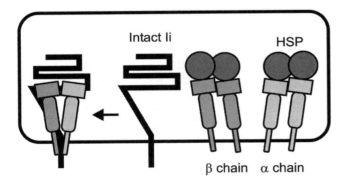

Figure 8. Invariant chain promotes assembly of class II heterodimers from free chains.

An **invariant (Ii) chain** is a nonpolymorphic 31kD glycoprotein that associates with class II histocompatibility molecules in the endoplasmic reticulum (Figure 8). It inhibits the linking of endogenous peptides with the class II molecule, conveying it to appropriate intracellular compartments. Truncation of the invariant chain stimulates a second signal that may function in the trans-Golgi network, prior to the conveyance of MHC class II molecules to the cell surface.

Desetope is a term derived from "determinant selection". It describes that region of class II histocompatibility molecules that reacts with the antigen during antigen presentation (Figures 9 and 10). Allelic variation permits these contact residues to vary, which is one of the factors in histocompatibility molecule selection of a particular epitope that is being presented.

An **agretope** refers to the region of a protein antigen that combines with a MHC class II molecule during antigen presentation. This is then recognized by the T cell receptor MHC class II complex. Amino acid sequences differ in their reactivity with MHC class II molecules. A **histotope** is the portion of an MHC class II histocompatibility molecule that reacts with a T lymphocyte receptor. A **restitope** is that segment of a T cell receptor that makes contact and interacts with a class II histocompatibility antigen molecule during antigen presentation.

A **superantigen** is an antigen such as a bacterial toxin that is capable of stimulating multiple T lymphocytes, especially CD4+ T cells leading to the release of relatively large quantities of cytokines. Selected bacterial toxins may stimulate all T lymphocytes in the body that contain a certain family of V β T cell receptor genes. Superantigens may induce proliferation of 10% of CD4+ T cells by combining with the T cell receptor V β and to the MHC HLA-DR α-1 domain. Superantigens are thymus-dependent (TD) antigens that do not require phagocytic processing. Instead of fitting into the T cell receptor (TCR) internal groove where a typical processed peptide antigen fits, superantigens bind to the external region of the αβ TCR and simultaneously link to DP, DQ, or DR molecules on antigen-presenting cells (Figure 11). Superantigens react with multiple TCR molecules whose peripheral structure is similar. Thus, they stimulate multiple T cells that augment a protective T and B cell antibody response. This enhanced responsiveness to antigens such as toxins produced by staphylococcci and streptococci is an important protective mechanism in the infected individual (Figure 12). **MHC-I antigen presentation** is discussed in Chapter IV; **ICAM-1, ICAM-2, ICAM-3, LFA-1,** and **LFA-3** are discussed in Chapter II.

A **granuloma** is a tissue reaction characterized by altered macrophages (epithelioid cells), lymphocytes and fibroblasts (Figure 13). These cells form microscopic masses of mononuclear cells. Giant cells form from some of these fused cells. Granulomas may be of the foreign body type, such as those surrounding silica or carbon particles, or of the immune type that encircle particulate antigens derived from microorganisms. Activated macrophages trap antigen, which may cause T cells to release lymphokines causing more macrophages to accumulate. This process isolates the microorganism. Granulomas appear in cases of tuberculosis and develop under the influence of helper T cells that react against *Mycobacterium tuberculosis*. Some macrophages

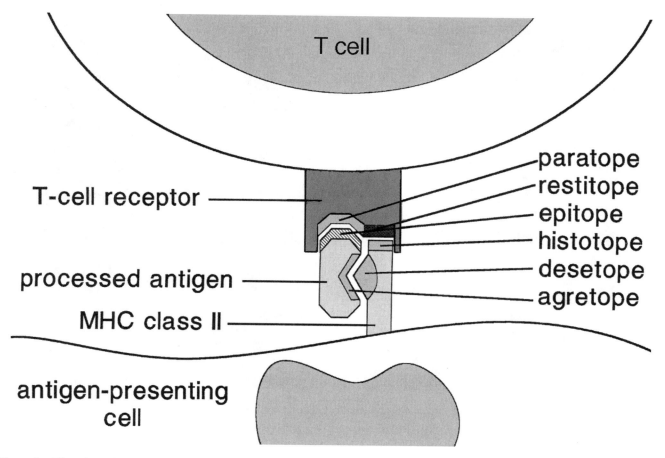

Figure 9. The schematic representation of the interaction of the class II MHC, processed peptide antigen and T cell receptor molecules during antigen presentation.

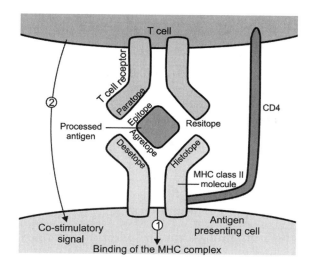

Figure 10. Co-stimulator for the activation of T cells.

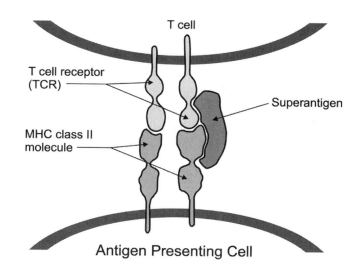

Figure 11. Superantigen.

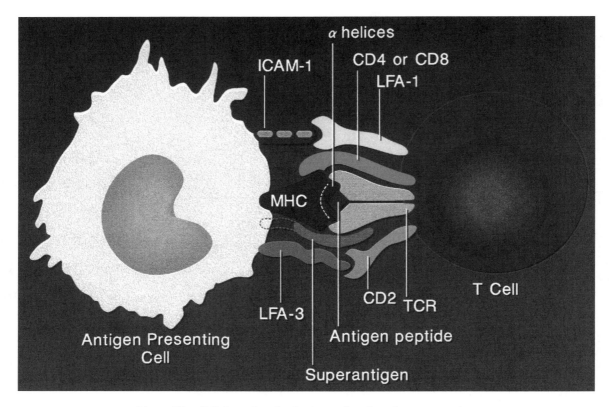

Figure 12.   Cellular and molecular interactions in antigen presentation.

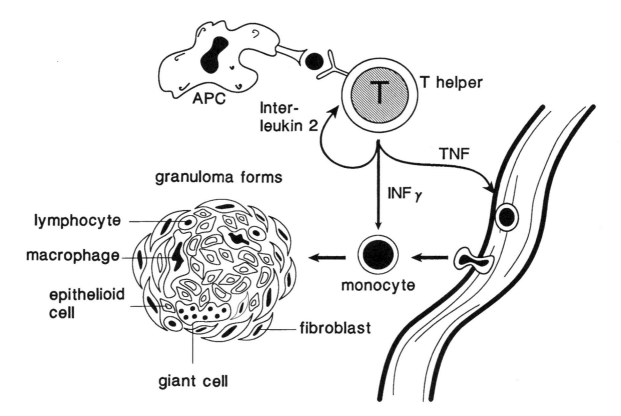

Figure 13.   Granuloma.

and epithelioid cells fuse to form multinucleated giant cells in immune granulomas. There may also be occasional neutrophils and eosinophils. Necrosis may develop.

T-B cell cooperation refers to B cell and helper T cell cooperation that leads to B cell proliferation and differentiation into plasma cells that synthesize and secrete specific antibody (Figure 14). B cell immunoglobulin receptors react with protein antigens. This is followed by endocytosis, antigen processing, and presentation to helper T lymphocytes. Their antigen-specific T cell receptors recognize processed antigens only in the context of MHC class II molecules on the B cell surface during antigen presentation. CD4+ helper T cells secrete lymphokines, including IL-2, that promote B cell growth and differentiation into plasma cells which secrete specific antibodies. T cells are required for B cells to be able to switch from forming IgM to synthesizing IgG or IgA. B and T lymphocytes recognize different antigens. B cells may recognize peptides, native proteins, or denatured proteins. T cells are more complex in their recognition system in that a peptide antigen can be presented to them only in the context of MHC class II or class I histocompatibility molecules. Hapten-carrier complexes have been successfully used in delineating the different responses of B and T cells to each part of this complex. Immunization of a rabbit or other animal with a particular hapten-carrier complex will induce a primary immune response, and a second injection of the same hapten-carrier conjugate will induce a secondary immune response. However, linkage of the same hapten to a different carrier elicits a much weaker secondary response in an animal primed with the original hapten-carrier complex. This is termed the carrier effect. B lymphocytes recognize the hapten and T lymphocytes the carrier.

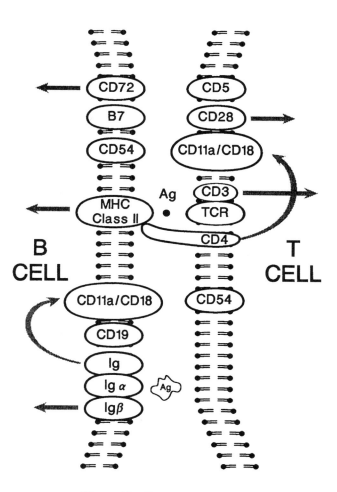

Figure 14. T-B cell interactions.

6

B Lymphocyte Development, Immunoglobulin Genes and Immunoglobulin Structure

Antibodies are glycoprotein substances produced by B lymphoid cells in response to stimulation with an immunogen. They possess the ability to react *in vitro* and *in vivo* specifically and selectively with the antigenic determinants or epitopes eliciting their production or with an antigenic determinant closely related to the homologous antigen. Antibody molecules are immunoglobulins found in the blood and body fluids. Thus, all antibodies are immunoglobulins formed in response to immunogens. Antibodies may be produced by hybridoma technology in which antibody secreting cells are fused by polyethylene glycol (PEG) treatment with a mutant myeloma cell line. Monoclonal antibodies are widely used in research, diagnostic medicine and have potential in therapy. Antibodies in the blood serum of any given animal species may be grouped according to their physicochemical properties and antigenic characteristics. Immunoglobulins are not restricted to the plasma but may be found in other body fluids or tissues, such as urine, spinal fluid, lymph nodes, spleen, etc. Immunoglobulins do not include the components of the complement system. Immunoglobulins (antibodies) constitute approximately 1 to 2% of the total serum proteins in health.

γ-globulins are serum proteins that show the lowest mobility toward the anode during electrophoresis when the pH is neutral. It is the most cationic of the serum globulins. Gammaglobulins comprise 11.2 to 20.1% of the total serum content in man. Antibodies are in the gamma globulin fraction of serum.

The **bursa of Fabricius** (Figure 1) is located near the terminal portion of the cloaca, and like the thymus, is a lymphoepithelial organ. The bursa begins to develop after the fifth day of incubation and becomes functional around the 10th–12th day. It has an asymmetric sac-like shape and a star-like lumen which is continuous with the cloacal cavity. The epithelium of the intestine covers the bursal lumen but lacks mucous cells. The bursa contains abundant lymphoid tissue forming nodules beneath the epithelium. The nodules show a central medullary region containing epithelial cells and project into the epithelial coating. The center of the medullary region is less structured and also contains macrophages, large lymphocytes, plasma cells and granulocytes. A basement membrane separates the medulla from the cor-

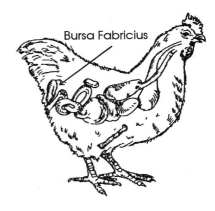

Figure 1. The bursa of Fabricius is an outpouching of the hindgut located near the cloaca in avian species that governs B cell ontogeny. This specific lymphoid organ is the site of migration and maturation of B lymphocytes.

tex; the latter comprises mostly small lymphocytes and plasma cells. The bursa is well developed at birth but begins to involute around the 4th month; it is vestigial at the end of the first year. There is a direct relationship between the hormonal status of the bird and involution of the bursa. Injections of testosterone may lead to premature regression or even lack of development, depending on the time of hormone administration. The lymphocytes in the bursa originate from the yolk sac and migrate there via the blood stream. They comprise B cells which undergo maturation to immunocompetent cells capable of antibody synthesis. Bursectomy at the 17th day of incubation induces agammaglobulinemia, with absence of germinal centers and plasma cells in peripheral lymphoid organs.

A **bursacyte** is a lymphocyte that undergoes maturation and differentiation under the influence of the bursa of Fabricius in avian species. This cell synthesizes antibodies which provides humoral immunity in this species. A bursacyte is a B lymphocyte.

The anatomical site in mammals and other nonavian species that resembles the bursa of Fabricius in controlling B cell ontogeny is termed a **bursa equivalent**. Mammals do not have a specialized lymphoid organ for maturation of B lymphocytes. Although lymphoid nodules are present along the gut, forming distinct structures called Peyer's patches, their role in B cell maturation is no different from that of lymphoid structures in other organs. After commitment to B cell lineage, the B cells of mammals leave the bone marrow in a relatively immature stage; likewise, after education in the thymus, T cells migrate from the thymus also in a relatively immature stage; both populations continue their maturation process away from the site of origin and are subject to influences originating in the environment in which they reside.

Bursectomy refers to the surgical removal or ablation of the bursa of Fabricius, an outpouching of the hindgut near the cloaca in birds. Surgical removal of the bursa prior to hatching or shortly thereafter followed by treatment with testosterone *in vivo* leads to failure of the B cell limb of the immune response responsible for antibody production.

Pre-B cells develop (Figures 2 and 3) from lymphoid stem cells in the bone marrow. These are large, immature lymphoid cells that express cytoplasmic T chains, but no light chains or surface immunoglobulin and are found in fetal liver and adult bone marrow. They are the earliest cells of the B cell lineage. Antigen is not required for early differentiation of the B cell series. Pre-B cells differentiate into immature B cells, followed by mature B cells that express surface immunoglobulin. Pre-B cell immunoglobulin genes contain heavy chain V, D, and J gene segments that are contiguous. No rearrangement of light chain gene segments has yet occurred. In addition to their cytoplasmic IgM, pre-B cells are positive for CD10, CD19, and HLA-DR markers.

B cells (Figure 4) are lymphocytes that derive from the fetal liver in the early embryonal stages of development and from the bone marrow thereafter. Plasma cells that synthesize antibody develop from precursor B cells.

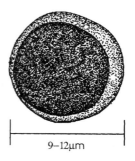

Figure 4.   B cell.

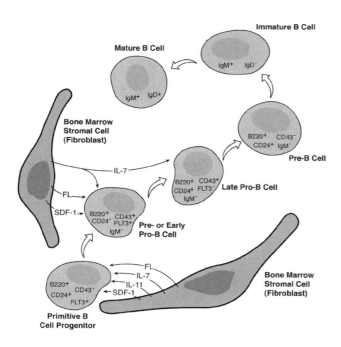

Figure 2.   FLT-3 and bone marrow B cell lymphopoiesis.

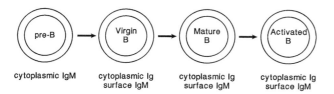

Figure 3.   Pre-B cell development.

B cell tolerance is manifested as a decreased number of antibody-secreting cells following antigenic stimulation, compared to a normal response. Hapten-specific tolerance can be induced by inoculation of deaggregated haptenated-gammaglobulins (Ig). Induction of tolerance requires membrane Ig cross-linking. Tolerance may have a duration of 2 months in B cells of the bone marrow and 6–8 months in T cells. Whereas prostaglandin E enhances tolerance induction, IL-1, LPS or 8-bromoguanosine block tolerance instead of an immunogenic signal. Tolerant mice carry a normal complement of hapten-specific B cells. Tolerance is not attributable to a diminished number or isotype of antigen receptor. It has also been shown that the six normal activation events related to membrane Ig turnover and expression do not occur in tolerant B cells. Whereas tolerant B cells possess a limited capacity to proliferate, they fail to do so in response to antigen. Antigenic challenge of tolerant B cells induces them to enlarge and increase expression, yet they are apparently deficient in a physiologic signal requisite for progression into a proliferative stage.

B Lymphocytes are cells of the B cell lineage that mature under influence of the bursa of Fabricus in birds and bursa-equivalent (bone marrow) in mammals. B cells occupy follicular areas in lymphoid tissues and account for 30% of the lymphocytes in the circulating blood. They synthesize antibodies and provide defense against microorganisms including bacteria and viruses. Surface and cytoplasmic markers reveal the stage of development and function of lymphocytes in the B cell lineage. Pre-B cells contain cytoplasmic immunoglobulins whereas mature B lymphocytes express surface immunoglobulins and complement receptors. B lymphocyte markers include CD9, CD19, CD20, CD24, Fc receptors, B1, BA-1, B4 and Ia.

A **B lymphocyte hybridoma** is a clone formed by the fusion of a B lymphocyte with a myeloma cell. Activated splenic B lymphocytes from a specifically immune mouse are fused with myeloma cells by polyethylene glycol. Thereafter, the cells are plated in multi-well tissue culture plates containing HAT medium. The only surviving cells are the hybrids since the myeloma cells employed are deficient in hypoxanthine-guanine phosphoribosyl transferase and fail to grow in HAT medium. Wells with hybridomas are screened for antibody synthesis. This is followed by cloning which is carried out by limiting dilution or in soft agar. The hybridomas are maintained either in tissue culture or through inoculation into the peritoneal cavity of a mouse that corresponds genetically to the cell strain. The antibody producing B lymphocyte confers specificity and the myeloma cell confers immortality upon the hybridoma. B lymphocyte hybridomas produce monoclonal antibodies.

B lymphocyte tolerance refers to the immunologic nonreactivity of B lymphocytes induced by relatively large doses of antigen. It is of relatively short duration. By contrast, T cell tolerance requires less antigen and is a longer duration. Exclusive B cell tolerance leaves T cells immunoreactive and unaffected.

The **B lymphocyte receptor** (Figure 5) is an immunoglobulin anchored to the B lymphocyte surface. Its combination with antigen leads to B lymphocyte division and differentiation into memory cells, lymphoblasts and plasma cells. The original antigen specificity of the immunoglobulin is maintained in the antibody molecules subsequently produced. B lymphocyte receptor immunoglobulins (Figure 6) are to be distinguished from those in the surrounding medium that adhere to the B cell surface through Fc receptors.

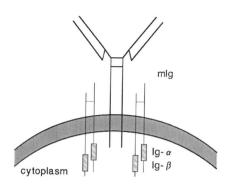

Figure 6. Schematic representation of Ig on a cell membrane.

A **B cell antigen receptor** (Figure 7) is an antibody expressed on antigen reactive B cells that is similar to secreted antibody but it is membrane-bound due to an extra domain at the Fc portion of the molecule. Upon antigen recognition by the membrane-bound immunoglobulin, noncovalently associated accessory molecules mediate transmembrane signaling to the B cell nucleus. The immunoglobulin and accessory molecule complex is similar in structure to the antigen receptor-CD3 complex of T lymphocytes.

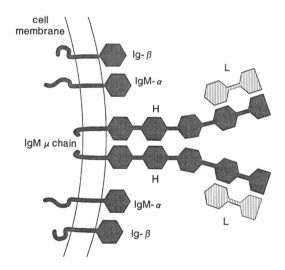

Figure 7. B cell antigen receptor.

A **B cell co-receptor** (Figure 8) is a three protein complex that consists of CR2, TAPA-1 (Figure 9), and CD19. CR2 unites not only with an activated component of complement, but also with CD23. TAPA-1 is a serpentine membrane protein. CD19's cytoplasmic tail is the mechanism through which the complex interacts with lyn, a tyrosine kinase. Activation of the co-receptor by ligand binding leads to union of phosphatidyl inositol-3′ kinase with CD19 resulting in activation. This produces intracellular signals that facilitated B cell receptor signal transduction.

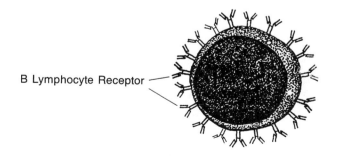

Figure 5. B lymphocyte receptor.

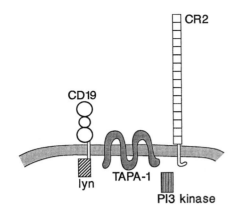

Figure 8. B cell co-receptor.

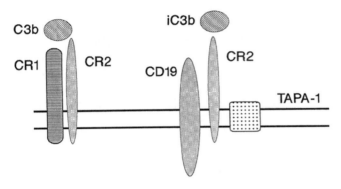

Figure 9. Complement receptor complexes on the surface of B cells include CR1, C3b, CR2, CD19, iC3b, CR2 (CD21) and TAPA-1. B cell markers that are used routinely for immunophenotyping by flow cytometry include CD19, CD20 and CD21.

CD19 (Figure 10) is an antigen with a MW of 90 kD that has been shown to be a transmembrane polypeptide with at least two immunoglobulin-like domains. The CD19 antigen is the most broadly expressed surface marker for B cells, appearing at the earliest stages of B cell differentiation. The CD19 antigen is expressed at all stages of B cell maturation, from the pro-B cell stage until just before the terminal differentiation to plasma cells. CD19 complexes with CD21 (CR2) and CD81 (TAPA-1). It is a co-receptor for B lymphocytes.

CD20 (Figure 11) is a B cell marker with a MW of 33, 35, 37 kD that appears relatively late in the B cell maturation (after the pro-B cell stage), and then persists for some time before the plasma cell stage. Its molecular structure resembles that of a transmembrane ion channel. The gene is on chromosome 11 at band q12-q13. It may be involved in regulating B cell activation.

CD21 (Figure 12) is an antigen with a MW of 145 kD that is expressed on B cells and, even more strongly, on follicular dendritic cells. It appears when surface Ig is expressed after the pre-B cell stage and is lost during early stages of terminal

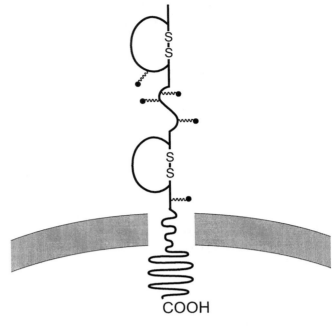

Figure 10. CD19.

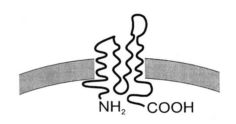

Figure 11. CD20.

B cell differentiation to the final plasma cell stage. CD21 is coded for by a gene found on chromosome 1 at band q32. The antigen functions as a receptor for the C3d complement component and also for Epstein-Barr virus. CD21, together with CD19 and CD81, constitutes the co-receptor for B cells. It is also termed CR2.

Plasma cells (Figures 13–15) are antibody producing cells. Immunoglobulins are present in their cytoplasm and secretion of immunoglobulin by plasma cells has been directly demonstrated *in vitro*. Increased levels of immunoglobulins in some pathologic conditions are associated with increased numbers of plasma cells and conversely, their number at antibody producing sites increases following immunization. Plasma cells develop from B cells and are large, spherical or ellipsoidal cells, 10–20 μ in size. Mature plasma cells have abundant cytoplasm, staining deep blue with Wright's stain, and have an eccentrically located, round or oval nucleus, usually surrounded by a well defined perinuclear clear zone. The nucleus contains coarse and clumped masses of chromatin, often arranged in a cartwheel fashion. The nuclei of normal, mature plasma cells have no nucleoli, but

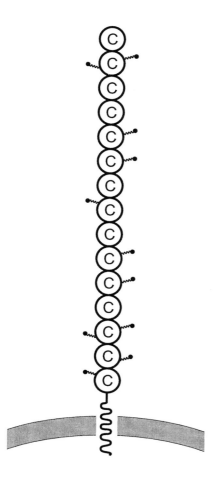

Figure 12.   CD21.

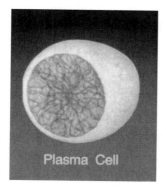

Figure 13.   Plasma Cell Diagram

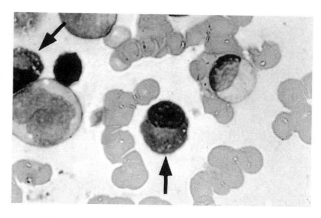

Figure 14.   Plasma cell in peripheral blood smear.

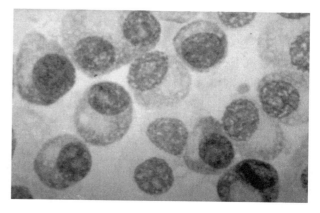

Figure 15.   Plasma cell cluster in peripheral blood smear.

those of neoplastic plasma cells, such as those seen in multiple myeloma, have conspicuous nucleoli. The cytoplasm of normal plasma cells has conspicuous Golgi complex and rough endoplasmic reticulum and frequently contains vacuoles. The nuclear to cytoplasmic ratio is 1:2. By electron microscopy, plasma cells show very abundant endoplasmic reticulum indicating extensive and active protein synthesis. Plasma cells do not express surface immunoglobulin or complement receptors which distinguishes them from B lymphocytes.

B Cell Activation (Figure 16) follows antigen binding to membrane immunoglobulin molecules on B lymphocytes surfaces. This interaction of antigen and membrane immunoglobulin may lead to two types of response. Either biochemical signals are conveyed to the cells via the B lymphocyte antigen receptor leading to lymphocyte activation, or antigen is taken into endosomal vesicles where protein antigens are processed and resulting peptides presented at the B lymphocyte surface to helper T cells. With respect to B lymphocyte antigen receptor signaling, the relatively short cytoplasmic tails of membrane IgM and IgD are unable to transduce signals caused by Ig clustering. Therefore, Igα and Igβ that are expressed on mature B cells in a noncovalent association with membrane Ig actually transduce signals (Figure 17).

Virgin B cells that have never interacted with antigen must have two separate types of signals to proliferate and differentiate. The antigen provides the first signal through interaction with surface membrane Ig molecules on specific B lymphocytes. Helper T cells and their lymphokines provide the second type of signal needed. Whereas, polysaccharides and lipids, as nonprotein antigens, induce IgM antibody responses without antigen-specific T cell help, protein antigens, which are helper T cell-dependent, lead to the production of immunoglobulin of more than one isotype and of

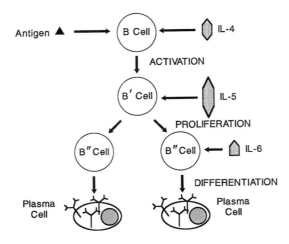

Figure 16. B cell activation.

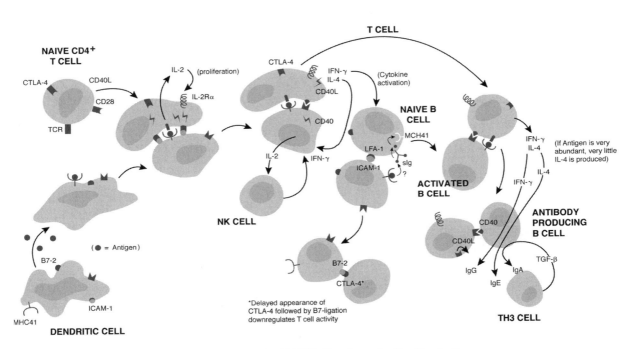

Figure 17. Hypothetical B7/CD40 pathway for B cell activation.

high affinity in addition to immunologic memory. Igα and Igβ together with membrane Ig molecules constitute the **B lymphocyte antigen receptor complex**. Igα and Igβ function in B lymphocytes as CD3 and proteins do in T cells. Requisite for signal transduction are the immunoreceptor tyrosine-based activation motifs (ITAMs) in the cytoplasmic domains of Igα and Igβ. Cross-linking of the B cell receptor complex by antigen leads to increased cell size and cytoplasmic ribonucleic acid with increased biosynthetic organelles including ribosomes as resting cells enter the G1 stage in the cell cycle. Class II molecules and B7-2 and B7-1 costimulators show increased expression. B cells stimulated by antigen are then able to activate helper T cells. Expression

of receptors for T cell cytokines increases, thereby facilitating the ability of antigen-specific B cells to receive T cell help. The effect of B cell receptors complex signaling on proliferation and differentiation depends in part on the type of antigen. Following activation as a result of combination with antigen, cell proliferation and differentiation are facilitated by interaction with helper T lymphocytes. Helper T cells must recognize antigen and there must be interaction between protein antigen-specific B cells and T lymphocytes for antibody to be formed. When B cells, acting as antigen-presenting cells, interact with helper T lymphocytes that are specific for the peptide being presented, there are numerous ligand-receptor interactions that facilitate transmission of signals to B cells that are requisite to generate a humoral immune response. Among these are B7 molecules:CD28 and CD40:CD40 ligand interactions. Cytokines play important roles in antibody production through switching from one heavy chain isotype to another and by providing amplification mechanisms through augmentation of B lymphocyte proliferation and differentiation. Germinal centers are the sites of synthesis of antibodies of high affinity and of memory B cells.

Patching (Figure 18) describes the accumulation of membrane receptor proteins cross-linked by antibodies or lectins on a lymphocyte surface prior to capping. The antigen-antibody complexes are internalized following capping which permits antigen processing and presentation in the context of MHC molecules. Membrane protein redistribution into patches is passive not requiring energy. The process depends on the lateral diffusion of membrane constituents in the plane of the membrane.

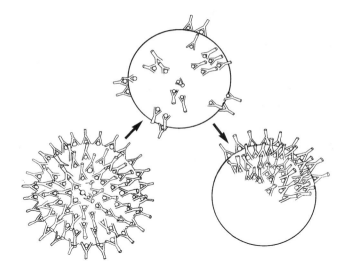

Figure 19. Capping.

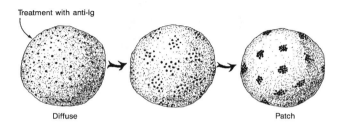

Figure 18. Patching.

Capping (Figure 19) refers to the migration of antigens on the cell surface to a cell pole following cross-linking of antigens by specific antibody. These antigen-antibody complexes coalesce or aggregate into a "cap" produced by interaction of antigen with cell surface IgM and IgD molecules at sites distant from each other, as revealed by immunofluorescence. Capping is followed by interiorization of antigen. Following internalization, the cell surface is left bereft of immunoglobulin receptors until they are re-expressed.

The **capping phenomenon** is the migration of surface membrane proteins toward one pole of a cell following cross-linking by specific antibody, antigen or mitogen. Bivalent or polyvalent ligands cause the surface molecules to aggregate into patches. This passive process is referred to as patching. The ligand-surface molecule aggregates in patches move to a pole of the cell where they form a cap. If a cell with patches becomes motile, the patches move to the rear forming a cluster of surface molecule-ligand aggregates that constitutes a cap. The process of capping requires energy and may involve interaction with microfilaments of the cytoskeleton. In addition to capping in lymphocytes, the process occurs in numerous other cells.

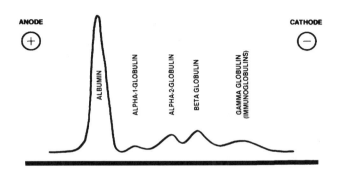

Figure 20. Electrophoresis of serum protein showing the gamma globulin region that contains the immunoglobulins.

Immunoglobulin genes (Figure 20) encode heavy and light polypeptide chains of antibody molecules and are found on different chromosomes, i.e., chromosome 14 for heavy chain, chromosome two for κ light chain and chromosome 22 for λ light chain. The DNA of the majority of cells does not contain one gene that encodes a complete immunoglobulin heavy or light polypeptide chain. Separate gene segments that are widely distributed in somatic cells and germ cells come together to form these genes. In B cells, gene rearrangement leads to creation of an antibody gene that codes for a specific protein. Somatic gene rearrangement also occurs with the genes that encode T cell antigen receptors. Gene rearrangement of this type permits the great versatility of the immune system in recognizing a vast array of epitopes. Three forms of gene segments join to form an immunoglobulin light chain gene. The three types include light chain variable region (V_L), joining (J_L) and constant region (C_L) gene segments. V_H, J_H, and C_H as well as D (diversity) gene segments assemble to encode the heavy chain. Heavy and light chain genes have a closely similar organizational structure. There are 100 to 300 V_κ genes, five

J_κ genes and one C_κ gene on chromosome 2's κ locus. There are 100 V_H genes, 30 D genes, six J_H genes and 11 C_H genes on chromosome 14's heavy chain locus. Several V_λ six J_λ and six C_λ genes are present on chromosome 22's λ locus in man. V_H and V_L genes are classified as V gene families depending on the sequence homology of their nucleotides or amino acids.

The **immunoglobulin superfamily** (Figure 21) is comprised of several molecules that participate in the immune response and show similarities in structure causing them to be named the immunoglobulin supergene family. Included are CD2, CD3, CD4, CD7, CD8, CD28, T cell receptor (TCR), MHC class I and MHC class II molecules, leukocyte function associated antigen 3 (LFA-3), the IgG receptor, and a dozen other proteins. These molecules share in common with each other an immunoglobulin-like domain, with a length of approximately 100 amino acid residues and a central disulfide bond that anchors and stabilizes antiparallel beta strands into a folded structure resembling immunoglobulin. Immunoglobulin superfamily members may share homology with

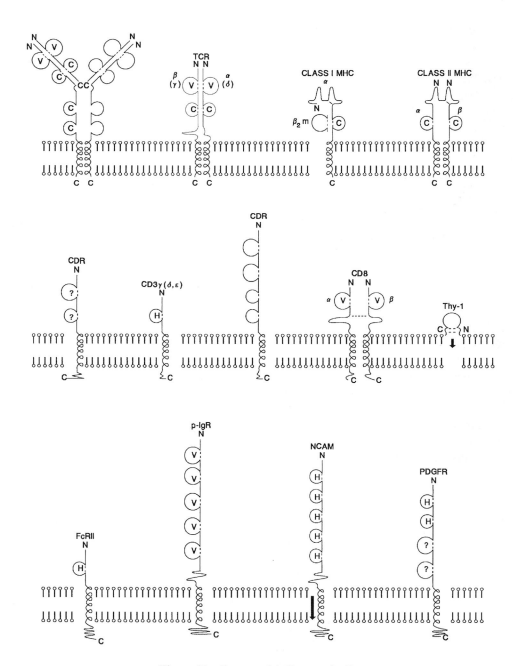

Figure 21.   Immunoglobulin superfamily.

constant or variable immunoglobulin domain regions. Various molecules of the cell surface with polypeptide chains whose folded structures are involved in cell to cell interactions belong in this category. Single gene and multigene members are included.

Immunoglobulins (Figure 22) are mature B cell products synthesized in response to stimulation by an antigen. Antibody molecules are immunoglobulins of defined specificity produced by plasma cells (Figure 23). The immunoglobulin molecule consists of heavy (H) and light (L) chains fastened together by disulfide bonds. The molecules are subdivided into classes and subclasses based on the antigenic specificity of the heavy chains. Heavy chains are designated by lower case Greek letters (μ, γ, α, δ, ε), and the immunoglobulins are designated IgM, IgG, IgA, IgD, and IgE, respectively. The three major classes are IgG, IgM, IgA and two minor classes are IgD and IgE which together comprise less than 1% of the total immunoglobulins. The two types of light chains (termed κ and λ) are present in all five immunoglobulin classes, although only one type is present in an individual molecule.

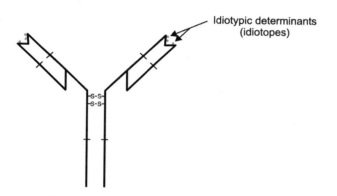

Figure 22. Schematic representation of idiotypes present on an immunoglobulin molecule.

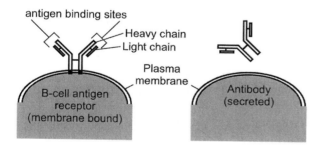

Figure 23. Schematic representation of an antigen receptor on the plasma membrane of a B-cell.

IgG, IgD, and IgE have two H and two L polypeptide chains, whereas IgM and IgA consist of multimers of this basic chain structure. Disulfide bridges and noncovalent forces stabilize immunoglobulin structure. The basic monomeric

unit is Y-shaped, with a hinge region rich in proline and susceptible to cleavage by proteolytic enzymes. Both H and L chains have a constant region at the carboxy terminus and a variable region at the amino terminus. The two heavy chains are alike, as are the two light chains in any individual immunoglobulin molecule. Approximately 60% of human immunoglobulin molecules have κ light chains and 40% have λ light chains. The five immunoglobulin classes are termed isotypes based on the heavy chain specificity of each immunoglobulin class. Two immunoglobulin classes, IgA and IgG have been further subdivided into subclasses based on H chain differences. There are four IgG subclasses designated as IgG1 through IgG4, and two IgA subclasses termed IgA1 and IgA2.

Digestion of IgG molecules with papain yields two Fab fragments and one Fc fragment. Each Fab fragment has one antigen-binding site. By contrast, the Fc fragment has no antigen-binding site but is responsible for fixation of complement and attachment of the molecule to a cell surface. Pepsin cleaves the molecule toward the carboxy-terminal end of the central disulfide bond yielding an $F(ab')_2$ fragment and a pFc' fragment. $F(ab')_2$ fragments have two antigen-binding sites. L chains have a single variable and constant domain, whereas H chains possess one variable and three to four constant domains.

Secretory IgA is found in body secretions such as saliva, milk, and intestinal and bronchial secretions. IgD and IgM are present as membrane bound immunoglobulins on B cells where they interact with antigen to activate B cells. IgE is associated with anaphylaxis and IgG, which is the only immunoglobulin capable of crossing the placenta, is the major human immunoglobulin.

An **immunoglobulin heavy chain** (Figure 24) is a 51kD to 71kD polypeptide chain present in immunoglobulin molecules and serves as the basis for dividing immunoglobulins into classes. The heavy chain is comprised of three to four

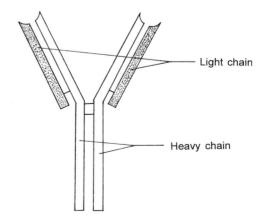

Figure 24. Immunoglobulin heavy chains that are fastened to each other or to light polypeptide chains by disulfide bonds.

constant domains, depending upon class, and one variable domain. In addition, a hinge region is present in some chains. There is approximately 30% homology with respect to amino acid sequence among the five classes of immunoglobulin heavy chain in man. The heavy chain of IgM is μ, of IgG is γ, of IgA is α, of IgD is δ and of IgE is ε. A **heavy chain** is a principal constituent of immunoglobulin molecules. Each immunoglobulin is comprised of at least one four-polypeptide chain monomer which consists of two heavy and two light polypeptide chains. The two heavy chains are identical in any one molecule as are the two light chains.

Immunoglobulin heavy chain binding protein (BiP) is a 77kD protein that combines with selected membrane and secretory proteins. It is believed to facilitate their passage through the endoplasmic reticulum.

A **light chain** (Figure 25) is a 22kD polypeptide chain found in all immunoglobulin molecules. Each four-chain immunoglobulin monomer contains two identical light polypeptide chains. They are joined to two like heavy chains by disulfide bonds. There are two types of light chains designated κ and λ. An individual immunoglobulin molecule possesses two light chains that are either κ or λ but never a mixture of the two. The types of light polypeptide chains occur in all five of the immunoglobulin classes. Each light chain has an N-terminal V region which constitutes part of the antigen-binding site of the antibody molecule. The C region or constant terminal reveals no variation except for the Inv and Oz allotype markers in humans. **Km** (formerly **Inv**) is the designation for the κ light chain allotype genetic markers.

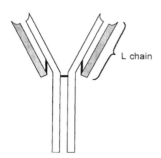

Figure 25. Light polypeptide chains of immunoglobulins that are fastened to heavy chains through disulfide bonds and are found in all classes of immunoglobulin.

Disulfide bonds (Figure 26) are the -S-S- chemical bonds between amino acids that link polypeptide chains together. Chemical reduction may break these bonds. Disulfide bonds in immunoglobulin molecules are either intrachain or interchain. The interchain disulfide bonds include linking heavy to heavy and heavy to light. The different types of bonds in immunoglobulin molecules differ in their ease of chemical reduction.

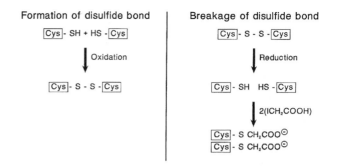

Figure 26. Depiction of the formation of disulfide bonds from the oxidation of two sulfhydryl groups as well as the breaking of disulfide bonds through reduction leading to sulfhydryl formation.

An **immunoglobulin domain** (Figure 27) is an immunoglobulin heavy or light polypeptide chain structural unit that is comprised of approximately 110 amino acid residues. Domains are loops that are linked by disulfide bonds on constant and variable regions of heavy and light chains. Immunoglobulin functions may be linked to certain domains. There is much primary and three dimensional structural homology among immunoglobulin domains. A particular exon may encode an immunoglobulin domain.

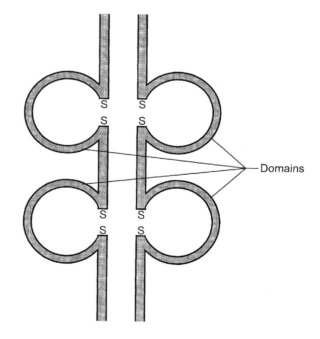

Figure 27. Domain structure of light or heavy polypeptide chains, the subunits of immunoglobulin molecules.

An **immunoglobulin fold** is an immunoglobulin domain's three dimensional configuration. An immunoglobulin fold has a sandwich-like structure comprised of two approximately parallel β-pleated sheets. There are four anti-parallel chain segments in one sheet and three in the other. Approximately 50% of the domain's amino acid residues are in the

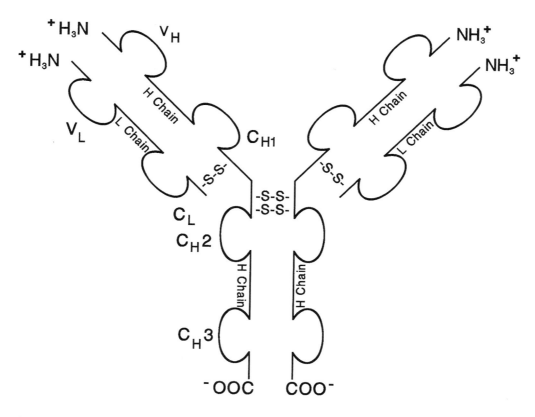

Figure 28. V_H and V_L regions on an antibody.

β-pleated sheets. The other 50% of the amino acid residues are situated in polypeptide chain loops and in terminal segments. The turns are sites of invariant glycine residues. Hydrophobic amino acid side chains are situated between the sheets.

The **V_H region** refers to the variable part of immunoglobulin heavy chain, which is the part of a variable region encoded for by the V_H gene segment (Figure 28). The V_L region describes the variable portion of an immunoglobulin light chain. The symbol may be used to designate the V_L gene encoded segment. V_κ is a variable region of an immunoglobulin κ light chain. This symbol may also be used to signify that part of a variable region encoded by the V_κ gene segment.

Hypervariable regions (Figure 29) constitute a minimum of four sites of great variability which are present throughout the H&L chain V regions. They govern the antigen binding site of an antibody molecule. Thus, grouping of these hypervariable residues into areas govern both conformation and specificity of the antigen-binding site upon folding of the protein molecule. Hypervariable residues are also responsible for variations in idiotypes between immunoglobulins produced by separate cell clones. Those parts of the variable region that are not hypervariable are termed the framework regions. Hypervariable regions are also called complementarity-determining regions (Figures 30 and 31).

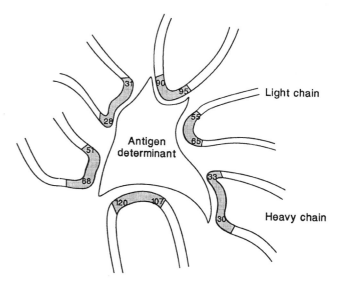

Figure 29.   Depiction of the structure of the six hypervariable regions of an antibody.

An **immunoglobulin λ chain** (Figure 32) is a 23kD 214 amino acid residue polypeptide chain with a single variable region and a single constant region (Figure 33). λ chains represent one of two light polypeptide chains comprising all five classes of immunoglobulin molecules. Approximately 40% of immu-

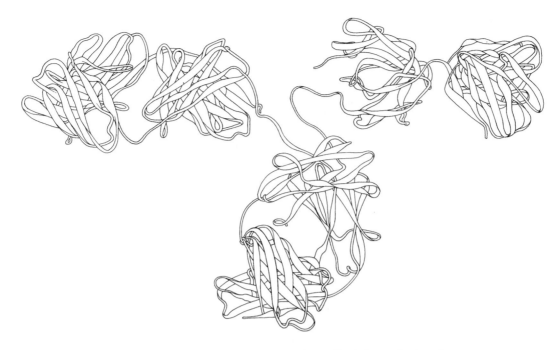

Figure 30.   Illustration of intact monoclonal antibody for canine lymphoma.

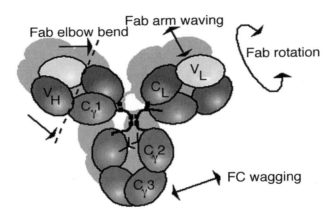

Figure 31.   Vitronectin.

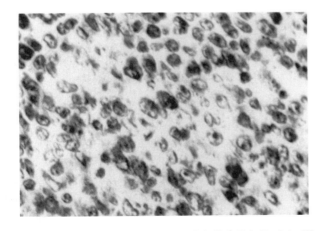

Figure 32.   Photomicrograph of immuglobulin λ light "staining" by immunnoperoxidase.

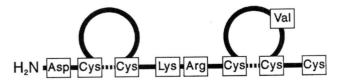

Figure 33.   Lambda light chain showing domain structure.

noglobulin light chains in man are λ. Wide variations in percentages are observed in other species. For example, the great majority of immunoglobulin light chains in horses and dogs are λ, whereas they constitute only 5% of murine light chains. Constant region differences among λ light chains of mice and man distinguish the molecules into four isotypes in humans. A different C gene segment encodes the separate constant regions defining each λ light chain isotype. The human λ light chain isotypes are designated Kern⁻Oz⁺, Kern⁺Oz⁻ and Mcg.

An **immunoglobulin κ chain** (Figure 34) is a 23kD 214 amino acid residue polypeptide chain that is comprised of a single variable region and a single constant region (Figure 35). It is one of the two types of light polypeptide chain present in all five immunoglobulin classes. Approximately 60% of light immunoglobulin chains in man are κ with wide variations of their percentages in other species. Whereas κ chains are virtually absent in immunoglobulins of dogs, they comprise the vast majority of murine immunoglobulin light chains. κ light chain allotypes in man are termed Km1, Km1,2, and Km3.

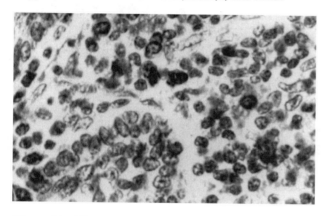

Figure 34.   Photomicrograph of immunoglobulin κ light chain "staining" by immunoperoxidase.

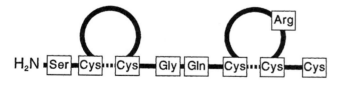

Figure 35.   Kappa light chain showing domain structure.

A **J chain** (Figure 36) is a 17.6kD polypeptide chain present in polymeric immunoglobulins that include both IgM and IgA. It links four-chain immunoglobulin monomers to produce the polymeric immunoglobulin structure. J chains are produced in plasma cells and are incorporated into IgM or IgA molecules prior to their secretion. Incorporation of the J chain appears essential for transcytosis of these immunoglobulin molecules to external secretions. The J chain comprises 2 to 4% of an IgM pentamer or a secretory IgA dimer. Tryptophan is absent from both mouse and human J chains. J chains are comprised of 137 amino acid residues and a single

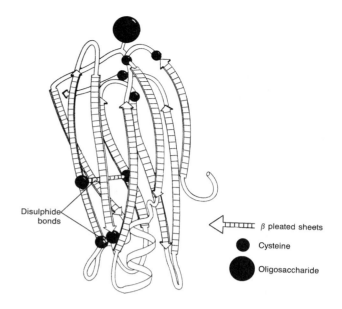

Figure 36.   Structure of J chain that occurs in secretory IgA and IgM molecules and facilitates polymerization.

complex N-linked oligosaccharide on asparagine. Human J chain contains three forms of the oligosaccharide which differ in sialic acid content. The J chain is fastened through disulfide bonds to penultimate cysteine residues of T or I heavy chains. The human J chain gene is located on chromosome 4q21, whereas the mouse J chain gene is located on chromosome 5.

An **immunoglobulin class** (Figure 37) is a subdivision of immunoglobulin molecules based on antigenic and structural differences in the Fc regions of their heavy polypeptide chains. Immunoglobulin molecules belonging to a particular class have at least one constant region isotypic determinant in common. The different classes, such as IgG, IgM and IgA, designate separate isotypes. Since the light chains of immunoglobulin molecules are one of two types, the heavy chains determine immunoglobulin class. There is about 30% homology of amino acid sequence among the five immunoglobulin heavy chain constant regions in man. Heavy chains (or isotypes), also differ in carbohydrate content. Immunization of a non-human species with human immunoglobulin provides antisera that may be used for class or isotype determination. Immunoglobulin G is divided into four subclasses and IgA is divided into two subclasses.

An **immunoglobulin subclass** (Figure 38) is a subdivision of immunoglobulin classes according to structural and antigenic differences in the constant regions of their heavy polypeptide chains. All molecules in an immunoglobulin subclass must express the isotypic antigenic determinants unique to that class, but in addition, they express other epitopes that render that subclass different from others. IgG has four subclasses designated IgG1, IgG2, IgG3 and IgG4. Whereas there is only 30% identity among the five immunoglobulin classes, there is three times that similarity among IgG subclasses. The IgA class is divisible into two sub-

Ig	IgG	IgM	IgA	IgD	IgE
Serum concentration (mg/dl)	800-1700	50-190	140-420	0.3-0.40	<0.001
Total Ig (%)	85	5-10	5-15	<1	<1
Complement fixation	+	++++	-	-	-
Principal biological effect	Resistance-opsonin; secondary response	Resistance-prepcipitin; primary response	Resistance prevents movement across mucous membranes	?	Anaphylaxis
Principal site of action	Serum	Serum	Secretions	?; receptor for B cells	Mast cells
Molecular weight (kd)	154	900	160 (+ dimer)	185	190
Serum half-life (days)	23	5	6	2-3	2-3
Antibacterial lysis	+	+++	+	?	?
Antiviral lysis	+	+	+++	?	?
H-chain class	γ	μ	α	μ	ε
Subclass	γ, γ, γ, γ,	μ, μ,	α, α,	μ, μ,	

Figure 37.   Table of human immunoglobulins and their properties.

classes, whereas the remaining three immunoglobulin classes have not been further subdivided into subclasses. The structural differences in subclasses are exemplified by the variations and number of inter-heavy chain disulfide bonds which the four IgG subclasses possess. The function of immunoglobulin molecules differs from one subclass to another as exemplified by the inability of IgG4 to fix complement.

Ig	IgG				IgM	IgA	IgE	IgD
H Chain Class	γ				μ	α	ε	δ
Subclass	γ_1	γ_2	γ_3	γ_4	μ_1 μ_2	α_1 α_2		

Figure 38.   Summary of the heavy chain designations of immunoglobulins that determine class and of their subdivisions that determine subclass.

Immunoglobulin G (IgG) (Figure 39) comprises approximately 85% of the immunoglobulins in adults. It has a molecular weight of 154kD based on two L chains of 22,000d each and two H chains of 55,000d each. It has the longest half-life (23 days) of the five immunoglobulin classes, crosses the placenta and is the principal antibody in the anamnestic or booster response. IgG (Figures 40–42) shows high avidity or binding capacity for antigen, fixes complement, stimulates chemotaxis and acts as an opsonin to facilitate phagocytosis (Figures 43 and 44).

The **immunoglobulin gamma (γ) chain** is a 51kD, 450 amino acid residue heavy polypeptide chain comprised of one variable V_H domain and a constant region with three domains designated C_H1, C_H2, and C_H3. The hinge region is situated between C_H1 and C_H2. There are four subclasses of IgG in man with four corresponding gamma chain isotypes designated $\gamma 1$, $\gamma 2$, $\gamma 3$ and $\gamma 4$. IgG1, IgG2, IgG3 and IgG4 have differences in their hinge regions and differ in the number and position of disulfide bonds that link the two K chains in each IgG molecule. There is only a 5% difference

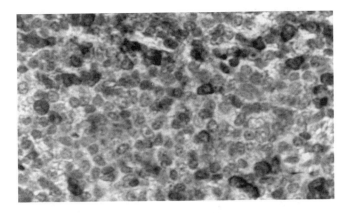

Figure 39.   Picture of Immunoglobulin — IgG

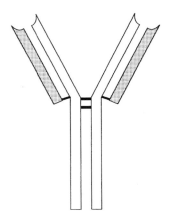

Figure 40.   IgG1.

in amino acid sequence among human γ chain isotypes, exclusive of the hinge region. Cysteine residues which makes it possible for inter-heavy (γ) chain disulfide bonds to form are found in the hinge area. IgG1 and IgG4 have

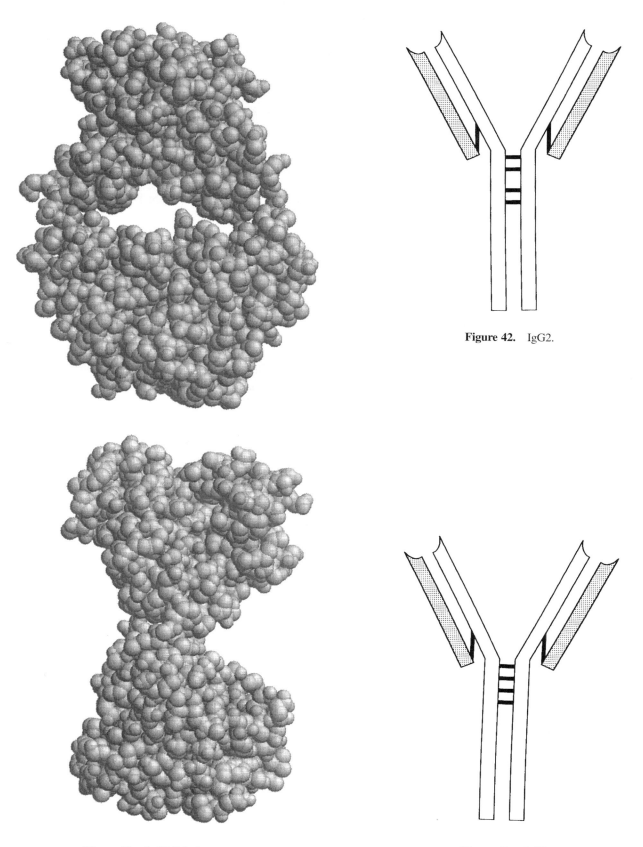

Figure 42. IgG2.

Figure 41. IgG1 Fab fragment.

Figure 43. IgG3.

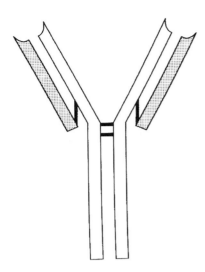

Figure 44. IgG4.

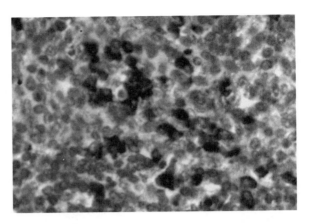

Figure 46. Picture of Immunoglobulin — IgM.

two inter-heavy chain disulfide bonds, IgG2 has four and IgG3 has eleven. Proteolytic enzymes, such as papain and pepsin, cleave an IgG molecule in the hinge region to produce Fab and $F(ab')_2$ and Fc fragments. Four murine isotypes have also been described. Two exons encode the carboxy-terminal region of membrane γ chain. Two γ chains together with two κ or λ light chains fastened together by disulfide bonds comprise an IgG molecule.

Immunoglobulin M (IgM) (Figure 45) comprises 5% to 10% of the total immunoglobulins in adults and has a half-life of five days. It is a pentameric molecule (Figures 46 and 47) with five 4-chain monomers joined by disulfide bonds and the J chain, with a total molecular weight of 900kD (Figure 48). Theoretically this immunoglobulin has

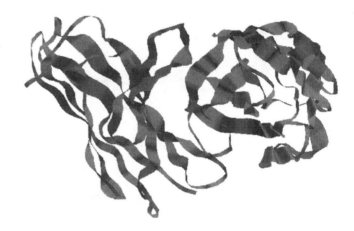

Figure 47. IgM Fv fragment.

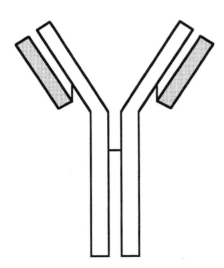

Figure 45. Monomeric IgM that contains two T chains and two κ or two λ light chains.

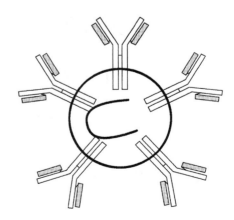

Figure 48. Pentameric IgM that consist of five 7S monomers comprised of two heavy and two light polypeptide chains each as well as one J chain per molecule.

ten antigen-binding sites. IgM is the most efficient immunoglobulin in fixing complement. A single IgM pentamer can activate the classic pathway. Monomeric IgM is found with IgD on the B lymphocyte cell surface where it serves as the receptor for antigen. Because IgM is relatively large, it is confined to intravascular locations. IgM is particularly important for immunity against polysaccharide antigens on the exterior of pathogenic microorganisms. It also promotes phagocytosis and bacteriolysis through its complement activation activity.

The **immunoglobulin mu (μ) chain** is a 72kD, 570 amino acid heavy polypeptide chain comprised of one variable region designated V_H and a four domain constant region designated C_H1, C_H2, C_H3 and C_H4. The μ chain does not have a hinge region. A "tail piece" is located at the carboxy-terminal end of the chain. It is comprised of 18 amino acid residues. A cysteine residue at the penultimate position of a carboxy-terminal region of the μ chain forms a disulfide bond that joins to the J chain. There are five N-linked oligosaccharides in the μ chain of man. Secreted IgM ($μ_s$) and membrane IgM ($μ_m$) μ chain differ only in the final 20 amino acid residues at the carboxy-terminal end. The membrane form of IgM has 41 different residues substituted for the final 20 residues in the secreted form. A 26 residue region of this carboxy-terminal section in the membrane form of IgM apparently represents the hydrophobic transmembrane part of the chain.

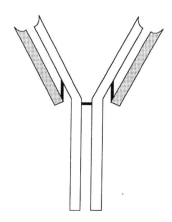

Figure 49. IgA1.

Immunoglobulin A (IgA) (Figure 49) comprises 5% to 15% of the serum immunoglobulins and has a half-life of 6 days. It has a molecular weight of 160kD and a basic four-chain monomeric structure. However, it can occur as monomers, dimers, trimers, and multimers. It contains α heavy chains and κ or λ light chains. There are two subclasses of IgA desingated IgA1 and IgA2 (Figure 50). In addition to serum IgA, a secretory or exocrine variety appears in body secretions and provides local immunity. For example, the Sabin oral polio vaccine stimulates secretory IgA antibodies in the gut, which provides effective immunity against poliomyelitis. IgA deficient individuals

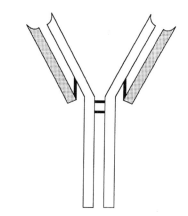

Figure 50. IgA2.

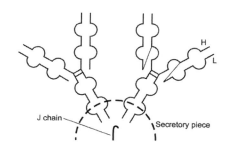

Figure 51. Secretory IgA that consists of two IgA monomers, a J chain and secretory piece that is believed to protect the molecule from enzymatic digestion in the gut.

have an increased incidence of respiratory infections associated with a lack of secretory IgA (Figure 51) in the respiratory system. Secretory or exocrine IgA appears in colostrum, intestinal and respiratory secretions, saliva, tears and other secretions.

The **immunoglobulin alpha (α) chain** is a 58kD, 470 amino acid residue heavy polypeptide chain that confers class specificity on immunoglobulin A molecules. The chain is divisible into three constant domains designated C_H1, C_H2 and C_H3 and one variable domain designated V_H. A hinge region is situated between C_H1 and C_H2 domains. An additional segment of 18 amino acid residues at the penultimate position of the chain contains a cysteine residue where the J chain can be linked through a disulfide bond. The IgA subclass is divisible into IgA1 and IgA2 subclasses, reflecting two separate alpha chain isotypes. The α2 chain has two allotypes designated A2m(1) and A2m(2) and does not have disulfide bonds linking H to L chains. Residues that are subclass specific are found in a number of positions in C_H1, the hinge region and C_H2 where α1 and α2 chains differ but α2 chains are the same. Differences in the two α chains are found in two C_H1 and five C_H3 positions. Thus, there are three varieties of α heavy chain in man.

Immunoglobulin class switching is the mechanism whereby an IgM producing B cell switches isotype to begin producing IgG molecules instead. Further differentiation may lead to a B cell producing IgA. However, the antigen-binding specificity of the antibody molecules with a different isotype remains unchanged.

Immunoglobulin D (IgD) (Figure 52), which has a molecular weight of 185kD, comprises less than 1% of serum immunoglobulins. It has the basic four-chain monomeric structure with two delta heavy chains (molecular weight 63,000d each) and either two kappa or two lambda light chains (molecular weight 22,000d each). The half life of IgD is only two to three days and the role of IgD in immunity remains elusive. Membrane IgD serves with IgM as an antigen receptor on B cell membranes.

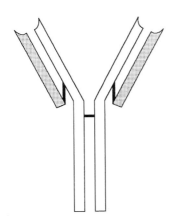

Figure 52.   IgD structure showing a four chain monomeric unit that consists of two δ heavy chains and either two κ or two λ light chain per molecule.

The **immunoglobulin delta (δ) chain** is a 64kD, 500 amino acid residue heavy polypeptide chain consisting of one variable region designated V_H and a three domain constant region designated C_H1, C_H2 and C_H3. There is also a 58 residue amino acid residue hinge region in δ chains of man. Two exons encode the hinge region. IgD is very susceptible to the action of proteolytic enzymes at its hinge region. Two separate exons encode the membrane component of δ chain. A distinct exon encodes the carboxy-terminal portion of the human δ chain that is secreted. The human δ chain contains three N-linked oligosaccharides. Two δ chains and two light chains, either κ or λ, fastened together by disulfide bonds constitute an IgD molecule.

Immunoglobulin E (IgE) (Figure 53) constitutes less than 1% of the total immunoglobulins and has a half life of approximately 2.5 days. This antibody has a four-chain unit structure with two epsilon heavy chains (molecular weight 75,000d each) and either two kappa or two lambda light chains per molecule (total molecular weight 190kD). IgE

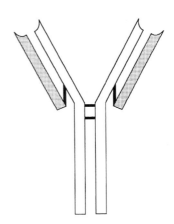

Figure 53.   IgE molecule

does not precipitate with antigen *in vitro* and is heat labile. IgE is responsible for anaphylactic hypersensitivity in man.

The **immunoglobulin epsilon (ε) chain** is a 72kD, 550 amino acid residue heavy polypeptide chain comprised of one variable region designated V_H and a four domain constant region designated C_H1, C_H2, C_H3, and C_H4. This heavy chain does not possess a hinge region. In man, the ε heavy chain has 428 amino acid residues in the constant region. There is no carboxy-terminal portion of the ε chains. Two ε heavy polypeptide chains and two κ or two λ light chains, fastened together by disulfide bonds comprise an IgE molecule.

In **pepsin digestion** (Figure 54) a proteolytic enzyme is used to cleave immunoglobulin molecules into $F(ab')_2$ fragments together with fragments of small peptides that represent what remains of the Fc fragment. Each immunoglobulin molecule yields only one $F(ab')_2$ fragment which is bivalent and may manifest many of the same antibody characteristics as intact IgG molecules such as anti-toxic activity in neutralizing bacterial toxins. Cleaving the Fc region from an IgG molecule deprives it of its ability to fix complement and bind to Fc receptors on cell surfaces. Pepsin digestion is useful in diminishing the immunogenicity of antitoxins. It converts them to $F(ab')_2$ fragments which retain antitoxin activity.

Papain (Figure 55) is a proteolytic enzyme extracted from *Carica papaya* that is used to digest each IgG immunoglobulin molecule into two Fab fragments and one crystallizable Fc fragment. This aided efforts to reveal the molecular structure of immunoglobulins. Papain cleaves the immunoglobulin G molecule on the opposite side of the central disulfide bond from pepsin, which cleaves the molecule to the C terminus side leading to the formation of 1 $F(ab')_2$ fragment, which is bivalent in contrast to the Fab fragments which are univalent. The Fc fragment of papain digestion has no antigen binding capacity although it does have complement fixing functions and attaches immunoglobulin molecules to Fc receptors on a cell membrane. The enzyme has also been

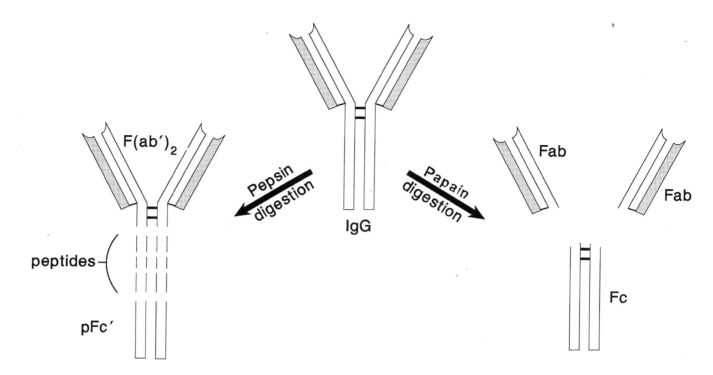

Figure 54.   Pepsin digestion

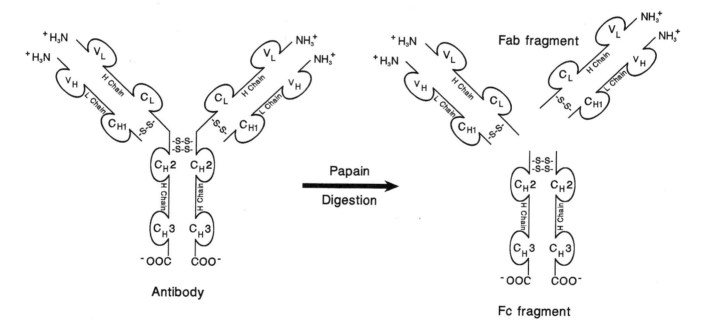

Figure 55.   Papain digestion of IgG molecules yielding two Fab and one Fc fragment per molecule.

used to render red blood cell surfaces susceptible to agglutination by incomplete antibody.

Immunoglobulin fragment is a term reserved for products that result from the action of proteolytic enzymes on immunoglobulin molecules. Intrachain disulfide bonds can be sev-

ered by reduction in the presence of denaturing agents such as urea, guanidine, or detergents. Peptide bonds in intact domains are not easily split by proteolytic enzymes. Light chains can be cleaved at the V-C junction giving rise to large segments that correspond to the V_L and C_L domains. Similar cleavage of the heavy chain is more difficult to achieve.

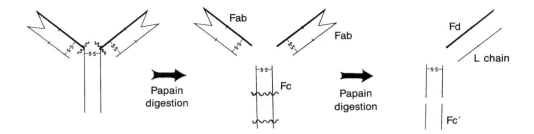

Figure 56. The Fab fragment is comprised of one light chain and the variable and CH1 regions of a heavy chain. They are united by disulfide bonds and have a single binding site for antigen. The heavy chain part of a Fab fragment is referred to as Fd. Further digestion with papain yields an Fc'.

Papain cleaves H chains at the N-terminus of the H-H disulfide bonds giving two individual portions of the terminus of the molecule, called Fab and the fragment of the C-terminus region, Fc, which is crystallizable. In contrast, pepsin cleaves H chains at the C-terminus of the H-H disulfide bonds. Thus, the two Fab fragments will remain joined and are called F(ab')$_2$. It degrades the C$_H$2 domains but splits the C$_H$3 domains which remain noncovalently bonded in dimeric form and are called pFc'. Further digestion of the pFc' with papain results in smaller dimeric fragments called Fc'. Plasmin has been found to cleave the immunoglobulin molecule between C$_H$2 and C$_H$3 giving rise to a fragment designated Facb. The heavy chain portion of the Fab, designated as Fd, and the heavy chain portion of the FabN fragment, termed Fd', results from the breakdown of an F(ab')$_2$ fragment produced by pepsin digestion of the IgG molecule. The Fv fragment consists of the variable domain of heavy and light chains on an immunoglobulin molecule where antigen binding occurs.

A **Fab fragment** (Figures 56 and 57) is a product of papain digestion of an IgG molecule. It is comprised of one light chain and the segment of heavy chain on the N-terminal side of the central disulfide bond. The light chain and heavy chain segment are linked by interchain disulfide bonds. It is 47kD and has a sedimentation coefficient of 3.5S. The Fab fragment has a single antigen-binding site. There are two Fab regions in each IgG molecule.

An **Fd fragment** consists of the heavy chain portion of a Fab fragment produced by papain digestion of an IgG molecule. It is on the N-terminal side of the papain digestion site.

The **Fv region** (Figure 58) consists of the N-terminal variable segments of both heavy and light chains in each Fab region of an immunoglobulin molecule with a four chain unit structure.

The **Wu-Kabat plot** (Figure 59) is a graph that demonstrates the extent of variability at individual amino acid residue positions in immunoglobulin and T cell receptor variable regions. Division of the different amino acid number at a given position by the frequency of the amino acid which

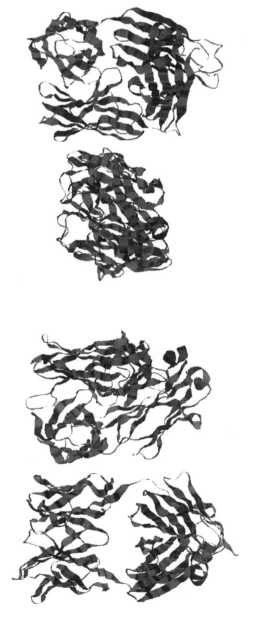

Figure 57. Fab fragment.

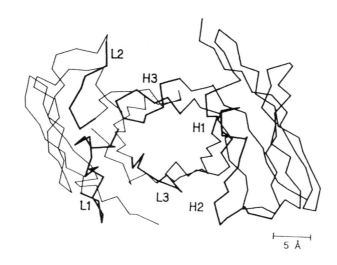

Figure 58.   Fv region.

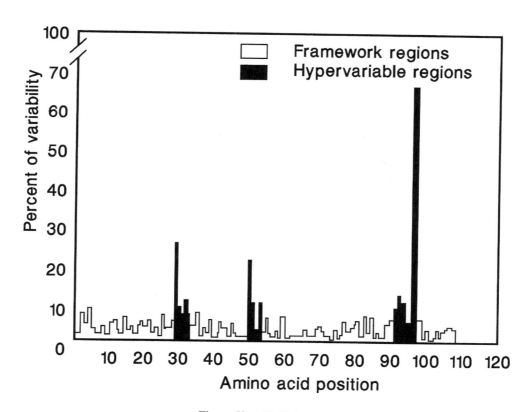

Figure 59.   Wu-Kabat plot.

occurs most commonly at that position gives the index of variability. The index varies between 1 and 400. To show the variability graphically, a biograph is prepared where the index is plotted at each residue position. This plot indicates the extent of variability at each position and is useful in localizing immunoglobulin and T cell receptor hypervariable regions.

The **Fc fragment (fragment crystallizable)** (Figure 60) is a product of papain digestion of an IgG molecule. It is comprised of two C-terminal heavy chain segments (C_H2, C_H3) and a portion of the hinge region linked by the central disulfide bond and noncovalent forces. This 50kD fragment is unable to bind antigen but has multiple other biological functions including complement fixation, interaction with Fc receptors on the cell surfaces and placental transmission of IgG. One Fc fragment is produced by papain digestion of each IgG molecule.

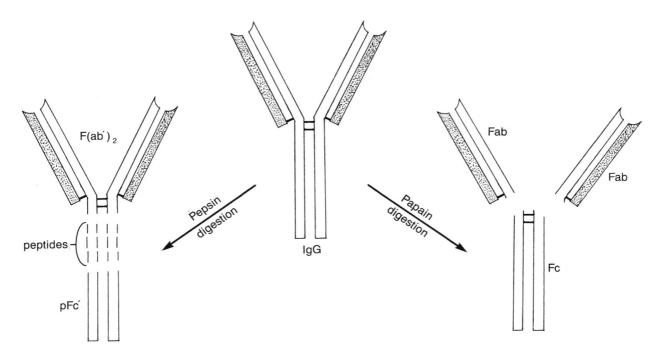

Figure 60.   Fc fragment.

The **Fc′ fragment** is a product of papain digestion of IgG. It is comprised of two non-covalently bonded C_H3 domains that lack the terminal 13 amino acids. This 24kD dimer consists of the region between the heavy chain amino acid residues 14 through 105 from the carboxy-terminal end. Normal human urine contains minute quantities of Fc′ fragment.

An **Fabc fragment** (Figure 61) is a 5S intermediate fragment produced by partial digestion of IgG by papain in which only one Fab fragment is cleaved from the parent molecule in the hinge region. This leaves the Fabc fragment which is comprised of a Fab region bound covalently to an Fc region and is functionally univalent.

A **Fab′ fragment** (Figure 62) is a product of reduction of an $F(ab')_2$ fragment that results from pepsin digestion of IgG. It is comprised of one light chain linked by disulfide

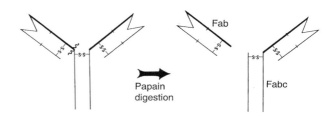

Figure 61.   Generation of an Fabc fragment by papain digestion of IgG in which one Fab region is cleaved leaving an Fabc fragment consisting of the Fc region and one Fab region of the molecule bearing a single antigen-binding site.

bonds to the N-terminal segment of heavy chain. The Fab′ fragment has a single antigen-binding site. There are two Fab′ fragments in each $F(ab')_2$ fragment.

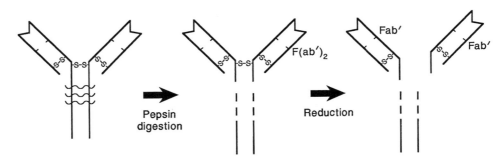

Figure 62.   Pepsin digestion of an IgG molecule leading to the formation of $F(ab')_2$ intermediate fragments and with reduction to the formation of Fab′ fragments.

An **F(ab′)₂ fragment** is a product of pepsin digestion of an IgG molecule. This 95kD immunoglobulin fragment has a valence, or antigen-binding capacity, of two which renders it capable of inducing aggutination or precipitation with homologous antigen. However, the functions associated with the intact IgG molecule's Fc region, such as complement fixation and attachment to Fc receptors on cell surfaces, are missing. Pepsin digestion occurs on the carboxy-terminal side of the central disulfide bond at the hinge region of the molecule which leaves the central disulfide bond intact. The C_H2 domain is converted to minute peptides, yet the C_H3 domain is left whole, and the two C_H3 domains comprise the pFc′ fragment.

An **Fd′ fragment** (Figure 63) is the heavy chain portion of an Fab′ fragment produced by reduction of the F(ab′)₂ fragment that results from pepsin digestion of IgG. It is comprised of V_H1, C_H1 and the heavy chain hinge region. Fd′ contains 235 amino acid residues.

The **Facb fragment** (Figure 64) is fragment antigen and complement-binding. The action of plasmin on IgG molecules denatured by acid cleaves C_H3 domains from both heavy chain constituents of the Fc region. This yields a bivalent fragment functionally capable of precipitation and agglutination with an Fc remnant still capable of fixing complement.

An **Fb fragment** (Figure 65) is the product of subtilisin digestion of IgG. It is comprised of the Fab fragment's C_H1 and C_L (constant) domains.

An **Fv fragment** (Figure 66) consists of the N-terminal variable segments of both heavy (V_H) and light (V_L) chain domains that are joined by noncovalent forces. The fragment has one antigen binding site.

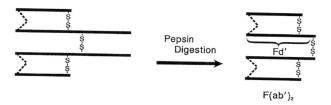

Figure 63.   F(ab′)₂ fragment containing 2 Fd′ heavy chain portions.

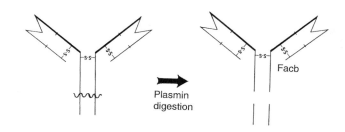

Figure 64.   Generation of Facb fragment through plasmin digestion of an IgG molecule.

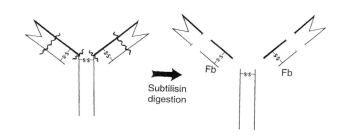

Figure 65.   Formation of Fb fragments by digestion of IgG molecules with subtilisin.

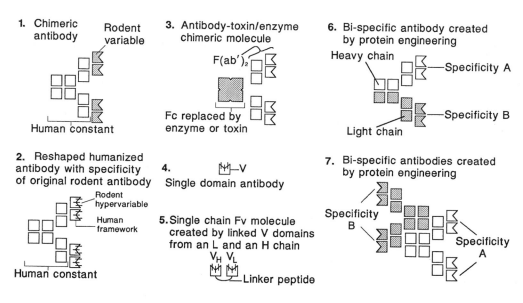

Figure 66.   Genetically engineered antibodies.

Isotype (Figure 67) refers to the antigens that determine the class or subclass of heavy chains or the type and subtype of light chains of immunoglobulin molecules. Every normal member of a species expresses each isotype. An immunoglobulin subtype is found in all normal individuals. Among the immunoglobulin classes, IgG and IgA have subclasses that are designated with Arabic numerals. They are distinguished according to domain number and size as well as the constant region's number of both intrachain and interchain disulfide bonds. The four isotypes of IgG are designated IgG1, IgG2, IgG3, and IgG4. The two IgA isotypes are designated IgA1 and IgA2. The μ, δ, and ε heavy chains and the κ and λ light chains each have one isotype.

Allotypes (Figure 68) originally were defined by antisera which differentiated allelic variants of Ig subclasses. The allotype is due to the existence of different alleles at the genetic locus which determines the expression of a given

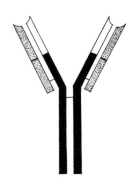

Figure 67. IgG showing that the isotype, designated in black, is determined by the heavy chain.

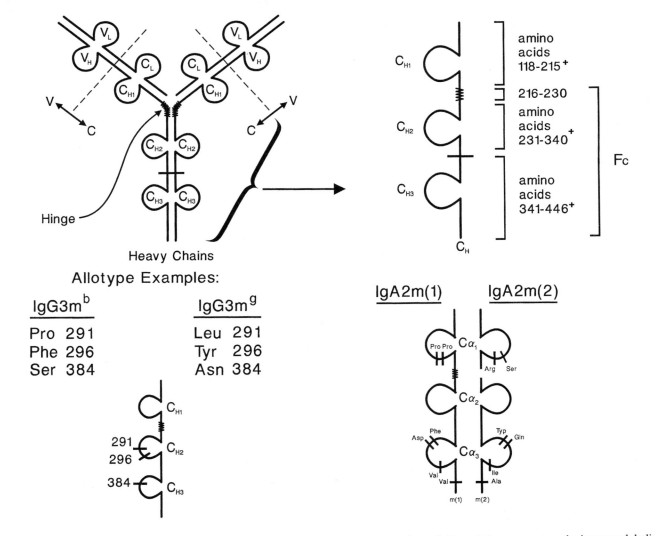

Figure 68. Allotype describes a distinct antigenic form of a serum protein that results from allelic variations present on the immunoglobulin heavy chain constant region.

determinant. Immunoglobulin allotypes have been extensively investigated in inbred rabbits. Currently, allotypes are usually defined by DNA techniques. To be designated as an official allotype, the polymorphism must be present in a reasonable subset of the population (approximately 1%) and follow Mendelian genetics. Allotype examples include the IgG3 Caucasian allotypes G3m^b and G3m^g. These two alleles vary at positions 291, 296, and 384. Another example is the allotype at the IgA2 locus. The IgA2m(1) allele is European/Near Eastern while IgA2m(2) is African/East Asian. The allotypic differences are in CI$_1$ and CI$_3$, and the IgA2m(2) allele has a shorter hinge than the IgA2m(1) allele. An allotope is an allotype's antigenic determinant.

Gm allotype (Figure 69) refers to a genetic variant determinant of the human IgG heavy chain. Allelic genes that encode the γ1, γ2 and γ3 heavy chain constant regions encode the Gm allotypes. They were recognized by the ability of blood sera from rheumatoid arthritis patients, which contain anti-IgG rheumatoid factor, to react with them. Gm allotypic determinants are associated with specific amino acid substitution in different γ chain constant regions in man. IgG subclasses are associated with certain Gm determinants. For example, IgG1 is associated with G1m(1) and G1m(4), and IgG3 is associated with G3m(5). Although the great majority of Gm allotypes are restricted to the IgG γ chain Fc region, a substitution at position 214 of C$_H$1 of arginine yields the G1m(4) allotype and a substitution at this same site of lysine yields G1m(17). For Gm expression, the light chain part of the molecule must be intact.

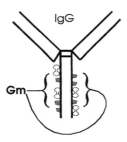

Figure 69. Illustration of the location of Gm marker specificities on the Fc region of an IgG molecule.

An **Am allotypic marker** (Figure 70) is an allotypic antigenic determinant located on the α heavy chain of the IgA molecule in man. Of the two IgA subclasses, the IgA1 subclass has no known allotypic determinant. The IgA2 subclass has two allotypic determinants designated A2m(1) and A2m(2) based on differences in α2 heavy chain primary structures. Allelic genes at the A2m locus encode these allotypes which are expressed on the α2 heavy chain constant regions.

Idiotype (Figure 71) refers to that segment of an immunoglobulin or antibody molecule that determines its specificity for antigen and is based upon the multiple combinations of

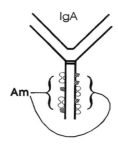

Figure 70. Illustration of the location of Am marker specificities on the Fc region of a serum IgA molecule.

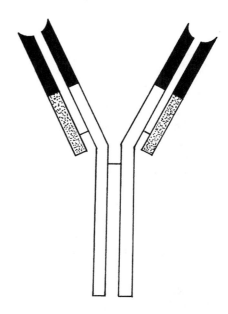

Figure 71. Idiotype which is determined by the variable regions of heavy and light chains of an immunoglobulin molecule.

variable (V), diversity (D) and joining (J) exons. The idiotype is located in the Fab region and its expression usually requires participation of the variable regions of both heavy and light chains, namely the Fv fragment which contains the antigen combining site.

The antigen-binding specificity of the combining site may imply that all antibodies produced by an animal in response to a given immunogen have the same idiotype. This is not true since the antibody response is heterogeneous. There will usually be a major idiotype representing 20–70% of the specific antibody response. The remainder carry different idiotypes that may cross react with the major idiotype. Crossreacting idiotypy represents the extent of heterogeneity among the antibodies of a given specificity.

The unique antigenic determinants that govern the idiotype (Id) of an immunoglobulin molecule occur on the products of either a single or several clones of cells synthesizing immunoglobulins (Figure 72). This unique idiotypic determinant is sometimes called a private idiotype which

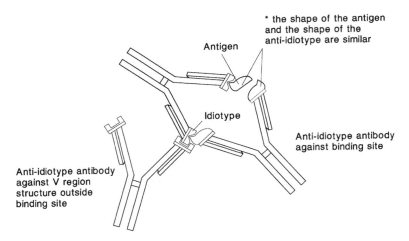

Figure 72. Idiotype network

appears in all V regions of immunoglobulin molecules whose amino acid sequences are the same. Shared idiotypes are also known as public idiotype determinants. These may appear in a relatively large number of immunoglobulin molecules produced by inbred strains of mice or other genetically identical animals in response to a specific antigen. The localization of idiotypes in the antigen-binding site of the molecule's V region is illustrated by the ability of haptens to block or inhibit the interaction of antiidiotypic antibodies with their homologous antigenic markers or determinants in the antigen-binding region of antibody molecules.

Jerne network theory (Figure 73) refers to the hypothesis that antibodies produced in response to a specific antigen would themselves induce a second group of antibodies which would in turn downregulate the original antibody-producing cells. The second antigen (Ab-2) would recognize epitopes of antibody 1's antibody-binding region. These would be antiidiotypic antibodies. Such antiidiotypic antibodies would also be

reactive with the antigen-binding region of T cell receptors for which they were specific. Thus, a network of antiantibodies would produce a homeostatic effect on the immune response to a particular antigen. This theory was subsequently proven and confirmed by numerous investigators.

Autobody (Figure 74) refers to an antibody that exhibits the internal image of antigen as well as a binding site for antigen. It manifests dual binding to both idiotope and epitope. It bears an idiotope that is complementary to its own antigen-binding site or paratope. Thus, it has self-binding potential. This type of anti-idiotypic antibody has features of Ab1 and Ab2 on the same molecule causing it to be designated Ab1-2 or "autobody". The name points to the potential for self-aggregation of the molecules and the potential participation of autobodies in autoimmune phenomena. Antibodies to phosphorylcholine (PC) epitope raised in Balb/c mice expressing the T15 idiotype self aggregate, i.e., bind to one another.

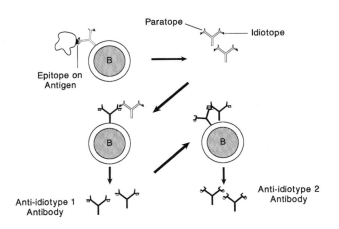

Figure 73. Jerne network theory.

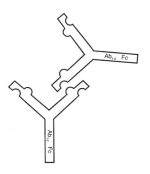

Figure 74. Autobody.

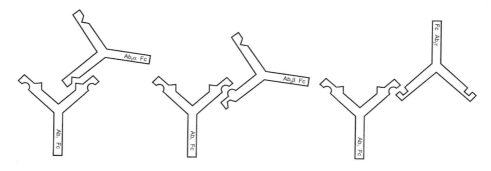

Figure 75.   Homobody.

Homobody (Figure 75) designates an idiotypic determinant of an antibody molecule whose three-dimensional structure resembles antigen. It is also called the internal image of antigen. For example, antiidiotypic antibodies, of this type, to insulin receptor may partially mimic the action of insulin.

Epibody refers to an anti-idiotypic antibody reactive with an idiotype of a monoclonal, human anti-IgG autoantibody as well as with human IgG Fc region (Figure 76). These antibodies identify an antigenic determinant associated with the sequence Ser-Ser-Ser. The ability of an epibody to identify an epitope shared by a rheumatoid factor idiotope and an Fc gamma epitope demonstrates that this variety of anti-idiotypic antibody may function as a rheumatoid factor.

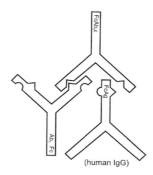

Figure 76.   Epibody

7

Immunoglobulin Synthesis, Properties, and Metabolism

Following enunciation of the clonal selection theory of antibody formation by Burnet in 1957, experimental evidence confirms the validity of this selective theory as opposed to the instructive theory of antibody formation which prevailed during the first half of the 20th century. As immunogeneticists attempted to explain the great diversity of antibodies encoded by finite quantities of DNA, Tonegawa offered a plausible explanation for the generation of antibody diversity in his studies of immunoglobulin gene C, V, J, and D regions and their rearrangement. It is necessary for those segments that encode genes and determine immunoglobulin H & L chains to undergo rearrangement prior to gene transcription and translation. Newly synthesized immunoglobulin molecules have different properties based upon their immunoglobulin class or isotype. Nevertheless, antigen-binding specificities reside in the Fab regions of antibody molecules, which governs their interactions with antigens *in vitro* and *in vivo*. By contrast, complement binding and activation capabilities, binding to cell surface, and transport through cells reside in the Fc region of the molecule. The fate of immunoglobulin molecules also differs according to the immunoglobulin class, each with its own characteristic half life. Only IgG is protected from catabolism by binding to a specific receptor.

Some antibodies are protective, others cross the placenta from mother to fetus, whereas others participate in hypersensitivity reactions that lead to adverse effects in target tissues. Antibodies are a diverse and unique category of proteins whose antigen-binding diversity is expressed in the 10^{20} antibody molecules synthesized from the 10^{12} B lymphocytes found in the human body.

The **template theory** (historical) is an instructive theory of antibody formation which requires antigen to be present during the process of antibody synthesis. According to the refolding template theory, uncommitted and specific globulins could become refolded on the antigen, serving as a template for it. The cell releases the complementary antibodies, which rigidly retain their shape through disulfide bonding. This theory was abandoned as it became clear that the specificity of antibodies is due to the particular arrangement of their primary amino acid sequence. The template

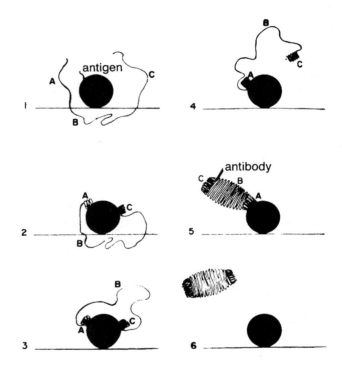

Figure 1. Instructive theory of antibody formation.

theory could not explain immunological tolerance or the anamnestic (memory) immune response.

The **instructive theory (of antibody formation)** was a hypothesis that postulated acquisition of antibody specificity after contact with specific antigen (Figure 1). According to one template theory of antibody formation, antigen must be present during the process of antibody synthesis. According to the refolding template theory, uncommitted and specific globulins could become refolded upon the antigen, serving as a template. The cell released the complementary antibodies, which rigidly retained their shape through disulfide bonding. This theory was abandoned when it was shown that the specificity of antibodies is due to the particular arrangement of their primary amino acid sequence. *de novo* synthesis template theories which recognized the necessity for antibodies to be synthesized by amino acids in the proper and predetermined order had to contend with the serious objection that proteins cannot serve as informational models for the synthesis of proteins. Instructive theories were abandoned when immunologic tolerance was demonstrated and when antigen was shown to be unnecessary for antibody synthesis to occur. The template theories have never explained the anamnestic (memory) immune response. Antibody specificity depends upon the variable-region amino acid sequence, especially the complementarity-determining or hypervariable regions.

The **selective theory** is a hypothesis that describes antibody synthesis as a process in which antigen selects cells expressing receptors specific for that antigen. The antigen-cell receptor interaction leads to proliferation and differentiation of that clone of cells which synthesizes significant quantities of antibodies of a single specificity. Selective theories included the side chain theory of Paul Ehrlich proposed in 1899, the natural selection theory proposed by Niels Jerne in 1955 and the cell selection theory proposed by Talmage and then Burnet in 1957. Burnet termed his version of the theory the clonal selection theory of acquired immunity. The basic tenets of the clonal selection theory have been substantiated by scientific evidence. The selective theories maintain that cells are genetically programmed to react to certain antigenic specificities prior to antigen exposure. This is in sharp contrast to the instructive theories which postulated that antigen was necessary to serve as a template around which polypeptide chains were folded to yield specific antibodies. This template theory was abandoned when antibody was demonstrated in the absence of antigen (Figure 2).

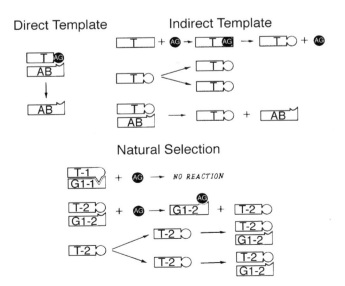

Figure 2. Comparison of template with natural selection theories of antibody synthesis.

The **clonal selection theory** is a selective theory of antibody formation proposed by F. M. Burnet who postulated the presence of numerous antibody-forming cells, each capable of synthesizing its own predetermined antibody (Figure 3). Cells selected by the best fitting antigen, multiply and form clones of cells which continue to synthesize the same antibody. Considering the existence of many different cells, each capable of synthesizing an antibody of a different specificity, all known facts of antibody formation are easily accounted for. An important element of the clonal selection theory is the hypothesis that many cells with different antibody specificities arise through random somatic mutations during a period of hypermutability early in life. Also early in life, the "forbidden" clones of antibody-forming cells (i.e., the cells that make antibody to the animal's own antigen) are destroyed after encountering these autoantigens. This process accounts for an animal's tolerance of its own antigens. Antigen would have no effect on most lymphoid cells but would selectively stimulate those cells already synthesizing the corresponding antibody at a low rate. The cell surface antibody serves as a receptor for antigen, allowing proliferation into clones of cells producing antibody of that specificity. Burnet introduced the "forbidden clone" concept to explain autoimmunity. Cells capable of forming antibody against normal self antigen are "forbidden" and eliminated during embryonic life. During fetal development, clones that react with self antigens are destroyed or suppressed. The subsequent activation of suppressed clones reactive with self antigens in later life may induce autoimmune disease. D. W. Talmadge proposed a cell selection theory of antibody formation which was the basis for Burnet's clonal selection theory.

Monoclonal antibody (MAb) is an antibody synthesized by a single clone of B lymphocytes or plasma cells (Figure 4). The first to be observed were produced by malignant plasma cells in patients with multiple myeloma and associated gammopathies. The identical copies of the antibody molecules produced contain only one class of heavy chain and one type of light chain. Kohler and Millstein in the mid-1970s developed B lymphocyte hybridomas by fusing an antibody-producing B lymphocyte with a mutant myeloma cell that was not secreting antibody. The B lymphocyte product provided the specificity, whereas the myeloma cell conferred immortality on the hybridoma clone. Today monoclonal antibodies (MAb) are produced in large quantities against a plethora of antigens for use in diagnosis and sometimes in treatment. MAb are homogeneous and are widely employed in immunoassays, single antigen identification in mixtures, delineation of cell surface molecules, assay of hormones and drugs in serum, among many other uses. Since the response to some immunogens is inadequate in mice, monoclonal antibodies have also been generated using rabbit cells. Monoclonal antibodies have been radioactively labeled and used to detect tumor metastasis, differentiate

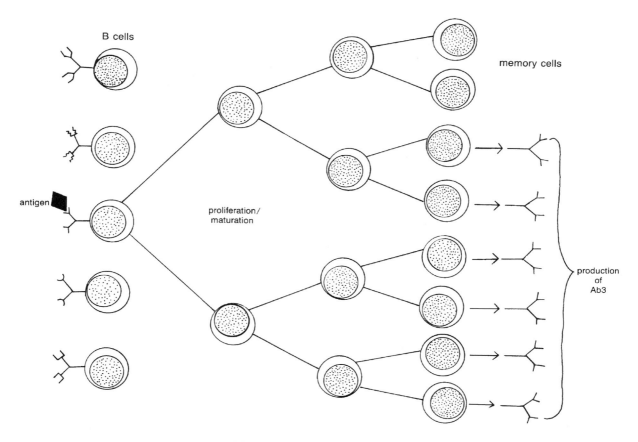

Figure 3.   Clonal selection theory.

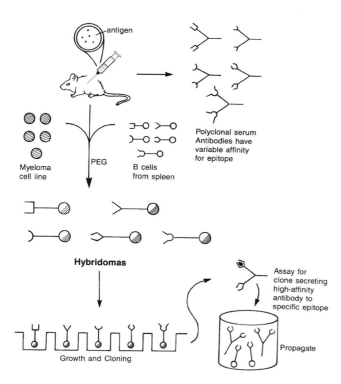

Figure 4.   Monoclonal antibody.

subtypes of tumors with monoclonal antibodies against membrane antigens or intermediate filaments, identify microbes in body fluids, and assay circulating hormones. MAb may be used to direct immunotoxins or radioisotopes to tumor targets with potential for tumor therapy.

A **B lymphocyte hybridoma** is a hybrid cell produced by the fusion of a splenic antibody secreting cell immunized against that particular antigen with a mutant myeloma cell from the same species that no longer secretes its own protein product (Figures 5 and 6). Polyethylene glycol is used to effect cell fusion. Antibody-synthesizing cells do not secrete hypoxanthine guanine phosphoribosyl transferase (HGPRT), an enzyme needed for DNA nucleotide synthesis, but do provide the ability to produce a specific monoclonal antibody. The mutant myeloma cell line confers immortality upon the hybridoma. If the nucleotide synthesis pathway is inhibited, the myeloma cells become HGPRT-dependent. The antibody synthesizing cells provide the HGPRT and the mutant myeloma cell enables endless reproduction. Once isolated through use of a selective medium such as HAT, hybridoma cell lines can be maintained for relatively long periods. Hybridomas produce specific monoclonal antibodies that may be collected in great quantities for use in diagnosis and selected types of therapy (Figures 7 and 8).

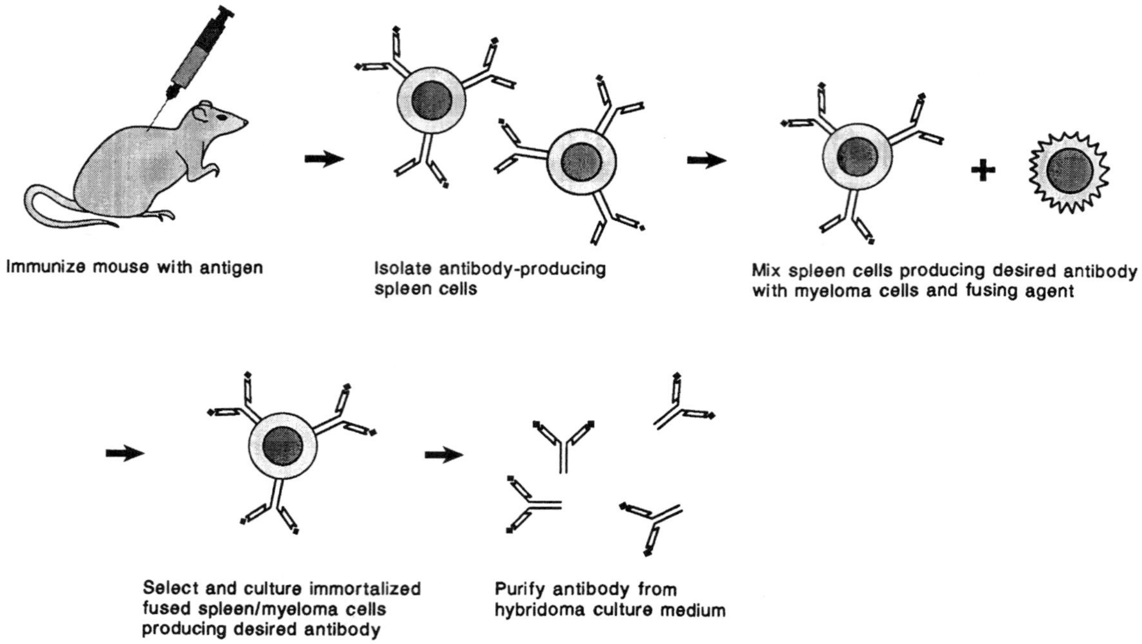

Immunize mouse with antigen
Isolate antibody-producing spleen cells
Mix spleen cells producing desired antibody with myeloma cells and fusing agent
Select and culture immortalized fused spleen/myeloma cells producing desired antibody
Purify antibody from hybridoma culture medium

Figure 5. Making of a hybridoma for monoclonal antibody production.

Antigen
Spleen
B cells
HGPRT- myeloma cells
PEG
to
HAT medium
B cells
Hybridoma
Myeloma
No Growth
Growth
No Growth

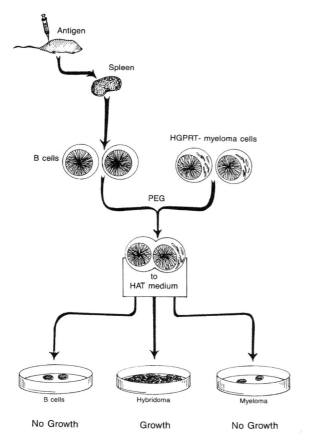

Figure 6. B lymphocyte hybridoma.

Polyclonal antibodies are multiple immunoglobulins responding to different epitopes on an antigen molecule. This multiple stimulation leads to the expansion of several antibody-forming clones whose products represent a mixture of immunoglobulins in contrast to proliferation of a single clone which would yield a homogeneous monoclonal antibody product. Thus, polyclonal antibodies represent the natural consequence of an immune response in contrast to monoclonal antibodies which occur *in vivo* in pathologic conditions such as multiple myeloma or are produced artificially by hybridoma technology against one of a variety of antigens.

The **doctrine of original antigenic sin** occurs when the immune system response against a virus to which an individual was previously exposed, such as a parental strain, is greater than it is against the immunizing agent, such as type A influenza virus variant (Figure 9). This concept is referred to as the "doctrine of original antigenic sin".

The **Brambell receptor**, named for F. W. R. Brambell, a pioneer in transmission of immunity, conserves IgG by binding to its Fc region and protects it from catabolism by lysosomes (Figure 10). The mechanism of binding is pH dependent. In the endosomes' low pH, the receptor FcRB binds to IgG. IgG is then transported to the luminal surface of the catabolic cell, where the neutral pH mediates release of the bound IgG (Figures 11 and 12). **Half life ($T_{1/2}$)** is the time required for a substance to be diminished to one half of its previous serum level by degradation or decay; by catabolism, as in biological half-life; or by elimination. In

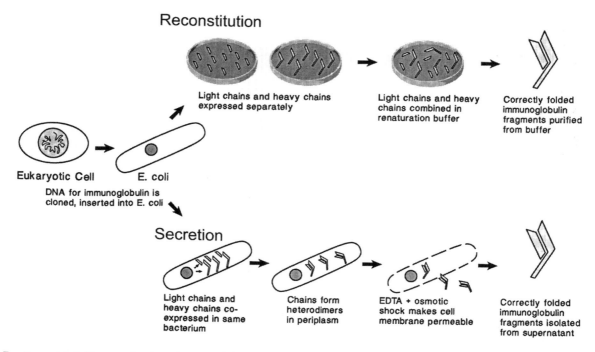

Figure 7. Beyond hybridoma technology, immunoglobulin subunits and fragments have been produced using cloned DNA expressed in bacteria.

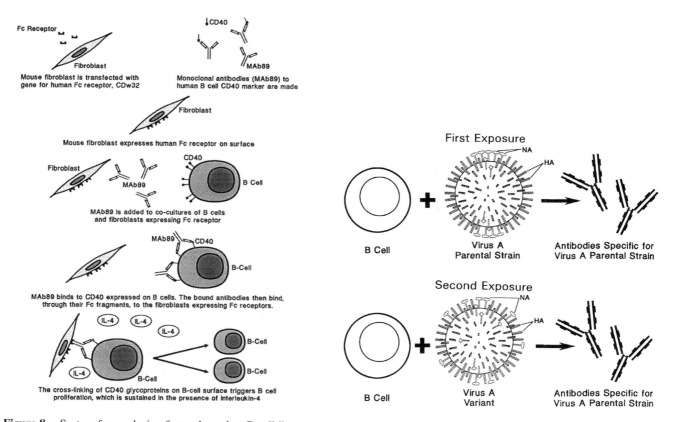

Figure 8. System for producing factor-dependent B cell lines.

Figure 9. Doctrine of original antigenic sin.

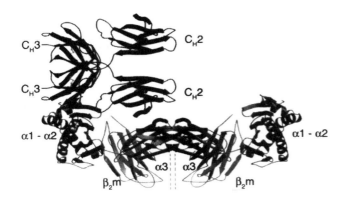

Figure 10.   Brambell receptor.

Low IgG

High IgG

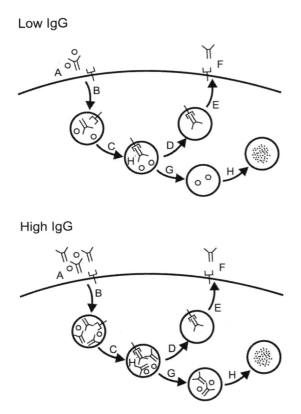

Figure 11.   Mechanism of γ-globulin protection from catabolism. IgG (Y) and plasma proteins (o) (A) are internalized into endosomes of endothelium (B), without prior binding. In the low pH (H⁺) of the endosome (C)), binding of IgG is promoted. (D, E, F) IgG retained by receptor recycles to the cell surface and dissociates in the neutral pH of the extracellular fluid, returning to circulation . (G,H). Unbound proteins are shunted to the lysosomes for degradation. With "low IgG," receptor efficiently "rescues" IgG from catabolism. With "high IgG," receptor is saturated and excess IgG passes to catabolism for a net acceleration of IgG catabolism.

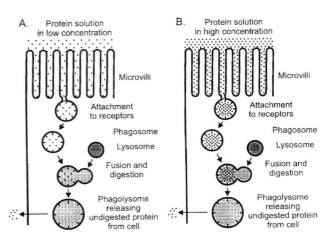

Figure 12.   Mechanism of γ-globulin transmission by the cell. (A) Concentration of γ-globulin is only a little more than sufficient to saturate the receptors and the proportion degraded is less than 40%. (B) Concentration is about four times that in (A) and hence over 80% is degraded. The amount released from the cell remains constant, irrespective of concentration.

immunology, $T_{1/2}$ refers to the time in which an immunoglobulin remains in the blood circulation. For IgG, the half life is 20 to 25 days; for IgA, 6 days; for IgM, 5 days; for IgD, two to eight days; and for IgE, one to five days. **Antibody-half life** is the mean survival of any particular antibody molecule after its formation. It refers to the time required to rid the body of one half of a known amount of antibody. Thus, antibody half-life differs according to the immunoglobulin family to which the antibody belongs. **Fractional catabolic rate** is the total immunoglobulin percentage that is catabolized each day, predicted from the half-life of plasma or from the excretion rate of catabolized immunoglobulin products in urine. IgG has the lowest catabolic rate of 8–20% per day while IgE has the highest catabolic rate of 74% per day.

Avidity refers to the strength of binding between an antibody and its specific antigen (Figure 13). The stability of this union is a reflection of the number of shared binding sites. Avidity is the binding force or intensity between multivalent antigen and multivalent antibody. Multiple binding sites on

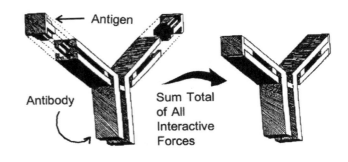

Figure 13.   Avidity.

both the antigen and the antibody, e.g., IgM, multiple antibodies interacting with various epitopes on the antigen, and reactions of high affinity between each of the antigens and its homologous antibody, all increase the avidity. Such nonspecific factors as ionic and hydrophobic interactions also increase avidity. Whereas affinity is described in thermodynamic terms, avidity is not, since it is described according to the assay procedure employed. The sum of the forces contributing to the avidity of an antigen and antibody interaction may be greater than the strength of binding of the individual antibody-antigen combinations contributing to the overall avidity of a particular interaction. K_a, the association constant for Ab+Ag = AbAg interaction, is frequently used to indicate avidity.

Antibody affinity is the force of one antibody molecule's paratope with its homologous epitope on the antigen molecule (Figure 14). It is a consequence of positive and negative portions affecting these molecular interactions.

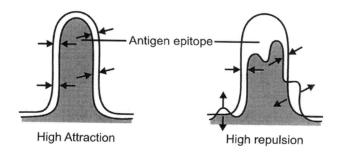

Figure 14. Antibody affinity.

Affinity maturation refers to the sustained increase in affinity of antibodies for antigen with time following immunization (Figure 15). The genes encoding the antibody variable regions undergo somatic hypermutation with the selection of B lymphocytes whose receptors express high affinity for antigen. The IgG antibodies that form following the early heterogeneous IgM response manifest greater specificity and less heterogeneity than do the IgM molecules.

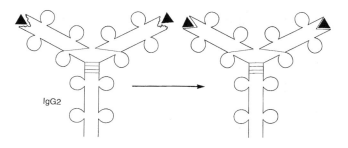

Figure 15. Affinity maturation.

Hybrid antibody is an immunoglobulin molecule with two antigen binding sites of different specificity, that may be prepared artificially, but never occurs in nature (Figure 16).

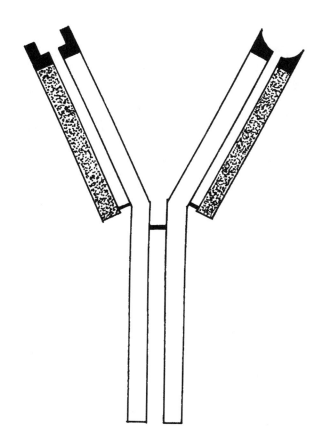

Figure 16. Hybrid antibody.

If whole IgG molecules or the F(ab′)₂ fragments prepared from them are subjected to mild reduction, the central disulfide bond is converted to sulfhydryl groups. A preparation of half molecules or Fab′ fragments is produced. If either of these is reoxidized, hybrid molecules will constitute some of the products. These can be purified by passing over immunoadsorbents containing bound antigen of the appropriate specificity. Hybrid antibodies are monovalent and do not induce precipitation. They can be used to label cell surface antigens in which one antigen-binding site of the molecule is specific for cell surface epitopes, and the other combines with a marker that renders the reaction product visible. **Bispecific antibodies** are molecules that have two separate antigen-binding specificities. They may be produced by either cell fusion or chemical techniques. An immunoglobulin molecule in which one of two antigen-binding sites is specific for one antigen-binding specificity, whereas the other antigen-binding site is specific for a different antigen specificity. This never occurs in nature, but it can be produced in vitro by treating two separate antibody specificities with mild reducing agents converting the central disulfide bonds of both antibody molecules to sulfhydryl groups, mixing the two specificities of half molecules together, and allowing them to reoxidize to form whole molecules, some of which will be bispecific.

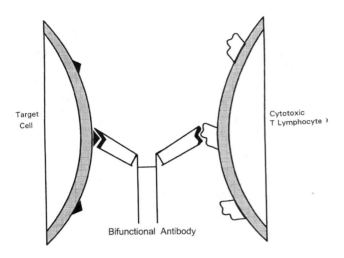

Figure 17.   Bifunctional antibody.

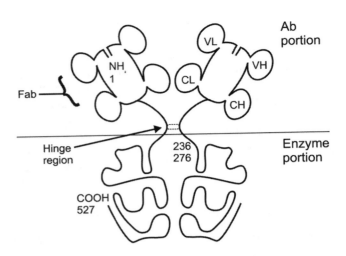

Figure 18.   Abzyme. (59D8-tPA)

A **bifunctional antibody** is an immunoglobulin molecule in which the Fab variable regions have different antigen binding specificities (Figure 17).

An **abzyme** is the union of antibody and enzyme molecules to form a hybrid catalytic molecule (Figure 18). Specificity for a target antigen is provided through the antibody portion, and catalytic function is provided through the enzyme portion. Thus, these molecules have numerous potential uses

such as catalyzing various chemical reactions, and may show great promise as protein-clearing antibodies, as in the dissolution of fibrin clots from occluded coronary arteries in myocardial infarction.

Designer antibody is a genetically engineered immunoglobulin needed for a specific purpose (Figure 19). The term has been used to refer to chimeric antibodies produced by linking mouse gene segments that encode the constant region

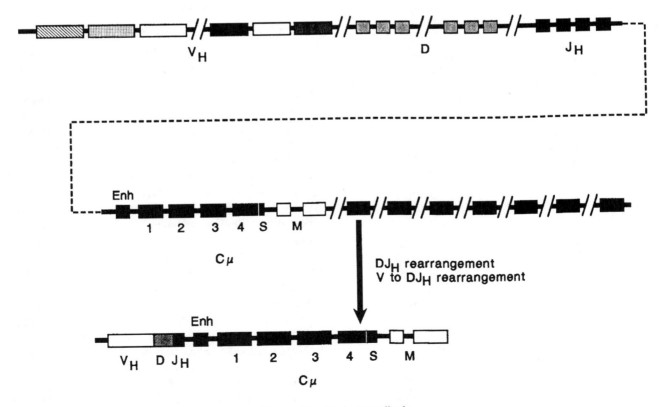

Figure 19.   Designer antibody.

of a human immunoglobulin. This technique provides the antigen specificity obtained from the mouse antibody, while substituting the less immunogenic Fc region of the molecule from a human source. This greatly diminishes the likelihood of an immune response in humans receiving the hybrid immunoglobulin molecules, since most of the mouse immunoglobulin Fc region epitopes have been eliminated through the human Fc substitution.

Passive immunization describes the transfer of specific antibody or sensitized lymphoid cells from an immune to a previously nonimmune recipient host (Figure 20). Unlike active immunity, which may be of relatively long duration, passive immunity is relatively brief and lasts only until the injected immunoglobulin or lymphoid cells have disappeared. Examples of passive immunization include: (1) the administration of gammaglobulin to immunodeficient individuals, and (2) the transfer of immunity from mother to young, i.e., antibodies across the placenta or the ingestion of colostrum containing antibodies.

Antibody feedback (Figure 21) is the negative feedback system whereby antigen-specific antibodies downregulate further immune responses to that antigen. Several mechanisms may be responsible for this, including:

1. Removal of the initiating stimulus by the antibody.
2. Binding of antigen/IgG antibody immune complexes to the Fcγ receptor of B cells.
3. Inhibition of T cell responses by antigen/antibody complexes.

The use of Rh immune globulin to prevent erythroblastosis fetalis in the infants of Rh negative mothers is an example of antibody feedback.

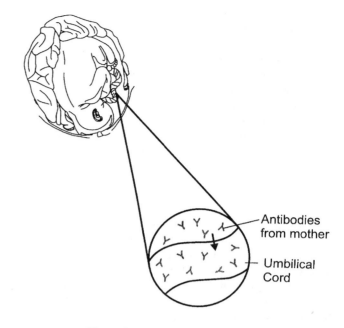

Figure 20. Passive immunization.

An **antiidiotypic antibody** is an antibody that interacts with antigenic determinants (idiotopes) at the variable N-terminus of the heavy and light chains comprising the paratope region of an antibody molecule where the antigen-binding site is located. The idiotope antigenic determinants may be situated either within the cleft of the antigen-binding region or on the periphery or outer edge of the variable region of heavy and light chain components.

An **antiidiotypic vaccine** is an immunizing preparation of antiidiotypic antibodies that are internal images of certain exogenous antigens. To develop an effective antiidiotypic vaccine, epitopes of an infectious agent that induce protective

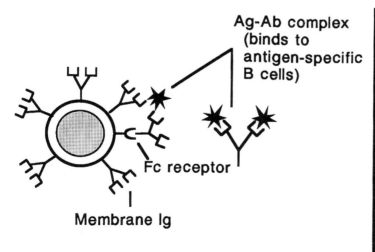
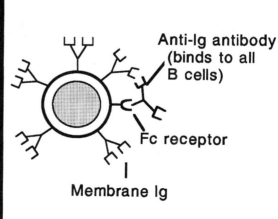

Figure 21. Antibody feedback.

immunity must be identified. Antibodies must be identified which confer passive immunity to this agent. An antiidiotypic antibody prepared using these protective antibodies as the immunogen, in some instances, can be used as an effective vaccine. Antiidiotypic vaccines have effectively induced protective immunity against such viruses as rabies, coronavirus, cytomegalovirus, and hepatitis B; such bacteria as *Listeria monocytogenes, Escherichia coli,* and *Streptococcus pneumoniae;* and such parasites as *Schistosoma mansoni* infections. Antiidiotypic vaccination is especially desirable when a recombinant vaccine is not feasible. Monoclonal antiidiotypic vaccines represent a uniform and reproducible source for an immunizing preparation.

A **blocking antibody** (Figure 22) is (1) An incomplete IgG antibody that, when diluted, may combine with red blood cell surface antigens and inhibit agglutination reactions used for erythrocyte antigen identification. This can lead to errors in blood grouping for Rh, K and k blood types. Pretreatment of red cells with enzymes may correct the problem; (2) An IgG antibody specifically induced by exposure of allergic subjects to specific allergens to which they are sensitive, in a form that favors IgG rather than IgE production. The IgG specific for the allergens to which they are sensitized, competes within IgE molecules bound to mast cell surfaces, thereby preventing their degranulation and inhibiting a type I hypersensitivity response; (3) A specific immunoglobulin molecule that may inhibit the combination of a competing antibody molecule with a particular epitope. Blocking antibodies may also interfere with the union of T cell receptors with an epitope for which they are specific, as occurs in some tumor-bearing patients with blocking antibodies that may inhibit the tumoricidal action of cytotoxic T lymphocytes.

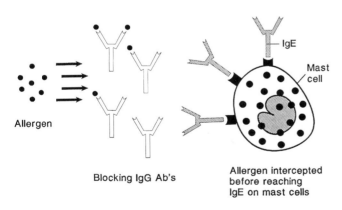

Figure 22.   Blocking antibody.

Monogamous bivalency is the binding of a bivalent antibody molecule such as IgG, with two identical antigenic determinants or epitopes on the same antigen molecule, in contrast to each Fab region of the IgG molecule uniting with an identical antigenic determinant on two separate antigen

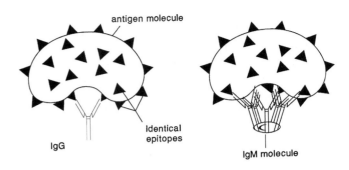

Figure 23.   Monogamous bivalency and monogamous multivalency.

molecules (Figure 23). For this monogamous binding to take place, the epitopes must be positioned on the surface of the antigen molecule in such a manner that the binding of one Fab region to an epitope can position the remaining Fab of the IgG molecule for easy interaction with an adjacent identical epitope. Interaction of this type represents high affinity of binding, which lends a stability to the antigen-antibody complex. The combination of one IgM molecule to multiple epitopes on a single molecule of antigen would represent **monogamous multivalency**.

The **Fc receptor** is a structure on the surface of some lymphocytes, macrophages or mast cells that specifically binds the Fc region of immunoglobulin, often when the Fc is aggregated. The Fc receptors for IgG are designated FcγR (Figure 24). Those for IgE are designated FcεR and those for IgA are designated FcαR (Figure 25). IgM and IgD Fc receptors have yet to be defined. Neutrophils, eosinophils, mononuclear phagocytes, B lymphocytes, selected T lymphocytes and accessory cells bear Fc receptors for IgG on their surfaces. When the Fc region of immunoglobulin binds to the cation permease Fc receptor, there is an influx of Na^+ or K^+ that activates phagocytosis, H_2O_2 formation and cell movement by macrophages. **Fc receptors** are found on 95% of human peripheral blood T lymphocytes. On about 75%

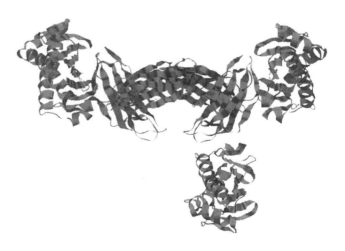

Figure 24.   Fc (IgG) receptor (neonatal).

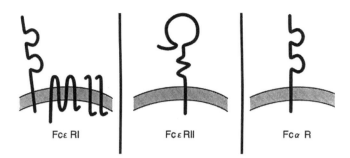

Figure 25. Fcα and Fcε receptors.

of the cells, the FcR are specific for IgM; the remaining 20% are specific for IgG. The FcR-bearing T cells are also designated T_M and T_G or Tμ and Tγ. The T_M cells act as helpers in B cell function. They are required for the B cell responses to pokeweed mitogen (PWM). In cultures of B cells with PWM, the T_M cells also proliferate, supporting the views on their helper effects. Binding of IgM to FcR of T_M cells is not a prerequisite for helper activity. In contrast to T_M cells, the T_G cells effectively suppress B cell differentiation. They act on the T_M cells, and their suppressive effect requires prior binding of their Fc-IgG receptors by IgG immune complexes. There are a number of other differences between T_M and T_G cells. Circulating T_G cells may be present in increased number, often accompanied by a reduction in the circulating number of T_M cells. Increased numbers of T_G cells are seen in cord blood and in some patients with hypogammaglobulinemia, sex-linked agammaglobulinemia, IgA deficiency, Hodgkin's disease and thymoma, to mention only a few.

Fcγ receptors (FcγR) are receptors for the Fc region of IgG (Figure 26). B and T lymphocytes, natural killer cells, polymorphonuclear leukocytes, mononuclear phagocytes and platelets contain FcγR. When these receptors bind immune complexes, the cell may produce leukotrienes, prostaglandins, modulate antibody synthesis, increase consumption of oxygen, activate oxygen metabolites and become phagocytic. The three types of Fcγ receptors include FcγRI, FcγRII (CD32), and FcγRIII (CD16). FcγRI represents a high-affinity receptor found on mononuclear phagocytes. In humans,

it binds IgG1 and IgG3. FcγRII and FcγRIII represent low-affinity IgG receptors. In humans, neutrophils, monocytes, eosinophils, platelets and B lymphocytes express FcγRII on their membranes. Neutrophils, natural killer cells, eosinophils, macrophages, and selected T lymphocytes express FcγRIII on their membranes and bind IgG1 and IgG3. Paroxysmal nocturnal hemoglobulinuria patients have deficient FcγRIII on their neutrophil membranes.

Fcε receptor (FcεR) is a receptor on mast cells and selected leukocytes for the Fc region of IgE. When immune complexes bind to Fcε receptors, the cell may respond by releasing the mediators of immediate hypersensitivity such as histamine and serotonin. Modulation of antibody synthesis may also occur. There are two varieties of Fcε receptors, designated FcεRI and FcεRII (CD23) (Figures 27 and 28). FcεRI represents a high-affinity receptor found on mast cells

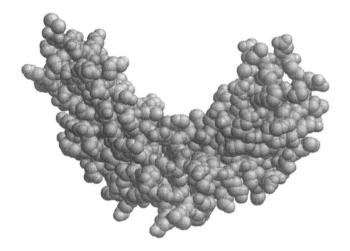

Figure 27. FcεRI.

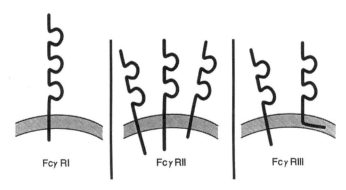

Figure 26. Fcγ receptors.

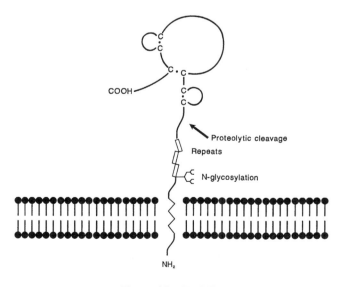

Figure 28. FcεRII.

and basophils. It anchors monomeric IgE to the cell surface. It possesses 1α, 1β and 2γ chains. FcεRII represents a low-affinity receptor. It is found on mononuclear phagocytes, B lymphocytes, eosinophils and platelets. Subjects with increased IgE in the serum have elevated numbers of FcεRII on their cells. It is a 321 amino acid single polypeptide chain that is homologous with asialoglycoprotein receptor.

The **polyimmunoglobulin receptor** is an attachment site for polymeric immunoglobulins located on epithelial cell and hepatocyte surfaces that facilitate polymeric IgA and IgM transcytosis to the secretions. After binding, the receptor-immunoglobulin complex is endocytosed and enclosed within vesicles for transport. Exocytosis takes place at the cell surface where the immunoglobulin is discharged into the intestinal lumen. A similar mechanism in the liver facilitates IgA transport into the bile. The receptor segment that is bound to the polymeric immunoglobulin is known as the secretory component which can only be used once in the transport process. A **genome** consists of all genetic information that is contained in a cell or in a gamete. **Genomic DNA** is the DNA found in the chromosomes. The **genetic code** includes the codons, i.e., nucleotide triplets, correlating with amino acid residues in protein synthesis. The nucleotide linear sequence in mRNA is translated into the amino acid

residue sequence. **Gene mapping** refers to gene localization or gene order. Gene localization can be in relationship to other genes or to a chromosomal band. The term may also refer to the ordering of gene segments.

Immunoglobulin genes encode heavy and light polypeptide chains of antibody molecules and are found on different chromosomes, i.e., chromosome 14 for heavy chain, chromosome 2 for κ light chain and chromosome 22 for λ light chain (Figures 29 and 30). The DNA of the majority of cells does not contain one gene that encodes a complete immunoglobulin heavy or light polypeptide chain. Separate gene segments that are widely distributed in somatic cells and germ cells come together to form these genes. In B cells, gene rearrangement leads to creation of an antibody gene that codes for a specific protein. Somatic gene rearrangement also occurs with the genes that encode T cell antigen receptors. Gene rearrangement of this type permits the great versatility of the immune system in recognizing a vast array of epitopes. Three forms of gene segments join to form an immunoglobulin light chain gene. The three types include light chain variable region (V_L), joining region (J_L), and constant region (C_L) gene segments. V_H, J_H, and C_H as well as D (diversity) gene segments assemble to encode the heavy

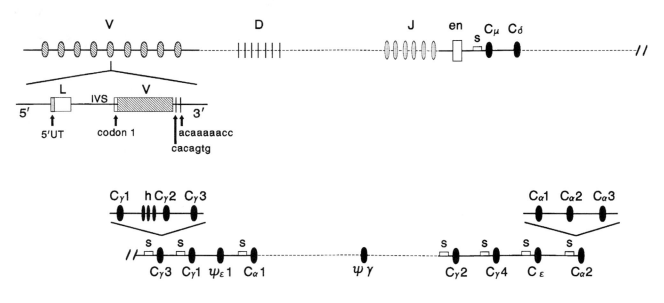

Figure 29.   Immunoglobulin gene.

Figure 30.   Mouse immunoglobulin gene

chain. Heavy and light chain genes have a closely similar organizational structure. There are 100 to 300 V_κ genes, five J_κ genes and one C_κ gene on chromosome 2's κ locus. There are 100 V_H genes, 30 D genes, six J_H genes and 11 C_H genes on chromosome 14's heavy chain locus. Several V_λ, six J_λ and six C_λ genes are present on chromosome 22's λ locus in man. V_H and V_L genes are classified as V gene families, depending on the sequence homology of their nucleotides or amino acids.

Gene diversity is the determination of the extent of an immune response to a particular antigen or immunogen as determined by mixing and matching of exons from variable, joining, diversity and constant region gene segments. S. Tonegawa received the Nobel prize for revealing the mechanism of the generation of diversity in antibody formation.

Restriction fragment length polymorphism (RFLP) is the genome diversity in DNA from different subjects revealed by restriction map comparisons. This is based on differences in restriction fragment lengths which are determined by sites of restriction endonuclease cleavage of the DNA molecules. This is revealed by preparing Southern blots using appropriate molecular hybridization probes. Polymorphisms may be demonstrated in exons, introns, flanking sequences or any DNA sequence. Variations in DNA sequence show Mendelian inheritance. Results are useful in linkage studies and can help to identify defective genes associated with inherited disease. The **gene conversion hypothesis** describes the method by which alternative sequences can be introduced into the MHC genes without reciprocal crossover events. This mechanism could account for the incredible polymorphism of alleles. The alternative sequences may include those found in the class I-like genes and pseudogenes present on chromosome 6. Hypothetically, gene conversion was an evolutionary event as well as an ongoing one, giving rise to new mutations, therefore new alleles, within a population. **Gene cloning** is the use of recombinant DNA technology to replicate genes or their fragments. **Gene bank** is a synonym for DNA library.

Isotype switching refers to the mechanism whereby a cell changes from synthesizing a heavy polypeptide chain of one isotype to that of another, as from μ chain to γ chain formation of B cells that have received a switch signal from a T cell (Figure 31). The **genetic switch hypothesis** is a concept that predicts a switch in the gene governing heavy chain synthesis by plasma cells during immune response ontogeny.

Gene rearrangement refers to genetic shuffling which results in elimination of introns and the joining of exons to produce mRNA (Figures 32–34). Gene rearrangement within a lymphocyte signifies its dedication to the formation of a single cell type, which may be immunoglobulin synthesis by B lymphocytes or production of a β chain receptor by T lymphocytes. Neoplastic transformation of lymphocytes may be followed by the expansion of a single clone of cells which

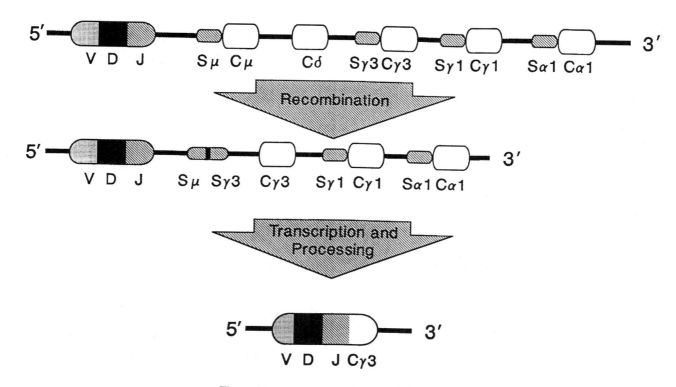

Figure 31.   Isotype switching (from IgM to IgG).

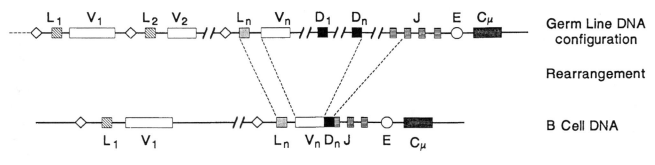

◇ = Promoter
L = Leader sequence
V = Variable region
D = Diversity regions
J = Junction regions
C = Constant region coding block
E = Enhancer sequence

Figure 32.   Immunoglobulin gene rearrangement.

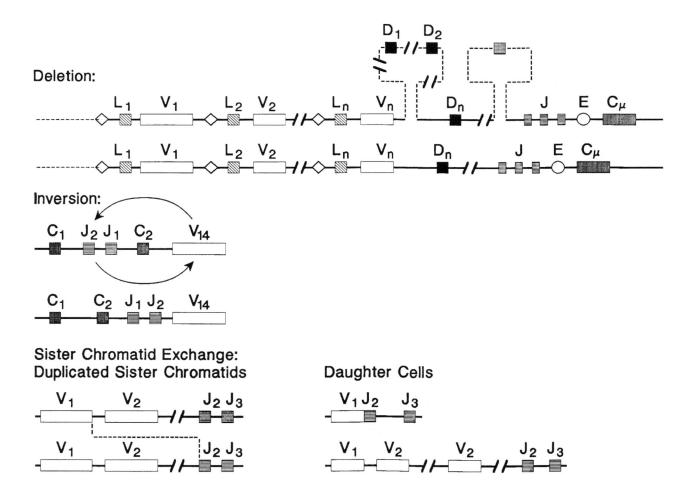

Figure 33.   Immunoglobulin gene rearrangement.

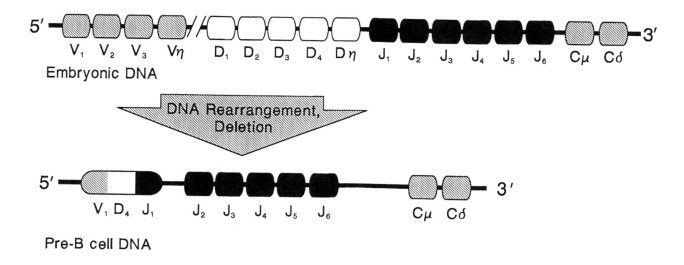

Figure 34.   Gene rearrangement.

is detectable by Southern blotting. **RNA splicing** is the method whereby RNA sequences that are nontranslatable (known as introns) are excised from the primary transcript of a split gene. The translatable sequences (known as exons) are united to produce a functional gene product.

Allelic exclusion occurs when one of two genes for which the animal is heterozygous is expressed, whereas the remaining gene is not (Figure 35). Immunoglobulin genes manifest this phenomenon. Allelic exclusion accounts for a B cell's ability to express only one immunoglobulin or a T cell's capacity to express a T cell receptor of a single specificity. Investigations of allotypes in rabbits established that individual immunoglobulin molecules have identical heavy chains and light chains. Immunoglobulin synthesizing cells produce only a single class of H chain and one type of light chain at a time. Thus, by allelic exclusion a cell that is synthesizing antibody expresses just one of two alleles encoding an immunoglobulin chain at a particular locus. **Isotypic exclusion** is the productive rearrangement of light-chain genes such as the rearrangement of the λ gene which occurs when both κ gene alleles are rearranged aberrantly.

Junctional diversity occurs when gene segments join imprecisely, the amino acid sequence may vary and affect variable region expression (Figure 36). This can alter codons at gene segment junctions. These include the V-J junction of the genes encoding immunoglobulin κ and γ light chains, the V-D, D-J, and D-D junctions of genes encoding immunoglobulin heavy chains, or the genes encoding T cell receptor β and δ chains.

D exon is a DNA sequence that encodes a portion of the immunoglobulin heavy chain's third hypervariable region (Figure 37). It is situated on the 5′ side of J exons. An intron lies between them. During lymphocyte differentiation, V-D-J sequences are produced that encode the complete variable region of the heavy chain. A **V gene** is a gene encoding the

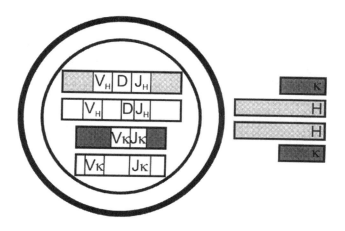

Figure 35.   Allelic exclusion.

variable region of immunoglobulin light or heavy chains. Although it is not in proximity to the C gene in germ-line DNA, the V gene lies near the 5′ end of the C gene from which it is separated by a single intron.

A **V gene segment** is a DNA segment encoding the first 95–100 amino acid residues of immunoglobulin and T cell polypeptide chain variable regions. There are two coding regions in the V gene segment which are separated by a 100–400 base pair intron. The first 5′ coding region is an exon that codes for a brief untranslated mRNA region and for the first 15–18 signal peptide residues. The second 3′ coding region is part of an exon that codes for the terminal 4 signal peptide residues and 95–100 variable region residues. A J gene segment encodes the rest of the variable region. A D gene segment is involved in the encoding of immunoglobulin heavy chains and T cell receptor β and δ chains. A **variable region** is that segment of an immunoglobulin molecule or antibody formed by the variable domain of a light

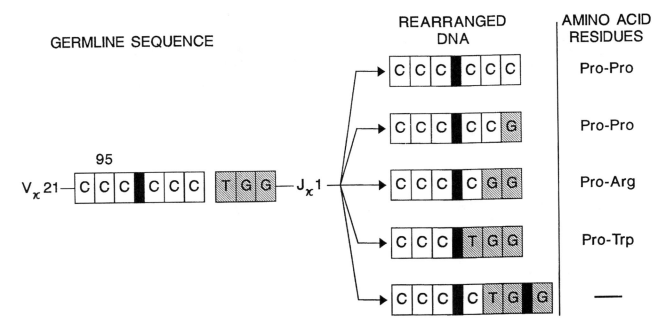

Figure 36. Junctional diversity.

Structure of Heavy Chain Gene From IgM- Producing Cell

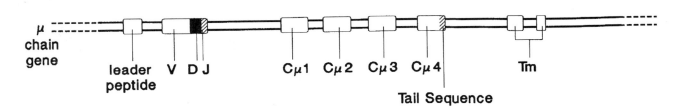

Figure 37. D exon and V segment.

polypeptide chain either κ or λ, or of a heavy polypeptide chain (α, γ, μ, δ, or ε). This is sometimes referred to as the Fv region and is encoded by the V gene.

V region subgroups are individual chain V region subdivisions based on significant homology in amino acid sequence.

Framework regions (FR) are the amino acid sequences in variable regions of heavy or light immunoglobulin chains other than the hypervariable sequences. There is much less variability in the framework region than in the hypervariable region. Two beta-pleated sheets opposing one another comprise the structural features of an antibody domain's framework regions. Polypeptide chain loops join the beta-pleated sheet strands. The framework regions contribute to the secondary and tertiary structure of the variable region domain, although they are less significant than the hypervariable regions for the antigen-binding site. The framework region forms the folding part of the immunoglobulin molecule. Light chain FRs are found at amino acid residues 1–28,

38–50, 56–89 and 97–107. Heavy chain FRs are present at amino acid residues 1–31, 35–49, 66–101, and 110–117.

Recombination activating genes RAG-1 and RAG-2 are genes that activate Ig gene recombination. Pre-B cells and immature T cells contain them. It remains to be determined whether RAG-1 and RAG-2 encode the recombinases or the regulatory proteins that control recombinase function. RAG-1 and RAG-2 gene products are requisite for rearrangements of both Ig and TCR genes. In the absence of these genes neither Ig nor T cell receptor proteins are produced. This blocks the production of mature T and B cells.

A **genotype** is an organism's genetic makeup. A **haplotype** consists of those phenotypic characteristics encoded by closely linked genes on one chromosome inherited from one parent. It frequently describes several major histocompatibility complex (MHC) alleles on a single chromosome. Selected haplotypes are in strong linkage disequilibrium between alleles of different loci. According to Mendelian genetics, 25% of siblings will share both haplotypes.

8
Antigen-Antibody Interaction

Serology is the study of the *in vitro* reaction of antibodies in blood serum with antigens, i.e., usually those of microorganisms inducing infectious disease. Precipitation, agglutination, and complement fixation are serological methods used in diagnosis and research.

Stimulation of B lymphoid cells by antigen leads to the formation of immunoglobulin molecules (antibodies) which may enter into a number of different types of immunological and chemical reactions. These have been classified into (1) primary, (2) secondary, and (3) tertiary reactions.

The **primary reaction** is the actual binding of antibody, via its Fab or antigen binding fragment, to its homologous antigen forming an antibody-antigen complex (Figure 1). After the two substances are brought into contact, their initial union takes place almost instantaneously (within millisec-

onds). **Secondary reactions** are those visible effects resulting from antibody-antigen binding such as precipitation, agglutination, flocculation, complement fixation, and so on.

Tertiary reactions, which may result from either primary or secondary interactions of antibody with antigen, include those *in vivo* biological manifestations of antibody reactivity. Some *in vitro* secondary interactions, such as cytophilic reactions (adherence of the antibody via its Fc to a cell surface) may, when occurring *in vivo*, give rise to tertiary manifestations. Because tertiary reactions occur *in vivo* they tend to be very complex and are subject to many variables.

In an immune response, antibodies are directed against specific conformational areas on the antigen molecule referred to as antigenic determinants. Antigens are macromolecules

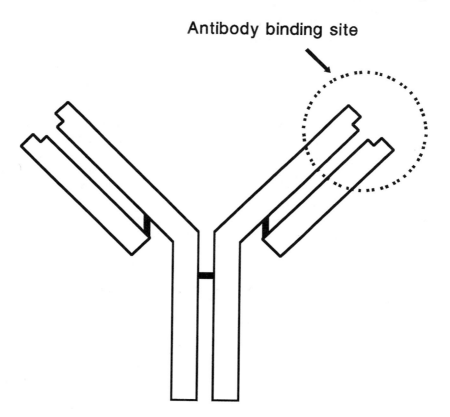

Figure 1. Antibody binding site.

which stimulate antibody production. Antibody populations directed against these macromolecules are notoriously heterogeneous with respect to their antibody specificity and affinity, since antibodies to many different antigenic determinants may be present simultaneously in the sera. Bivalent and multivalent antibodies directed against multideterminant antigens result in the formation of large antibody-antigen aggregates of the type $(Ab)_x (Ag)_y$ varying in size, complexity, and solubility.

Landsteiner devised a method whereby an immune response could be directed against small molecules of known structure. He referred to these substances as "haptens" which by themselves were too small to initiate an immune response, but were capable of reacting with the products of an immune response. He chemically coupled these "haptens" to large biological macromolecules, such as ovalbumin, which he termed carriers, producing conjugated antigens capable of stimulating an immune response. The nonvalent hapten in pure form, together with the serum antibodies, could then be used to study antibody-hapten interactions without the complications of multideterminant macromolecular antigens. These antibody populations were still heterogeneous with respect to structure, class, subclass, and so on. Isolation of monoclonal antibodies derived from the blood sera of multiple myeloma patients led to sequencing and X-ray diffraction studies on homogeneous antibody populations. Recently, hybridoma technology has provided a mechanism to produce monoclonal homogeneous antibodies *in vitro*.

The **noncovalent forces** of the antibody-antigen complex include hydrogen bonding, ionic or Coulombic bonding, Van der Waals interactions, hydrophobic bonding, and steric repulsion forces which are extremely sensitive to the distance between the interacting groups. Although charge on the antigen is not required for antigen-antibody binding, it may play a very important role in determining the stability of the antigen-antibody complex. There are discrepancies in the literature as to whether charged antigens elicit antibodies of reciprocal charge. It appears that the charge effect per se is exerted by the microenvironment of the antigen and antibody molecules (such as pH, ionic strength of solution, etc.) and not so much by the net charge of the molecules as a whole.

Ionic or **Coulombic forces** of attraction result from the interaction between oppositely charged ionic groups on the antigen and antibody molecules (Figure 2). As can be seen from the equation of Coulomb:

$$F = \frac{Q^+ Q^-}{\varepsilon r^2}$$

where ε is the dielectric constant of the medium, Q^+ and Q^- are the positive and negative charges in electrostatic units, respectively, and r is the distance between the centers of the

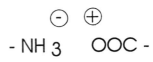

Figure 2. Electrostatic forces.

charged sites, the Coulombic force of attraction is inversely proportional to the square of the distances between antigen and antibody.

Apolar or **hydrophobic bonding** is of considerable importance in the antigen-antibody complex when it is in an aqueous environment and may contribute greatly to its stabilization. A net attractive force results from a decrease in energy is that obtained from the preference of apolar or hydrophobic regions of the interacting molecules to associate with themselves rather than with solvent molecules (H_2O). The reaction is endothermic ($\Delta H > 0$); in order for it to be spontaneous ($\Delta H < 0$) it must occur through a concomitant increase in entropy through an entropy driven reaction. This can be reviewed from the following thermodynamic relationship:

$$\Delta G = \Delta H - T\Delta S$$

where ΔG is the free energy change, ΔH is the enthalpy change, ΔS is the entropy charge, and T is the absolute temperature. When $\Delta H > 0$ (endothermic reaction) a positive ΔS is needed for an overall energy decrease ($\Delta G < 0$) resulting in the attractive force. The binding of this attractive force increases (ΔG becomes more negative) as ΔH decreases and as the temperature T increases.

Hydrogen bonds are formed between hydrogen atoms covalently linked to an electronegative atom and a second electronegative atom containing an unshared pair of electrons (Figure 3). The hydrogen atom becomes electron deficient through polarization of its electron cloud towards the electronegative atom covalently bonded to it, allowing for an electrostatic attraction to a relatively negative second electronegative atom. The contribution of hydrogen bonding to the stability of the complex is minor compared to the other forces involved and decreases with the sixth power of the distance between interaction groups.

The **Van der Waals forces** (or **London forces**) contribute somewhat to the stabilization of the antigen-antibody complex that results from attraction of oscillating dipoles of atoms and molecules moving their electrons from one side to another (Figure 4). Dispersion forces occur only when the two molecules are very close together and decrease with the sixth power of the distance between interaction sites.

The major attractive forces involved in the antigen-antibody complex have been described and are all inversely proportional to the distance between interacting groups. **Steric repulsion**, on the other hand, results in a repulsive force and

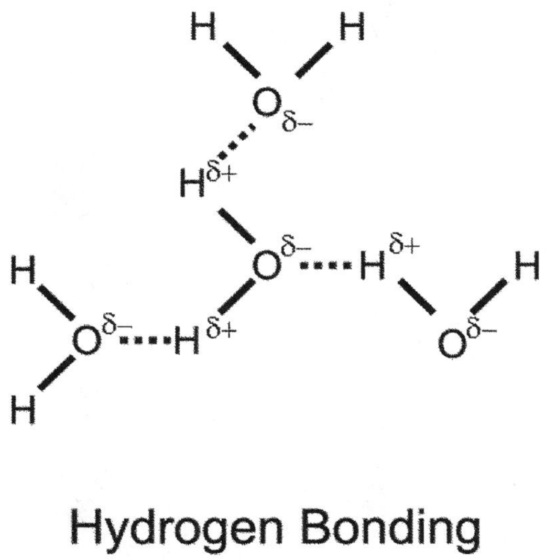

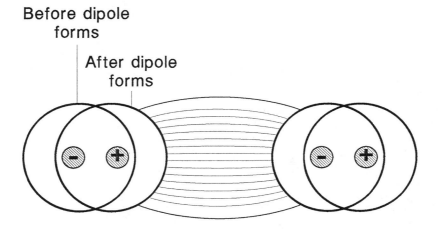

Hydrogen Bonding

Figure 3. The hydrogen bonds are shown in dotted lines.

Figure 4. Van der Waals forces.

tends to decrease the stability of the complex. This repulsive force results from the interpenetration of the electron clouds of the antigenic determinant and the antigen binding region of the antibody. When the electron clouds of the antigenic determinant and the homologous antigen binding site on the antibody molecule are not complementary, the steric repulsion between the two becomes great and decreases the stability of the complex. By contrast, when complementary electron clouds come together, steric repulsion forces are minimized. This permits a closer association between the two interacting molecules and increases the attractive forces described above, leading to formation of a stable complex. Thus, steric repulsion provides the basis for the antigenic specificity of the antigen-antibody reaction.

In summary, the forces that account for the stability of an antigen-antibody complex are the following: (1) attractive forces resulting in increased binding or stability and (2) repulsive forces resulting in decreased binding or stability (Figure 5).

The stability of the antigen-antibody complex, expressed as antibody affinity, is actually a sum of all attractive and repulsive forces acting at a given time (Figure 6).

When attractive forces exceed repulsive forces, an antigen-antibody complex may result if given sufficient time for interaction. Measurement of the quantity of complexes formed with respect to time (kinetically derived quantity) is referred to as avidity. Avidity may be measured by determining the

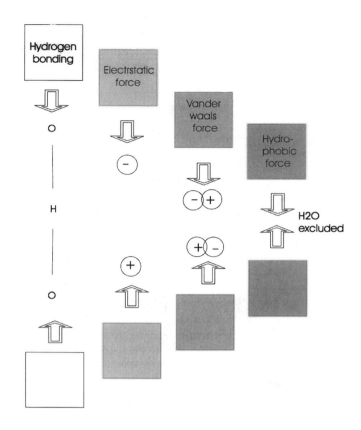

Figure 5. Attractive forces binding antigen to antibody.

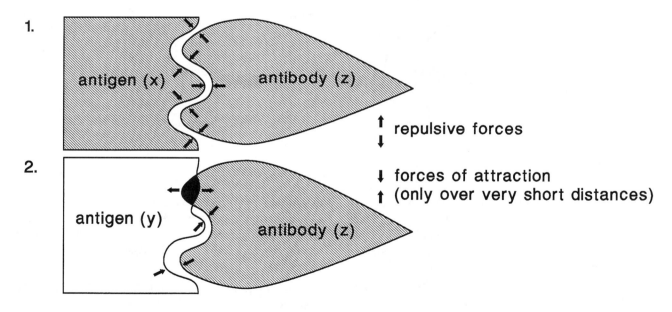

Figure 6. Antibody affinity.

time it takes for a given amount of radiolabeled antigen to dissociate from antibody. Differences in avidity of various antisera can be seen from a comparison of their precipitation curves (Figure 7).

In order for the classical laws of thermodynamics to apply, the following two assumptions must be made: (1) the reactants, both antigen and antibody, must be pure and in solution and (2) the reactants must be homogeneous with regard to

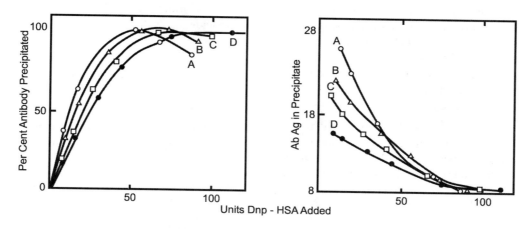

Figure 7. Precipitation curves showing differences in avidity of four antisera for the same antigen. The order of avidity of the sera is A>B>C>D.

antigen binding sites and antigenic determinants. Though antibodies are extremely heterogeneous with respect to structure as well as multivalent with respect to antigen binding sites, measurements can be performed when purified antibodies to define monovalent haptens are used.

Using univalent haptens (H) and antibodies (Ab), the elementary reversible antibody-hapten reaction that gives rise to complexes of the AbH can be written as follows:

$$Ab + H \underset{k_r}{\overset{k_f}{\rightleftharpoons}} AbH$$

where k_f is the rate constant for the association reaction and k_r is the rate constant for the dissociation reaction, assuming that all antibody binding sites are identical and independent of each other. By applying the law of mass action, the equilibrium constant K, also called antibody affinity for reaction can be derived as follows:

$$k_f[Ab][H] = k_r[AbH]$$

$$K = \frac{k_f}{k_r} = \frac{[AbH]}{[Ab][H]}$$

where [Ab], [H], [AbH] are the free antibody concentration, free hapten concentration, and the antibody-hapten complex concentration (or the concentration of bound hapten or antibody sites occupied), respectively. Standard free energy change $\Delta G°$ for the association reaction of hapten and antibody is related to the equilibrium constant K by the following:

$$\Delta G° = -RT \ln K$$

where R is the gas constant and T the temperature in degrees Kelvin. Affinity is a thermodynamically derived quantity which may be expressed by either K, which becomes more positive as affinity increases, or $\Delta G°$, which becomes more negative as affinity increases. Antibody affinity may be interpreted as measuring either (1) the strength of binding of the antibody to its homologous antigenic determinant or (2) the stability of the hapten-antibody complex. Avidity is really a measure of the "stickiness" of antibody toward hapten and is not, in actuality, a thermodynamically derived quantity as is affinity.

Having calculated the equilibrium constant, or antibody affinity K, standard enthalpy change $\Delta H°$ for the reaction can be calculated from the Van't Hoff equation which expresses the change in K as a function of T.

$$\frac{d(\ln K)}{dT} = \frac{-\Delta H°}{RT^2}$$

Integration of equation 4 from T_1 to T_2 gives:

$$\int_{T_1}^{T_2} d(\ln K) = \int_{T_1}^{T_2} \frac{-\Delta H°}{RT^2} dT$$

which yields:

$$\ln \frac{K_2}{K_1} = \frac{\Delta H°}{R} \frac{(T_2 - T_1)}{(T_2 T_1)}$$

where K_2 and K_1 are the equilibrium constants at T_2 and T_1 respectively. Algebraic rearrangement gives the following expression for $\Delta H°$:

$$\Delta H° = \frac{\ln K_2 - \ln K_1}{\frac{1}{T_1} - \frac{1}{T_2}}$$

Application of the Langmuir adsorption isotherm equation to antibody-hapten reactions has been shown to be useful in affinity measurements as well as in calculations of antibody valency. In an antibody-hapten solution where [H] is the concentration of free hapten, let d equal the fraction of antigen binding sites occupied and (1-d) equal the fraction of available antigen binding sites.

Since the rate of reaction is directly proportional to the number of available antigen binding sites, the rate of the forward reaction, rate f, and the rate of the reverse reaction, rate r, at a given temperature T may be written as follows:

$$\text{rate f} = K_f(1-d)[H]$$

$$\text{rate r} = K_r(d)$$

At equilibrium the forward and reverse rates are equal, therefore,

$$\text{rate f} = \text{rate r}$$
$$K_f(1-d)[H] = K_r(d) \tag{1}$$

Solving for d gives the Langmuir adsorption isotherm equation as applied to the antigen-hapten reaction for univalent antibody and hapten:

$$d = \frac{K[H]}{1+K[H]} \tag{2}$$

For antibody of valency n, the following also can be shown:

$$\frac{d}{n} = \frac{K[H]}{1+K[H]} \tag{3}$$

Algebraic rearrangement of the Langmuir adsorption isotherm yields the Scatchard Equation (4)

$$\frac{d}{[Ag]} = nK - dK \tag{4}$$

from which a plot of d/[Ag] vs. d for the ideal antibody-hapten system over a range of free hapten concentrations [H] gives a straight line with slope –K (Figure 8).

Extrapolation to the x-axis gives antibody valency n. The Scatchard plot allows for the calculation of antibody affinity and valency from the concentration of antigen and antigen-antibody complex. It can be shown from the Scatchard equation that when half the antigen binding sites in bivalent antibody (n = 2) are hapten bound (d = 1), K is equal to 1/[Ag].

$$K_0 = 2K - K = \frac{1}{[H]} \tag{5}$$

The average intrinsic association constant K_0 is thus defined as the reciprocal of free hapten concentration at equilibrium when half of the antigen binding sites on antibody molecules are bound by hapten.

Another method for obtaining antibody affinity and valency is the Langmuir plot using the following rearrangement of equation 3

$$\frac{1}{d} = \frac{1}{n} \cdot \frac{1}{[H]} \cdot \frac{1}{K} + \frac{1}{n} \tag{6}$$

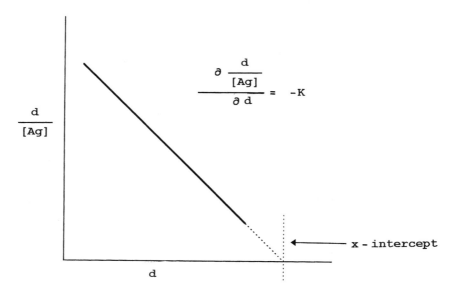

Figure 8.   Scatchard plot.

A plot of 1/d vs. reciprocal hapten concentration, the Langmuir plot, results in a slope of 1/nK and y-intercept of 1/n (Figure 9).

The following method may also be employed for calculation of antibody affinity which only requires the measurement of free and bound hapten concentrations. This is done by solving equation 3 with respect to the antibody-hapten complex. In the following derivation, [AbH] is the hapten-antibody complex concentration or the concentration of bound antibody combining sites and $[Ab_t]$ is the concentration of total antibody combining sites.

$$\frac{d}{n} = \frac{K[H]}{1 + K[H]} \tag{7}$$

then becomes

$$\frac{[AbH]}{[Ab_t]} = \frac{K[H]}{1 + K[H]} \tag{8}$$

Rearrangement to a more suitable form for plotting gives

$$\frac{1}{[AbH]} = \frac{1}{[Ab_t]K[H]} + \frac{1}{[Ab_t]} \tag{9}$$

A plot of 1/[AbH] vs. 1/[H] gives a line with a y-intercept of $1[Ab_t]$ and slope for $1/K[Ab_t]$. Thus antibody affinity is equal to the product of the y-intercept and the reciprocal of the slope (Figure 10).

Both the Scatchard and Langmuir plots theoretically give rise to linear relationships when applied to ideal antigen-antibody reactions. In reality, however, the plots may deviate considerably from linearity due to the heterogeneity of antibody affinities within an antibody population. Antibody heterogeneity has long been known and was originally described in terms of the Gaussian distribution function by Heidelberger and Kendall in 1935. A more modern approach to quantification of this affinity distribution uses the logarithmic transformation of the Sipsian distribution function,

$$\log \frac{d}{n-d} = a \log K_0 + a \log[Ag]$$

where d represents the moles of antigen or hapten bound per mole of antibody, k_0 the average intrinsic association constant, and a the index of heterogeneity. A plot of log d/(n-d) vs. log[Ag] yields a line of slope a (Figure 11).

The antibody population approaches homogeneity with respect to K as the heterogeneity index approaches unity. In addition, K_0 can be obtained from the graph by extrapolation, since K_0 is equal to 1/[Ag] when the log d/(n-d) is equal to 0 and represents the peak of the distribution.

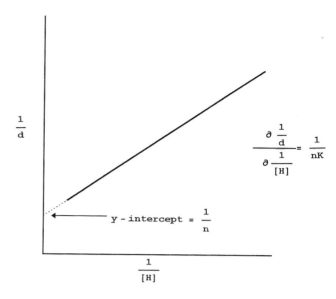

Figure 9. Langmuir Plot.

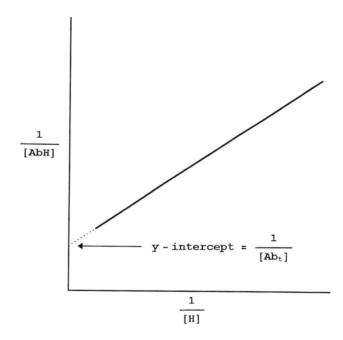

Figure 10. Modification of Langmuir plot.

Actual data can be obtained in the lab. An adequate means of measuring such quantities as bound and unbound hapten concentrations must be available for calculations. The following three methods have been popular in the study of primary interaction between antibody and antigen.

Equilibrium dialysis was developed for the study of primary antibody-hapten interactions (Figure 12). The basis for the technique is as follows. Two cells are separated by a semipermeable membrane allowing free passage of hapten

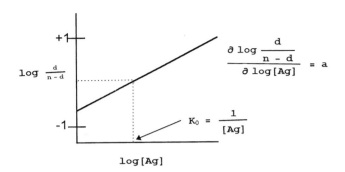

Figure 11. Plot of Sipsian distribution function.

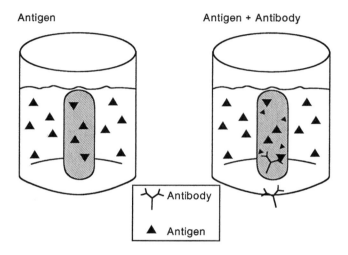

Figure 12. Equilibrium dialysis.

molecules but not larger antibody molecules. At time zero (t_0), there is a known concentration of hapten in cell A and antibody in cell B. Hapten from cell A diffuses across the membrane into cell B until, at equilibrium, the concentration of free hapten is the same in both cells A and B; that is, the rate of diffusion of hapten from cell A to B is the same as that from cell B to A. Though the concentrations of free hapten are the same in both cells, the total amount of hapten in cell B is greater because some of the hapten is bound to the antibody molecules. In order to obtain d and [H], a series of experiments are performed which varies the starting amount of hapten concentration while keeping antibody concentration constant.

The **ammonium sulfate method** is a means of measuring the primary antigen-binding capacity of antisera and detects both precipitating and nonprecipitating antibodies. It offers an advantage over equilibrium dialysis in that large, nondializable protein antigens may be used. This assay is based on the principle that certain proteins are soluble in 50% saturated ammonium sulfate, whereas antigen-antibody complexes are not. Complexes may be separated from unbound antigen. Spontaneous precipitation will occur if precipitating-type antibody is used, until a point of antigen excess is reached where complex aggregation no longer occurs and soluble complexes form. Upon the addition of an equal volume of saturated ammonium sulfate solution (SAS), these complexes become insoluble leaving radiolabeled antigen in solution. SAS fractionation does not significantly alter the stoichiometry of the antibody-antigen reaction and inhibits the release or exchange of bound antigen. The radioactivity of this "induced" precipitate is a measure of the antigen-binding capacity of the antisera as opposed to a measure of the amount of antigen or antibody spontaneously precipitated.

Fluorescence quenching is a method used to ascertain association constants of antibody molecules interacting with ligands. Fluorescence quenching results from excitation energy transfer where certain electronically excited residues in protein molecules, such as tryptophan and tyrosine, transfer energy to a second molecule that is bound to the protein. Maximum emission is a wavelength of approximately 345 nm. The attachment of the acceptor molecule need not be covalent. This transfer of energy occurs when the absorbance spectrum of the acceptor molecule overlaps with that of the emission spectrum of the donor and takes place via resonance interaction (Figure 13).

There is no need for direct contact between the two molecules for energy transfer. If the acceptor molecule is nonfluorescent, diminution of energy occurs through non-radiation processes. On the other hand, if the acceptor molecule is fluorescent, the transfer of radiation results in its own fluorescence (sensitized fluorescence). Fluorescence quenching techniques can provide very sensitive quantitative data on antibody-hapten interactions.

Following the union of soluble macromolecular antigen with homologous antibody in the presence of electrolytes *in vitro* or *in vivo*, complexes of increasing density form within seconds after contact, in a lattice arrangement and settle out of solution as the **precipitation** or **precipitation reaction**. The materials needed for a precipitation reaction include antigen, antibody, and electrolyte. The reaction of soluble antigen and antibody in the precipitation test may be observed in liquid or in gel media. The reaction in liquid media may be qualitative or quantitative. Following the discovery of the precipitation reaction by Kraus in 1897, only qualitative and semiquantitative measurement of precipitate could be made. The term precipitinogen sometimes is used to designate the antigen and precipitin is the antibody in a precipitation reaction.

The **ring precipitation test** is a qualitative precipitin test used for more than a century, in which soluble antigen (or antibody) is layered onto an antibody (or antigen) solution in a serological or capillary tube without agitating or mixing the two layers. If the antigen and antibody are specific for one another, a ring of precipitate will form at the interface.

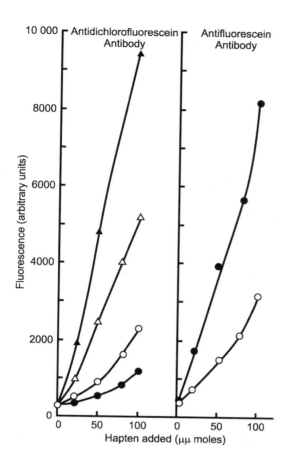

Quenching of Fluorescein (○) and Di-chlorofluorescein (●) Fluorescence by Homologous and Cross-reacting Rabbit Antibody. Dichloro-fluorescein (▲) and Fluorescein Fluorescence (△) in Buffer Alone Are Shown in the Left-hand Figure.

Figure 13. Titration curves using fluorescence quenching.

This simple technique was among the first antigen-antibody tests performed (Figure 14).

Quantitative precipitin reaction is an immunochemical assay based on the formation of an antigen-antibody precipitate

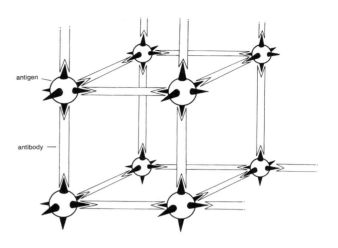

Figure 14. Precipition test.

in serial dilutions of the reactants, permitting combination of antigen and antibody in various proportions. The ratio of antibody to antigen is graded sequentially from one tube to the next. The optimal proportion of antigen and antibody present in the tube shows the most rapid flocculation and yields the greatest amount of precipitate. After washing, the precipitate can be analyzed for protein content through such procedures as the micro-Kjeldahl analysis to ascertain nitrogen content, spectrophotometric assay or other techniques. Heidelberger and Kendall used the technique extensively, employing pneumococcus polysaccharide antigen and precipitating antibody to show that nitrogen determinations reflected a quantitative measure of antibody content. The classic precipitin reaction may be illustrated using the serum of a rabbit immunized with egg albumin (Figure 15).

In this technique, a constant volume and concentration of rabbit antibody is placed in a row of serological tubes. Varying amounts of the egg albumin antigen are added and the tubes incubated. Let's say there is no precipitate in tube 1, a slight quantity in tube 2, a heavy amount in tubes 3, 4, 5, a slight quantity in tube 6 and none in tube 7. All tubes are centrifuged and the supernatants tested for both unreacted antigen and antibody. There is excess antigen but no free

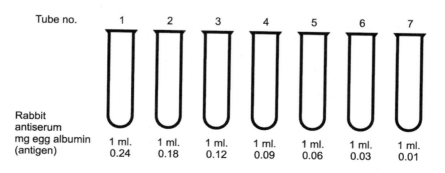

Tube no.	1	2	3	4	5	6	7
Rabbit antiserum mg egg albumin (antigen)	1 ml. 0.24	1 ml. 0.18	1 ml. 0.12	1 ml. 0.09	1 ml. 0.06	1 ml. 0.03	1 ml. 0.01

Figure 15. Precipitation reaction in liquid media.

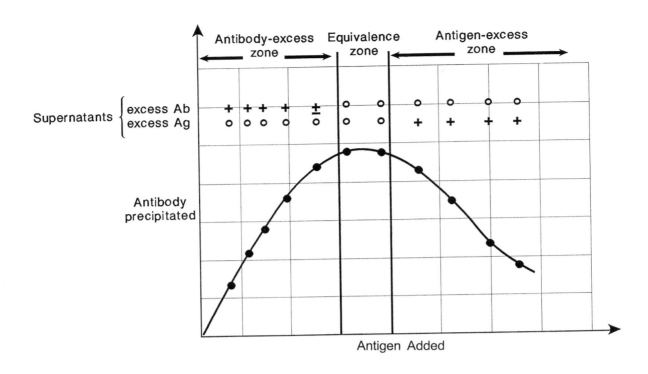

Figure 16. Precipitation curve.

antibody in tubes 1, 2, and 3. In the supernatant of tube 4 there is neither antigen nor antibody, therefore this tube is called the equivalence tube, where antigen and antibody are in identical proportions and completely reacted. In the supernatants of tubes 5, 6 and 7 there is antibody but no antigen. Why was there no precipitate in tubes 1 and 7? Both tubes contained antigen as well as antibody which reacted but did not form aggregates large enough to precipitate out of solution. Therefore, an excess of either antigen or antibody may inhibit precipitation, particularly an excess of antigen.

Milligrams of antibody in the precipitate are plotted on the ordinate and the milligrams of antigen added are plotted on the abscissa of a graph (Figure 16). The **precipitin curve** contains an ascending and a descending limb and zones of antibody excess, equivalence, and antigen excess. By testing with the homologous reagents, unreacted antibodies and antigens can be detected in the supernatants. If antigen is homogeneous, or if antibodies specific for only one of a mixture of antigens are studied by the precipitin reaction, then none of the supernatants contain both unreacted antibodies and unreacted antigens that can be detected.

The ascending limb of the precipitation curve represents the zone of antibody excess where free antibody molecules are present in the supernatants. The descending limb represents the zone of antigen excess where free antigen is present in the supernatants. Maximum precipitation occurs in the zone of equivalence (or equivalence point) where neither antigen nor antibody can be detected in the supernatants (Figure 17).

In contrast to the nonspecific system described above, the presence of more than one antigen-antibody system in the reaction medium can be revealed by the demonstration of unreacted antibody and antigen in certain supernatants. This occurs when there is an overlap between the zone of antigen excess in one antigen-antibody combination with the zone of antibody excess of a separate antigen-antibody system (Figure 18).

The **lattice theory** (Figure 19) proposed by Marrack, explains how multivalent antigen molecules and bivalent antibodies combine to yield antigen–antibody ratios that differ from one precipitate to another, depending upon the zone of the precipitin reaction in which they are formed. When the ratio of antibody to antigen is above 1.0, a visible precipitate forms. However, when the ratio is less than 1.0, soluble complexes result and remain in the supernatant. These soluble complexes are associated with the precipitin curve's descending limb.

The incremental addition of antigen to an optimal amount of antibody precipitates only 78% of the antibody amount precipitated by one step addition to the antigen. This demonstrates the presence of both precipitating and nonprecipitating antibodies. Although the nonprecipitating variety cannot lead to the formation of insoluble antigen-antibody complexes, they can be assimilated into precipitates that correspond to their specificity. Rather than being univalent as was once believed, they may merely have a relatively low affinity for the homologous antigen. Monogamous bivalency, which describes the combination of high affinity

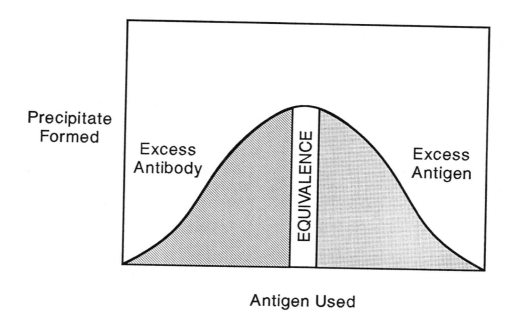

Figure 17.   Precipitate formed verses antigen used.

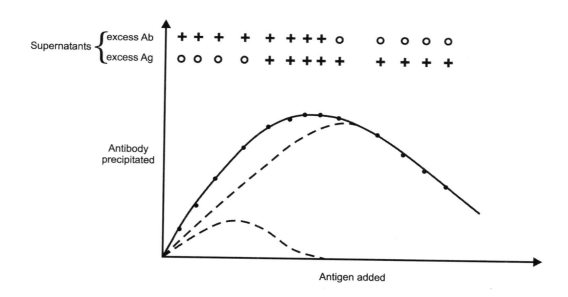

Precipitin Curve for a Multi-specific System.
The Precipitation Observed (——) is the
Sum of Two or More Precipitin Reactions (----).

Figure 18.   Precipitin curve for a multi-specific system.

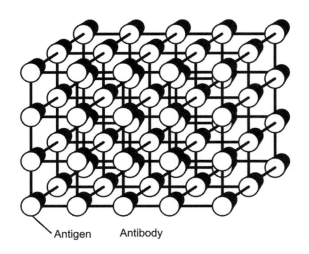

Antigen   Antibody

Figure 19.   Antigen-antibody lattice formation.

antibody with two antigenic determinants on the same antigen particle, represents an alternative explanation of the failure of these molecules to participate with their homologous antigen. The formation of nonprecipitating antibodies, which usually represents 10 to 15% of the antibody population produced, is dependent upon such variables as heterogeneity of the antigen, characteristics of the antibody, and animal species.

Factors that affect the precipitin reaction are pH, salt concentration (ionic strength), temperature, the presence of complement in the sera used, and time curve, respectively. The precipitin reaction usually remains unaffected by changes of pH in the range of 6.6 to 8.5. Synthetic antigens are the most sensitive to changes in pH and the greater the number of charged amino acids, the greater their sensitivity.

Electrolytes contribute to the stabilization of the reaction. The overall charge of the molecules used as antigens should be considered. Avian antisera show an anomalous behavior,

in that more precipitation is obtained in high NaCl concentration than occurs in physiological saline.

Generally, the amount of antibody precipitated at 4°C is greater than at 37°C. Here again, synthetic polypeptides are the most sensitive to the temperature changes, but the individual variations should be determined experimentally. Small amounts of complement may be present and may persist for many months at 4°C. By binding to immune complexes, complement augments the specific precipitates and shifts the solubility equilibrium. It precipitates antigen-antibody complexes in the antigen excess zone. The error is greater with rabbit and guinea pig sera than with human sera.

The time required for the formation of a precipitate varies with the system and contrasts with the rapidity of antigen and antibody interaction. Generally, it depends on the ratio of antigen to antibody and is more rapid at the equivalence zone. The precipitin reaction should be viewed as a series of competing biomolecular reactions. Some antigens and antibodies require longer times for precipitation (for example, gelatin-antigelatin system requires 10 days).

Other factors such as the storage of serum, volumes, washing of the complexes, use of diluents, presence of active enzymes in serum, and state of aggregation of antigen may affect the course of the precipitation reaction.

Flocculation differs from the classic precipitin reaction in that insoluble aggregates are not formed until a greater amount of antigen is added than would be required in a typical precipitin reaction (Figure 20). If the antibody (or total protein) precipitated is plotted vs. antigen added, the plot does not extrapolate to the origin. In flocculation reactions, excess antibody as well as excess antigen inhibits precipitation. Precipitation occurs only over a narrow range of antibody to antigen ratios. Soluble antigen-antibody complexes are formed in both antigen and antibody excess.

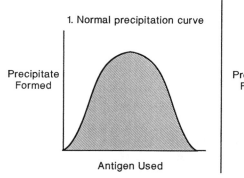

1. Normal precipitation curve

Precipitate Formed

Antigen Used

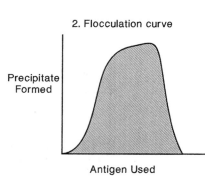

2. Flocculation curve

Precipitate Formed

Antigen Used

Figure 20.   Flocculation.

Horse antisera commonly give flocculation reactions (for example, antisera to diphtheria and certain streptococcal toxins). The peculiar aspects of the flocculation reaction must be attributed to the reacting antibodies as opposed to the antigen, which gives a typical precipitin reaction with rabbit antisera. For many years this reaction was known as the toxin-antitoxin type of curve because it was observed with horse antibodies against diphtheria and tetanus toxins. In recent years it has been observed with blood sera from some patients with Hashimoto's thyroiditis. These patients develop autoantibodies against human thyroglobulin. This antithyroglobulin antibody may give a classic precipitin curve, but some individuals develop a flocculation type of antibody response against the antigen.

How do the flocculation and precipitin curves differ? In flocculation, soluble antigen-antibody complexes form in antigen as well as in antibody excess regions. In the precipitin reaction, precipitate is developed with even minute quantities of antigen, causing the curve to pass through the origin (Figure 21). The graph is a classic flocculation curve based on the data of Pappenheimer and Robinson.

Roitt and associates demonstrated that one human antiserum to thyroglobulin gave a precipitin curve (Figure 22).

They also showed a flocculation curve (Figure 23).

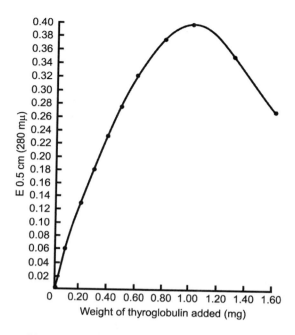

Figure 22. Precipitation curve with human thyroglobulin and homologous antibody.

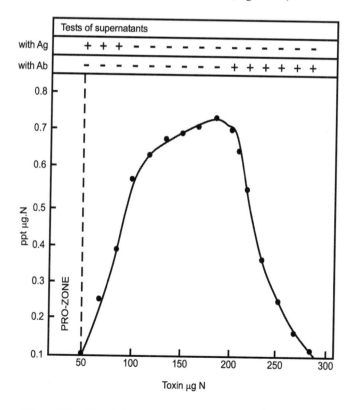

Figure 21. Floculation curve of Pappenheimer and Robinson.

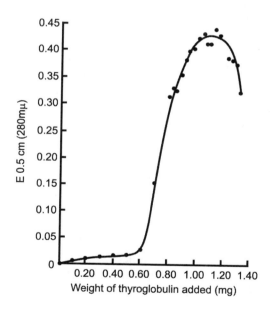

Figure 23. Flocculation curve with human thyroglobulin and homologous antibody.

Although no satisfactory explanation has yet been offered for the flocculation curve, it may be attributable in part to such variables as antibody heterogeneity or the relative binding affinities of flocculating antibodies compared with those of precipitins. Different antigenic determinants may be involved in flocculation and precipitation.

$$T + A \xrightleftharpoons{} TA \xrightleftharpoons{} (TA)_w \quad \text{(soluble)}$$

$$TA + A \xrightleftharpoons{} TA_2 \xrightleftharpoons{} (TA_2)_x \quad \text{(insoluble)}$$

$$TA_2 + A \xrightleftharpoons{} TA_3 \xrightleftharpoons{} (TA_3)_y \quad \text{(insoluble)}$$

$$TA_3 + A \xrightleftharpoons{} TA_4 \xrightleftharpoons{} (TA_4)_z \quad \text{(soluble in presence of excess antigen)}$$

The addition of toxin to the homologous antitoxin in several fractions with appropriate time intervals between them results in greater toxicity of the mixture than would occur if all the samples of toxin were added at once. Therefore, a greater amount of antitoxin is required for neutralization if toxin is added in divided doses than if all toxin is added at one time. Or less toxin is required to neutralize the given quantity of antitoxin if all toxin is added at one time than if it is added in divided doses with time intervals between. This form of reaction has been called the **Danysz phenomenon** or **Danysz effect**. Neutralization in the above instances is tested by injection of the toxin-antitoxin mixture into experimental animals. This phenomenon is attributed to the combination of toxin and antitoxin in multiple proportions. The addition of one fraction of toxin to excess antitoxin leads to maximal binding of antitoxin by toxin molecules. When a second fraction of toxin is added, insufficient antitoxin is available to bring about neutralization. Therefore, the mixture is toxic due to uncombined excess toxin. Equilibrium is reached after an appropriate time interval. The interaction between toxin and antitoxin is considered to occur in two steps: (1) rapid combination of toxin and antitoxin and (2) slower aggregation of the molecules. These reactions are outlined in the steps shown above.

Nephelometry is a technique used to assay proteins and other biological materials through the formation of a precipitate of antigen and homologous antibody (Figure 24). The assay depends on the turbidity or cloudiness of a suspension. It is based on determination of the degree to which light is scattered when a helium-neon laser beam is directed through the suspension. Antigen concentration is ascertained using a standard curve devised from the light scatter produced by solutions of known antigen concentration. This method is used by many clinical immunology laboratories for the quantification of complement components and immunoglobulins in patients' sera or other body fluids.

Oudin in 1946 overlaid antibody incorporated in agar in a test tube with the homologous antigen. A band of precipitation appeared in the gel where the antigen-antibody interaction occurred. Mixtures of antibodies of several specificities

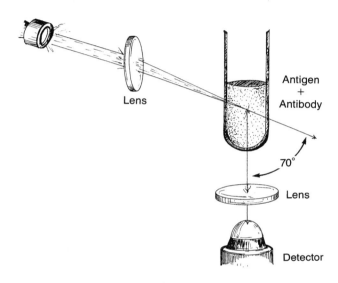

Figure 24. Nephelometry.

were overlaid with a mixture of the homologous antigens and a distinct band for each resulted. Oudin's technique involves simple (or single) diffusion in one dimension (Figure 25). Oakley and Fulthorpe (1953) placed antiserum incorporated into agar in the bottom of a tube, covered this with a layer of plain agar which was permitted to solidify and then added antigen. This was double diffusion in one dimension. Double diffusion in two dimensions was developed by Ouchterlony and independently by Elek in 1948. Agar is poured on a flat glass surface such as a microscope slide, glass plate, or Petri dish. Wells or troughs are cut in the agar and these are filled with antigen and antibody solutions under study. Multiple component systems may be analyzed by use of this method and cross-reactivities detected. Double diffusion in agar is a useful method to demonstrate similarity among structurally related antigens. Equidistant holes are punched in agar gel containing electrolytes. Antigen is placed in one well, antiserum in an adjacent well, and the plates are observed the following day for a precipitation line where antigen and antibody have migrated toward one another and reached equivalent concentrations. A single line

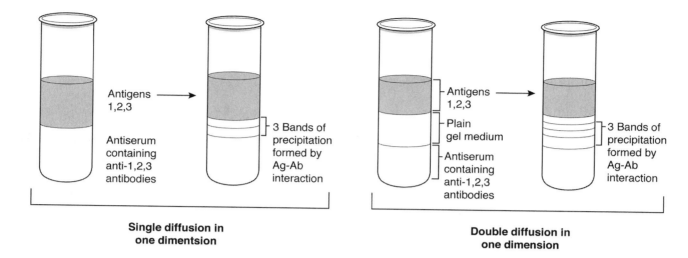

Figure 25.   Precipitation in gel media.

implies a single antigen-antibody system. If agar plates containing one central well with others cut equidistant from it at the periphery are employed, a reaction of identity may be demonstrated by placing antibody in the central well and the homologous antigen in the adjacent peripheral wells.

A confluent line of precipitate is produced in the shape of an arc. This implies that the antigen preparations in adjacent peripheral wells are identical (**reaction of identity**); they have the same antigenic determinants (Figure 26). If antibodies against two unrelated antigen preparations are combined and placed in the central well and their homologous antigens placed in separate adjacent peripheral wells, a line of precipitation is produced by each antigen-antibody reaction to give the appearance of crossed sword points. This constitutes a **reaction of nonidentity** (Figure 27).

It implies that the antigenic determinants are different in each of the two samples of antigen. A third pattern known as a **reaction of partial identity** occurs when two antigen preparations that are related but not the same are placed in separate adjacent wells with an antibody preparation that crossreacts with both of them placed in a central well (Figure 28).

The precipitation lines between each antigen-antibody system converge, but a spur or extension of one of the precipitation lines occurs. This reaction of partial identity with spur formation implies that the antigen preparations are similar, but that one has an antigenic determinant(s) not present in the other. A reaction of identity and nonidentity may be observed simultaneously, implying that two separate antigen preparations have both common and different antigenic determinants.

Mancini in 1965, developed a quantitative technique employing single radial diffusion to quantify antigens. Plates are poured in which specific antibody is incorporated into agar. Wells are cut and precise quantities of antigen are

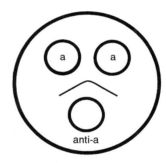

Figure 26.   Reaction of identity.

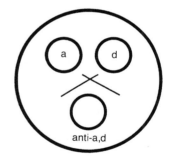

Figure 27.   Reaction of nonidentity.

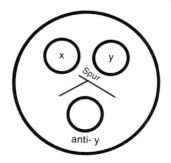

Figure 28.   Reaction of partial identity.

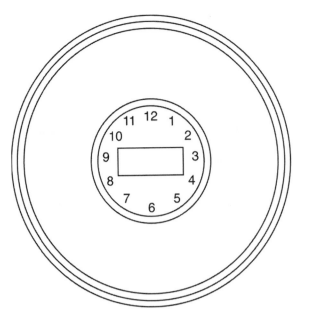

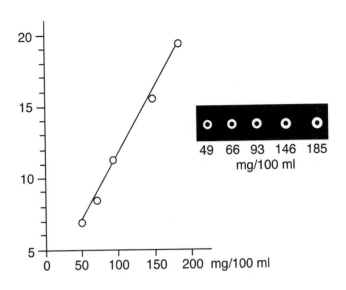

Figure 29.   Radial immunodiffusion.

placed over time. The antigen is permitted to diffuse into the agar containing antibody and produce a ring of precipitation where they interact (Figure 29). The precipitation ring encloses an area proportional to the concentration of antigen measured 48 to 72 hours following diffusion. Standard curves are employed using known antigen standards and the antigen concentration is reflected by the diameter of the ring ascertained. The Mancini technique can detect as little as 1 to 3 micrograms per milliliter of antigen.

Agglutination is the combination of soluble antibody with particulate antigens in an aqueous medium containing electrolytes, such as erythrocytes, latex particles bearing antigen or bacterial cells to form an aggregate which may be viewed either microscopically or macroscopically (Figure 30). If antibody is linked to insoluble beads or particles, they may be agglutinated by soluble antigen by reverse agglutination. Agglutination is the basis for multiple serological reactions including blood grouping, diagnosis of infectious diseases, rheumatoid arthritis (RA) test, etc. To carry out an agglutination reaction, serial dilutions of antibody are prepared and

a constant quantity of particulate antigen is added to each antibody dilution. Red blood cells may serve as carriers for adsorbed antigen, e.g., tanned red cell or bis-diazotized red cell technique. Like precipitation, agglutination is a secondary manifestation of antigen-antibody interaction. As specific antibody crosslinks particulate antigens, aggregates form that become macroscopically visible and settle out of suspension. The agglutination reaction has a sensitivity 10 to 500 times greater than that of the precipitin test with respect to antibody detection. Agglutination permits phagocytic cells to engulf invading macroorganisms. This is a major role of agglutinin in the immune reaction (Figure 31).

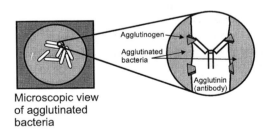

Figure 31.   Bacterial agglutination.

However, massive agglutination may occur without immunization. Antibodies alone are not enough and phagocytes must be present to remove the precipitate in these circumstances. **Titer** is the quantity of a substance required to produce a reaction with a given volume of another substance. An **agglutination titer** is the highest dilution of a serum which causes clumping of particles such as bacteria. Titer is an approximation of the antibody activity in each unit volume of a serum sample. The term is used in serological

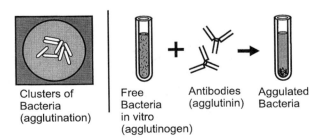

Figure 30.   Agglutination.

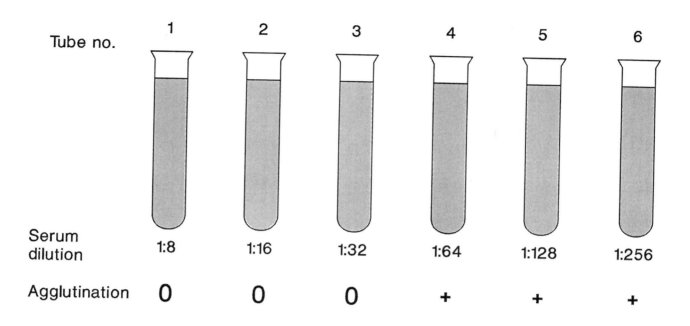

Figure 32. Prozone effect.

reactions and is determined by preparing serial dilutions of antibody to which a constant amount of antigen is added. The end point is the highest dilution of antiserum in which a visible reaction with antigen, e.g., agglutination, can be detected. The titer is expressed as the reciprocal of the serum dilution which defines the end point. If agglutination occurs in the tube containing a 1:240 dilution, the antibody titer is said to be 240. Thus, the serum would contain approximately 240 units of antibody per milliliter of antiserum. The titer only provides an estimate of antibody activity. For absolute amounts of antibody, quantitative precipitation or other methods must be employed.

The **prozone** is that portion of the dilution range in which an immune serum of high agglutinin titer fails to agglutinate the homologues (Figure 32).

Antigens and antibodies agglutinate because of plus and minus charges (Figure 33). Antigen-antibody reactions are therefore surface phenomena. The antibody is the mirror image of the antigen.

Factors that affect the agglutination test are electrolytes, pH, and temperature, respectively. Salt decreases the potential difference between antigen particles and the surrounding liquid medium in which they are suspended. It also decreases cohesive forces between antigen particles. Agglutination occurs when the potential drops below 15 millivolts. As the salt concentration is increased the potential drops, favoring agglutination; but the cohesive forces between particles also drops which is unfavorable to agglutination. Finally, a salt concentration is reached where no agglutination occurs. A concentration near 0.15 M is ideal.

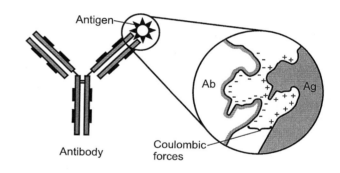

Figure 33. Antigen-antibody complex. Role of positive and negative charges in agglutination of antigen by antibody.

With sera of high antibody titer, complete agglutination occurs over a wide pH range. Upon lowering the titer, the optimal pH also drops until acid agglutination occurs around a pH of 4. This acid agglutination is nonspecific, since even normal serum will agglutinate cells at this low pH. This type of nonspecific agglutination is not antibody dependent.

The rate of agglutination increases rapidly from 0 to 30°C. Above that temperature it is less rapid and above 56°C the antibody molecules are injured by heat. Shaking or stirring accelerates agglutination.

Certain conditions must be established in the reacting medium for agglutination to take place. These include ionic strength and pH. Optimally, agglutination reactions are carried out in neutral dilute salt solution, such as 0.15 M sodium chloride. The significance of ionic strength is demonstrated by agglutination without antibodies at neutral pH or by bacteria bearing a negative surface charge following the addition of enough salt to induce damping of these charges. Low salt concentration below 10^{-3} M NaCl, may prevent agglutination of bacteria or other particulate antigens with antibody already attached to their surfaces. It appears necessary to dampen the highly negative surface charge of cells by counter ions to permit close enough contact between cells for bivalent antibody molecules to form specific connecting bridges between them.

9

The Thymus and T Lymphocytes

Stem cells in the bone marrow that are destined to develop into T cells migrate to the thymus where they undergo maturation and development. These precursors of T cells possess unrearranged TCR genes and express neither CD4 nor CD8 markers. Thymocytes, the developing T cells, are found first in the outer cortex where their numbers increase, the TCR genes are rearranged and CD3, CD4, CD8 and T cell receptor molecules are expressed on the surface. During maturation, these cells pass from the cortex to the medulla. As maturation proceeds, CD4−CD8− (double-negative) T cells develop into CD4+CD8+ (double-positive) cells that then become either CD4−CD8− or CD4−CD8+ single positive T cells. Somatic rearrangement of variable, diversity (β) and joining gene segments in the area of C gene segments lead to the production of functional genes that encode TCR α and β polypeptides. Many T cell specificities result from the numerous combinations possible for joining of separate gene segments in addition to various mechanisms for junctional diversity. Somatic mutation and affinity maturation do not take place in TCR genes, in contrast to their occurrence in Ig genes. Somatic rearrangement of germ line genes is also responsible for the functional genes that encode TCR γ and δ polypeptides.

Even though there are fewer V genes in the γ and δ loci and greater junction diversity, the mechanisms to produce γδ diversity resemble those for the αβ receptor. A few cortical thymocytes express γδ receptors. Thereafter, a line of developing T lymphocytes express numerous αβ TCR receptors. Beta chains appear first followed by α chains of the TCR. The β chain associates itself with an invariant pre-T α surrogate alpha chain. Signals transduced by the pTαβ receptor facilitate expression of CD4 and CD8 and facilitate expansion of immature thymocytes. CD4+CD8+ cortical thymocytes first express αβ receptors. Self MHC restriction and self-tolerance develop as a consequence of the interaction between cortical epithelial cells and non-lymphoid cells derived from the bone marrow that both express MHC. This leads to selection of those T cells that are to be saved. During positive selection, CD4+CD8+ TCR αβ thymocytes recognize peptide-MHC complexes on thymic epithelial cells with low avidity. This saves them from programmed cell death or apoptosis. Recognition of self peptide-MHC complexes on thymic antigen presenting cells with high avidity by CD4+CD8+ TCR αβ+ thymocytes leads to apoptosis. The majority of cortical thymocytes are killed during selection

processes. Those αβ TCR thymocytes that remain undergo maturation and proceed to the medulla where they become single positive cells that are either CD4+CD8− or CD4−CD8+. During residence in the medulla, these cells become either helper or cytolytic cells prior to their journey to the peripheral lymphoid tissues where they function as self MHC-restricted helper T cells or pre-cytotoxic T lymphocytes capable of responding to foreign antigen.

The **thymus** is a triangular bilobed structure enclosed in a thin fibrous capsule and located retrosternally (Figures 1 and 2). Each lobe is subdivided by prominent trabeculae into interconnecting lobules and each lobule comprises two histologically and functionally distinct areas, cortex and medulla (Figure 3). The cortex consists of a mesh of epithelial reticular cells enclosing densely packed large lymphocytes (called thymocytes). It has no germinal centers. The lymphoid cells are of mesenchymal origin; the epithelial cell component is of endodermal origin. The thymic cortex contains three types of epithelial reticular cells: type I, type II, and type III. Type I epithelial reticular cells are found at the outer part of the cortex isolating the thymus from the body. The middle of the cortex houses the type II epithelial reticular cells. They compartmentalize the cortex into small areas of lymphocytes. Deep in the cortex and at the corticomedullary junction are the type III reticular epithelial cells. Like type II cells these also compartmentalize the cortex. They also isolate the cortex from the medulla. The isolation provided by the type I and III epithelial reticular cells keep the thymocytes from coming in contact with foreign antigen. The prothymocytes, which migrate from the bone marrow to the subcapsular regions of the cortex, are influenced by this microenvironment which directs their further development. The process of education is exerted by hormonal substances produced by the thymic epithelial cells. The cortical cells proliferate extensively. Some of these cells are short-lived and die. The surviving cells acquire characteristics of thymocytes (Figure 4). The cortical cells migrate to the medulla (Figure 5) and from there to the peripheral lymphoid organs, sites of their main residence. The medullary areas of the thymus contain loosely packed thymocytes and many epithelial reticular cells (Figure 6). Like the cortex, the medulla also consists of three types of epithelial reticular cells: type IV, type V, and type VI. Type IV cells are found at the corticomedullary junction and are associated with type III cells. The middle section of the medulla is composed of

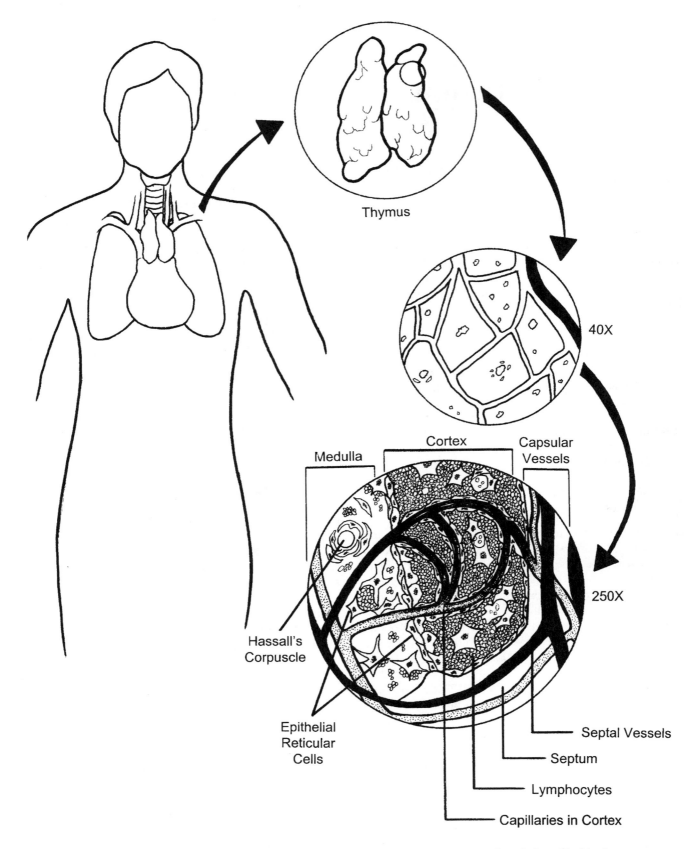

Figure 1.   Diagram showing the location of the thymus in the human body with an enlarged view of its histology.

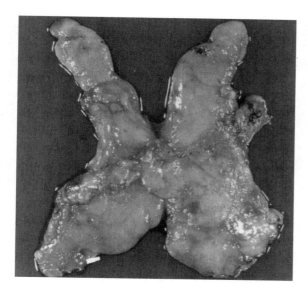

Figure 2. Normal adult thymus. The thymus often shows an X- or H-shaped configuration.

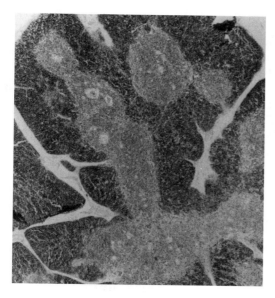

Figure 3. Normal thymus. The normal thymus in this infant shows the lobulation and sharp separation of cortex from the stalklike medulla (x40).

type V epithelial reticular cells. The most characteristic feature of the medulla, the Hassall's corpuscles (Figures 7 and 8), are formed by the type VI epithelial reticular cells. These remnants of epithelial islands are histologically identifiable and are markers for thymic tissue. The thymocytes are small cells ready to exit the thymus. The blood supply to the cortex comes from capillaries that form anastomosing arcades. Drainage is mainly through veins; the thymus has no lymphatic vessels.

The thymus develops from the branchial pouches of the pharynx at about six weeks of embryonal age. The parathyroid

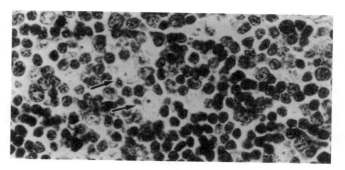

Figure 4. Thymic epithelial cells: cortex. Epithelial cells of the cortical type have large, round to oval, clear nuclei and conspicuous nucleoli.

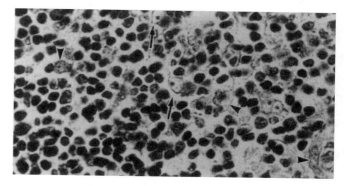

Figure 5. Thymic epithelial cells: cortico-medullary junction. Epithelial cells of cortical type (arrows) and medullary type (arrowheads) are intermingled.

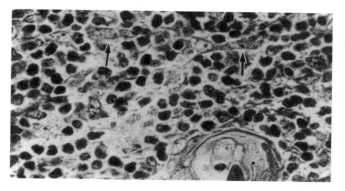

Figure 6. Thymic epithelial cells: medulla. Fusiform epithelial cells have spindle-shaped nucleus, coarse chromatin structure, and interconnecting cell processes. A Hassall's corpuscle is seen in the right lower part.

glands and other tissues with epithelial cells also develop from pharyngeal pouches. In most species the thymus is fully developed at birth. In humans, the weight of the thymus at birth is 10–15g. It continues to increase in size reaching a maximum (30–40g) at puberty. It begins to involute with increasing age, but the adult gland is still functional. The medulla involutes first with pyknosis and beading of the nuclei of small lymphocytes giving a false impression of an

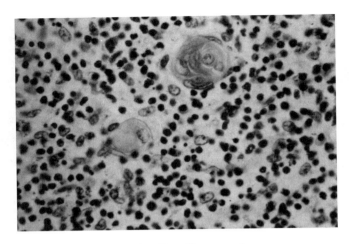

Figure 7. Hassall's corpuscle.

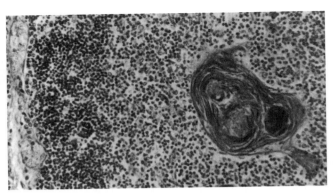

Figure 8. Normal thymus. This child's thymus shows the dense cortex composed predominantly of lymphocytes and the less dense medulla with fewer lymphocytes. Note the Hassall's corpuscle.

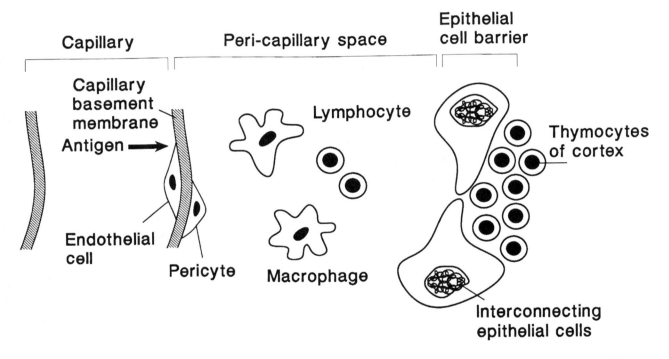

Figure 9. Three levels of lymphocyte protection which form the blood-thymus barrier: capillary wall, macrophages in pericapillary space, and a wall of epithelial cells.

increased number of Hassall's corpuscles. The cortex atrophies progressively.

The **blood-thymus barrier** protects thymocytes from contact with antigen (Figure 9). Lymphocytes reaching the thymus are prevented from contact with antigen by a physical barrier. The first level is represented by the capillary wall with endothelial cells inside the pericytes outside of the lumen. Potential antigenic molecules which escape the first level of control are taken over by macrophages present in the pericapillary space. Further protection is provided by a third level, represented by the mesh of interconnecting epithelial

cells which enclose the thymocyte population. The effects of thymus and thymic hormones on the differentiation of T cells is demonstrable in animals congenitally lacking the thymus gland (nu/nu animals), neonatally or adult thymectomized animals, and in subjects with immunodeficiencies involving T cell function. Differentiation is associated with surface markers whose presence or disappearance characterizes the different stages of cell differentiation. There is extensive proliferation of the subcapsular thymocytes. The largest proportion of these cells die but the remaining cells continue to differentiate. The differentiating cells become smaller in size and move through interstices in the thymic medulla. The fully developed thymocytes pass through the walls of the post-capillary venules to reach the systemic circulation and seed in the peripheral lymphoid organs. Some of them recirculate but do not return to the thymus.

Thymic epithelial cells are present in the cortex (Figure 10) and in the medulla (Figure 11) of the thymus, and are derived from the third and fourth pharyngeal pouches. They affect maturation and differentiation of thymocytes through the secretion of thymopoietin, thymosins, and serum thymic factors. Thymic epithelial cells express both MHC class I and class II molecules.

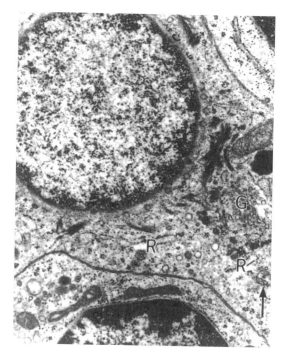

Figure 10. Type 2 "pale" epithelial cell in outer cortex. R: profiles of RER; G: a Golgi complex; arrow: multivesicular body (x9000).

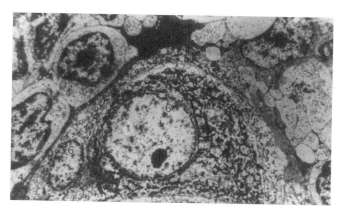

Figure 11. Two type 6 "large medullary" epithelial cells (6) adjacent to a hassall's corpuscle and two type 4 epithelial cells (4) in the medulla (x7000).

Thymic nurse cells are relatively large epithelial cells that are very near thymic lymphocytes and are believed to have a significant role in T lymphocyte maturation and differentiation.

A **thymocyte** is a lymphocyte in the thymus gland.

A **thymus dependent (TD) antigen** is an immunogen that requires T lymphocyte cooperation for B cells to synthesize specific antibodies. Presentation of thymus-dependent antigen to T cells must be in the context of MHC class II molecules. Thymus-dependent antigens include proteins, polypeptides, hapten-carrier complexes, erythrocytes, and many other antigens that have diverse epitopes.

Thymus dependent areas are regions of peripheral lymphoid tissues occupied by T lymphocytes. Specifically, these include the paracortical areas of lymph nodes, the zone between nodules and Peyer's patches, and the center of splenic Malpighian corpuscles. These regions contain small lymphocytes derived from the circulating cells that reach these areas by passage through high endothelial venules. Proof that these anatomical sites are thymus-dependent areas is provided by the demonstration that animals thymectomized as neonates do not have lymphocytes in these areas. Likewise, humans or animals with thymic hypoplasia or congenital aplasia of the thymus reveal no T cells in these areas.

Thymus-dependent cells are lymphoid cells that mature only under the influence of the thymus.

A **thymus-independent (TI) antigen** is an immunogen that can stimulate B cells to synthesize antibodies without participation by T cells. These antigens are less complex than thymus-dependent antigens. They are often polysaccharides that contain repeating epitopes or lipopolysaccharides (LPS) derived from Gram-negative microorganisms. Thymus-independent antigens induce IgM synthesis by B lymphcytes without cooperation by T cells. They also do not stimulate immunological memory. Murine TI antigens are classified as either TI-1 or TI-2 antigens. LPS, which activate murine B cells without participation by T or other cells, are typical TI-1 antigens. Low concentrations of LPS stimulate synthesis of specific antigen, whereas high concentrations activate essentially all B cells to grow and differentiate. TI-2 antigens include polysaccharides, glycolipids, and nucleic acids. When T lymphocytes and macrophages are depleted, no antibody response develops against them.

Cells leaving the thymus migrate to all peripheral lymphoid organs and seed in the T-dependent regions of the lymph nodes, spleen and the periphery of the lymphoid follicles (Figure 12). The rate of release of thymocytes from the thymus is markedly increased following antigenic stimulation. The patterns of migration of thymus cells (as well as

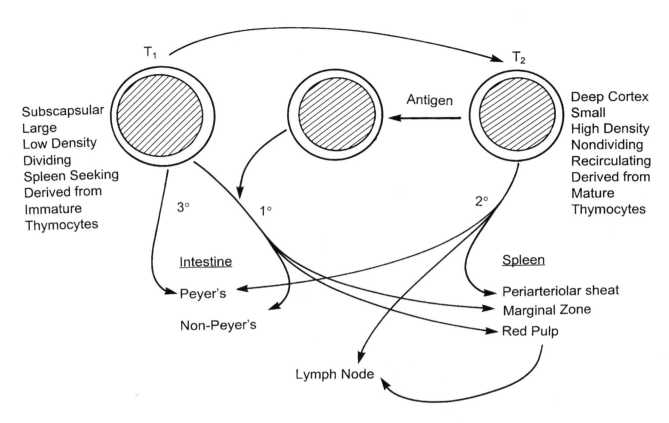

Figure 12.   Migration patterns of thymus cells.

of B cells) have been studied by adoptive transfer of labeled purified cells into irradiated syngeneic mice matched for age and sex.

Class II-restricted CD4 T cell repertoire development is shaped by two distinct subsets of thymic epithelium: cortical epithelium and a fucose bearing subset of medullary epithelium. The cortical epithelium appears to be solely responsible for positive selection. The medullary epithelium is specialized for negative selection. There are two types of medullary epithelium involved. UEA-1+ MEC are capable of immediate negative selection only. Bone marrow derived dendritic cells are the most effective antigen presenting cells and the most potent cells involved in the induction of intrathymic negative selection (Figure 13).

Negative selection is the process whereby those thymocytes that recognize "*self antigens*" in the context of self MHC undergo clonal deletion (apoptosis) or clonal anergy (inactivation). The resulting cell population is self MHC restricted and self antigen tolerant.

Positive selection is the survival of those thymocytes that recognize *self MHC* as well as self or foreign antigen, and the death of those that do not recognize self MHC. The resulting cell population is self MHC restricted and capable of interacting with both self and foreign antigens.

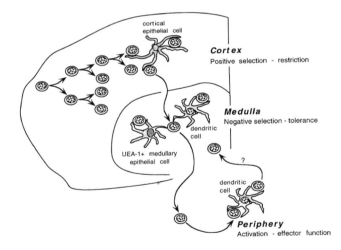

Figure 13.   A model for the thymic compartment specialization.

A pro-T cell is the earliest identifiable thymocyte and is recognized by expression of cell surface antigens such as CD2, CD7, or CD3 M protein in the cytoplasm. Rearrangement of δ, γ, and β TCR genes accompanies differentiation of pro-T cells into pre-T cells.

Pre-T cells are developed from pro-T cells through gene rearrangement (Figure 14). They give rise to γδ TCR-bearing cells through rearrangement and expression of γ and δ TCR

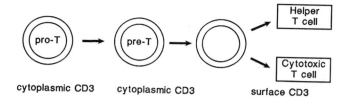

Figure 14. Schematic of pre-T cells.

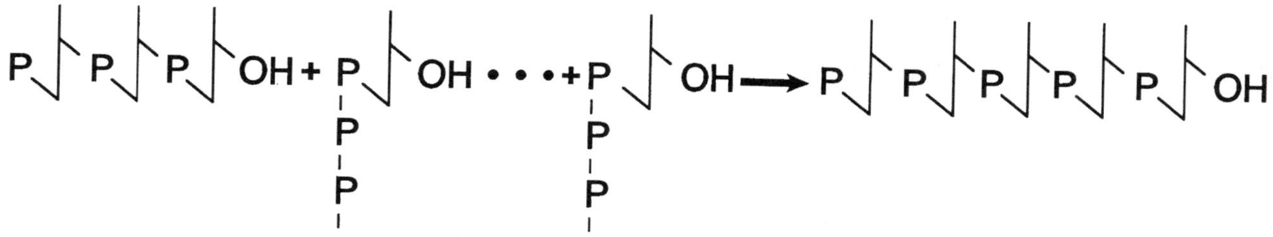

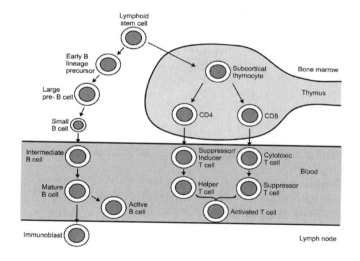

Figure 15. Activity of Terminal Deoxynucleotidyl Transferase (TdT).

genes. Pre-T cells that give rise to T lymphocytes expressing the αß T cell receptor rearrange α TRC genes, and delete the δ TCR genes situated on the chromosome between the Vα and Cα genes

A **prothymocyte** is a hematopoeitic stem cell from the bone marrow which migrates to the thymus by the blood circulation and enters through the epithelial cell lining of the cortex. Prothymocytes (pre-T cells) differentiate in the thymus microenvironment. The prothymocytes are educated in the thymus to function as T cells. There are four thymic peptide hormones termed thymulin, thymosin α, thymosin β, and thymopoietin. These hormones are significant in T lymphocyte proliferation and differentiation. Direct interaction with the thymus epithelium, which expresses HLA antigens, is necessary for forming functional T lymphocytes and for learning to recognize major histocompatibility complex (MHC) antigens. Prothymocytes proliferate and migrate from the cortex to the medulla. Some of them are short-lived and die. The long-lived cells acquire new characteristics and are called thymocytes. They exit the thymus as immature cells and seed to specific areas of the peripheral lymphoid organs where they continue to differentiate through a process driven by an antigen. From these areas, they recirculate throughout the body.

DNA nucleotidylexotransferase [terminal deoxynucleotidyltransferase (TdT)] is a DNA polymerase that randomly catalyzes deoxynucleotide addition to the 3′-OH end of a DNA strand in the absence of a template (Figure 15). It can also be employed to add homopolymer tails. Immature T and B lymphocytes contain TdT. The thymus is rich in TdT, which is also present in the bone marrow. TdT inserts a few nucleotides in T cell receptor genes and immunoglobulin

Figure 16. T cell maturation.

gene segments at the V-D, D-J, and V-J junctions. This enhances sequence diversity.

Thymus cell differentiation is stem cell maturation and differentiation into mature T lymphocytes (Figures 16 and 17). This is accompanied by the appearance and disappearance of specific surface CD antigens (Figure 18). In humans, the differentiation of CD38 positive stem cells into early thymocytes is signaled by the appearance of CD2 and CD7, followed by the transferrin receptor marker. This is followed by expression of CD1, which identifies thymocytes in the mid-stage of differentiation, when T cell receptor genes γ, δ, and later α and β rearrange. This is followed by the expression of CD3, CD4, and CD8 surface antigens by thy-

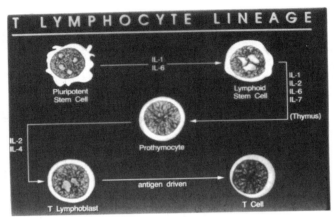

Figure 17. Differentiation of a stem cell into a mature T cell.

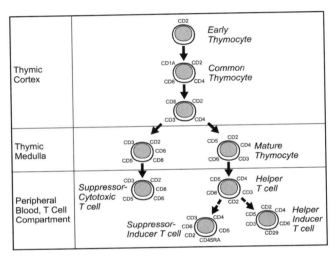

Figure 18. Diagram of T cell maturation showing addition of CD (cluster of differentiation) markers and the position of the T cell (in thymus or periphery) when the marker is added.

mocytes, yet CD1 usually disappears at this time. Ultimately, the CD4+CD8−, and the CD4−CD8+ subpopulations which both express the CD3 pan-T cell marker appear. An analogous maturation of T cells takes place in mice. Thymus cell differentiation is also called **thymus cell education**.

A **T cell-dependent (TD) antigen** is an immunogen that is much more complex than the T cell-independent (TI) antigens. They are usually proteins, protein-nuclear protein conjugates, glycoproteins, or lipoproteins. They stimulate all five classes of immunoglobulin, elicit an anamnestic or memory response, and are present in most pathogenic microorganisms. These properties ensure that an effective immune response can be generated in a host infected with these pathogens.

T cell domains are specific areas in lymph nodes and other lymphoid organs where T lymphocytes localize preferentially.

A **T cell-independent (TI) antigen** is an immunogen that is simple in structure, often a polysaccharide such as the polysaccharide of the pneumococcus, a dextran polyvinyl hooter, or a bacterial lipopolysaccharide. They elicit an IgM response only, and fail to stimulate an anamnestic response. They are not found in most pathogenic microbes.

Cluster of differentiation (CD) is the term given to cell surface molecules comprising epitopes, identifiable by monoclonal antibodies, on the surfaces of hematopoietic (blood) cells in man, as well as in mice and other animals. CD markers are given numerical designations in man, but separate designations equivalent to the human CD numbers are given to animal determinants. Some individuals use the CD designation to refer to the antibodies which identify a particular antigen.

Pan-T cell markers are surface epitopes found on all normal T lymphocytes. These include the 50kD CD2 molecule that is the sheep erythrocyte rosette marker and is found exclusively on T lymphocytes, the 41kD CD7 moleucle, CD1 present on peripheral T lymphocytes and cortical thymocytes, the mature T lymphocyte marker CD3, and CD5.

CD2 (Figure 19) is a T cell antigen that is the receptor molecule for sheep red cells and is also referred to as the T11 antigen or the leukocyte function associated antigen-2 (LFA-2). The molecule has a MW of 50kD. The antigen also seems to be involved in cell adherence, probably binding LFA-3 as its ligand. CD2 can activate T lymphocytes.

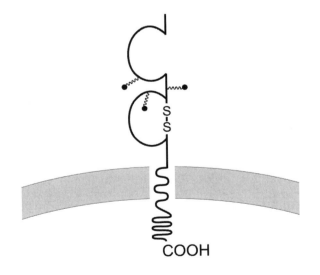

Figure 19. Structure of CD2.

A **rosette** consists of cells of one type surrounding a single cell of another type. In immunology, it was used as an early method to enumerate T cells. E rosettes form when CD2 markers (LFA-2) on human T lymphocytes adhere to LFA-3

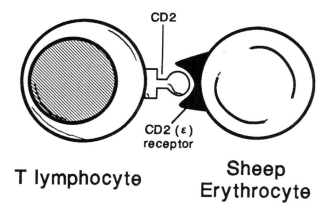

Figure 20.   Adhesion of a T lymphocyte and sheep red blood cell.

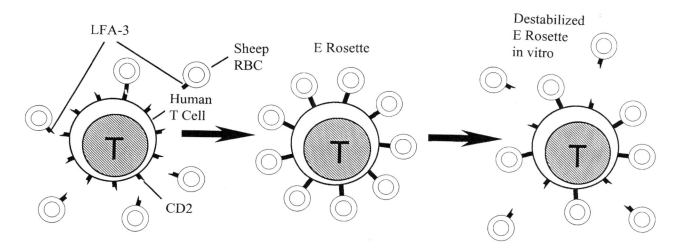

Figure 21.   Formation of a rosette.

molecules on sheep red cells surrounding them to give a rosette arrangement (Figures 20 and 21). This method is useful because sheep red cells do not form spontaneous rosettes with human B lymphocytes. CD2⁻ T cells are now enumerated by the use of monoclonal antibodies and flow cytometry.

CD1 (Figure 22) is an antigen that is a cortical thymocyte marker which disappears at later stages of T cell maturation. The antigen is also found on interdigitating cells, fetal B cells, and Langerhans cells. These chains are associated with β_2-microglobulin. The antigen is thus analogous to classical histocompatibility antigens, but coded for by a different chromosome. More recent studies have shown that the molecule is coded for by at least five genes on chromosome 1, three of which produce recognized polypeptide products. CD1 may participate in antigen presentation.

CD4 (Figures 23–26) is a single chain glycoprotein, also referred to as the T4 antigen, that has a MW of 56kD and

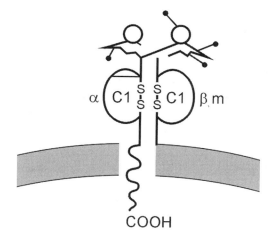

Figure 22.   Structure of CD1.

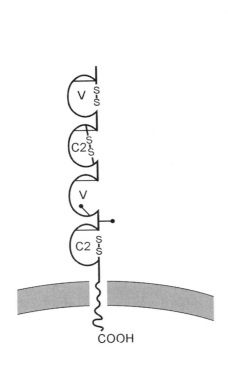

Figure 23. Structure of CD4.

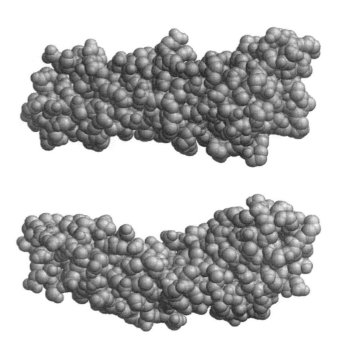

Figure 25. Space filling model of CD4 type I crystal form. Human recombinant form expressed in Chinese hamster ovary cells.

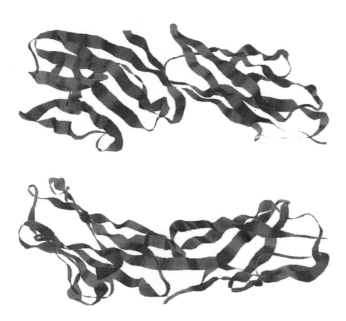

Figure 24. Ribbon structure of T cell surface glycoprotein CD4.

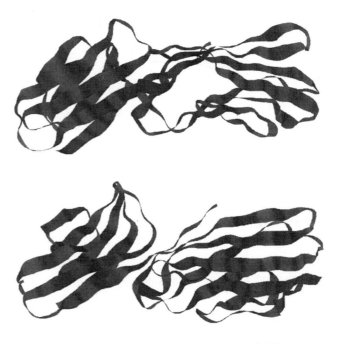

Figure 26. Ribbon structure of CD4 domains 3 and 4. Rat recombinant form expressed in Chinese hamster ovary cells.

is present on approximately two-thirds of circulating human T cells, including most T cells of the helper/inducer type. The antigen is also found on human monocytes and macrophages. The molecule is a receptor for gp120 of HIV-1 and HIV-2 (AIDS viruses). This antigen binds to class II

MHC molecules on antigen-presenting cells (APC), and may stabilize APC/T cell interactions. It is physically associated with the intracellular tyrosine protein kinase, known as p56[lck], which phosphorylates nearby proteins. This antigen is thereby relaying a signal to the cells. Cross-linking of

CD4 may induce activation of this enzyme and phosphorylation of CD3.

Helper T cells are CD4$^+$ helper/inducer T lymphocytes. They represent a subset of T cells which are critical for induction of an immune response to a foreign antigen. Antigen is presented by an antigen-presenting cell such as the macrophage in the context of self MHC class II antigen and IL-1. Once activated, the CD4$^-$ T cells express IL-2 receptors and produce IL-2 molecules which act in an autocrine fashion by combining with the IL-2 receptors and stimulating the CD4$^-$ cells to proliferate. Differentiated CD4$^-$ lymphocytes synthesize and secrete lymphokines that affect the function of other cells of the immune system such as CD8$^-$ cells, B cells, and NK cells. B cells differentiate into plasma cells that synthesize antibody. Activated macrophages participate in delayed-type hypersensitivity (type IV) reactions. Cytotoxic T cells also develop. Murine monoclonal antibodies are used to enumerate CD4$^-$ T lymphocytes by flow cytometry.

A **nonspecific T lymphocyte helper factor** is a soluble factor released by CD4$^-$ helper T lymphocytes that nonspecifically activates other lymphocytes.

T cell nonantigen-specific helper factor is a substance that provides nonspecific help to T lymphocytes.

T$_H$0 cells are a subset of CD4$^-$ cells in both humans and mice based on cytokine production and effector functions. T$_H$0 cells synthesize multiple cytokines. They are responsible for effects intermediate between those of T$_H$1 and T$_H$2 cells, based on the cytokines synthesized and the responding cells. T$_H$0 cells may be precursors of T$_H$1 and T$_H$2 cells (Figure 27).

T$_H$1 cells are a subset of CD4$^-$ cells which synthesize interferon-gamma (INF-γ), IL-2, and tumor necrosis factor (TNF)-β. They are mainly responsible for cellular immunity against intracellular microorganisms and for delayed-type hypersensitivity reactions. They affect IgG2a antibody synthesis and antibody-dependent cell-mediated cytotoxicity. T$_H$1 cells activate host defenses mediated by phagocytes. Intracellular microbial infections induce T$_H$1 cell development which facilitates elimination of the microorganisms by phagocytosis. T$_H$1 cells induce synthesis of antibody that activates complement and serves as an opsonin that facilitates phagocytosis. The IFN-γ they synthesized enhances macrophage activation (Figure 27).

T$_H$2 cells are a subset of CD4$^-$ cells which synthesize IL-4, IL-5, IL-6, IL-9, IL-10, and IL-13. They greatly facilitate IgE and IgG1 antibody responses by synthesis of mast cell and eosinophil growth and differentiation factors, and mucosal immunity by facilitation of IgA synthesis. IL-4 facilitates IgE antibody synthesis. IL-5 is an eosinophil activating substance. IL-10, IL-13, and IL-4 suppress cell-mediated immunity. T$_H$2 cells are principally responsible for host

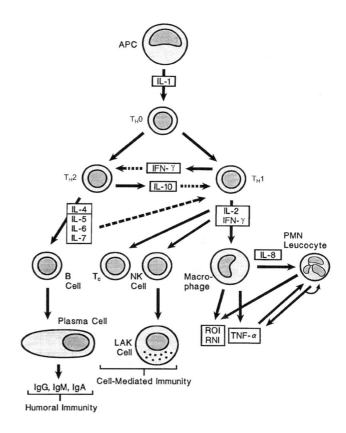

Figure 27. Functions of T$_H$1 and T$_H$2 cells in the immune response via the release of cytokines.

defense exclusive of phagocytes. They are crucial for the IgE and eosinophil response to helminths and for allergy attributable to activation of basophils and mast cells through IgE (Figure 27).

An **inducer T lymphocyte** is a cell required for the initiation of an immune response. The inducer T lymphocyte recognizes antigens in the context of MHC class II histocompatibility molecules. It stimulates helper, cytotoxic, and suppressor T lymphocytes, whereas helper T cells activate B cells. The human leukocyte common antigen variant, termed 2H4, occurs on the inducer T cell surface, and 4B4 surface molecules are present on CD4$^-$ helper T cells. CD4$^-$ T lymphocytes must be positive for either 4B4 or for 2H4.

L3T4 is a CD4 marker on mouse lymphocytes that signifies the T helper/inducer cell. It is detectable by specific monoclonal antibodies and is equivalent to the CD4$^-$ lymphoctye in man.

L3T4$^-$ T lymphocytes are murine CD4$^-$ T cells.

CD8 (Figures 28–30) is an antigen, also referred to as the T8 antigen, that has a MW of 32–34 kD. The CD8 antigen consists of two polypeptide chains, α and β, which may exist in the combination α/α homodimer or α/β heterodimer. Most antibodies are against the α-chain. This antigen binds to

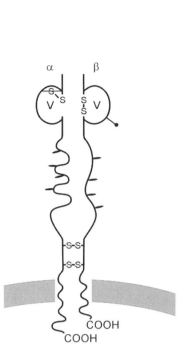

Figure 28.   Structure of CD8.

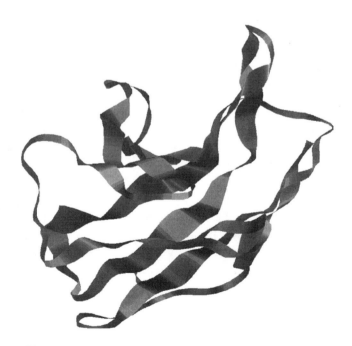

Figure 29.   Ribbon structure of a human CD8 T cell receptor.

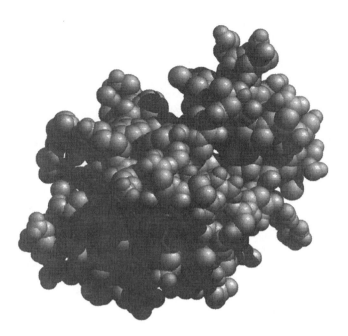

Figure 30.   Space filling model of a human CD8 T cell receptor.

class I MHC molecules on antigen presenting cells (APC), and may stabilize APC/class I cell interactions. Like CD4, it appears to be physically associated with the p56[lck] protein tyrosine kinase which phosphorylates nearby proteins. This antigen is thereby relaying a signal to the cell. It is widely used as a marker for the subpopulation of T cells that includes suppressor/cytotoxic cells. The antigen is also present on splenic sinusoidal lining cells.

Cytotoxic T lymphocytes (CTLs) are specifically sensitized T lymphocytes that are usually CD8[+] and recognize antigens through the T cell receptor on cells of the host infected by viruses or that have become neoplastic. CD8[+] cell recognition of the target is in the context of MHC class I histocompatibility molecules. Following recognition and binding, death of the target cell occurs a few hours later. CTLs secrete lymphokines that attract other lymphocytes to the area and release serine proteases and perforins that produce ion channels in the membrane of the target leading to cell lysis (Figure 31). Interleukin-2, produced by CD4[+] T cells, activates cytotoxic T cell precursors. Interferon-γ generated from CTLs activates macrophages. CTLs have a significant role in the

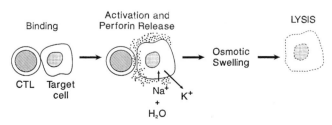

Figure 31.   CTL-mediated Target Cell Lysis.

rejection of allografts and in tumor immunity. A minor population of CD4+ lymphocytes may also be cytotoxic, but they recognize target cell antigens in the context of MHC class II molecules.

A **suppressor cell** is part of a lymphoid cell subpopulation that is able to diminish or suppress the immune reactivity of other cells. An example is the CD8+ suppressor T lymphocyte subpopulation detectable by monoclonal antibodies and flow cytometry in peripheral blood lymphocytes.

Suppressor/inducer T lymphocytes are a subpopulation of T lymphocytes which fail to induce immunosuppression themselves, but are claimed to activate suppressor T lymphocytes.

The **suppressor T cell factor (TSF)** is a soluble substance synthesized by suppressor T lymphocytes that diminishes or suppresses the function of other lymphoid cells. The suppressor factor downregulates immune reactivity. T_sF is also used as an abbreviation for suppresor T cell factor.

A **T cell antigen-specific suppressor factor** is a soluble substance that is produced by a suppressor T cell after it has been activated. This suppressor factor may bind antigen and cause the immune response to be suppressed in a manner that is antigen specific.

A **nonspecific T cell suppressor factor** is a CD8+ suppressor T lymphocyte soluble substance that nonspecifically suppresses the immune response.

Suppressor T cells (Ts cells) are a T lymphocyte subpopulation that diminishes or suppresses antibody formation by B cells or downregulates the ability of T lymphocytes to mount a cellular immune response. Ts cells may induce suppression that is specific for antigen, idiotype, or nonspecific suppression. Some CD8+ T lymphocytes diminish T helper CD4+ lymphocyte responsiveness to both endogenous and exogenous antigens. This leads to suppression of the immune response. An overall immune response may be a consequence of the balance between helper T lymphocyte and suppressor T lymphocyte stimulation. Suppressor T cells are significant in the establishment of immunologic tolerance and are particularly active in response to unprocessed antigen. The inability to confirm the presence of receptor molecules on suppressor cells has cast a doubt as to the existence of the suppressor cell; however, functional suppressor cell effects are indisputable. Some suppressor T lymphocytes are antigen specific and are important in the regulation of T helper cell function. Like cytotoxic T cells, T suppressor cells are MHC class I rectricted.

Lyt antigens are murine T cell surface alloantigens that distinguish T lymphocyte subpopulation designated as helper (Lyt1) and suppressor (Lyt2 and Lyt3 antigens). Corresponding epitopes on B cells are termed Ly.

Lyt 1,2,3 is a category of murine T lymphocyte surface antigens that subdivide cells into helper T cells (Lyt1) and suppressor T cells (Lyt2 and Lyt3).

Thy (Θ) are epitopes found on murine thymocytes and the majority of murine T lymphocytes.

Thy-1 is a murine and rat thymocyte surface glycoprotein that is also found in neuron membranes of several species. Thy-1 was originally termed the Θ alloantigen. Thy.1 and Thy.2 are the two allelic forms. A substitution of one amino acid, arginine or glutamine, at position 89 represents the difference between Thy1.1 and Thy1.2. Mature T cells and thymocytes in the mouse express Thy-1. The genes encoding Thy-1 are present on chromosome 9 in the mouse. Whereas few human lymphocytes express Thy-1, it is present on the surfaces of neurons and fibroblasts.

Thy-1 antigen is a murine isoantigen present on the surface of thymic lymphocytes and on thymus-derived lymphocytes found in peripheral lymphoid tissues. Central nervous system tissues may also expess Thy-1 antigen.

Thy-1+ dendritic cells are cells derived from the T lymphocyte lineage found within the epithelium of the mouse epidermis.

Thymic stromal-derived lymphopoietin (TSLP) is a cytokine isolated from a murine thymic stromal cell line that possesses a primary sequence distinct from other known cytokines. The cDNA encodes a 140-amino acid protein that includes a 19 amino acid signal sequence. TSLP stimulates B220+ bone marrow cells to proliferate and express surface μ. TSLP synergizes with other signals to induce thymocyte and peripheral T cell proliferation but is not mitogenic for T cells alone.

Thymulin is a nonapeptide (Glu-Ala-Lys-Ser-Gln-gly-Ser-Asn) extracted from blood sera of human, pig, and calf thymuses. Thymulin shows a strong binding affinity for the T cell receptor on the lymphocyte membrane. Its zinc-binding property is associated with biological activity. Thymulin's enhancing action is reserved exclusively for T lymphocytes. It facilitates the function of several T lymphocyte subpopulations, but mainly enhances T suppressor lymphocyte activity. Thymulin was formerly called FTS.

Contrasuppression is a part of the immunoregulatory circuit that prevents suppressor effects in a feedback loop (Figure 32). This is a postulated mechanism to counteract the function of suppressor cells in a feedback-type mechanism. Proof of contrasuppressor and suppressor cell circuits awaits confirmation by molecular biologic techniques. A contrasuppressor cell is a T cell that opposes the action of a suppressor T lymphocyte.

CD3 is a molecule, also referred to as the T3 antigen, that consists of five different polypeptide chains with MWs ranging from 16–28 kD. The five chains are designated γ, δ, ε,

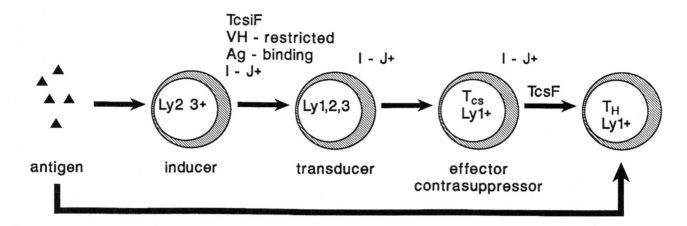

Figure 32.   Contrasuppression.

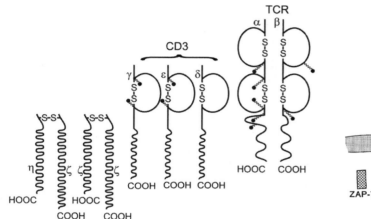

Figure 33.   Structure of CD3/TCR complex.

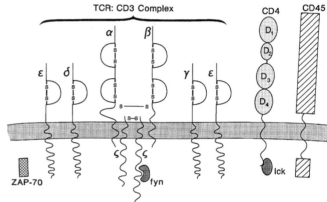

Figure 34.   Structure of TCR/CD3 complex showing the lck, fyn, and ZAP phosphotyrosine kinases.

ξ, and η, with most CD3 antibodies being against the 20 kD ε-chain. Physically, they are closely associated with each other and also with the T cell antigen receptor in the T cell membrane (Figure 33). Incubation of T cells with CD3 antibodies induces calcium flux and proliferation. This group of molecules may therefore transmit a signal to the cell interior following binding of antigen to the antigen receptor.

Lck, fyn, and **ZAP (phosphotyrosine kinases in T cells)** are the PTKs associated with early signal transduction in T cell activation (Figure 34). Lck is a src type PTK. It is found on T cells in physical association with CD4 and CD8 cytoplasmic regions. Deficiency of lck results in decreased stimulation of T cells and decreased T cell growth. Fyn is also a src PTK; however, it is found on hematopoietic cells. Increased fyn results in enhanced T cell activaition, but a deficiency of fyn has not been shown to decrease T cell growth. Fyn deficiency inhibits T cell activation in only some T cell subsets. ZAP or ξ associated protein kinase is like the syk PTK in B cells. It is found only on T cells and NK cells.

Activity of the enzyme is dependent on association of ZAP with the ξ chain following TCR activation.

ZAP-70 is a 70kD kinase present in the cytosol that is believed to participate in maintaining T lymphocyte receptor signaling. It is similar to syk in B lymphocytes.

There are two types of **T lymphocyte antigen receptors (TCRs)**: TCR1, which appears first in ontogeny, and TCR2 (Figure 35). TCR2 is a heterodimer of two polypeptides (α and β); TCR1 consists of γ and δ polypeptides (refer to Figure 36). Each of the two polypeptides comprising each receptor has a constant and a variable region (similar to immunoglobulin). Reminiscent of the diversity of antibody molecules, T cell antigen receptors can likewise identify a tremendous number of antigenic specificities (estimated to be able to recognize 10^{15} epitopes).

The TCR is a structure comprised of a minimum of seven receptor subunits whose production is encoded by six separate genes. Following transcription, these subunits are

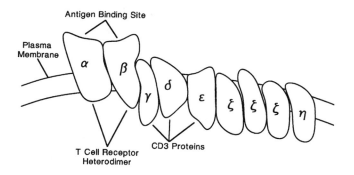

Figure 35. T lymphocyte receptor.

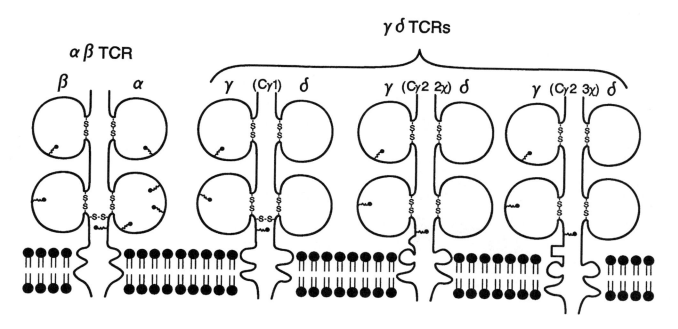

Figure 36. Structure of T receptors showing αβ and γδ receptors.

assembled precisely. Assimilation of the complete receptor complex is requisite for surface expression of TCR subunits. Numerous biochemical events are associated with activation of a cell through the TCR receptor. These events ultimately lead to receptor subunit phosphorylation.

T cells may be activated by the interaction of antigen, in the context of MHC, with the T cell receptor. This involves transmission of a signal to the interior through the CD3 protein to activate the cell.

The γδ T **cell receptor** is a far less common receptor than the αβ TCR. It is comprised of γ and δ chains and occurs on the surface of early thymocytes and less than 1% on peripheral blood lymphocytes. The γδ TCR appears on double-negative CD4⁻CD8⁻ cells. Thus, the γδ heterodimer resembles its αβ counterpart in possessing both V and C regions, but has less diversity. TCR specificity and diversity are attributable to the multiplicity of germ line V gene seg-

ments subjected to somatic recombination in T cell ontogeny, leading to a complete TCR gene. Cells bearing the γδ receptor often manifest target cell killing that is not MHC restricted. Monoclonal antibodies to specific TCR V regions are being investigated for possible use in the future treatment of autoimmune diseases. γδ T cells are sometimes found in association with selected epithelial surfaces, especially in the gut.

There are four separate sets of **T cell receptor genes** that encode the antigen-MHC binding region. Most (approximately 95%) peripheral T lymphocytes express α and β gene sets. Approximately 5% of circulating peripheral blood T cells and a subset of T lymphocytes in the thymus express γ and δ genes. The αβ chains or the γδ chains, encoded by their respective genes, form an intact T cell receptor and are associated with γ, δ, ε, ζ, and η chains that comprise the CD3 molecular complex. The arrangement of TCR genes resembles that of genes which encode immunoglobulin heavy chains. The TCR δ genes are located in the center of the α genes. V, D, and J segment recombination permits TCR gene diversity. Rearrangement of a Vα segment to a Jα segment yields an intact variable region. There are two sets of D, J, and C genes at the β locus. During joining, marked diversity is achieved by V-J, V-D-D-J, and V-D-J rearrangements. Humans have eight Vγ, three Jγ, and an initial Cγ gene. Before reaching Cγ2, there are two more Jγ genes. The δ locus contains five Vδ, two Dδ, and six Jδ genes. TCR gene recombination takes place by mechanisms that resemble those of B cell genes. B and T lymphocytes have essentially the same rearrangement enzymes. TCR genes do not undergo somatic mutation, which is essential to immunoglobulin diversity.

αβ T cells are T lymphocytes that express αβ chain heterodimers on their surface. The vast majority of T cells are of the αβ variety (Figure 37).

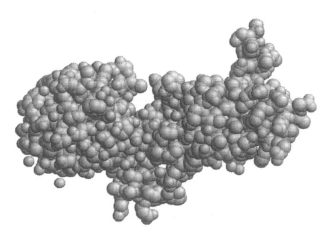

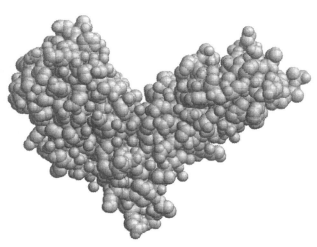

Figure 37. β chain of a T cell antigen receptor of a mouse.

A **"silencer sequence"** blocks transcription of the T cell receptor α chain. This sequence is found 5′ to the α chain enhancer in non-T cells and in those with γδ receptors.

γδ T cells are early T lymphocytes that express γ and δ chains comprising the T cell receptor of the cell surface. They comprise only 5% of the normal circulating T cells in healthy adults. γδ T cells "home" to the lamina propria of the gut. Their function is not fully understood.

Tp44 (CD29) is a T lymphocyte receptor that regulates cytokine synthesis, thereby controlling responsiveness to antigen. Its significance in regulating activation of T lymphocytes is demonstrated by the ability of monoclonal antibody against CD28 receptor to block T cell stimulation by specific antigen. During antigen-specific activation of lymphocytes, stimulation of the CD28 receptor occurs when it combines with the B7/BB1 coreceptor during the interaction between T and B lymphocytes. CD28 is a T lymphocyte differentiation antigen that four-fifths of CD3/Ti positive lymphocytes express. It is a member of the immunoglobulin superfamily. CD28 is found only on T lymphocytes and on plasma cells. There are 134 extracellular amino acids with a transmembrane domain and a brief cytoplasmic tail in each CD28 monomer.

CD5 (Figure 38), also referred to as the T1 antigen, is a single chain glycopolypeptide with a MW of 67 kD, and is present on the majority of human T cells. Its density increases with maturation of T cells. It is also found on a subpopulation of B cells. Sensitive immunohistochemical techniques have demonstrated its presence on immature B cells in the fetus and at low levels on mantle zone B cells in adult human lymphoid tissue. The majority of cases of B cell chronic lymphocytic leukemia expresses easily detectable levels of CD5. CD5 binds to CD72.

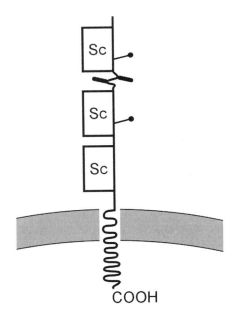

Figure 38. Structure of CD5

CD6 is a molecule sometimes referred to as the T12 antigen. It is a single chain glycopolypeptide with a MW of 105kD and is present on the majority of human T cells (similar in distribution to CD3). It stains some B cells weakly.

CD7 is an antigen with a MW of 40kD which is present on the majority of T cells. It is useful as a marker for T cell neoplasms when other T cell antigens are absent. The CD7 antigen is probably a Fc receptor for IgM.

CD45 (Figure 39) is an antigen that is a single chain glycoprotein, referred to as the leukocyte common antigen (or "T200"). It consists of at least five high molecular weight glycoproteins present on the surface of the majority of human leukocytes (MWs: 180, 190, 205, 220 kD). The different isoforms arise from a single gene via alternative mRNA splicing. The variation between the isoforms is all in the extracellular region. The larger (700 amino acid) intracellular portion is identical in all isoforms and has protein tyrosine phosphatase activity. It can potentially interact with intracellular protein kinases such as p56^{lck}, which may be involved in triggering cell activation. By dephosphorylating proteins, CD45's actions oppose that of a protein kinase. It facilitates signaling through B cell and T cell antigen receptors.

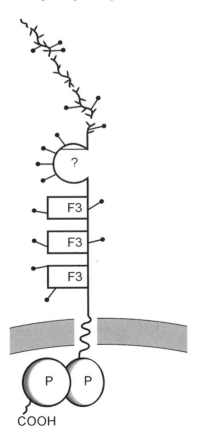

Figure 39. Structure of CD45. Also known as leukocyte common antigen.

Leukocyte common antigen (LCA) is an antigen shared in common by both T and B lymphocytes and expressed to a lesser degree by histiocytes and plasma cells. By immunoperoxidase staining, it can be demonstrated in sections of paraffin-embedded tissues containing these cell types. It is a valuable marker to distinguish lymphoreticular neoplasms from carcinomas and sarcomas. LCA is also called CD45. T200 is an obsolete term for leukocyte common antigen (LCA).

A **T lymphocyte (T cell)** is a thymus-derived lymphocyte that confers cell-mediated immunity (Figure 40). They cooperate with B lymphocytes enabling them to synthesize antibody specific for thymus-dependent antigens, including switching from IgM to IgG and/or IgA production. T lymphocytes exiting the thymus recirculate in the blood, lymph, and in the peripheral lymphoid organs. They migrate to the deep cortex of lymph nodes. Those in the blood may attach to post capillary venule endothelial cells of lymph nodes and to the marginal sinus in the spleen. After passing across the venules into the splenic white pulp or lymph node cortex, they reside there for 12 to 24 hours and exit by the efferent lymphatics. They proceed to the thoracic duct and from there to the left subclavian vein where they enter the blood circulation.

Mature T cells are classified on the basis of their surface markers, such as CD4 and CD8. CD4+ T lymphocytes recognize antigens in the context of MHC class II histocompatibility molecules whereas CD8+ T lymphocytes recognize antigen in the context of class I MHC histocompatibility molecules. The CD4+ T cells participate in the afferent limb of the immune response to exogenous antigen, which is presented to them by antigen-presenting cells. This stimulates the synthesis of IL-2 which activates CD8+ T cells, NK cells and B cells, thereby orchestrating an immune response to the antigen. Thus, they are termed helper T lymphocytes. They also mediate delayed-type hypersensitivity reactions. CD8+ T lymphocytes include cytotoxic and suppressor cell populations. They react to endogenous antigen and often express their effector function by a cytotoxic mechanism, e.g., against a virus-infected cell. Other molecules on mature T cells in humans includes the E rosette receptor CD2 molecule, the T cell receptor, the pan T cell marker termed CD3, and transferrin receptors.

T cells are derived from hematopoietic precursors that migrate to the thymus where they undergo differentiation which continues thereafter to completion in the various lymphoid tissues throughout the body or during their circulation to and from these sites. The T cells are primarily involved in the control of the immune responses by providing specific cells capable of helping or suppressing these responses. They also have a number of other functions related to cell-mediated immune phenomena.

A **T lymphocyte clone** is a daughter cell of one T lymphocyte derived from the blood or spleen that is added to culture

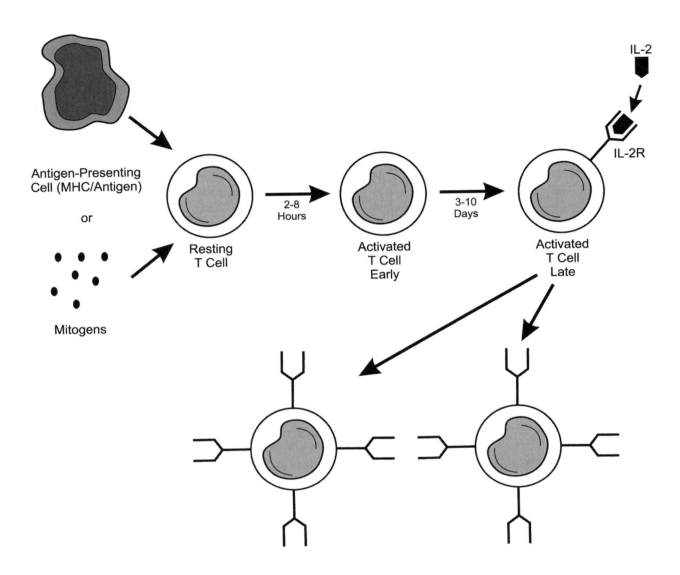

Figure 40. T cell activation.

medium and activated by antigen. Those T cells that are stimulated by antigen form blasts which can be separated from the remaining T cells by density gradient centrifugation. The T cells that have responded to antigen are diluted, and aliquots are dispensed into tissue culture plates to which antigen and IL-2 are added. Each well contains a single lymphocyte. This method provides individual T cell clones.

A **T lymphocyte subpopulation** is a subset of T cells that have a specific function and express a specific cluster of differentiation (CD) markers or other antigens on their surface. Examples include the CD4+ helper T lymphocyte subset and the CD8+ suppressor/cytotoxic T lymphoctye subset.

Calcineurin is a protein phosphatase that is serine/threonine-specific. Activation of T cells apparently requires deletion of phosphates from serine or threonine residues (Figures 41 and 42). Its action is inhibited by the immuno-

suppressive drugs cyclosporin-A and FK506. Cyclosporin-A and FK-506 combine with immunophilin intracellular molecules to form a complex that combines with calcineurin and inhibits its activity.

Phorbol esters (Figure 43) are esters of phorbol alcohol (4,9,12-beta,13,20-pentahydroxy-1,6-tigliadien-3-on) found in croton oil and myristic acid. Phorbol myristate acetate (PMA), which is of interest to immunologists, is a phorbol ester that is 12-O-tetradecanoylphorbol-13-acetate (TPA). This is a powerful tumor promoter that also exerts pleotrophic effects on cells in culture such as stimulation of macromolecular synthesis and cell proliferation, induction of prostaglandin formation, alteration in the morphology, and permeability of cells and disappearance of surface fibronectin. PMA also acts on leukocytes. It links to and stimulates protein kinase C leading to threonine and serine residue phosphorylation in the transmembrane protein

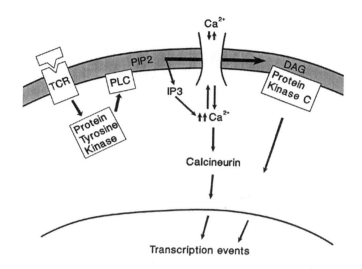

Figure 41. Schematic representation of cellular events upon binding of an activated T cell to the T cell receptor.

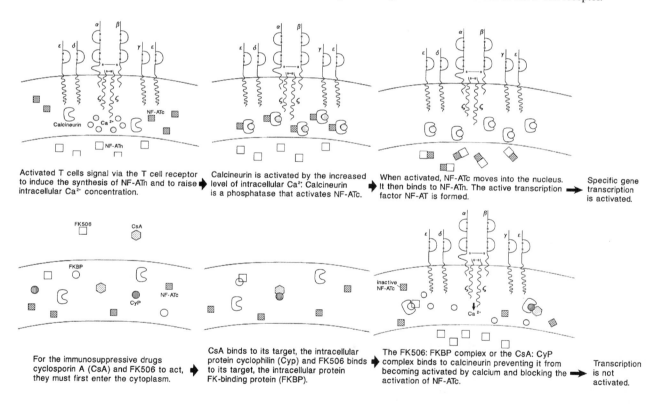

Activated T cells signal via the T cell receptor to induce the synthesis of NF-ATn and to raise intracellular Ca²⁺ concentration.

Calcineurin is activated by the increased level of intracellular Ca²: Calcineurin is a phosphatase that activates NF-ATc.

When activated, NF-ATc moves into the nucleus. It then binds to NF-ATn. The active transcription factor NF-AT is formed.

Specific gene transcription is activated.

For the immunosuppressive drugs cyclosporin A (CsA) and FK506 to act, they must first enter the cytoplasm.

CsA binds to its target, the intracellular protein cyclophilin (Cyp) and FK506 binds to its target, the intracellular protein FK-binding protein (FKBP).

The FK506: FKBP complex or the CsA: CyP complex binds to calcineurin preventing it from becoming activated by calcium and blocking the activation of NF-ATc.

Transcription is not activated.

Figure 42. Calcineurin.

cytoplasmic domains such as in the CD2 and CD3 molecules. These events enhance interleukin-2 receptor expression on T cells and facilitate their proliferation in the presence of interleukin-1 as well as TPA. Mast cells, polymorphonuclear leukocytes and platelets may all degranulate in the presence of TPA.

Protein kinase C (Figure 44) is an enzyme that Ca²⁺ activates in the cytoplasm of cells. As a receptor for phorbol ester, it participates in cell activation, signal transduction leading to hormone secretion, enzyme secretion, neurotransmitter release, and mediation of inflammation. It is also involved in lipogenesis and gluconeogenesis. PKC also participates in differentiation of cells and tumor promotion.

By light microscopy, **resting lymphocytes** (Figure 45) appear as a distant and homogeneous population of round cells, each with a large, spherical or slightly kidney-shaped

Phorbol 12,13-dibutyrate (PDBu)

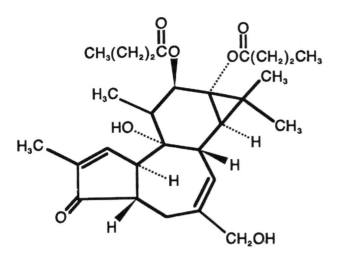

Figure 43.   Structure of phorbol ester.

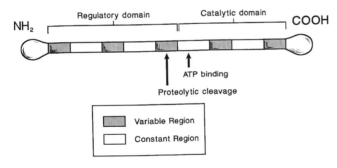

Figure 44.   Protein kinase C.

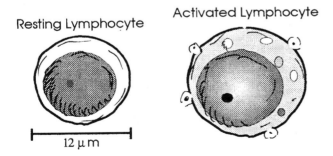

Figure 45.   Comparison of a resting and an activated lymphocyte.

indentation and contains densely packed chromatin. Occasionally, nucleoli can be distinguished. The small lymphocyte variant, which is the predominant morphologic form, is slightly larger than an erythrocyte. Larger lymphocytes, ranging between 10–20 μm in diameter, are difficult to differentiate from monocytes. They have more cytoplasm and may show azurophilic granules. Intermediate-size forms between the two have been described. By phase contrast microscopy, living lymphocytes demonstrate a feeble motility with ameboid movements which give the cells a hand mirror shape. The mirror handle is called a uropod. In large lymphocytes, mitochondria and lysosomes are better visualized; some cells show a spherical, birefringent, 0.5 μm diameter inclusion called a Gall body. Lymphocytes do not spread on surfaces. The different classes of lymphocytes cannot be distinguished by light microscopy. By scanning electron microscopy, B lymphocytes sometimes show a hairy (rough) surface, but this is apparently an artifact. Electron microscopy does not provide additional information except for visualization of the cellular organelles which are not abundant. This suggests that the small, resting lymphocytes are end-stage cells. With appropriate stimulation, however, they are capable of considerable morphologic changes.

Activated lymphocytes are cells with surface receptors that interact with specific antigens or mitogens such as phytohemagglutinin, concanavalin A, or staphylococcal protein A. The morphologic appearance of activated (or stimulated) lymphocytes is characteristic, and in this form the cells are called immunoblasts. These cells increase in size from 15 to 30 μm in diameter, show increased cytoplasmic basophilia, and develop vacuoles, lysosomes, and ribosomal aggregates. Pinocytotic vesicles are present on the cell membrane. The nucleus contains little chromatin which is limited to a thin marginal layer, and the nucleolus becomes conspicuous. The array of changes that follows stimulation is called transformation. Such cells are called transformed cells. An activated B lymphocyte may synthesize antibody molecules, whereas an activated T cell may mediate a cellular immune reaction.

A **sensitized lymphocyte** is a primed lymphocyte that has been previously exposed to a specific antigen.

Tac is a cell suface protein on T lymphocytes that binds IL-2. It is a 55kD polypeptide that is expressed on activated T lymphocytes. Tac is an abbreviation of T activation. The p55 Tac polypeptide combines with IL-2 with a kD of about 10^{-8} M. Interaction of IL-2 with p55 alone does not lead to activation. IL-2 binds to a second protein termed p70 or p75 that has a higher affinity of binding to p55. T cells expressing p70 or p75 alone are stimulated by IL-2. However, cells that express both receptor molecules bind IL-2 more securely and can be stimulated with a relatively lower IL-2 concentration. Anti-Tac monoclonal antibody can inhibit T cell proliferation. Tac antigen is CD25.

nucleus which occupies most of the cell. The nucleus surrounded by a narrow rim of basophilic cytoplasm with occasional vacuoles. It usually has a poorly visible single

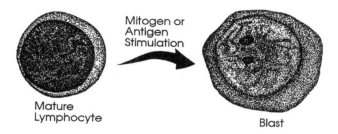

Figure 46. Blastogenesis.

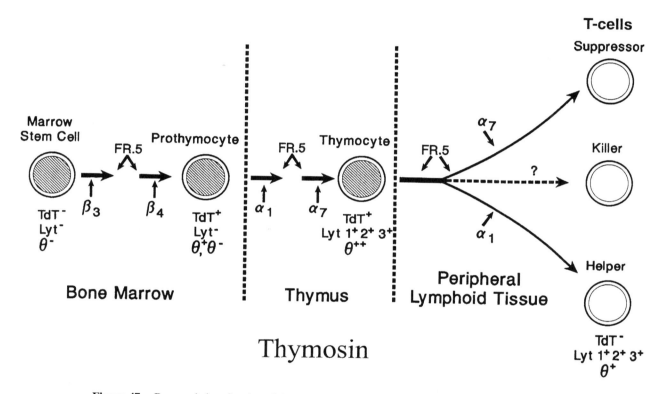

Figure 47. Proposed site of action of thymosin polypeptides on maturation of T-cell subpopulations.

Blastogenesis (Figure 46), or blast transformation, is the activation of small lymphocytes to form blast cells. A blast cell is a relatively large cell that is greater than 8 μm in diameter with abundant RNA in the cytoplasm, a nucleus containing loosely arranged chromatin, and a prominent nucleolus. Blast cells are active in synthesizing DNA and contain numerous polyribosomes in the cytoplasm.

Thymic hormones are soluble substances synthesized by thymic epithelial cells that promote thymocyte differentiation. They include thymopoietin and thymosins, peptides which help to regulate differentiation of T lymphocytes.

Thymic humoral factors (THFs) are soluble substances such as thymosins, thymopoietin, serum thymic factor, etc. which are synthesized by the thymus and govern differentiation and functiuon of lymphocytes.

Thymosin (Figure 47) is a 12kD protein hormone produced by the thymus gland that provides T lymphocyte immune function in animals that have been thymectomized.

Thymosin α-1 (thymopoietin) is a hormone produced by the thymus that stimulates T lymphocyte helper activity (Figure 48). It induces production of lymphokines such as interferon and macrophage inhibiting factor. It also enhances Thy-1.2 and Lyt-1-2-3 antigens of T lymphocytes. It may also alter thymocyte TdT concentrations.

Thymopoietin is a 49-amino acid polypeptide thymic hormone secreted by epithelial cells in the thymus. It affects neuromuscular transmission, induces early T lymphocyte differentiation, and affects immune regulation. Thymopoietin functions biologically to normalize immune imbalances related to either hypo- or hyperresponsiveness. These could

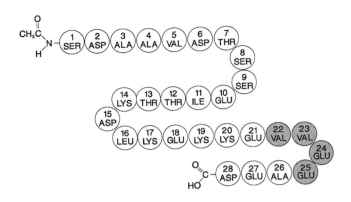

Figure 48.   Structure of thymosin α-1

be related to thymic involution with age, thymectomy, or other factors that result in immunologic imbalance. It is a 7-kD protein that facilitates the expression of Thy-1 antigen on T lymphocytes, possibly interfering with neuromuscular transmission, which has often been implicated in myasthenia gravis patients who develop thymoma.

Thymopentin (TP-5) is a synthetic pentapeptide, Arg-Lys-Asp-Val-Tyr, which corresponds to amino acid residues 32–36 of the thymic hormone thymopoietin. Thymopentin is the minimal fragment that can produce the biological activities of thymopoietin, i.e., thymopentin is the active site of thymopoietin (Figure 49).

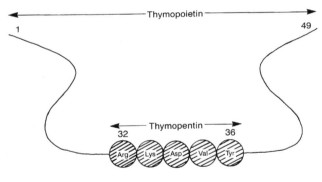

Figure 49.   Structure of thymopoietin and thymopentin.

Thymin is a hormone extracted from the thymus that has an activity resembling that of thymopoietin.

Athymic mice are a strain which lack a thymus and have no hair (Figure 50). T lymphocytes are absent; therefore, no manifestations of T cell immunity are present, i.e., they do not produce antibodies against thymus-dependent antigens and fail to reject allografts. They possess a normal complement of B cells and NK cells. These nude or *nu/nu* mice are homozygous for a mutation, *v*, on chromosome 11 which is inherited as an autosomal recessive trait. These features make the strain useful in studies evaluatingthymic-independent immune responses.

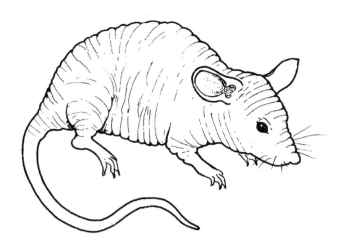

Figure 50.   Athymic (nude) mouse.

A **thymectomy** is the surgical removal of the thymus. Mice thymectomized as neonates fail to develop cell-mediated immunity and humoral immunity to thymus-dependent antigens.

Neonatal thymectomy in mice also leads to a chronic and eventually fatal disease called wasting disease which is characterized by lymphoid atrophy and weight loss. Wasting disease is also called runt disease or runting syndrome. Animals may develop ruffled fur, diarrhea, and a hunched appearance. Gnotobiotic (germ-free) animals fail to develop wasting disease following neonatal thymectomy. Thus, thymectomy of animals that are not germ free may lead to fatal infection as a consequence of greatly decreased cell-mediated immunity. Wasting may appear in immunodeficiencies such as AIDS as well as in graft vs. host (GVH) reactions.

Runt disease also results when neonatal mice of one strain are injected with lymph node or splenic lymphocytes from a different strain. It is accompanied by weight loss, failure to thrive, diarrhea, splenomegaly, and can lead to death. The immune system of the neonatal animal is immature and reactivity against donor cells is weak or absent. Runt disease is an example of graft vs. host reaction.

Apoptosis (Figures 51 and 52) is programmed cell death in which the chromatin becomes condensed and the DNA is degraded. The immune system employs apoptosis for clonal deletion of cortical thymocytes by antigen in immunologic tolerance. Contrary to necrosis, programmed cell death occurs to regulate steady-state levels of hematopoietic cells that undergo cellular division and differentiation. No local inflammatory response is induced with apoptosis because cellular contents which stimulate inflammation are not released. Regulatory genes which control apoptosis have been identified. These include:

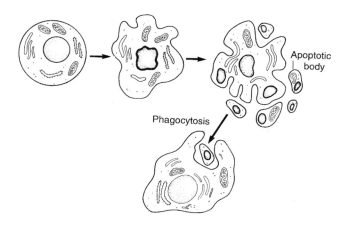

Figure 51.   Apoptosis with phagocytosis.

bcl-2	prevents apoptosis
bax	promotes apoptosis by opposing *bcl-2*
bcl-Xl	prevents apoptosis
bcl-Xs	promotes apoptosis by opposing *bcl-Xl*
ICE	promotes apoptosis by encoding enzyme IL-1b convertase
fas/apo-1	promotes apoptosis

Apoptosis regulates the number of active immune cells in circulation so unnecessarily activated lymphocytes are eliminated once an antigenic response has ended. As the response subsides, signals promoting apoptosis appear. For instance,

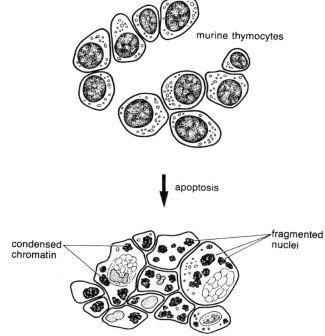

Figure 52   Apoptosis.

B-cell activation induces increased cytokine receptors and decreased bcl-2 expression. This makes the cell more susceptible to apoptosis than naive B-cells or memory cells.

10
Cytokines

Leukocytes or other types of cells produce soluble proteins or glycoproteins termed cytokines that serve as chemical communicators from one cell to another. Cytokines are usually secreted, although some may be expressed on a cell membrane or maintained in reservoirs in the extracellular matrix. Cytokines combine with surface receptors on target cells that are linked to intracellular signal transduction and second messenger pathways. Their effects may be autocrine, acting on cells that produce them, or paracrine acting on neighboring cells and only rarely endocrine, acting on cells at distant sites.

Cytokines are immune system proteins that are biological response modifiers. They coordinate antibody and T cell immune system interactions, and amplify immune reactivity. Cytokines include monokines synthesized by macrophages and lymphokines produced by activated T lymphocytes and natural killer cells. Monokines include interleukin-1, tumor necrosis factor, α and β interferons and colony stimulating factors. Lymphokines include interleukins-2-6, γ interferon, granulocyte-macrophage colony-stimulating factor and lymphotoxin. Endothelial cells and fibroblasts and selected other cell types may also synthesize cytokines (Figure 1).

Lymphokine research can be traced to the 1960s when macrophage migration inhibitory factor was described. It is believed to be due to more than one cytokine in lymphocyte supernatants. Lymphotoxin was described in activated lymphocyte culture supernatants in the late 1960s and lymphokines were recognized as cell-free soluble factors formed when sensitized lymphocytes react with specific antigen. These substances were considered responsible for cell-mediated immune reactions. Interleukin-2 was described as T cell growth factor. Tumor necrosis factor (TNF) was the first monocyte/macrophage-derived cytokine or monokine to be recognized. Other cytokines derived from monocytes include lymphocyte activation factors (LAF), later named interleukin 1. It was found to be mitogenic for thymocytes. Whereas, immunologists described lymphokines and monokines, virologists described interferons. Interferon is a factor formed by virus-infected cells that is able to induce resistance of cells to infection with homologous or heterologous viruses. Subsequently, interferon-γ, synthesized by T lymphocytes activated by mitogen, was found to be distinct from interferons-α and -β and to be formed by a variety of cell types. Colony stimulating factors (CSFs) were described

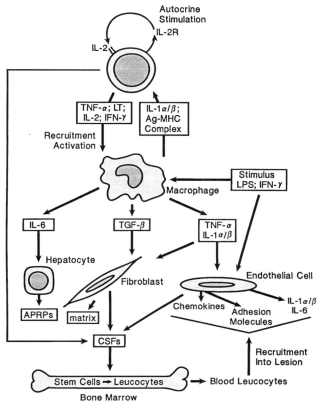

CSF = Colony Stimulating Factor
APRP = Acute-Phase Reactant Protein

Figure 1. Generation of cytokines by endothelial cells, fibroblasts, T-helper lymphocytes, and monocyte/macrophages.

as proteins capable of promoting proliferation and differentiation of hematopoietic cells. CSFs promote granulocyte or monocyte colony formation in semisolid media. Proteins that facilitate the growth of nonhematopoietic cells are not usually included with the cytokines. Transforming growth factor β has an important role in inflammation and immunoregulation as well as immunosuppressive actions on T cells.

Classes of cytokine receptors include the immunoglobulin receptor superfamily, the hematopoietin/cytokine receptor superfamily, the nerve-growth factor receptor superfamily, the G-protein coupled receptor superfamily and the other receptor tyrosine or serine kinases plus unclassified group.

Cytokine receptor families is a classification system of cytokine receptors according to conserved sequences or folding motifs. Type I receptors share a tryptophan-serine-X-tryptophan-serine, or WSXWS sequence, on the proximal extracellular domains. Type I receptors recognize cytokines with a structure of four α-helical strands, including IL-2 and G-CSF. Type II receptors are defined by the sequence pattern of Type I and Type II interferon receptors. Type III receptors are those found as receptors for TNF (p55 and p75). CD40, nerve growth factor receptor and Fas protein have sequences homologous to those of Type III receptors. A fourth family of receptors has extracellular domains of the Ig superfamily. IL-1 receptors as well as some growth factors and colony stimulating factors have Ig domains. The fifth family of receptors displays a seven transmembrane α-helical structure. This motif is shared by many of the receptors linked to GTP-binding proteins.

A principal feature of cytokines is that their effects are pleiotropic and redundant. Cytokines do not exert a specific effect on one type of target cell. Most of them have a broad spectrum of biological effects on more than one type of tissue and cell. Various cytokines may interact with the same cell type to produce similar effects. Cytokine receptors are grouped into two classes. Class I receptors include those that bind a number of interleukins, including IL-2, IL-3, IL-4, IL-6, IL-7, IL-9, IL-11, IL-12 and IL-15. Other type I receptors are those for erythropoietin (EPO), growth hormone (GH), granulocyte-colony-stimulating (G-CSF), granulocyte-macrophage colony stimulating factor (GM-CSF), leukemia inhibitory factor (LIF) and ciliary neurotrophic factor (CNTF). Class II receptors include those that bind interferon (IFN) α/β, IFNγ and IL-10. Cytokine receptors are usually comprised of multipeptide complexes with a specific ligand binding subunit and a signal transducer subunit that is class specific. Receptors for IL-3, IL-5 and GM-CSF possess a unique a component and a common b signal transducer subunit which accounts for the redundant effects these molecules have on hematopoietic cells. IL-6, CNTF, LIF, Oncostatin M (OM) and interleukin 11 (IL-11) belong to a family of receptors that share a gp130 signal transducer subunit in common, which explains some of the similar functions these molecules have on various tissues. In the IL-2 receptor system, which is comprised of three peptide chains, α, β and γ, a β and γ gene heterodimer accounts for IL-2 signal transduction with respect to T cell growth. IL-4, IL-7, and IL-15 also promote growth of T cells. IL-4, IL-7 and IL-15 use the IL-2 receptor γ chain which accounts for the redundant functions of these cytokines as T cell growth factors.

Cytokines have been named on the basis of the cell of origin or of the bioassay used to define them. This system has lead to misnomers such as tumor necrosis factor which is more appropriately termed an immunomodulator and pro-inflammatory cytokine. The interleukins now number 17, even though IL-8 is in fact a member of the chemokine cytokine family. The chemokines share a minimum of 25% amino acid homology, are similar in structure and bind to 7 rhodopsin superfamily transmembrane spanning receptors. The chemokines are comprised of the CXC or α chemokines encoded by genes on chromosome 4 in humans and the CC or β chemokines encoded by genes on chromosome 17. CXC chemokines attract neutrophils whereas CC chemokines attracts monocytes.

A **lymphokine** is a nonimmunoglobulin polypeptide substance synthesized mainly by T lymphocytes that affects the function of other cells. It may either enhance or suppress an immune response. Lymphokines may facilitate cell proliferation, growth and differentiation, and they may act on gene transcription to regulate cell function. Lymphokines have either a paracrine or autocrine effect. Many lymphokines have now been described. Well known examples of lymphokines include interleukin 2, interleukin 3, migration inhibitory factor (MIF) and gamma interferon. The term cytokine includes lymphokines, soluble products produced by lymphocytes, as well as monokines and soluble products produced by monocytes.

A **monokine** is a cytokine produced by monocytes. Any one of a group of biologically active factors secreted by monocytes and macrophages that has a regulatory effect on the function of other cells such as lymphocytes. Examples include interleukin-1 and tumor necrosis factor.

MIF (macrophage/monocyte migration inhibitory factor) is a substance synthesized by T lymphocytes in response to immunogenic challenge that inhibits the migration of macrophages. MIF is a 25kD lymphokine. Its mechanism of action is by elevating intracellular cAMP, polymerizing microtubules and stopping macrophage migration. MIF may increase the adhesive properties of macrophages, thereby inhibiting their migration. The two types of the protein MIF include one that is 65kD with a pI of 3–4 and another that is 25kD with a pI of approximately 5.

Recombinant DNA technology has permitted the preparation of relatively large quantities of cytokines enabling investigators to perform X-ray and NMR studies to determine molecular structure. Other investigations of gene organization, chromosomal location and receptor usage have permitted the classification of cytokines into six separate families.

Chemokines are a family of 8 to 10kD chemotactic cytokines that share structural homology. They are chemokinetic and chemotactic, stimulating leukocyte movement and directed movement. Two internal disulfide loops are present in chemokine molecules, that may be subdivided according to the position of the two amino terminal cysteine residues, i.e., adjacent (cys-cys) or separated by a single amino acid (cys-X-cys). Activated mononuclear phagocytes as well as fibroblasts, endothelium and megakaryocytes synthesize cys-X-cys chemokines, including interleukin-8, that act mainly on polymorphonuclear neutrophils as acute inflammatory mediators. Activated T lymphocytes synthesize cys-cys chemokines that act principally on mononuclear inflammatory cell subpopulations. Cys-X-cys and cys-cys chemokines combine with heparan sulfate proteoglycans on endothelial cell surfaces. They may activate chemokinesis of leukocytes that adhere to endothelium via adhesion molecules. Chemokine receptors are being characterized, and selected ones interact with more than one chemokine.

Intercrine cytokines is a family comprised of a minimum of 8–10kD cytokines that share 20–45% amino acid sequence homology. All are believed to be basic heparin-binding polypeptides with proinflammatory and reparative properties. Their cDNA has conserved single open reading frames, 5′ region typical signal sequences, and 3′ untranslated regions that are rich in AP sequences. Human cytokines that include interleukin-8, platelet factor 4, β thromboglobulin, IP-10 and melanoma growth stimulating factor or GRO comprise a subfamily encoded by genes on chromosome 4. They possess a unique structure. LD78, ACT-2, I-309, RANTES and macrophage chemotactic and activating factor (MCAF) comprise a second subset and are encoded by genes on chromosome 17 of man. Human chromosome 4 bears the intercrine α genes and chromosome 17 bears the intercrine β genes. Four cysteines are found in the intercrine family. Adjacent cysteines are present in the intercrine beta subfamily that includes huMCAF, huBLD-78, huACT-II, huRANTES, muTCA-III, muJE, muMIP-1α and muMIP-1β. One amino acid separates cysteines of the intercrines alpha-subfamily which is comprised of huPF-4, hubetaTG, huIL-8, ch9E3, huGRO, huIP-10 and muMIP-2. The cysteines are significant for tertiary structure and for intercrine binding to receptors.

Interleukin(s) IL are a group of cytokines synthesized by lymphocytes, monocytes and selected other cells that promote growth of T cells, B cells, hematopoietic stem cells and have various other biological functions.

Interleukin-1 (IL-1) is a cytokine synthesized by activated mononuclear phagocytes that have been stimulated by ribopolysaccharide or by interaction with CD4+ T lymphocytes. It is a monokine and is a mediator of inflammation, sharing many properties in common with tumor necrosis factors (TNF). IL-1 is comprised of two principal polypeptides of 17kD each with isoelectric points of 5.0 and 7.0. They are designated IL-1α and IL-1β, respectively. Genes found on chromosome 2 encode these two molecular species. They have the same biological activities and bind to the same receptor on cell surfaces. Both IL-1α and IL-1β are derived by proteolytic cleavage of 33kD precursor molecules. IL-1α acts as a membrane associated substance, whereas IL-1β is found free in the circulation. IL-1 receptors are present on numerous cell types. IL-1 may either activate adenylate cyclase elevating cAMP levels and then activating protein kinase A, or it may induce nuclear factors that serve as cellular gene transcriptional activators. IL-1 may induce synthesis of enzymes that generate prostaglandins which

may in turn induce fever, a well known action of IL-1. IL-1's actions differ according to whether it is produced in lower or in higher concentrations. At low concentrations, the effects are mainly immunoregulatory. IL-1 acts with polyclonal activators to facilitate CD4+ T lymphocyte proliferation as well as B lymphocyte growth and differentiation. IL-1 stimulates multiple cells to act as immune or inflammatory response effector cells. It also induces further synthesis of itself as well as of IL-6 by mononuclear phagocytes and vascular endothelium. It resembles tumor necrosis factor (TNF) in inflammatory properties. IL-1 secreted in greater amounts produces endocrine effects as it courses through the peripheral blood circulation. For example, it produces fever and promotes the formation of acute phase plasma proteins in the liver. It also induces cachexia. Natural inhibitors of IL-1 may be produced by mononuclear phagocytes activated by immune complexes in humans. The inhibitor is biologically inactive and prevents the action of IL-1 by binding with its receptor serving as a competitive inhibitor. Corticosteroids and prostaglandins suppress IL-1 secretion. IL-1 was formerly called lymphocyte activating factor (LAF).

Interleukin-1 (IL-1) receptor (Figure 2) is a 80kD receptor on T lymphocytes, chondrocytes, osteoblasts and fibroblasts that binds IL-1α and IL-1β (Figure 3). Helper/inducer CD4+ T lymphocytes are richer in IL-1 receptors than are suppressor/cytotoxic (CD8+) T cells. The IL-1 receptor has an extracellular portion that binds ligand and contains all N-linked glycosylation sites. A 217 amino acid segment, apparently confined to the cytoplasm, could be involved in signal transduction. Further studies of ligand-binding have been facilitated through development of a soluble form of the cloned IL-1 receptor molecule which contains the extracellular part but not the transmembrane cytoplasmic region of the molecule. IL-1α and IL-1β molecules bind with equivalent affinities. The IL-1 receptor has been claimed to have more than one subunit. This is based on the demonstration of bands such as a 100kD band, in addition to that characteristic of the receptor which is 80kD. The recombinant IL-1 receptor functions in signal transduction. When the cytoplasmic part of the IL-1 receptor is depleted, the molecule does not function. The human T cell IL-1 receptor has now been cloned and found to be quite similar to its murine counterpart. Two affinity classes of binding sites for IL-1 have been described (Figures 4 and 5).

Interleukin-1 receptor antagonist protein (IRAP) (Figure 6) is a substance on T lymphocytes and endothelial cells that inhibits IL-1 activity.

Interleukin-1 receptor deficiency refers to CD4+ T cells deficient in IL-1 receptors in affected individuals. They fail to undergo mitosis when stimulated and fail to generate interleukin-2. This leads to a lack of immune responsiveness and constitutes a type of combined immunodeficiency. Opportunistic infections are increased in affected children who have inherited the condition as an autosomal recessive trait.

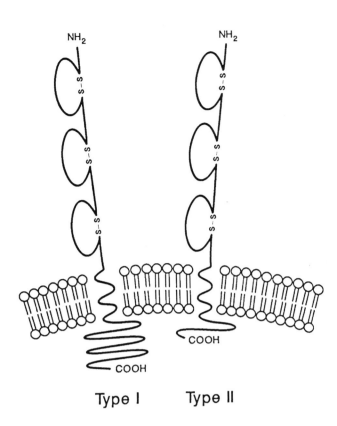

Figure 2. IL-1 receptors, type I and type II.

Interleukin-2 (IL-2) (Figure 7) is a 15.5kD glycoprotein synthesized by CD4+ T helper lymphocytes. It was formerly called T cell growth factor. IL-2 has an autocrine effect acting on the CD4+ T cells that produce it. Although mainly produced by CD4+ T cells, a small amount is produced by CD8+ T cells. Physiologic amounts of IL-2 do not have an endocrine effect since it acts on the cells producing it or on those nearby acting as a paracrine growth factor. IL-2's main effects are on lymphocytes. The amount of IL-2 which CD4+ T lymphocytes synthesize is a principal factor in determining the strength of an immune response. It also facilitates formation of other cytokines produced by T lymphocytes including interferon-γ and lymphotoxins. Inadequate IL-2 synthesis can lead to antigen-specific T lymphocyte anergy. IL-2 interacts with T lymphocytes by reacting with IL-2 receptors. IL-2 also promotes NK cell growth and potentiates the cytolytic action of NK cells through generation of lymphokine-activated killer (LAK) cells. Although NK cells do not have the p55 lower affinity receptor, they do express the high affinity p70 receptor and thus require high IL-2 concentrations for their activation. IL-2 is a human B cell growth factor and promotes synthesis of antibody by these cells. However, IL-2 does not induce isotype switching. IL-2 promotes the improved responsiveness of immature bone marrow cells to other cytokines. In the thymus, it may promote immature T cell growth. The IL-2 gene is located on

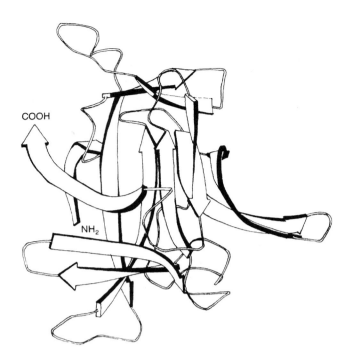

Figure 3. Tube structure of backbone of interleukin-1α. Resolution. 2.3 angstroms. This entry contains only α carbon coordinates. Interleukin-2 complex (human). Theoretical model. This interleukin-2 complex was generated by homology modelling. This is a shape-filling diagram.

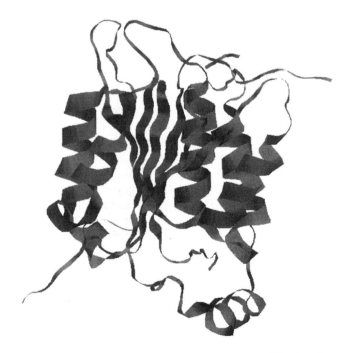

Figure 4. Human IL-1β converting enzyme. X-ray diffraction. Resolution. 2.6 angstroms.

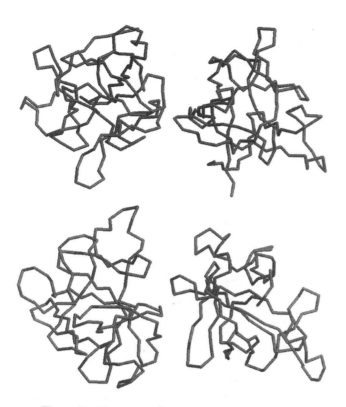

Figure 5. Human IL-1β. NMR. Backbone structure.

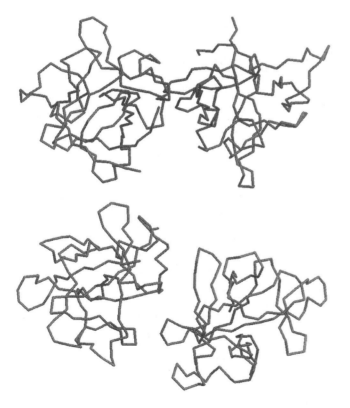

Figure 6. IL-1 receptor antagonist protein. Resolution. 3.2 angstroms.

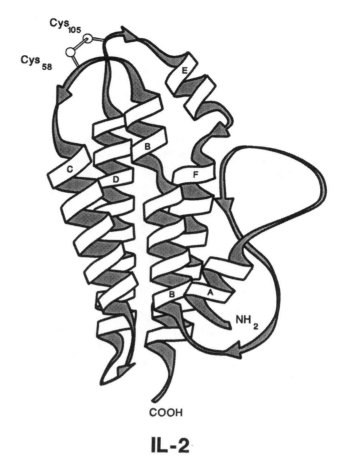

IL-2

Figure 7. Schematic representation of IL-2.

chromosome 4 in man. Corticosteroids, cyclosporin A and prostaglandins inhibit IL-2 synthesis and secretions.

Interleukin-2 receptor (IL-2R) is known also as CD25. Il-2R is a structure on the surface of T lymphocytes, natural killer and B lymphocytes characterized by the presence of a 55kD polypeptide, p55, and a 70kD polypeptide termed p70, which interacts with IL-2 molecules at the cell surface. The p55 polypeptide chain is referred to as Tac antigen, an abbreviation for T activation. The expression of both p55 and p70 permits a cell to bind IL-2 securely with a K_d of about 10^{-8}. p55, the low affinity receptor, apparently complexes with p70, the high affinity receptor, to accentuate the p70 receptor's affinity for IL-2. This permits increased binding in cells expressing both receptors. In addition, lesser quantities of IL-2 than would otherwise be required for stimulation are effective when both receptors are present on the cell surface. Antibodies against p55 or p70 can block IL-2 binding. Powerful antigenic stimulation such as in transplant rejection may lead to the shedding of p55 IL-2 receptors into the serum. The gene encoding the p55 chain is located on chromosome 10p14 in man. IL-2, IL-1, IL-6, IL-4 and TNF may induce IL-2 receptor expression.

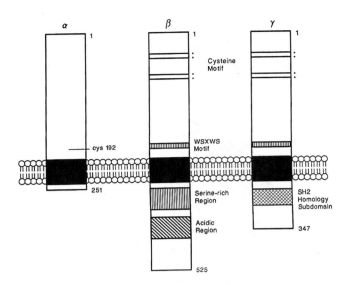

Figure 8. Schematic representation of interleukin-2 receptor αβγ subunit (IL-2Rαβγ).

Interleukin-2 receptor α subunit (IL-2Rα) (Figure 8) is a 55kD polypeptide subunit of the IL-2R with a K_d of 10^{-8} M. The α subunit is responsible for increasing the affinity between cytokine and receptor, however it has no role in signal transduction. It is expressed only on antigen stimulation of T cells, usually within 2 hours. Following long-term T cell activation the α subunit is shed, making it a potential candidate for a serum marker of strong or prolonged antigen stimulation. The gene encoding IL-2Rα is located on chromosome 10p14 in man.

Interleukin-2 receptor β subunit (IL-2Rβ) (Figure 8) is a 70–74 kD subunit of IL-2R with a K_d of 10^{-9} M. The β subunit is a member of the cytokine receptor family Type I due to its tryptophan serine-x-tryptophan-serine (WSXWS) domain. It is a constitutive membrane protein co-ordinately expressed with IL-2Rγ.

Interleukin-2 receptor βγ subunit (IL-2Rβγ) is a heterodimer found on resting T cells. Only those T cells expressing IL-2Rβγ are capable of growth in response to IL-2, as this is the portion of the receptor responsible for signal transduction.

Interleukin-2 receptor γ subunit (IL-2Rγ) subunit (Figure 8) is also a type I (WSXWS) receptor that is associated with IL-4 and IL-7 receptors as well as IL-2Rγ. Mutations in the γ subunit have been found in some SCIDS cases with X-linked inheritance, resulting in decreased proliferation of B and T cells.

Interleukin-2 receptor αβγ subunit (IL-2Rαβγ) is a complete IL-2 receptor. It consists of two distinct polypeptides, IL-2α, which is induced upon activation, and IL-2βγ, which is present on resting T cells. Upon expression of all three proteins affinity increases to 10^{-11}M and very low (physiologic)

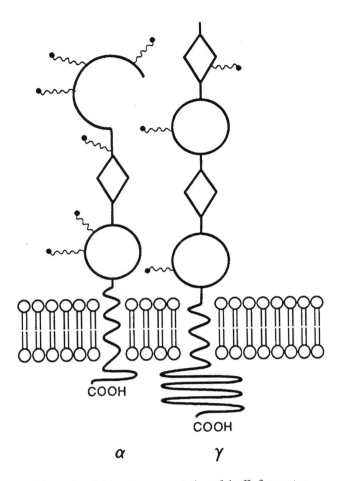

Figure 9. Schematic representation of the IL-3 receptor.

levels of IL-2 are capable of stimulating the cell. IL-2R is found on T lymphocytes, natural killer cells and B lymphocytes although natural killer cells do not express IL-2Rα. IL-2, IL-1, IL-6, IL-4, and TNF may induce IL-2R expression.

Interleukin-3 (IL-3) is a 20kD lymphokine synthesized by activated CD4+ T helper lymphocytes that acts as a colony stimulating factor by facilitating proliferation of some hematopoietic cells and promoting proliferation and differentiation of other lymphocytes. It acts by binding to high and low affinity receptors, inducing tyrosine phosphorylation and inducing colony formation of erythroid, myeloid, megakaryocytic and lymphoid hematopoietic cells. It also facilitates mast cell proliferation and the release of histamine. It facilitates T lymphocyte maturation through induction of 20α-hydroxysteroid dehydrogenase. The gene encoding IL-3 is situated on the long arm of chromosome 5.

Interleukin-3 receptor (IL-3R) (Figure 9) is a low affinity IL-3-binding α subunit (IL-3Rα) (CD123) that associates with a β subunit to produce a high affinity IL-3 receptor. The IL-3Rα subunit has an N-terminal region consisting of 100 amino acid residue, a cytokine receptor domain and a fibronectin III domain containing the WSXWS motif. The

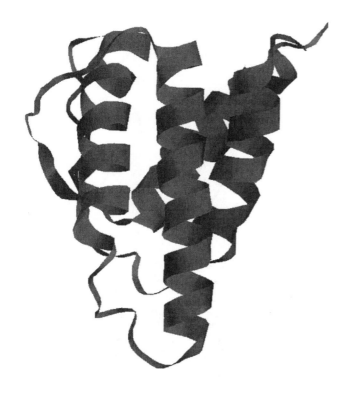

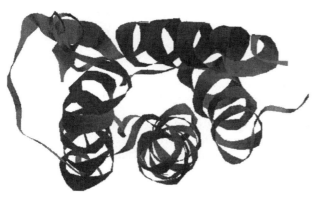

Figure 10.   Human IL-4. NMR.

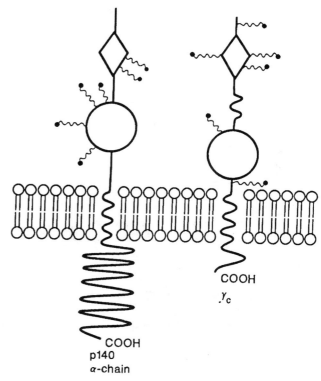

Figure 11.   Schematic representation of the IL-4 receptor.

truncated cytoplastic domain is associated with the inability to signal. There are two homologous segments in the β subunit's extracellular region. A cytokine receptor domain followed by a fibronectin domain is present in each of these segments. The human alpha chain contains six potential N-linked glycosylation sites whereas the β chain has three. Tyrosine and serine/threonine phosphorylation of numerous cellular proteins occurs rapidly following union of IL-3 with its receptor. The β subunit is requisite for signal transduction.

Interleukin-4 (IL-4)(B cell growth factor) (Figures 10 and 11) is a 20kD cytokine produced by CD4+ T lymphocytes mainly but also by activated mast cells. Most studies of IL-4 have been in mice where it serves as a growth and differen-

tiation factor for B cells and is a switch factor for synthesis of IgE (Figure 12). It also promotes growth of a cloned CD4+ T cell subset. Further properties of murine IL--4 include its function as a growth factor for mast cells and activating factor for macrophages. It also causes resting B lymphocytes to enlarge and enhances class II MHC molecule expression. IL-4 was previously termed B cell growth factor I (BCGF-I) and also termed B cell stimulating factor 1 (BSF-1). In man, CD4+ T lymphocytes also produce IL-4 but the human variety has not been shown to serve as a B cell or mast cell growth factor. Human IL-4 also fails to activate macrophages. Both murine and human IL-4 both induce switching of B lymphocytes to synthesize IgE. Thus, IL-4 may be significant in allergies. Human IL-4 also induces CD23 expression by B lymphocytes and macrophages in man. IL-4 may have some role in cell-mediated immunity.

Interleukin-5 (IL-5) (eosinophil differentiation factor) (Figure 13) is a 20kD cytokine synthesized by some activated CD4+ T lymphocytes and by activated mast cells. Formerly it was called T cell replacing factor or B cell growth factor II. It facilitates B cell growth and differentiation into cells that secrete IgA. It is a costimulator with IL-2 and IL-4 of B cell growth and differentiation. IL-5 also stimulates eosinophil growth and differentiation. It activates mature eosinophils to render them capable of killing helminths. Through IL-5, T lymphocytes exert a regulatory effect on inflammation mediated by eosinophils. Because of its

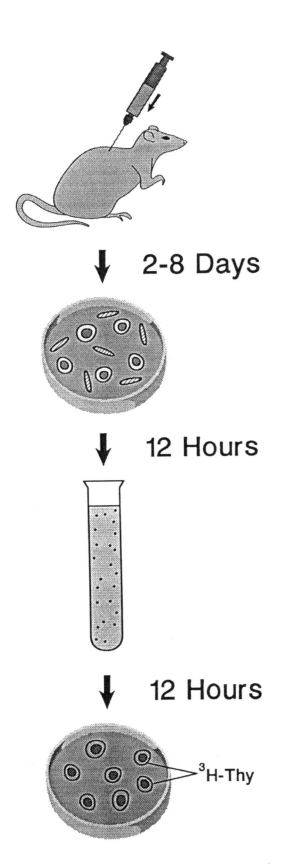

Figure 12. Induction of IL-4 response in short-term culture

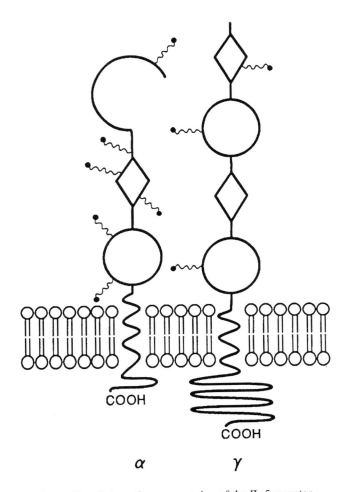

Figure 13. Schematic representation of the IL-5 receptor.

action in promoting eosinophil differentiation, it has been called eosinophil differentiation factor (EDF). IL-5 can facilitate B cell differentiation into plaque-forming cells of the IgM and IgG classes. In parasitic diseases, IL-5 leads to eosinophilia.

Interleukin-6 (IL-6) (Figures 14–16) is a 26kD cytokine produced by vascular endothelial cells, mononuclear phagocytes, fibroblasts, activated T lymphocytes and various neoplasms such as cardiac myxomas, bladder cancer and cervical cancer. It is secreted in response to IL-1 or TNF. Its main actions are on hepatocytes and B cells. Although it acts on many types of cells, a significant function is its ability to cause B lymphocytes to differentiate into cells that synthesize antibodies. IL-6 induces hepatocytes to form acute phase proteins that include fibrinogen. It is the main growth factor for activated B lymphocytes late in B cell differentiation. IL-6 is a growth factor for plasmacytoma cells which produce it. IL-6 also acts as a costimulator of T lymphocytes and of thymocytes. It acts in concert with other cytokines that promote the growth of early bone marrow hematopoietic stem cells. It acts together with IL-1 to costimulate activation of T_H cells. IL-6 was formerly termed B cell differentiation

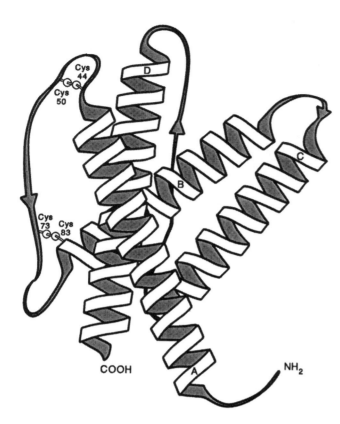

Figure 14.   Schematic represenation of IL-6.

factor (BCDF) and B cell stimulating factor 2 (BSF-2). It has also been implicated in the pathogenesis of plaques in psoriasis (Figure 17).

Interleukin-7 (IL-7) (Figure 18) facilitates lymphoid stem cell differentiation into progenitor B cells. Principally a T lymphocyte growth factor synthesized by bone marrow stromal cells. It promotes lymphopoiesis governing stem cell differentiation into early pre-T and B cells. It is also formed by thymic stroma and promotes the growth and activation of T cells and activates macrophages. It also enhances fetal and adult thymocyte proliferation.

Interleukin-8 (IL-8) (neutrophil activating protein-1) is an 8kD protein of 72 residues produced by macrophages and endothelial cells. It has a powerful chemotactic effect on T lymphocytes and neutrophils and up-regulates the binding properties of leukocyte adhesion receptor CD11b/CD18. IL-8 regulates expression of its own receptor on neutrophils and that has antiviral, immunomodulatory and antiproliferative properties. It prevents adhesion of neutrophils to endothelial cells activated by cytokines thereby blocking neutrophil-mediated injury. It participates in inflammation and the migration of cells. It facilitates neutrophil adherence to endothelial cells. It accomplishes this through the induction of β_2 integrins by neutrophils. (Figures 19–21)

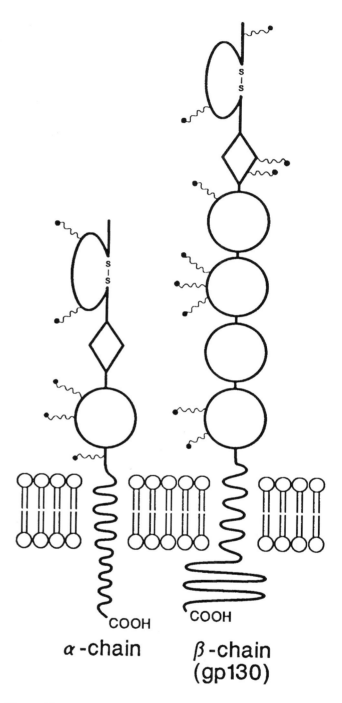

α-chain   β-chain (gp130)

Figure 15.   Schematic representation of the IL-6 receptor. IL-6 receptors of high affinity are comprised of two subunits that are noncovalently associated. There is low affinity binding of IL-6 to the IL-6R α chain but no signal is produced. The gp130 extracellular domain is comprised of an IgSF C to set domain at the N-terminus. The cytokine receptor-SF domain and four fibronectin III domain follow. The WSXWS motif is present only in the first of the fibronectin III domain. There are five potential N-linked glycosylation sites in the human IL-6R α chain and 10 in the GP130. IL-6 receptor.

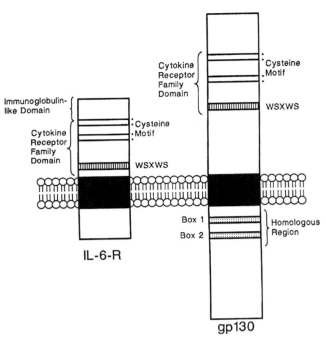

Figure 16. Schematic representation of the IL-6 receptor.

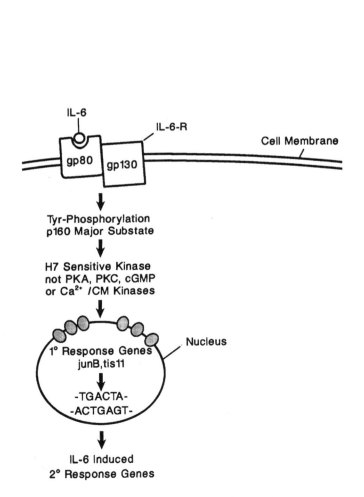

Figure 17. Pathway of IL-6 induction and signaling.

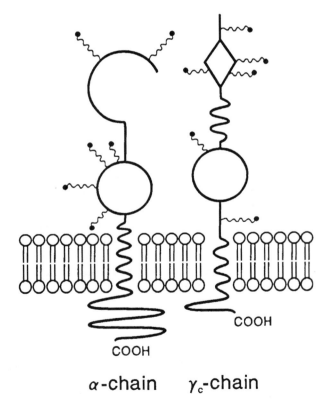

Figure 18. Schematic representation of the IL-7 receptor that is comprised of an IL-7 binding chain designated CD127 and the γ chain of the IL-2R. Following a 100 amino acid N-terminal region, there is a fibronectin III domain with a WSXWS motif in the IL-7R binding chain. The IL-7R functional constituent is the IL-2R γ chain that augments IL-7 binding. In the human form of the IL-7 receptor, there are five potential N-linked glycosylation sites.

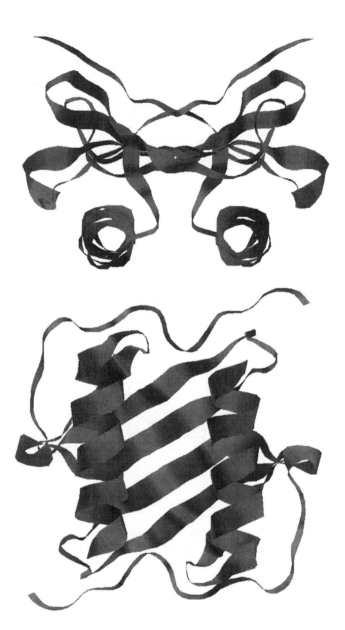

Figure 19.   Human IL-8. NMR.

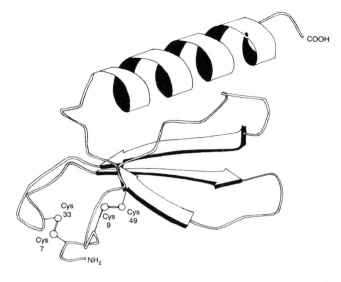

Interleukin-8 (IL-8)

Figure 20.   A three dimensional minimized mean structure, derived by NMR, of the polypeptide backbone structure of human recombinant interleukin-8.

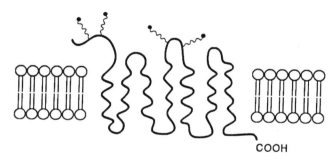

Figure 21.   Schematic representation of the IL-8 receptor, which may be of either high or of low affinity. These receptors are seven transmembrane spanning and are G-protein linked. They belong to the rhodopsin superfamily. Whereas the high affinity receptor binds IL-8 exclusively, the low affinity receptor also shows specificity for NAP-2 and GRO/MPSA.

Interleukin-9 (IL-9) (Figures 22 and 23) is a cytokine that facilitates the growth of some T helper cell clones but not of clones of cytolytic T lymphocyte clones. It is encoded by genes comprised of 5 exons in a 4kb segment of DNA in both mice and humans. In the presence of erythropoietin, IL-9 supports erythroid colony formation. In conjunction with IL-2, IL-3, IL-4 and erythropoietin, IL-9 may enhance hematopoiesis *in vivo*. It may facilitate bone marrow-derived mast cell growth stimulated by IL-3 and fetal thymocyte growth in response to IL-2. T_H2 cells preferentially express IL-9 following stimulation with ConA or by antigen presented on syngeneic antigen presenting cells.

Interleukin-9 (murine growth factor P40, T cell growth factor III) is a hematopoietic growth factor glycoprotein derived from a megakaryoblastic leukemia. Selected human T lymphocyte lines and peripheral lymphocytes activated by mitogen express it. IL-9 is related to mast cell growth-enhancing activity both structurally and functionally. The genes encoding IL-9 is located on chromosomes 5 and 13.

Interleukin-10 (IL-10)(cytokine synthesis inhibitory factor) (Figures 24 and 25) is an 18kD polypeptide devoid of carbohydrate, in humans, that acts as a cytokine synthesis inhibitory factor. It is expressed by CD4+ and CD8+ T lymphocytes, monocytes, macrophages, activated B lymphocytes,

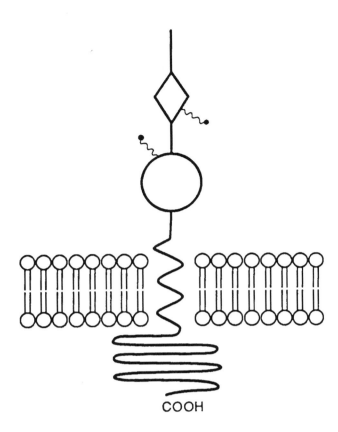

COOH

Figures 22. Schematic representation of the IL-9 receptor, only one type of which has been found on murine T cell lines. Investigation of the recombinant murine receptor has demonstrated association between the IL-2R gamma chain and the IL-9R. Macrophages, some T cell tumors and mast cell lines have been shown to express IL-9 receptors.

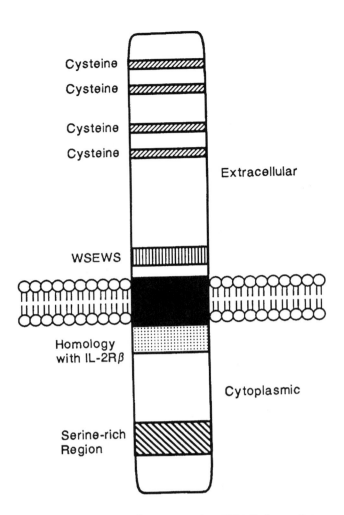

Figures 23. Schematic representation of the IL-9 receptor.

B lymphoma cells and keratinocytes. It inhibits some immune responses and facilitates others. It inhibits cytokine synthesis by T_H1 cells, blocks antigen presentation and the formation of interferon-γ. It also inhibits the macrophage's ability to present antigen and to form IL-1, IL-6 and TNFα. It also participates in IgE regulation. Although IL-10 suppresses cell-mediated immunity, it stimulates B lymphocytes, IL-2 and IL-4 T lymphocyte responsiveness *in vitro*, and murine mast cells exposed to IL-3 and IL-4. IL-10 might have future value in suppressing T lymphocyte autoimmunity in multiple sclerosis, type I diabetes mellitus and in facilitating allograft survival. T_H2 cells of murine T-clones secrete IL-10 which suppresses synthesis of cytokines by T_H1 cells.

Interleukin-11 (IL-11) is a cytokine produced by stromal cells derived from the bone marrow of primates. It is a growth factor that induces IL-6-dependent murine plasmacytoma cells to proliferate. IL-11 has several biological actions that include its hematopoietic effect. In man, the genomic sequence and gene encoding IL-11 is comprised of five exons and four introns. The gene is located at band

19q13.3-13.4 on the long arm of chromosome 19. It may facilitate plasmacytoma establishment, possibly representing an important role for IL-11 in tumorigenesis. In combination with IL-3, IL-11 can potentiate megakaryocyte growth, producing increased numbers, size and ploidy values. It may be important in formation of platelets. In the presence of functional T lymphocytes, IL-11 can stimulate the production of B cells that secrete IgG. It has a synergistic effect in primitive hematopoietic cell proliferation that is IL-3 dependent.

Interleukin-12 (IL-12) is a heterodimeric molecule comprised of 35kD and 40kD chains linked by disulfide bonds. It acts on T cells as a cytotoxic lymphocyte maturation factor (CLMF). It also serves as a natural killer (NK) cell stimulatory factor (NKSF). IL-12 is a growth factor for activated CD4+ and CD8+ T lymphocytes and for NK cells. It facilitates NK cell and LAK cell lytic action exclusive of IL-2. It can induce resting peripheral blood mononuclear cells to form interferon gamma *in vitro*. IL-12 may act synergistically with IL-2 to increase responses by cytotoxic lymphocytes. It

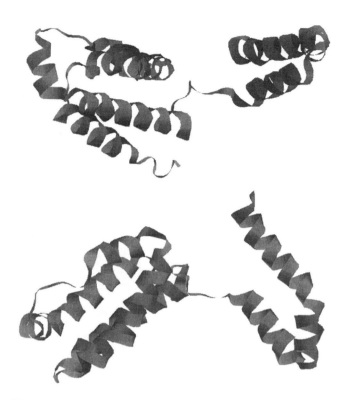

Figure 24. IL-10. By X-ray diffraction. Resolution. 1.8 angstroms.

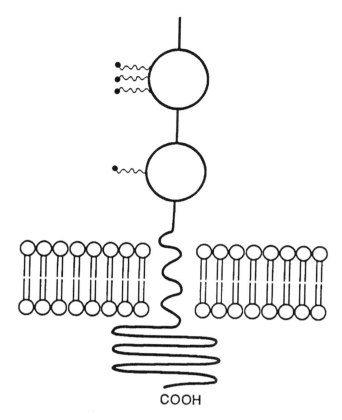

Figure 25. Schematic representation of the IL-10 receptor that is a class II cytokine receptor family molecule. There are two homologous fibronectin III domains in the 220 amino acid extracellular region. There are two conserved tryptophans and one pair of conserved cysteines in the first fibronectin domain and a disulfide loop produced from a second pair of conserved cysteines. However, there is no WSXWS motif, which is found in class I cytokine receptors. The human IL-10 receptor has six potential N-linked glycosylation sites. Signal transduction is believed to involve the JAK family of kinases, but this remains to be elucidated.

may have potential as a therapeutic agent in the treatment of tumors or infections, especially if used in combination with IL-2.

Interleukin-13 (IL-13) (Figure 26) is a cytokine expressed by activated T cells that inhibits inflammatory cytokine production induced by lipopolysaccharide in human peripheral blood monocytes. It synergizes with interleukin-2 to regulate the synthesis of interferon-γ in large granular lymphocytes. Mapping reveals that the IL-13 gene is linked closely to the IL-4 gene. IL-13 could be considered a modulator of B cell responses. It stimulates B cell proliferation with ant-Ig and anti-CD40 antibodies as well as promotes IgE synthesis. It also induces resting B cells to express CD23/FcεRII and class II MHC antigens. The biological activities of IL-13 are similar to those of IL-4. Therefore, both IL-13 and IL-4 may contribute much to the development of allergies. Although IL-13 and IL-4 affect B cells similarly, they have different functions. IL-13 induces less IgE and IgG4 production than does IL-4. IL-13 does not act on T cells or T cell clones; it also fails to induce expression of CD8α on CD4+ T cell clones and has no T cell growth promoting activity.

IL-13 suppresses cell-mediated immunity. It suppresses the cytotoxic functions of monocytes/macrophages and the generation of proinflammatory cytokines. IL-13 has a pleitrophic action on monocytes/macrophages, neutrophils and B cells. It usually produces an inhibitory effect on monocytes/macrophages and down-regulates Fcγ receptors and

secretion of inflammatory cytokines and nitric oxide induced by lipopolysaccharide. IL-13 inhibits macrophage function in cell-mediated immunity. It induces neutrophils to form IL-1 receptor antagonist and IL-1 receptor II. This leads to inhibition of IL-1, a central inflammatory mediator, which is in accord with the anti-inflammatory function of IL-13.

Interleukin-14 (IL-14) formerly was known as high-molecular-weight B cell growth factor (HMW-BCGF). IL-14 is a cytokine produced by follicular dendritic cells, germinal center T cells and some malignant B cells. Normal and malignant B cells, notably germinal center B cells and NHL-B cells respectively, express receptors for IL-14. Its predominant activity is to enhance the proliferation of B cells and to induce memory B cell production and maintenance. Work with NHL-B cell lines has shown that inhibition of the expression of the IL-14 gene results in diminished cell growth and eventual cell death.

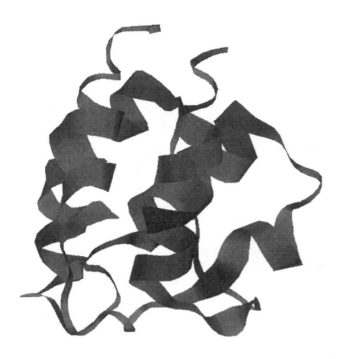

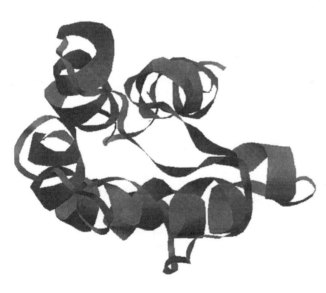

Figure 26. A ribbon diagram of IL-13 that constitutes a theoretical model of human IL-13. This represents the first of two alternative structures of IL-13 generated by homology modeling.

Interleukin-15 (IL-15) is a T cell growth factor that shares many of the biological properties of IL-2. IL-15 enhances peripheral blood T cell proliferation, and *in vitro* studies demonstrate its ability to induce cytotoxic T cells. IL-15 mRNA has not been found in activated peripheral T cells, but monocyte enriched peripheral blood cell lines as well as placental and skeletal muscle tissues do express IL-15. The IL-2 receptor and IL-15 receptor also share a common component.

Interleukin-16 (IL-16) is a 13.2kD protein containing 130 amino acid residues. It is also called lymphocyte chemoattractant (LCA). It activates a migratory response in CD4+ T cells and CD4+ monocytes and eosinophil. Human IL-16 also induces IL-2 receptor expression by T lymphocytes. rIL-16 has been found to suppress T cell proliferation in mixed lymphocyte reactions.

Interleukin-17 (IL-17) is a glycoprotein of 155 amino acids secreted as a homodimer by activated memory CD4+ T cells. It is also called cytotoxic T lymphocyte associated antigen 8. It is believed to share 57% amino acid identity with the protein predicted from ORF13, an open reading frame of Herpes virus saimiri. hIL-17 has no direct effect on cells of hematopoietic origin but does stimulate epithelial, endothelial, and fibroblastic cells to secrete cytokines such as IL-6, IL-8 and granulocyte-colony-stimulating factor as well as prostaglandin E2. hIL-17 may be an early initiator of T cell-dependent inflammatory reactions and part of the cytokine network linking the immune system to hematopoiesis.

Interferons (IFNs) are a group of immunoregulatory proteins synthesized by T lymphocytes, fibroblasts and other types of cells following stimulation with viruses, antigens, mitogens, double-stranded DNA or lectins. Interferons are classified as α and β, that have antiviral properties, and as γ that is known as immune interferon. α and β share a common receptor but γ has its own. Interferons have immunomodulatory functions. They enhance the ability of macrophages to destroy tumor cells, viruses and bacteria. Interferons α and β were formerly classified as type I interferons. They are acid-stable and synthesized mainly by leukocytes and fibroblasts. Interferon-γ is acid-labile and is formed mainly by T lymphocytes stimulated by antigen or mitogen. This immune interferon has been termed type II interferon in the past. Whereas the ability of interferon to prevent infection of noninfected cells is species specific, it is not virus specific. Essentially all viruses are subject to its inhibitory action. Interferons induce formation of a second inhibitory protein that prevents viral messenger RNA translation. In addition to gamma interferon formation by T cells activated with mitogen, natural killer cells also secrete it. Interferons are not themselves viricidal.

Interferon α (IFN-α) (Figure 27) contains at least 13 immunomodulatory 189 amino acid residue glycoproteins synthesized by macrophages and B cells that are able to prevent the replication of viruses, are antiproliferative and are pyrogenic, inducing fever. IFN-α stimulates natural killer cells and induces expression of class I MHC antigens. It also has an immunoregulatory effect through alteration of antibody responsiveness. The 14 genes that encode IFN-α are positioned on the short arm of chromosome 9 in man. Polyribonucleotides as well as RNA or DNA viruses may induce IFN-α secretion. Recombinant IFN-α has been prepared and

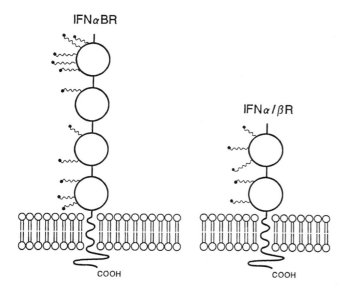

IFNαBR

IFNα/βR

COOH   COOH

Figure 27. Three dimensional crystal structure of recombinant murine interferon α. There is overall similarity of the basic polypeptide chain folding among all the interferon α and interferon β molecules from various sources.

used in the treatment of hairy cell leukemia, Kaposi's sarcoma, chronic myeloid leukemia, human papilloma virus related lesions, renal cell carcinoma, chronic hepatitis and selected other conditions. Patients may experience severe flu-like symptoms as long as the drug is administered. They also have malaise, headache, depression, supraventricular tachycardia and may possibly develop congestive heart failure. Bone marrow suppression has been reported in some patients.

Interferon β (IFN-β) is an antiviral, 20kD protein comprised of 187 amino acid residues. It is produced by fibroblasts and prevents replication of viruses. It has 30% amino acid sequence homology with interferon-α. RNA or DNA viruses or polyribonucleotides can induce its secretion. The gene encoding it is located on chromosome 9 in man.

Interferon γ (IFN-γ) is a glycoprotein that is a 21–24kD homodimer synthesized by activated T lymphocytes and natural killer (NK) cells causing it to be classified as a lymphokine. IFN-γ has antiproliferative and antiviral properties. It is a powerful activator of mononuclear phagocytes increasing their ability to destroy intracellular microorganisms and tumor cells. It causes many types of cells to express class II MHC molecules and can also increase expression of class I. It facilitates differentiation of both B and T lymphocytes. IFN-γ is a powerful activator of NK cells and also activates neutrophils and vascular endothelial cells. It is decreased in chronic lymphocytic leukemia, lymphoma and IgA deficiency as well as those infected with rubella, Epstein-Barr virus and cytomegalovirus. Recombinant IFN has been used for treatment of a variety of conditions including chronic lymphocytic leukemia, mycosis fungoides, Hodgkin's disease and

various other disorders. It has been found effective in decreasing synthesis of collagen by fibroblasts and might have potential in the treatment of connective tissue diseases. Persons receiving it may develop headache, chills, rash or even acute renal failure. The one gene that encodes IFN-γ in man is found on the long arm of chromosome 12.

Interferon-γ receptor (Figure 28) is a 90kD glycoprotein receptor comprised of one polypeptide chain. The only cells found lacking this receptor are erythrocytes. It is encoded by a gene on chromosome 6q in man.

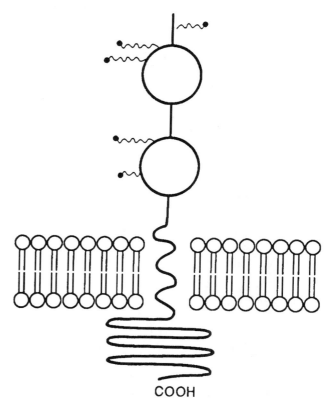

COOH

Figure 28. A preliminary three-dimensional structure of human interferon γ (recombinant form). Resolution. 3.5 Angstroms.

Tumor necrosis factor α (TNFα) (Figure 29) is a cytotoxic monokine produced by macrophages stimulated with bacterial endotoxin. TNF-α participates in inflammation, wound healing, and remodeling of tissue. TNF-α, which is also called cachectin, can induce septic shock and cachexia. It is a cytokine comprised of 157 amino acid residues. It is produced by numerous types of cells including monocytes, macrophages, T lymphocytes, B lymphocytes, NK cells, and other types of cells stimulated by endotoxin or other microbial products. The genes encoding TNF-α and TNF-β (lymphotoxin) are located on the short arm of chromosome 6 in man in the MHC region. High levels of TNF-α are detectable in the blood circulation very soon following administration of endotoxin or microorganisms. The administration of

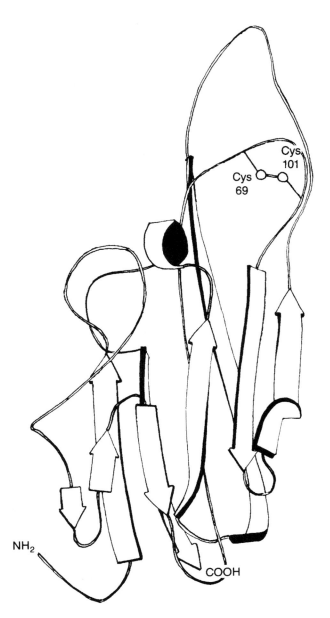

Figure 29. Molecular model of tumor necrosis factor-α (cachectin) (human recombinant form). Resolution 2.6 Angstroms. The molecule exists as a trimer in which the three subunits are related by approximately three-fold symmetry.

recombinant TNF-α induces shock, organ failure, hemorrhagic necrosis of tissues in experimental animals including rodents, dogs, sheep and rabbits, closely resembling the effects of lethal endotoxemia. TNF-α is produced during the first three days of wound healing. It facilitates leukocyte recruitment, induces angiogenesis and promotes fibroblast proliferation. It can combine with receptors on selected tumor cells and induce their lysis. TNF mediates the antitumor action of murine natural cytotoxic (NC) cells, which distinguishes their function from that of natural killer (NK) and cytotoxic T cells. TNF-α was termed cachectin because

of its ability to induce wasting and anemia when administered on a chronic basis to experimental animals. Thus it mimics the action in cancer patients and those with chronic infection with human immunodeficiency virus or other pathogenic microorganisms. It can induce anorexia which may lead to death from malnutrition.

Tumor necrosis factor-β (TNF-β) is a 25kD protein synthesized by activated lymphocytes. It can kill tumor cells in culture, induce expression of genes, stimulate proliferation of fibroblasts and mimics most of the actions of tumor necrosis factor α (cachectin). It participates in inflammation and graft rejection and was previously termed lymphotoxin. TNF-β and TNF-α have approximately equivalent affinity for TNF receptors. Both 55kD and 80kD TNF receptors bind TNF-β. TNF-β has diverse effects that include killing of some cells and causing proliferation of others. It is the mediator whereby cytolytic T cells, natural killer cells, lymphokine-activated killer cells and "helper-killer" T cells induce fatal injury to their targets. TNF-β and TNF-α have been suggested to play a role in AIDS, possibly contributing to its pathogenesis.

Tumor necrosis factor receptor (Figures 30 and 31) is a receptor for tumor necrosis factor that is comprised of 461 amino acid residues and possesses an extracellular domain that is rich in cysteine.

Lymphotoxin is a T lymphocyte lymphokine that is a heterodimeric glycoprotein comprised of a 5kD and a 15kD protein fragment. This cytokine is inhibitory to the growth of tumors either *in vitro* or *in vivo,* and it also blocks chemical-, carcinogen-, or ultraviolet light-induced transformation of cells. Lymphotoxin has cytolytic or cytostatic properties for tumor cells that are sensitive to it. Approximately three quarters of the amino acid sequence is identical between human and mouse lymphotoxin. Human lymphotoxin has 205 amino acid residues, whereas the mouse variety has 202 amino residues. Lymphotoxin does not produce membrane pores in its target cells such as those produced by perforin or complement, but is taken into cells after it is bound to their surface and subsequently interferes with metabolism. Lymphotoxin is also called tumor necrosis factor β (TNFβ).

Colony stimulating factors (CSF) (Figures 32 and 33) are glycoproteins that govern the formation, differentiation and function of granulocytes and mono-macrophage system cells. CSF promotes the growth, maturation and differentiation of stem cells to produce progenitor cell colonies. They facilitate the development of functional end-stage cells. They act on cells through specific receptors on the target cell surface. T cells, fibroblasts and endothelial cells produce CSF factors. Different colony stimulating factors act on cell line progenitors that include CFU-E (red blood cell precursors), GM-CFC (granulocyte-macrophage colony forming cells) (Figure 32), MEG-CFC (megakaryocyte-colony forming

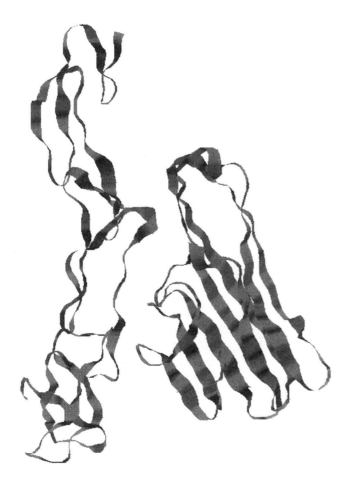

Figure 30. TNF receptor. Resolution. 2.85 angstroms.

cells), EO-CFC (eosinophil-leukocyte colony forming cells), T cells and B cells. Colony stimulating factors promote the clonal growth of cells. Colony stimulating factors include granulocyte-CSF that is synthesized by endothelial cells, macrophages, and fibroblasts. It activates the formation of granulocytes and is synergistic with IL-3 in the generation of megakaraocytes, and granulocytes-macrophages. Endothelial cells, T lymphocytes, and fibroblasts form granulocyte-macrophage-CSF which stimulates granulocyte and macrophage colony formation. It also stimulates megakaryocyte blast cells. Colony stimulating factor-1 is produced by endothelial cells, macrophages and fibroblasts and induces the generation of macrophage colonies. Multi-CSF (interleukin-3) is produced by T lymphocytes and activates the generation of granulocytes, macrophages, eosinophils and mast cells colonies. It is synergistic with other factors in activating hematopoietic precursor cells. Renal interstitial cells synthesize erythropoietin that activates erythroid colony formation.

M-CSF (Figures 34–36) facilitates growth, differentiation, survival and serves as an activating mechanism for macrophages and their precursors. It is derived from numerous

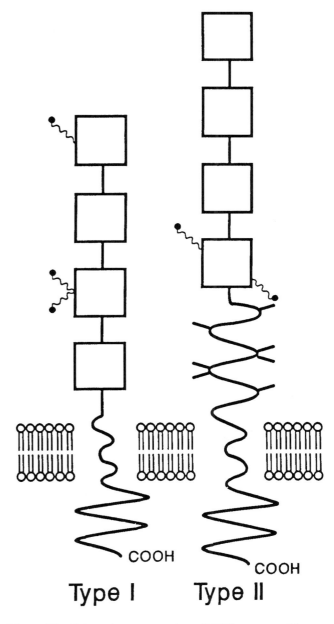

Figure 31. Schematic representation of TNF receptors. The two receptors for TNF are designated type I (CD120a) and type II (CD120b). The 55kD type I receptor and the 75kD type II receptor both bind TNFα and TNFβ (lymphotoxin). These two receptors belong to the NGFR/TNFR superfamily. The extracellular domain contains four cys-rich repeat. The two TNF receptors have essentially no homology in their intracellular domains. Soluble forms of both receptors have been described in urine and serum. With the exception of erythrocytes and resting T cells, TNF receptors are found on most all types of cells. Whereas, the type I p55 receptor is widely distributed on various cell types, the type II p75 receptor appears confined to hematopoietic cells. Whereas, there are three potential N-linked glycosylation sites in human p55 type I TNF receptors, there are two in the p75 type II form.

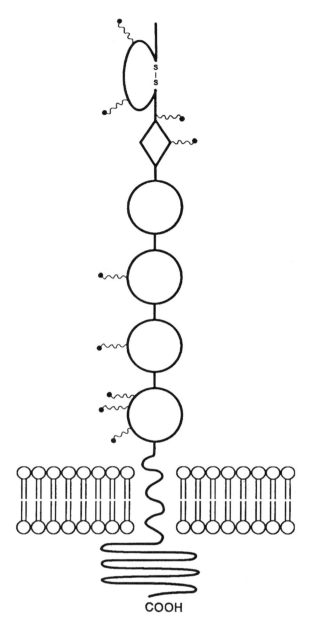

Figure 32. Schematic representation of the G-CSF receptor which is comprised of an immunoglobulin domain, a hematopoietin domain and three fibronectin III domains. There are two forms of the human receptor, i.e., the 25.1 form that has a C kinase phosphorylation site, and a second form in which the transmembrane region has been deleted. The mouse receptor, which shares 62.5% homology with the human receptor, is similar to the 25.1 form. The human G-CSF receptor has 46.3% sequence homology with IL-6 receptor's gp130 chain. The hematopoietin domain contains the binding site for G-CSF, yet proliferative signal transduction requires the membrane proximal 57 amino acids. Acute phase protein induction mediated by G-CSF involves residues 57-96. G-CSF receptors are found on neutrophils, platelets, myeloid leukemia cells, endothelium and placenta. The human form contains 9 potential N-linked glycosylation sites. It is believed that the receptor binds and mediates autophosphorylation of JAK-2 kinase.

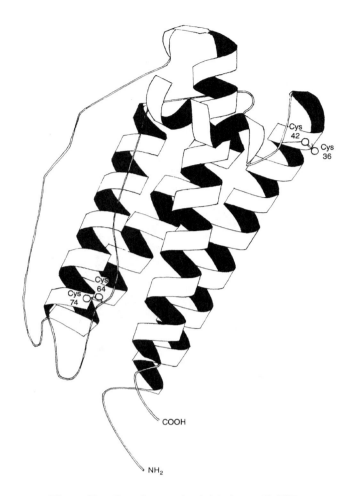

Figure 33.   Granulocyte stimulating factor (G-CSF).

sources such as lymphocytes, monocytes, endothelial cells, fibroblasts, epithelial cells, osteoblasts and myoblasts. X-ray crystallography of recombinant CSF reveals a structure in which four α helices are placed end to end in two bundles. Human and mouse M-CSF share 82% homology in the N-terminal 227 amino acids of the mature sequence, but there is only 47% homology in the remainder of the molecular structure. M-CSF derived from humans and from mice has been previously termed colony stimulating factor (CSF-1).

Transfer factor (TF) is a substance in extracts of leukocytes, that were as effective as viable lymphoid cells in transferring delayed-type hypersensitivity. The active principle is not destroyed by treatment with DNAase or RNAase. Originally described by H. S. Lawrence, transfer factor has been the subject of numerous investigations. Transfer factor is dialyzable and is less than 10kD. It has been separated on Sephadex. Following demonstration of its role in humans, transfer factor was later shown to transfer delayed-type hypersensitivity in laboratory animals. It was shown capable of also transferring cell-mediated immunity as well as delayed-type hypersensitivity between members of numerous animal species. It also became possible to transfer

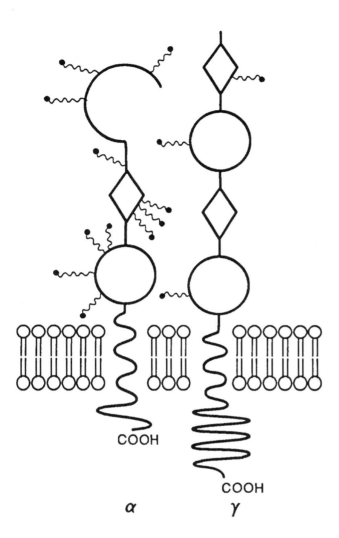

Figure 34. Schematic representation of a macrophage colony stimulating factor.

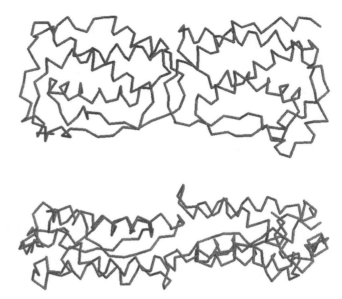

Figure 35. Human macrophage colony stimulating factor. Resolution. 2.5 angstroms.

delayed-type hypersensitivity across species barriers using transfer factor. Attempts to identify purified transfer factor have remained a major challenge. However, it has now been shown that transfer factor combines with specific antigen. Urea treatment of a solid phase immunosorbent permits its recovery. Thus, specific transfer factor is generated in an animal that has been immunized with a specific antigen. T helper lymphocytes produce transfer factor. It combines with T suppressor cells as well as with Ia antigen on B lymphocytes and macrophages. It also interacts with antibody specific for V-region antigenic determinants. It may be a fragment of the T cell receptor for antigen. Transfer factor has been used as an immunotherapeutic agent for many years to treat patients with immunodeficiencies of various types. It produces clinical improvement in numerous infectious diseases caused by viruses and fungi. Transfer factor improves cell-mediated immunity and delayed-type hypersensitivity response, i.e., it restores decreased cellular immunity to some degree.

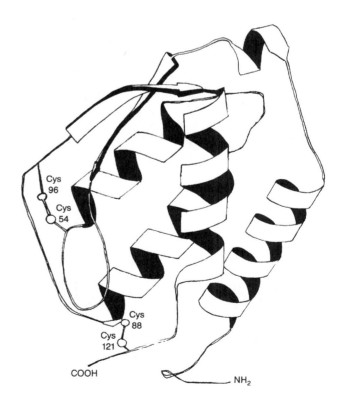

Figure 36. Human macrophage colony stimulating factor (α form, soluble) (human protein recombinant form). Three-dimensional structure of dimeric human recombinant macrophage colony stimulating factor. Resolution 2.5 Angstroms.

Insulin-like growth factors (IGFs) (Figure 37) consist of IGF-I and IGF-II which are prohormones with M_r of 9K and 14K respectively. IGF-I is a 7.6kD side-chain polypeptide hormone that resembles proinsulin structurally. It is formed by the liver and by fibroblasts. IGF-I is the sole effector of growth hormone activity. It is a primary growth regulator that is age dependent. It is expressed in juvenile life and is detectable in the circulating blood plasma. Levels of IGF-I increase in the circulation during juvenile life but decline after puberty. Circulating IGFs are not free in the plasma but are associated with binding proteins that may have the function of limiting the bioavailability of circulating IGFs, which may be a means of controlling growth factor activity. IGF-II is present mainly during the embryonic and fetal stages of mammalian development in various tissues. It is also present in the circulating plasma in association with binding proteins reaching its highest level in the fetal circulation and declining following birth. IGF-II is important for growth of the whole organism.

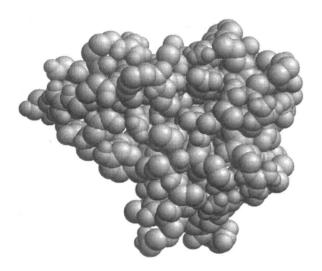

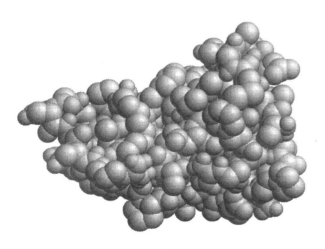

Figure 37.   Insulin-like growth factors (IGFs).

TGF-α (transforming growth factor-α)   A polypeptide produced by transformed cells (Figure 38). It shares approximately one-third of its 50 amino acid sequence with epidermal growth factor (EGF). TGF-α has a powerful stimulatory effect on cell growth and promotes capillary formation. A 5.5kD protein comprised of 50 amino acid residues (human form). This polypeptide growth factor induces proliferation of many types of epidermal and epithelial cells. It facilitates growth of selected transformed cells.

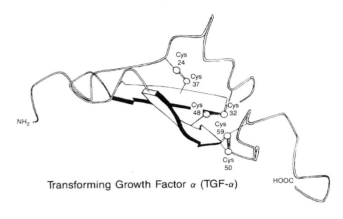

Transforming Growth Factor α (TGF-α)

Figure 38.   Transforming growth factor-α (NMR minimized average structure). The structure was determined by a combination of two-dimensional NMR distance geometry and restrained molecular dynamics using the program (GROMOS). United atoms were used for all non-polar hydrogen atoms, and so are not included in this coordinate entry.

There are five **TGF-βs (transforming growth factor-βs)** that are structurally similar in the C-terminal region of the protein. They are designated TGF-β1 through TGF-β5 and have similar functions with respect to their regulation of cellular growth and differentiation. After being formed as secretory precursor polypeptides, TGF-β1, TGF-β2 (Figure 39) and TGF-β3 molecules are altered to form a 25kD homodimeric peptide. The ability of TGF-β to regulate growth depends on the type of cell and whether or not other growth factors are also present. It also regulates deposition of extracellular matrix and cell attachment to it. It induces fibronectin, chondroitin/dermatin sulfate proteoglycans, collagen and glycosaminoglycans. TGF-β also promotes the formation and secretion of protease inhibitors. It has been shown to increase the rate of wound healing and induces granulation tissue. It also stimulates proliferation of osteoblasts and chondrocytes. TGF-β inhibits bone marrow cell proliferation and also blocks interferon-α-induced activation of natural killer (NK) cells. It diminishes IL-2 activation of lymphokine activated killer cells. TGF-β decreases cytokine-induced proliferation of thymocytes and also decreases IL-2-induced proliferation and activation of mature T lymphocytes. It inhibits T cell precursor differentiation into cytotoxic T lymphocytes. TGF-β may reverse the activation of

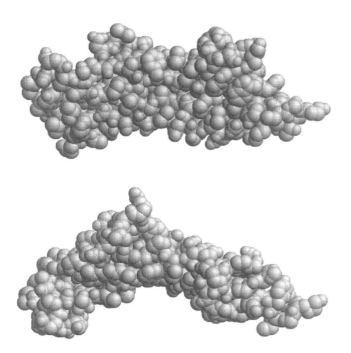

Figure 39. Human TGF-β2. Resolution. 1.8 angstroms.

macrophages by preventing the development of cytotoxic activity and superoxide anion formation that is needed for antimicrobial effects. In addition to suppressing macrophage activation, TGF may diminish MHC class II molecule expression. It also decreases Fc, receptor expression in allergic reactions. TGF-β has potential value as an immunosuppressant in tissue and organ transplantation. It may protect bone marrow stem cells from the injurious effects of chemotherapy. It may also have use as an antiinflammatory agent based on its ability to inhibit the growth of both T and B cells. It has potential as a possible treatment for selected autoimmune diseases. It diminishes myocardial damage associated with coronary occlusion, promotes wound healing and may be of value in restoring collagen and promoting formation of bone in osteoporosis patients.

Leukocyte inhibitory factor (LIF) is a lymphokine that prevents polymorphonuclear leukocyte migration. T lymphocytes activated *in vitro* may produce this lymphokine, which can interfere with the migration of polymorphonuclear neutrophils from a capillary tube as observed in a special chamber devised for the laboratory demonstration of this substance. Serine esterase inhibitors inhibit LIF activity, although they do not have this effect on migration inhibitory factor (MIF). This inhibitor is released by normal lymphocytes stimulated with the lectin concanavalin A or by sensitized lymphocytes challenged with the specific antigen. LIF is a 65 to 70kD protein.

Leukemia inhibitory factor (LIF) (Figures 40 and 41) is a lymphoid factor that facilitates maintenance of embryonic stem cells through suppression of spontaneous generation.

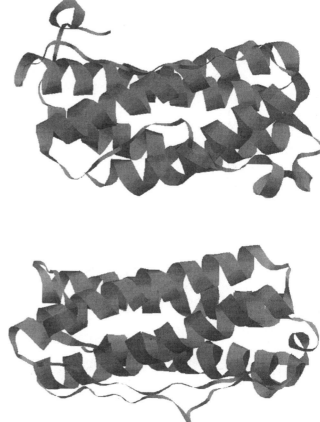

Figure 40. Leukemia inhibitory factor. Resolution 2.0 angstroms.

It also induces mitogenesis of selected cell lines, stimulation of bone remodeling, facilitation of megakaryocyte formation *in vivo* and suppression of cellular differentiation in culture. The recombinant form is a 20kD protein comprised of 180 amino acid residues.

Macrophage inflammatory protein-1-α (MIP-1α) (Figure 42) is an endogenous fever-inducing substance that binds heparin and is resistant to cyclooxygenase inhibition. Macrophages stimulated by endotoxin may secrete this protein, termed MIP-1, which differs from tumor necrosis factor (TNF) and IL-1, as well as other endogenous pyrogens because its action is not associated with prostaglandin synthesis. It appears indistinguishable from hematopoietic stem cell inhibitor and may function in growth regulation of hematopoietic cells.

The MIP-1α receptor is a seven membrane spanning structure. There is 32% homology between the receptor for MIP-1α and those for IL-8. A calcium flux occurs when MIP-1α binds to its receptor. Murine T cells, macrophages and eosinophils have been shown to express a receptor for MIP-1α. The human MIP-1α receptor has one potential

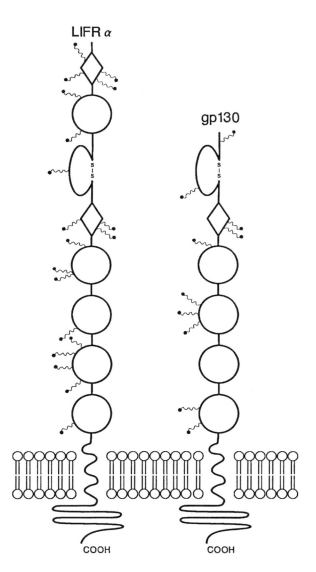

Figure 41.   Schematic representation of the leukemia inhibitory factor.

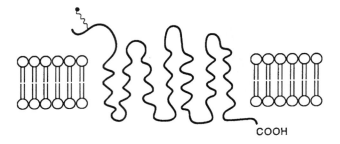

Figure 42.   Schematic representation of MIP-1α.

N-linked glycosylation site. The gene for the MIP-1α receptor in humans is found on chromosome 3p21.

MIP-1β is a cytokine produced by monocytes and lymphocytes and stimulates growth of myelopoietic cells and promotes leukocyte chemoattraction. This molecule belongs to the CC family of chemokine-intercrine cytokines and is related to MIP-1α. Human and murine forms of MIP-1β share 70% homology. T lymphocytes, B cells and macrophages represent sources of this chemokine. Human MIP-1β chemoattracts memory T lymphocytes. The major classes of cytokine receptors are arranged according to their corresponding superfamilies.

Cytokines play a significant role in the homeostasis of normal tissues and cells as well as in the induction and perpetuation of pathologic processes. Thus, much pharmaceutical industry research has been aimed at blocking the synthesis or action of one or more cytokine. Various methods have been tested to block cytokines. Studies have revealed that suppression of transcription of some cytokines can render experimental animals susceptible to life-threatening inflammatory conditions. Thus, prolonged treatment with a cytokine-blocking agent might produce pathologic changes. Modulating cytokines as therapeutic procedures must be approached with caution and require further study. Nevertheless, cytokines are major therapeutic targets in many human diseases. Thus, ways are being sought to modulate them to produce a desired therapeutic effect. The four major approaches to modulation of cytokines include: (1) inhibition cytokine synthesis, (2) inhibition of cytokine release, (3) inhibition of cytokine action, or (4) inhibition of cytokine intracellular signaling pathways.

Therapeutic cytokines that include γ interferon, α interferon, erythropoietin and colony-stimulating factor are already being used clinically. In the future, cytokine modulators will hopefully be used to downregulate the action of selected cytokines. One such approach would be the therapy of septic shock in which anti-endotoxin or anti-cytokine agents might be used for therapeutic purposes. Rheumatoid arthritis and other chronic diseases may also be treated by anti-cytokine therapies. Approaches will probably include blocking single cytokines by cloned chimerized antibodies or soluble receptor-antibody complexes to diminish tissue pathology. It remains to be determined whether pathologic changes induced by cytokines can be diminished by the use of agents that neutralize or inhibit synthesis of individual cytokines. Nevertheless, blocking the pathology of many diseases may depend upon targeting specific cytokines in the future.

11

The Complement System

Throughout the ages man has been fascinated and at times obsessed by the marvelous, mysterious and even baffling qualities of the blood. In 1889, Hans Buchner described a heat-labile bactericidal principle in the blood which was later identified as the complement system. In 1894, Jules Bordet working at the Pasteur Institute in Metchnikoff's laboratory discovered that the lytic or bactericidal action of freshly drawn blood, which had been destroyed by heating, was promptly restored by the addition of fresh, normal, unheated serum. Paul Ehrlich called Bordet's "alexine" das Komplement. In 1901, Bordet and Gengou developed the complement fixation test to measure antigen-antibody reactions. Ferrata in 1907 recognized complement to be a multiple component system, a complex of protein substances of mixed globulin composition present in normal sera of many animal species.

The classical pathway of complement activation was described first by investigators using sheep red blood cells sensitized with specific antibody and lysed with guinea pig or human complement. In addition to immune lysis, complement has many other functions and is important in the biological amplification mechanism that is significant in resistance against infectious disease agents. Complement's mechanism of action in the various biological reactions in which it participates has occupied the attention of a host of investigators. In 1954, Pillemer *et al.* suggested the existence of a nonantibody-dependent protein in the serum which is

significant for early defense of the host against bacteria and viruses. This protein was named properdin. It acts in combination with certain inorganic ions and complement components that make up the so-called properdin system which constitutes a part of the natural defense mechanism of the blood.

Multiple plasma proteins may be activated during inflammation. Immune complexes activate the classic pathway of complement whereas bacterial products activate the alternative pathway without participation by specific antibody. Many antimicrobial effects are produced by complement. C5a, C5b67 and C3a induce chemotaxis of leukocytes. C3b has opsonic properties. The membrane attack complex leads to lysis of bacterial cells. Complement also facilitates the antimicrobial effects of PMNs and macrophages through the alternative pathway (Figure 1).

Complement (C) is a system of 20 soluble plasma and other body fluid proteins together with cellular receptors for many of them and regulatory proteins found on blood and other tissue cells. These proteins play a critical role in aiding phagocytosis of immune complexes, which activate the complement system. These molecules and their fragments resulting from the activation process are significant in the regulation of cellular immune responsiveness. Once complement proteins identify and combine with target substance, serine proteases are activated. This leads ultimately to the

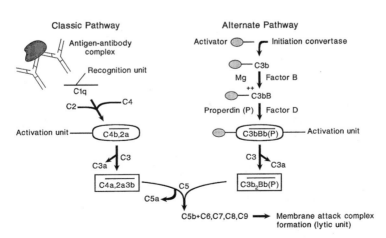

Figure 1. The classical and alternative pathways of the complement system.

207

assembly of C3 convertase, a protease on the surface of the target substance. The enzyme cleaves C3 yielding a C3b fragment that is bound to the target through a covalent linkage. C3b or C3bi bound to phagocytic cell surfaces become ligands for C3 receptors as well as binding sites for C5. The union of C5b with C6, C7, C8 and C9 generates the membrane attack complex (MAC) which may associate with the cell's lipid bilayer membrane to produce lysis, which is critical in resistance against certain species of bacteria. The complement proteins are significant, nonspecific mediators of humoral immunity. Multiple substances may trigger the complement system. There are two pathways of complement activation designated the classical pathway in which an antigen, e.g., red blood cell, and antibody combine and fix the first subcomponent designated C1q. This is followed in sequence as follows: C1qrs,4,2,3,5,6,7,8,9 to produce lysis. The alternative pathway does not utilize C1, 4 and 2 components. Bacterial products such as endotoxin and other agents may activate this pathway through C3. There are numerous biological activities associated with complement besides immune lysis. These include the formation of anaphylatoxin, chemotaxis, opsonization, phagocytosis, bacteriolysis, hemolysis and other amplification mechanisms.

The **classic pathway of complement** (Figure 2) is a mechanism to activate C3 through participation by the serum proteins C1, C4 and C2. Either IgM or a doublet of IgG may bind the C1 subcomponent C1q. Following subsequent activation of C1r and C1s, the two C1s substrates, C4 and C2 are cleaved. This yields C4b and C2a fragments that produce C4b2a known as C3 convertase. It activates opsonization, chemotaxis of leukocytes, increased permeability of vessels and cell lysis. Activators of the classic pathway include IgM, IgG, staphylococcal protein A, C-reactive protein and DNA. C1 inhibitor blocks the classical pathway by separating C1r and C1s from C1q. C4 binding protein also blocks the classical pathway by linking to C4b, separating it from C2a and permitting Factor I to split the C4b heavy chain to yield C4bi, which is unable to unite with C2a thereby inhibiting the classical pathway.

The first complement component designated C1 consists of a complex of three separate proteins designated C1q, C1r and C1s. The addition of an asterisk indicates activation. The formation of an active fragment following proteolysis of a component such as C3 is designated by a lower case letter such as C3a and C3b (Figure 3). Active fragments degrade either spontaneously or by the action of serum proteases. Inactive fragments are designated by i such as iC3b. The interaction of antibody with antigen forms antigen-antibody complexes that initiate the classical pathway. One molecule each of C1q and of C1s together with two molecules of C1r comprise the C1 complex or **recognition unit**. C1q facilitates recognition unit binding to cell surface antigen-antibody complexes. To launch the classical complement cascade, C1q must link to two IgG antibodies through their

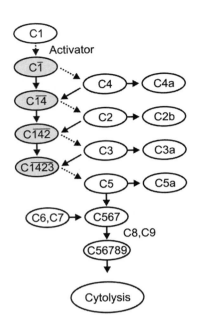

Figure 2.   The classical pathway of complement activation.

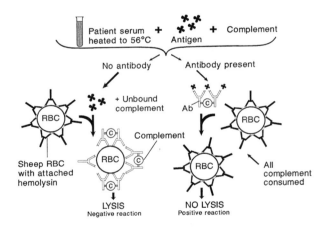

Figure 3.   Complement split products in an inflammatory response.

Fc regions. By contrast, one pentameric IgM molecule attached to a cell surface may interact with C1q to initiate the classical pathway. Binding of C1q activates C1r to become activated C1r*. This, in turn, activates C1s.

To create the **activation unit**, C1s* splits C4 to produce C4a and C4b and C2 to form C2a and C2b. The ability of a single recognition unit to split numerous C2 and C4 molecules represents an amplification mechanism in the cascade. The union of C4b and C2a produces C4b2a which is known as **C3 convertase**. C4b2a binds to the cell membrane and splits C3 into C3a and C3b fragments. The ability of C4b2a to cleave multiple C3 molecules represents another amplification mechanism. The interaction of C3b with C4b2a bound to the cell membrane produces a complete activation unit,

C4b2a3b, which is termed **C5 convertase**. It splits C5 into C5a and C5b fragments and represents yet another amplification mechanism because a single molecule of C5 convertase may cleave multiple C5 molecules.

The terminal stage of the classical pathway involves creation of the **membrane attack unit**, which is also called the lytic unit exclusive of the recognition and activation units, C5b binds to the cell membrane. This is followed by the successive interaction of single molecules of C6, C7 and C8 with the membrane-bound C5b. Finally, further interaction with several C9 molecules finishes formation of the lytic unit through non-covalent interactions without enzymatic alteration. Formation of a membrane attack unit or membrane attack complex *(MAC)* leads to a cell membrane lesion that permits loss of K^+ and ingress of Na^+ and water leading to hypotonic lysis of cells.

Not all C3b produced in classic complement activation unites with C4b2a to produce C5 convertase. Some of it binds directly to the cell membrane and acts as an opsonin which makes the cell especially delectable to phagocytes such as neutrophils and macrophages that have receptors for C3b.

Complement fragments C3a and C5a serve as powerful anaphalatoxins that stimulate mast cells to release histamine that enhances vascular permeability and smooth muscle contraction. Neutrophils release hydrolytic enzymes and platelet aggregate leading to microthrombosis, blood stasis, edema formation and local tissue injury/destruction. C5a not only acts as an anaphylatoxin but is also chemotactic for PMNs and macrophages.

Nonimmunologic classical pathway activators are selected microorganisms such as *Escherichia coli* and low virulence *Salmonella* strains as well as certain viruses such as parainfluenza react with Clq leading to C1 activation without antibody. Thus, this represents classical pathway activation which facilitates defense mechanisms. Various other substances such as myelin basic protein, denatured bacterial endotoxin, heparin and urate crystal surfaces may also directly activate the classical complement pathway.

C1 (Figure 4) is a 750kD multimeric molecule comprised of one C1q subcomponent, two C1r and two C1s subcomponents. The classical pathway of complement activation begins with binding of C1q to IgM or IgG molecules. C1q, C1r and C1s form a macromolecular complex in a Ca^{2+}-dependent manner. The 400kD C1q molecule possesses three separate polypeptide chains that unite into a heterotrimeric structure that resembles stems which contain an amino terminal in triple helix and a globular structure at the carboxy-terminus that resembles a tulip. Six of these tulip-like structures with globular heads and stems form a circular and symmetric molecular complex in the C1q molecule. There is a central core. The serine esterase molecules designated

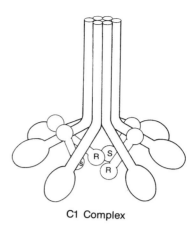

C1 Complex

Figure 4.   The subcomponents of C1 designated C1qrs.

C1r and C1s are needed for the complement cascade to progress. These 85kD proteins that are single chains unite, in the presence of calcium, to produce a tetramer comprised of two C1r and two C1s subcomponents to form a structure that is flexible and has a C1s-C1r-C1r-C1s sequence. When at least two C1q globular regions bind to IgM or IgG molecules, the C1r in a tetramer associated with the C1q molecule becomes activated leading to splitting of the $\overline{C1r}$ molecules in the tetramer with formation of a 57kD chain and a 28kD chain. The latter, termed C1r, functions as a serine esterase splitting the C1s molecules into 57kD and 28kD chains. The 28kD chain derived from the cleavage of C1s molecules, designated $\overline{C1s}$, also functions as a serine esterase, cleaving C4 and C2, causing progression of the classical complement pathway cascade.

C1 esterase inhibitor is a serum protein that counteracts activated C1. This diminishes generation of C2b that facilitates development of edema. **C1 inhibitor (C1 INH)** is a 478 amino acid residue single polypeptide chain protein in the serum. It blocks C1r activation, prevents $\overline{C1r}$ cleavage of $\overline{C1s}$ and inhibits $\overline{C1s}$ splitting of C4 and C2. The molecule is highly glycosylated with carbohydrate making up approximately one-half of its content. It contains 7 O-linked oligosaccharides linked to serine and 6 N-linked oligosaccharides tethered to an asparagine residue. Besides its effects on the complement system, C1 INH blocks factors in the blood clotting system that include kallikrein, plasmin, Factor XIa and XIIa. C1 INH is an α_2 globulin and is a normal serum constituent which inhibits serine protease. The 104kD C1 INH interacts with activated C1r or C1s to produce a stable complex. This prevents these serine protease molecules from splitting their usual substrates. Either $\overline{C1s}$ or $\overline{C1r}$ can split C1 INH to uncover an active site in the inhibitor which becomes bound to the proteases through a covalent ester bond. By binding to most of the C1 in the blood, C1 INH blocks the spontaneous activation of C1. C1 INH binding blocks conformational alterations that would lead to spontaneous activation of C1. When an antigen-antibody complex binds C1, C1 INH's inhibitory influence on C1 is relinquished. Genes on chromosome 11 in man encode C1 INH. C1r and C1s subcomponents disengage from C1q following their interaction with C1 INH. In hereditary angioneurotic edema, C1 INH formation is defective. In acquired C1 inhibitor deficiency, there is elevated catabolism of C1 INH.

C1q (Figure 5) is an 18 polypeptide chain subcomponent of C1, the first component of complement. It commences the classical complement pathway. The three types of polypeptide chain are designated A chain, B chain and C chain. Disulfide bonds link these chains. The C1q molecule's triple helix structures are parallel and resemble the stems of six tulips in the amino-terminal half of their structure. They then separate into six globular regions that resemble the heads of a tulip. The molecule is arranged in a heterotrimeric rod-like configuration bearing a collagen-like triple helix at its amino terminus and a tulip-like globular region at its carboxyl terminus. The combination of six of the rod-shaped structures leads to a symmetric molecular arrangement comprised of three helices at one terminus and the globular (tulip-like) heads at the other terminus. The binding of antibody to C1q initiates the classic complement pathway. It is the globular C-terminal region of the molecule that binds to either IgM or IgG molecules. A tetramer comprised of two molecules of C1r and two molecules of C1s bind by Ca^{2+} to the collagen-like part of the stem. C1q A chain and C1q B chain are coded for by genes on chromosome 1p in man. The interaction of C1q with antigen-antibody complexes represents the basis for assays for immune complexes in patients' serum. IgM, IgG1, IgG2 and IgG3 bind C1q whereas IgG4, IgE, IgA and IgD do not.

C1q receptors (C1q-R) binds the collagen segment of C1q fixed to antigen-antibody complexes. The C1q globular head is the site of binding of immunoglobulin's Fc region. Thus, the C1q-R can facilitate the attachment of antigen-antibody complexes to cells expressing C1q-R and Fc receptors. Neutrophils, B cells, monocytes, macrophages, NK cells, endothelial cells, platelets and fibroblasts all express C1q-R. C1q-R stimulation on neutrophils may lead to a respiratory burst.

C1r is a subcomponent of C1, the first component of complement in the classical activation pathway. It is a serine esterase. Ca^{2+} binds C1r molecules to the stem of a C1q molecule. Following binding of at least two globular regions of C1q with IgM or IgG, C1r is split into 189 a 463-amino-acid residue I chain, the N-terminal fragment and a 243-amino-acid residue carboxy-terminal β chain fragment where the active site is situated. C1s becomes activated when C1r splits its arginine-isoleucine bond.

C1s is a serine esterase that is a subcomponent of C1, the first component of complement in the classical activation pathway. Ca^{2+} binds two C1s molecules to the C1q stalk. Following activation, C1̄r̄ splits the single chain 85kD C1s

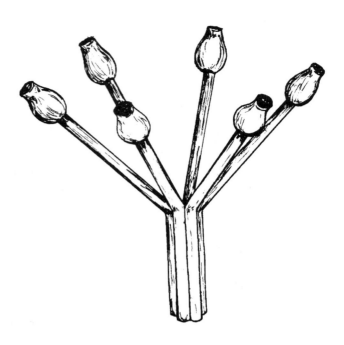

Figure 5. C1q.

molecule into a 431-amino-acid residue A chain and a 243-amino-acid residue B chain where the active site is located. C1̄s̄ splits a C4 arginine-alanine bond and a C2 arginine-lysine bond.

C2 (complement component 2) is the third complement protein to participate in the classical complement pathway activation. C2 is a 110kD single polypeptide chain that unites with C4b molecules on the cell surface in the presence of Mg^{2+}. C1̄s̄ splits C2 following its combination with C4b at the cell surface. This yields a 35kD C2b molecule and a 75kD C2a fragment. Whereas C2b may leave the cell surface, C2a continues to be associated with surface C4b. The complex of C4̄b̄2̄ā constitutes classical pathway C3 convertase. This enzyme is able to bind and split C3. C4b facilitates combination with C3. C2b catalyzes the enzymatic cleavage. C2a contains the active site of classical pathway C3 convertase (C4̄b̄2̄ā). C2 is encoded by genes on the short arm of chromosome of 6 in man. *C2A*, *C2B* and *C2C* alleles encode human C2. Murine C2 is encoded by genes at the S region of chromosome 17.

C2a is the principal substance produced by C1̄s̄ cleavage of C2. N-linked oligosaccharides may combine with C2a at 6 sites. The 509 carboxy-terminal amino acid residues of C2 constitute C2a. The catalytic site for C3 and C5 cleavage is located in the 287 residue carboxy-terminal sequence. The association of C2a with C4b yields the C3 convertase (C4̄b̄2̄ā) of the classical pathway.

C2b is a 223-amino-acid terminal residue of C2 that represents a lesser product of C1̄s̄ cleavage of C2. There are three abbreviated 68-amino-acid residue homologous repeats in

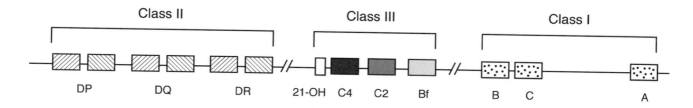

Figure 6. *C2* and *B* genes are situated within the MHC locus on the short arm of chromosome 6.

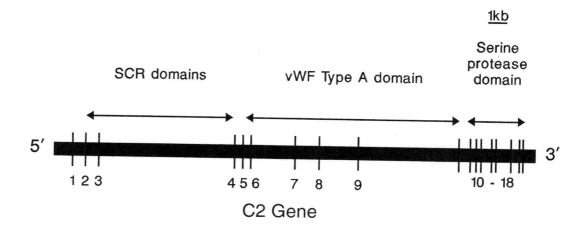

Figure 7.   Schematic representation of the exon/intron organization of the human *C2* gene. Exons, represented by vertical bars, are numbered.

C2b that are present in C3 or C4 binding proteins. N-linked oligosaccharides combine with C2b at two sites. A peptide split from the carboxy-terminus of C2b by plasmin has been implicated in the formation of edema in hereditary angio-neurotic edema patients.

C2 and ***B*** (Figures 6 and 7) genes are situated within the MHC locus on the short arm of chromosome 6. They are termed MHC class III genes. *TNF-α* and *TNF-β* genes are situated between the *C2* and *HLA-B* genes. Another gene designated *FD* lies between the *Bf* and *C4a* genes. C2 and B complete primary structures have been deduced from cDNA and protein sequences. C2 is comprised of 732 residues and is an 81kD molecule, whereas B contains 739 residues and is an 83kD molecule. Both proteins have a three-domain globular structure. During C3 convertase formation, the amino-terminal domains, C2b or Ba, are split off. They contain consensus repeats that are present in CR1, CR2, H, DAF, and C4bp, which all combine with C3 and/or C4 fragments and regulate C3 convertases. The amino acid sequences of the C2 and B consensus repeats are known. C2b contains site(s) significant for C2 binding to C4b. Ba, resembling C2b, manifests binding site(s) significant in C3 convertase assembly. Available evidence indicates that C2b possesses a C4b binding site and that Ba contains a corresponding C3b binding site.

In considering assembly and decay of C3 convertases, initial binding of the 3-domain structures C2 or B to activator-bound C4b or C3b, respectively, requires one affinity site on the C2b/Ba domain and another on one of the remaining two domains. A transient change in C2a and Bb conformation results from C2 or B cleavage by C1s or D. This leads to greater binding affinity, Mg^{+2} sequestration and acquisition of proteolytic activity for C3, C2a or Bb dissociation leads to C3 convertase decay. Numerous serum-soluble and membrane-associated regulatory proteins control the rate of formation and association of C3 convertases.

C3 (complement component 3) is a 195kD glycoprotein heterodimer that is linked by disulfide bonds. It is the fourth complement component to react in the classical pathway, and it is also a reactant in the alternative complement pathway. C3 contains α and β polypeptide chains and has an internal thioester bond which permits it to link covalently with surfaces of cells and proteins. Much of the C3 gene structure has now been elucidated. It is believed to contain approximately 41 exons. Eighteen of 36 introns have now been sequenced. The C3 gene of man is located on chromosome 19. Hepatocytes, monocytes, fibroblasts, and endothelial cells can synthesize C3. More than 90% of serum C3 is synthesized in the liver. The concentration of C3 in serum exceeds that of any other complement component. Human

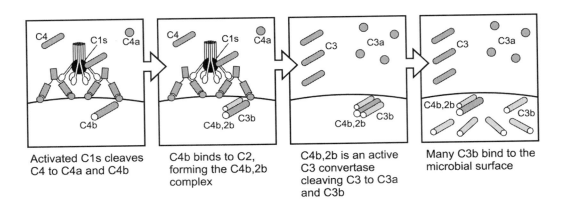

Figure 8.   The classical pathway of complement activation generates a C3 convertase.

C3 is generated as a single chain precursor which is cleaved into the two-chain mature state. C3 molecules are identical antigenically, structurally, and functionally regardless of cell source. Hepatocytes and monocytes synthesize greater quantities of C3 than do epithelial and endothelial cells. C3 convertases split a 9kD C3a fragment from C3's a chain. The other product of the reaction is C3b which is referred to as metastable C3b and has an exposed thioester bond. Approximately 90% of the metastable C3b thioester bonds interact with H_2O to form inactive C3b byproducts that have no role in the complement sequence. 10% of C3b molecules may bind to cell substances through covalent bonds or with the immunoglobulin bound to C4b2a. This interaction leads to the formation of $C\overline{4b2a3b}$, which is classical pathway C5 convertase, and serves as a catalyst in the enzymatic splitting of C5 that initiates membrane attack complex (MAC) formation. When C3b, in the classical complement pathway, interacts with E (erythocyte), A (antibody), C1 (complement 1) and 4b2a, EAC14b2a3b is produced. As many as 500 C3b molecules may be deposited at a single EAC14b2a complex on an erythrocyte surface. *C3S* (slow electrophoretic mobility) and *C3F* (fast electrophoretic mobility) alleles on chromosome 19 in man encode 99% of C3 in man with rare alleles accounting for the remainder. C3 has the highest concentration in serum of any complement system protein with a range of 0.552 to 1.2mg/ml. Following splitting of the internal thioester bond it can form a covalent link to amino or hydroxyl groups on erythrocytes, microorganisms or other substances. C3 is an excellent opsonin. C3 was known in the past as β_1C globulin.

C3 convertase (Figure 8) is an enzyme that splits C3 into C3b and C3a. There are two types, one in the classical pathway designated $C\overline{4b2a}$ and one in alternative pathway of complement activation termed $C\overline{3bBb}$. An amplification loop with a positive feedback is stimulated by alternative pathway C3 convertase. Each of the two types of C3 convertase lacks stability leading to ready disassociation of their constitutents. However, C3 nephritic factor can stabilize both classical and alternative pathway C3 convertases. Properdin may stabilize alternative pathway C3 convertase. C2a and Bb contain the catalytic sites.

C3a is a low molecular weight (9kD) peptide fragment of complement component C3. It is comprised of the 77 N-terminal end residues of C3 a chain. This biologically active anaphylatoxin, that induces histamine release from mast cells and causes smooth muscle contraction, is produced by the cleavage of C3 by either classical pathway C3 convertase, i.e., $C\overline{4b2a}$, or alternative complement pathway C3 convertase, i.e., $C\overline{3bBb}$. Anaphylatoxin inactivator, a carboxy-peptidase N, can inactivate C3a by digesting the C-terminal arginine of C3a. The **C3a receptor (C3a-R)** is a protein on the surface membrane of mast cells and basophils. It serves as a C3a anaphylatoxin receptor.

C3b is a principal fragment produced when complement component C3 is split by either classical or alternative pathway convertases is, i.e., $C\overline{4b2a}$ or $C\overline{3bBb}$, respectively. It results from C3 convertase digestion of C3's α chain. It is an active fragment as revealed by its combination with Factor B to produce $C\overline{3bBb}$, which is the alternative pathway C3 convertase. Classical complement pathway C5 convertase is produced when C3b combines with $C\overline{4b2a}$ to yield $C\overline{4b2a3b}$. Factor I splits the arginine-serine bonds in C3b, if Factor H is present, to yield C3bi. This produces the C3f peptide. Particle-bound C3b interacts with complement receptor 1. C3b interacts with C3b receptors on macrophages, B lymphocytes, polymorphonuclear neutrophils (PMNs) and possiblly T cells. It promotes phagocytosis, immune adherence and may function as an opsonin.

C4 (complement component 4) is a 210kD molecule comprised of α, β and δ chains. The α chain has an internal thioester bond linking a cysteine residue and adjacent glutamate residue. C4 reacts immediately following C1 in the classical pathway of complement activation. $C\overline{1s}$ splits the α chain of C4 at position 76–77 where an arginine-alanine bond is located. This yields a 8.6kD C4a fragment, an anaphylatoxin, and C4b, which is a larger molecule. C4b remains linked to C1. Many C4b molecules can be formed through the action of a single C$\overline{1s}$ molecule. Enzymatic cleavage renders α chain thioester bond of C4b fragment very unstable. The molecule's chemically active form is termed metastable C4b. C4bi intermediates form when C4b thioester bonds and water molecules react. C4b molecules may become bound covalently to cell surfaces when selected C4b thioester bonds undergo transesterification producing covalent amide or ester bonds with proteins or carbohydrates on the cell surface. This enables complement activation to take place on the surfaces of cells where antibodies bind. C4b may also link covalently with antibody. C4 is first formed as a 1700-amino-acid residue chain that contains β chain, α chain and γ chain components joined through connecting peptides. *C4A* and *C4B* genes located at the major histocompatibility complex on the short arm of chromosome 6 in man encode C4. *Slp* and *Ss* genes located on chromosome 17 in the mouse encode murine C4.

C4b is the principal molecule produced when C$\overline{1s}$ splits C4. C4b is that part of the C4 molecule that remains after C4a has been split off by enzymatic digestion. C4b unites with C2a to produce C$\overline{4b2a}$, an enzyme which is known as the classical pathway C3 convertase. Factor I splits the arginine-asparagine bond of C4b at position 1318-1319 to yield C4bi, if C4b binding protein is present. C4b linked to particulate substances reacts with complement receptor 1.

C3a/C4a receptor (C3a/C4a-R) is a common receptor on mast cells. When a C-terminal arginine is removed from C3a and C4a by serum carboxypeptidase N (SCPN), these anaphylatoxins lose their ability to activate cellular responses. Thus, C3a$_{\text{des Arg}}$ and C4a$_{\text{des Arg}}$ lose their ability to induce spasmogenic responses. C3a-R has been demonstrated on guinea pig platelets. Eosinophils have been found to bind C3a.

C5 (complement component 5) is a component comprised of an α and β polypeptide chains linked by disulfide bonds that react in the complement cascade following C1, C4b, C2a and C3b fixation to complexes of antibody and antigen. The 190kD dimeric C5 molecule shares homology with C3 and C4 but does not possess an internal thioester bond. C5 combines with C3b of C5 convertase of either the classical or the alternative pathway. C5 convertases split the α chain at an arginine-leucine bond at position 74–75 producing an 11kD C5a fragment, which has both chemotactic action for neutrophils and anaphylatoxin acitvity. It also produces a 180kD C5b fragment that remains anchored to the cell surface. C5b maintains a structure that is able to bind with C6. C5 is a β$_1$F globulin in man. C5b complexes with C6, C7, C8 and C9 to form the membrane attack complex (MAC) which mediates immune lysis of cells. Murine C5 is encoded by genes on chromosome 2.

C5a is a peptide split from C5 through the action of C5 convertases, C$\overline{4b2a3b}$ or C$\overline{3bBb3b}$. It is comprised of the C5 α chain's 74 amino terminal residues. It is a powerful chemotactic factor and is an anaphylatoxin, inducing mast cells and basophils to release histamine. It also causes smooth muscle contraction. It promotes the production of superoxide in polymorphonuclear neutrophils (PMNs) and accentuates CR3 and Tp150,95 expression in their membranes. In addition to chemotaxis it may facilitate PMN degranulation. Human serum contains anaphylatoxin inactivator that has carboxypeptidase-N properties. It deletes C5a's C-terminal arginine which yields C5a$_{\text{des Arg}}$. Although deprived of anaphylatoxin properties, C5a$_{\text{des Arg}}$ demonstrates limited chemotactic properties.

C5a$_{\text{74des Arg}}$ is that part of C5a that remains following deletion of the carboxy-terminal arginine through the action of anaphylatoxin inactivator. Although deprived of C5a's anaphylatoxin function, C5a$_{\text{74des Arg}}$ demonstrates limited chemotactic properties. This very uncommon deficiency of C2 protein in the serum has an autosomal recessive mode of inheritance. Affected persons have an increased likelihood of developing type III hypersensitivity disorders mediated by immune complexes, such as systemic lupus erythematosus. Whereas affected individuals possess the C2 gene, mRNA for C2 is apparently absent. Individuals who are heterozygous possess 50% of normal serum levels of C2 and manifest no associated clinical illness.

C5a receptor (C5a-R) is a receptor found on phagocytes and mast cells that binds the anaphylatoxin C5a, which plays an important role in inflammation. Serum carboxypeptidase N (SCPN) controls C5a function by eliminating the C-terminal arginine. This produces C5a$_{\text{des Arg}}$. Neutrophils are sites of C5a catabolism. C5a-R is a 150-200kD oligomer comprised of multiple 40-47kD C5a binding components. C5a-R mediates chemotaxis and other leukocyte reactions.

C5b is the principal molecular product that remains after C5a has been split off by the action of C5 convertase on C5. It has a binding site for C6 and complexes with it to begin generation of the membrane attack complex (MAC) of complement that leads to cell membrane injury and lysis.

C5 convertase is a molecular complex that splits C5 into C5a and C5b in both the classical and the alternative pathway of complement activation. Classical pathways C5 convertase is comprised of C$\overline{4b2a3b}$, whereas alternative pathway C5 convertase is comprised of C$\overline{3bBb3b}$. C2a and Bb contain the catalytic sites.

C6 (complement component 6) is a 128kD single polypeptide chain that participates in the membrane attack complex (MAC). It is encoded by *C6A* and *C6B* alleles. It is a b$_2$ globulin.

C7 (complement component 7) is an 843-amino-acid residue polypeptide chain that is a β$_2$ globulin. C5b67 is formed when C7 binds to C5b and C6. The complex has the appearance of a stalk with a leaf type of structure. C5b constitutes the leaf and the stalk consists of C6 and C7. The stalk facilitates introduction of the C5b67 complex into the cell membrane although no transmembrane perforation is produced. C5b67 anchored to the cell membrane provides a binding site for C8 and C9 in formation of the membrane attack complex (MAC). N-linked oligosaccharides bind to asparagine at positions 180 and 732 in C7.

C8 (complement component 8) is a 155kD molecule comprised of a 64kD α chain, a 64kD β chain and a 22kD γ chain. The α chain and γ chain are joined by disulfide bonds. Non-covalent bonds link α and γ chains to the β chain. The C5b678 complex becomes anchored to the cell surface when the γ chain inserts into the membrane's lipid bilayer. When the C8 β chain combines with C5b in C5b67 complexes, the α chain regions change in conformation from β-pleated sheets to α helices. The C5b678 complex has a limited capacity to lyse the cell to which it is anchored, since the complex can produce a transmembrane channel. The α chain of C8 combines with a single molecule of C9, thereby inducing C9 polymerization in the membrane attack complex (MAC). Genes at three different loci encode C8 α, γ and β chains. One-third of the amino acid sequences are identical between C8 α and β chains. These chains share identity of one-quarter of their amino acid sequences with C7 and C9. C8 is a $β_1$ globulin. In humans the C8 concentration is 10-20 μ/ml.

C9 (complement component 9) is a 535-amino-acid residue, single chain protein that binds to the C5b678 complex on the cell surface. It links to this complex through the a chain of C8, changes in conformation, significantly increases its length and reveals hydrophobic regions that can react with the cell membrane lipid bilayer. With Zn^{2+} present, a dozen C9 molecules polymerize to produce 100nm diameter hollow tubes that are positioned in the cell membrane to produce transmembrane channels. 12 to 15 C9 molecules interact with one C5b678 complex to produce the MAC. When viewed by an electron microscope, the pores in the plasma membrane produced by the poly-C9 have a 110-Å internal diameter, a 115-Å stalk anchored in the membrane's lipid bilayer and a 100-Å structure above the membrane that gives an appearance of a doughnut when viewed from above. Similar pores are produced by proteins released from cytotoxic T lymphocytes and natural killer cells called perforin or cytolysin. Sodium and water quickly enter cells through these pores leading to cell swelling and lysis. C9 shares one-quarter amino acid sequence identity with C7 and C8's α and β chains. It resembles perforin structurally. No polymorphism is found in C9, which is encoded by genes on chromosome 5 in man.

The **Membrane Attack Complex (MAC)** (Figures 9–11) consists of the five terminal proteins, i.e., C5, C6, C7, C8 and C9, associate into a membrane attack complex (MAC)

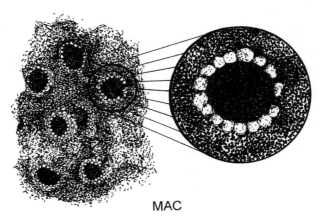

MAC

Figure 9. Membrane perforations resulting from membrane attack complex (MHC) action.

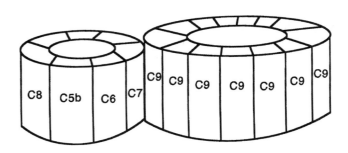

Figure 10. Membrane attack complex.

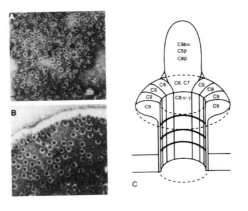

Figure 11. A. Electron micrograph of complement lesions (approximately 100 C) in evythrocyte membranes formed by poly C9 tubular complexes. B. Electron micrograph of complement lesions (approximately 160 C) induced on a target cell by a clone cytolytic T lymphocyte (CTL) line. CTL and natural killer (NK) induced membranes lesions are formed by tubular complexes of perforin which is homologous to C9. Therefore, except for the larger internal diameter, the morphology of the lesions is similar to that of complement-mediated lesions. C. Model of the MAC subunit arrangement.

on a target cell membrane to mediate injury. Initiation of MAC assembly begins with C5 cleavage into C5a and C5b fragments. A $(C5b, 6, 7, 8)_1(C9)_n$ complex then forms either on natural membranes or in their absence may combine with such plasma inhibitors as lipoproteins, antithrombin III and S protein. cDNA sequencing reveals the primary structure of all five related complement proteins. C9 is believed to have a five domain structure. C9 and C8 alpha proteins resemble each other not only structurally but also in sequence homologies. Both bind calcium and furnish domains that bind lipid enabling MAC to attach to the membrane.

Mechanisms proposed for complement-mediated cytolysis include extrinsic protein channel incorporation into the plasma membrane or membrane deformation and destruction. Only scant data is available concerning the domains or segments that link the MAC or its precursors to the membrane. Central regions of C6, C7, C8α, C8β and C9 have been postulated to contain amphilic structures which may be membrane anchors.

A single C9 molecule per C5b-8 (Figure 12) leads to erythrocyte lysis. C8 polymerization is not required. Gram-negative bacteria, which have both outer and inner membranes, resist complement action by lengthening surface carbohydrate content, which interferes with MAC binding. MAC assembly and insertion into the outer membrane is requisite for lysis of bacteria.

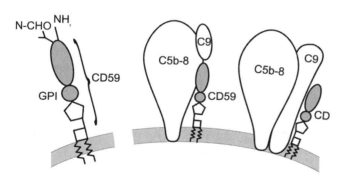

Figure 12. CD59.

Nucleated cells may rid their surfaces of MAC through endocytosis or exocytosis. Platelets have provided much data concerning sublytic actions of C5b-9 proteins.

Control proteins acting at different levels may inhibit killing of homologous cells mediated by MAC. Besides C8-binding protein or homologous restriction factor (HRF) found on human erythrocyte membranes, the functionally similar but smaller phosphatidylinositol glycan (PIG)-tailed membrane protein harnesses complement-induced cell lysis. In summary, the sublytic actions of MAC may be of greater consequence for host cells than are its cytotoxic effects.

Anaphylatoxins (Figure 13) are substances generated by the activation of complement that lead to increased vascular permeability as a consequence of the degranulation of mast cells with the release of pharmacologically active mediators of immediate hypersensitivity. These biologically active peptides of low molecular weight are derived from C3, C4, and C5. They are generated in serum during fixation of complement by Ag-Ab complexes, immunoglobulin aggregates, etc. Small blood vessels, mast cells, smooth muscle, and leukocytes in perpheral blood are targets of their action. Much is known about their primary structures. These complement fragments are designated C3a, C4a and C5a. They cause smooth muscle contraction, mast cell degranulation with histamine release, increased vascular permeability and the triple response in skin. They induce anaphylactic-like symptoms upon parenteral inoculation.

Anaphylatoxins

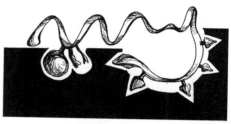

C3a/C3a57-77 --
Receptor interactions

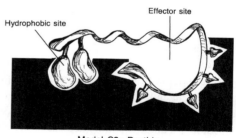

Figure 13. Anaphylatoxin-receptor interactions.

Anaphylatoxin inhibitor (AnaINH) is a 300kD α globulin. A carboxy peptidase that cleaves anaphylatoxin's carboxy terminal arginine. The enzyme acts on all three forms including C3a, C4a and C5a, inactivating rather than inhibiting them.

The **alternative complement pathway** (Figure 14) is a nonantibody dependent pathway for complement activation in which the early components C1, C2 and C4 are not required. It involves the protein properdin factor D, properdin factor B and C3b leading to C3 activation and continuing

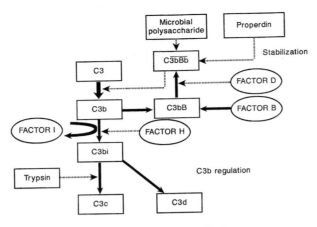

Alternative Complement Pathway

Figure 14.   Alternative complement pathway.

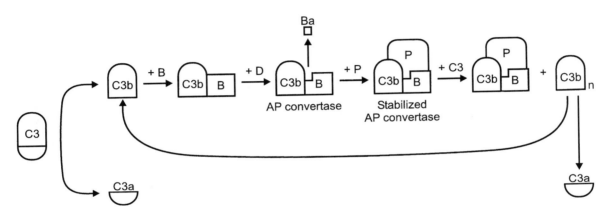

Figure 15.   The feedback loop of the alternative pathway.

to C9 in a manner identical to that which takes place in the activation of complement by the classical pathway. Substances such as endotoxin, human IgA, microbial polysaccharides and other agents may activate complement by the alternative pathway. The C3bB complex forms as C3b combined with Factor B. Factor D splits Factor B in the complex to yield the Bb active fragment that remains linked to C3b and Ba which is inactive and is split off. C3bBb, the alternative pathway C3 convertase splits C3 into C3b and C3a, thereby producing more C3bBb, which represents a positive feedback loop (Figure 15). Factor I, when accompanied by Factor H, splits C3b's heavy chain to yield C3bi which is unable to anchor Bb, thereby inhibiting the alternative pathway. Properdin and C3 nephritic factor stabilize C3bBb. C3 convertase stabilized by properdin activates complement's late components resulting in opsonization, chemotaxis of leukocytes, enhanced permeability and cytolysis. Properdin, IgA, IgG, lipopolysaccharide and snake venom can initiate the alternate pathway. Trypsin-related enzymes can activate both pathways.

Properdin (Factor P) is a globulin in normal serum that has a central role in activation of the alternative complement pathway activation. Additional factors such as magnesium ions are requisite for properdin activity. It is an alternative complement pathway protein that has a significant role in resistance against infection. It combines with and stabilizes the C3 convertase of the alternate pathway which is designated C3bBb. It is a 441 amino acid residue polypeptide chain with two points where N-linked oligosaccharides may become attached. Electron microscopy reveals it to have a cyclic oligomer conformation. Molecules comprised of six repeating 60 residue motifs which are homologous to 60 amino acids at C7, C8α and C8β amino, carboxy terminal ends and the C9 amino terminal end.

Alternative pathway C3 convertase (Figure 16) is an alternate unstable C3bB complex that splits C3 into C3a and C3b. Factor P, also known as properdin, stabilizes C3bB to yield C3bBbP. C3 nephritic factor can also stabilize C3bB.

C3bi (iC3b) (Figure 17) is the principal molecular product of C3b cleavage by Factor I. If complement receptor 1 or

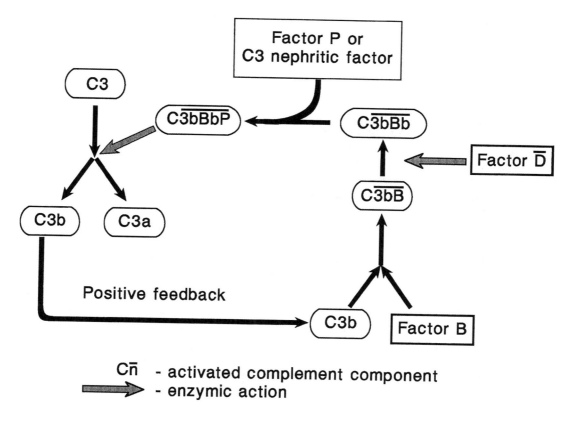

Cn̄ — activated complement component

⇒ — enzymic action

Alternative Pathway C3 Convertase

Figure 16.   Alternative pathway C3 convertase.

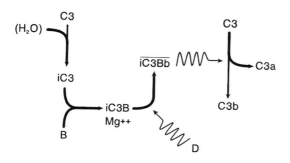

Tick-Over Mechanism

Figure 17.   Through the C3 tickover mechanism alternative pathway C3 convertase perpetually generates C3b. C3 internal thioester bond hydrolysis is the initiating event.

Factor H is present, Factor I can split C3bi's arginine-glutamic acid bond at position 954–955 to yield C3c and C3dg. C3bi attached to particles promotes phagocytosis when combined with complement receptor 3 on the surface of polymorphonuclear neutrophils (PMNs) and monocytes.

It also promotes phagocytosis by binding to conglutinin in the serum of cows.

C3c is the principal molecule that results from Factor I cleavage of C3bi when Factor H or complement receptor 1 is present. C3c is comprised of 27kD and 43kD α chain fragments linked through disulfide bonds to a whole β chain.

C3d is a 33kD B cell growth factor that is formed by proteolytic enzyme splitting of a lysine-histidine bond in C3dg at position 1001–1002. C3d is comprised of the carboxy-terminal 301-amino-acid residues of C3dg. It interacts with complement receptor 2 on the surface of B cells. C3d contains the C3 a chain's thioester.

C3dg is a 41kD, 349-amino-acid residue molecule formed by the cleavage of C3bi with factor H or complement receptor 1 present. Polymorphonuclear neutrophil leukocytes express complement receptor 4 which is reactive with C3dg. Complement receptor 2 on B cells is also a C3dg receptor.

C3e is a C3c α chain nonapeptide that causes leukocytosis. The peptide is comprised of Thr-Leu-Asp-Pro-Glu-Arg-Leu-Gly-Arg.

C3f is a 17 amino-acid-residue peptide split from the α chain of C3b by Factor I with Factor H or complement receptor 1 present.

C3g is an 8kD molecule comprised of the amino-terminal 47 amino acid residues of C3dg. Trypsin digestion of C3dg yields C3g, whose function is unknown.

C3 nephritic factor (C3NeF) is an IgG autoantibody to the alternate complement pathway C3 convertase that mimics the action of properdin. C3NeF is present in the serum of patients with membranoproliferative glomerulonephritis type II (dense deposit disease). It stabilizes the alternate pathway C3 convertase, thereby enhancing the breakdown of C3 and produces hypocomplementemia. Rarely, C3NeF may be IgG autoantibodies to C3 convertase (C4b2a) of the classical pathway. Systemic lupus erythematosus patients may contain antibodies against C4b2a that stabilizes the classical pathway C3 convertase leading to increased *in vivo* cleavage of C3.

Factor P (properdin) is a key participant in the alternative pathway of complement activation. It is a gammaglobulin, but not an immunoglobulin, that combines with C3b and stabilizes alternative pathway C3 convertase (C3bB) to produce C3bBbP. Factor P is a 3 or 4 polypeptide chain structure.

Factor B is an alternative complement pathway component. It is a 739 amino acid residue single polypeptide chain which combines with C3b and is cleaved by Factor D to produce alternative pathway C3 convertase. Cleavage by Factor D is at an arginine-lysine bond at position 234–235 to yield an amino-terminal fragment Ba. The carboxy-terminal fragment termed Bb remains attached to C3b. C3bBb is C3 convertase, and C3bBb3b is C5 convertase of the alternative complement pathway. The Bb fragment is the enzyme's active site. There are three short homologous, 60-amino-acid-residue repeats in Factor B, and it possesses four attachment sites for N-linked oligosaccharides. Alleles for human Factor B include *BfS* and *BfF*. The Factor B gene is located in the major histocompatibility complex situated on the short arm of chromosome 6 in humans and on chromosome 17 in mice. Also called C3 proactivator.

Factor D is a serine esterase of the alternative pathway of complement activation. It splits Factor B to produce Ba and Bb fragments. It is also called C3 activator convertase.

Factor D deficiency is an extremely rare genetic deficiency of Factor D which has an X-linked or autosomal recessive pattern of inheritance. There is only 1% of physiologic amounts of Factor D in the serum of affected patients, which renders them susceptible to repeated infection by *Neisseria* microorganisms. There are half the physiologic levels of Factor D in the serum of heterozygotes who have no clinical symptoms related to this deficiency.

Factor H is a regulator of complement in the blood under physiologic conditions. Factor H is a glycoprotein in serum that unites with C3b and facilitates dissociation of alternative complement pathway C3 convertase designated C3bBb, into C3b and Bb. Factor I splits C3b if Factor H is present. In man, Factor H is a 1231 amino acid residue single polypeptide chain. It is comprised of 20 short homologous repeats comprised of about 60 residues present in proteins that interact with C3 or C4. Factor H is an inhibitor of the alternative complement pathway. Previously called β-1H globulin.

Factor H deficiency is an extremely rare genetic deficiency of Factor H which has an autosomal recessive mode of inheritance. Only 1% of the physiologic level of Factor H is present in the serum of affected individuals, which renders them susceptible to recurrent infections by pyogenic microorganisms. Persons who are heterozygotes contain 50% of normal levels of Factor H in their serum and show no clinical effects.

Factor I (Figure 18) is a serine protease that splits the a chain of C3b to produce C3bi and the α chain of C4b to yield C4bi. Factor I splits a 17-amino-acid-residue peptide termed C3f, if Factor H or complement receptor 1 are present, from the C3b α chain to yield C3bi. Factor I splits the C3bi, if complement receptor I or Factor H is present, to yield C3c and C3dg. Factor I splits the C4b α chain, if C4 binding protein is present, to yield C4bi. C4c and C4d are produced by a second splitting of the a chain of C4bi. Factor I is a heterodimeric molecule. It is also called C3b/C4b inactivator.

Factor I deficiency is a very uncommon genetic deficiency of C3b inactivator. It has an autosomal recessive pattern of inheritance. There is less than 1% of the physiologic level of Factor I in the serum of affected subjects, which renders them susceptible to repeated infections by pyogenic microorganisms. These individuals also reveal deficiencies of Factor B and C3 in their serum since these components are normally split *in vivo* by alternative pathway C3 convertase (C3bBb), which factors I and H inhibit under physiologic conditions. These patients may develop urticaria because of the formation of C3a that induces release of histamine.

C4b binding protein (C4bp) is a 600kD protein in serum capable of binding six C4b molecules at once by means of seven spokes extending from a core at the center. C4bP halts progression of complement activation. Factor I splits C4b molecules captured by C4bp. C4bp belongs to the regulators of complement activity molecules. C4bp interferes with C2a association with C4b. It also promotes C4b2a dissociation into C4b and C2a. It is also needed for the action of Factor I in splitting C4b to C4bi and of C4bi into C4c and C4d. The C4bp gene is located on chromosome 1q3.2.

C4bi (iC4b) is the principal product of the reaction when Factor I splits. When C4b binding protein is present, C4bi splits an α chain arginine-threonine bond to yield C4c and C4d.

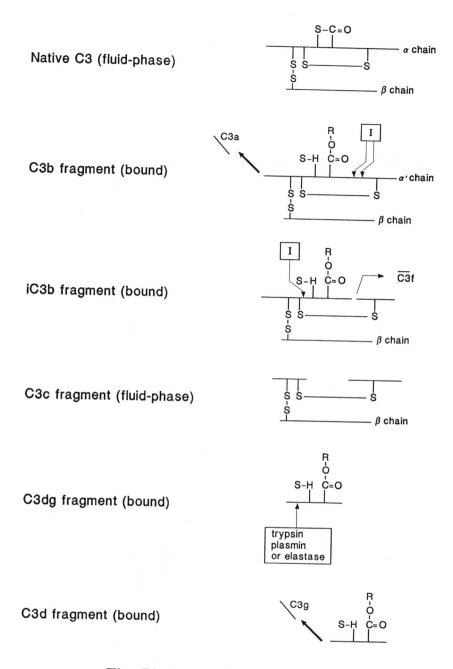

The Binding of Factor I to C3b

Figure 18.   The binding of Factor I to C3b.

C4c is the principal product of Factor I cleavage of C4bi, when C4b binding protein is present. This 145kD molecule, of unknown function, is comprised of β and γ chains of C4 and two α chain fragments.

C4d is a 45kD molecule produced by factor I cleavage of C4bi when C4b binding protein is present. C4d is the molecule where Chido and Rogers epitopes are located. It is also the location of the C4 α chain's internal thioester bond.

Complement inhibitors are protein inhibitors that occur naturally and block the action of complement components include factor H, factor I, C1 inhibitor and C4 binding protein (C4bp). Also included among complement inhibitors are heating to 56°C to inactivate C1 and C2, combination with hydrazine and ammonia to block the action of C3 and C4, and the addition of zymosan or cobra venom factor to induce alternate pathway activation of C3 which consumes C3 in the plasma.

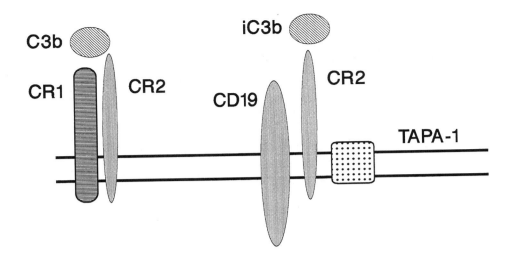

Complement Receptor Complexes on the Surface of B cells

Figure 19.   Complement receptor complexes on the surface of B cells.

Complement receptors (Figure 19) are receptors for products of complement reactions. Proteolytic cleavage of human complement component C3 takes place following activation of either the classical or the alternative complement pathway. Following the generation of C3a and C3b, the C3b covalently binds to bacteria, immune complexes or some other target and then unites with a high-affinity receptor termed the C3b/C4b receptor currently known as CR1. Subsequent proteolytic cleavage of the bound C3b is attributable to factor I and a cofactor. This action yields C3bi, C3d, g, and C3c, which interact with specific receptors. CR2 is the C3dg receptor and CR3 is the C3bi receptor.

Membrane complement receptors are receptors expressed on blood cells and tissue macrophages of man. These include C1q-R (C1q receptor), CR1 (C3b/C4b receptor; CD35), CR2 (C3d/Epstein-Barr virus (EBV) receptor; CD21), CR3 (iC3b receptor; CD11b/CD18), CR4 (C3bi receptor; CD11c/CD18), CR5 (C3dg-dimer receptor), fH-R (factor H receptor), C5a-R (C5a receptor) and C3a/C4a-R (C3a/C4a receptor). Ligands for C receptors generated by either the classic or alternate pathways include fluid-phase activation peptides of C3, C4 and C5 designated C3a, C4a and C5a, which are anaphylatoxins that interact with either C3a/C4a-R or C5a-R, and participate in inflammation. Other ligands for C receptors include complement proteins deposited on immune complexes that are either soluble or particulate. Fixed C4 and C3 fragments (C4b, C3b, C3bi, C3dg and C3d), C1q and factor H constitute these ligands. These receptors play a major role in facilitating improved recognition of pathogenic substances. They aid the elimination of bacteria and soluble immune complexes.

Neutrophils, monocytes, and macrophages express C3 receptors on their surface. Neutrophils and erythrocytes express immune adherence receptors, termed CR1, on their surface. Four other receptors for C3 are designated CR2, CR3, CR4 and CR5. Additional receptors for complement components other than C3 and a receptor for C3a are termed C1q-R (C1q receptor), C5a-R (C5a receptor), C3a-R (C3a receptor) and fH-R (factor H receptor).

Complement receptor-1 (CR1) is a CR1 membrane glycoprotein found on human erythrocytes, monocytes, polymorphonuclear leukocytes, B cells, a T cell subset, mast cells and glomerular podocytes. On red cells, CR1 binds C3b or C4b components of immune complexes facilitating their transport to the mononuclear phagocyte system. CR1 facilitates attachment, endocytosis and phagocytosis of C3b/C4b containing complexes to macrophages or neutrophils and may serve as a cofactor for factor I-mediated C3 cleavage. The identification of CR1 cDNA has made possible molecular analysis of CR1 biological properties.

Complement receptor-2 (CR2) is a receptor for C3 fragments that also serves as a binding site for Epstein-Barr virus (EBV). It is a receptor for C3bi, C3dg and C3d based on its specificity for their C3d structure. B cells, follicular dendritic cells of lymph nodes, thymocytes and pharyngeal epithelial cells but not T cells express CR2. EBV enters B lymphocytes by way of CR2. The gene encoding CR2 is linked closely with that of CR1. A 140kD single polypeptide chain makes up CR2, which has an SCR structure similar to that of CR1. CR2 may be active in B cell activation. Its expression appears restricted to late pre-B and to mature B cells. CR2 function is associated with membrane IgM. Analysis of cDNA clones has provided CR2's primary structure.

Complement receptor-3 (CR3) is a principal opsonin receptor expressed by monocytes, macrophages and neutrophils. It plays an important role in the removal of bacteria. CR3 binds fixed C3bi in the presence of divalent cations. It also binds bacterial lipopolysaccharides and b-glucans of yeast cell walls. The latter are significant in the ability of granulocytes to identify bacteria and yeast cells. CR3 is an integrin type of adhesion molecule that facilitates the binding of neutrophils to endothelial cells in inflammation. CR3 enables phagocytic cells to attach to bacteria or yeast cells with fixed C3bi, β-glucans or lipopolysaccharide on their surface. This facilitates phagocytosis and the respiratory burst. CR3 is comprised of a 165kD α-glycoprotein chain and a 95kD β-glycoprotein chain. 2 CR3 appears related to LFA-1 and P150,95 molecules and shares a β chain with them. All three of these molecules are of critical significance in antigen-independent cellular adhesion which confines leukocytes to inflammatory areas, among other functions. Deficient surface expression of these molecules occurs in leukocyte adhesion deficiency (LAD) in which patients experience repeated bacterial infections. The primary defect appears associated with the common β chain. Besides C3bi binding, CR3 is of critical significance in IgG- and CR1-facilitated phagocytosis by neutrophils and monocytes. CR3 has a more diverse function than does either CR1 or CR2.

Complement receptor 4 (CR4) is a glycoprotein membrane receptor for C3dg on polymorphonuclear neutrophils (PMNs), monocytes and platelets. CR4 facilitates Fc receptor-mediated phagocytosis and mediates Fc-independent phagocytosis. It consists of a 150kD α chain and a 95kD β chain. Chromosome 16 is the site of genes that encode the α chain whereas chromosome 21 is the site of genes that encode the β chain. Tissue macrophages express CR4. It is an integrin with a β chain in common with CR3 and LFA-1.

Complement receptor-5 (CR5) is a receptor that binds C3bi, C3dg and C3d fragments based on its specificity for their C3d component. Reactivity is only in the fluid phase and not when the fragments are fixed. CR5 is the C3dg-dimer receptor. Neutrophils and platelets manifest CR5 activity.

Decay-accelerating factor (DAF) (Figure 20) is a 70kD membrane glycoprotein of normal human erythrocytes, leukocytes and platelets but absent from the red blood cells of paroxysmal nocturnal hemaglobulinuria patients. It facilitates dissociation of classical complement pathway C3 convertase (C4b2a) into C4b and C2a. It also promotes the association of alternative complement pathway C3 convertase (C3bBb) into C3b and Bb. DAF is found on selected mucosal epithelial cells and endothelial cells. It prevents complement cascade amplification on the surfaces of cells

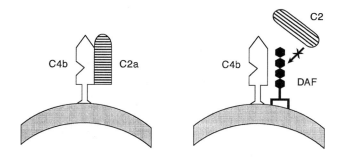

Figure 20. Decay acceleration factor.

to protect them from injury by autologous complement. DAF's physiologic function may be to protect cells from lysis by serum. DAF competes with C2 for linkage with C4b to block C3 convertase synthesis in the classical pathway. The DAF molecule consists of a single chain bound to the cell membrane by phosphatidyl inositol. Paroxysmal nocturnal hemoglobulinuria develops as a consequence of DAF deficiency.

Homologous restriction factor (HRF) is an eythrocyte surface protein that prevents cell lysis by homologous complement on its surface. It bears a structural resemblance to C8 and C9.

Paroxysmal nocturnal hemoglobulinuria (PNH) is a rare form of hemolytic anemia in which the red blood cells, as well as neutrophils and platelets manifest strikingly increased sensitivity to complement lysis. PNH red blood cell membranes are deficient in decay accelerating factor (DAF), LFA-3 and FcγRIII. Without DAF, which protects the cell membranes from complement lysis by classic pathway C5 convertase and decreases membrane attack complex formation, the erythrocytes and lymphocytes are highly susceptible to lysis by complement. Interaction of these PNH erythrocytes with activated complement results in excessive C3b binding which leads to formation of more C3b through the alternate complement pathway by way of factors B and D. Intravascular hemolysis follows activation of C5 convertase in the C5-9 membrane attack complex (MHC). The blood platelets and myelocytes in affected subjects are also DAF deficient and are readily lysed by complement. There is leukopenia, thrombocytopenia, iron deficiency and diminished leukocyte alkaline phosphatase. The Coombs' test is negative and there is also very low acetylcholine esterase activity in the red cell membrane. No antibody participating in this process has been found in either the serum or on the erythrocytes. The disease is suggested by episodes of intravascular hemolysis, iron deficiency and hemosiderin in the urine. It is confirmed by hemolysis in acid medium, termed the HAM test.

Complement fixation (Figure 21) is a primary union of antigen with antibody in the complement fixation reaction takes place almost instantaneously and is invisible. A measured

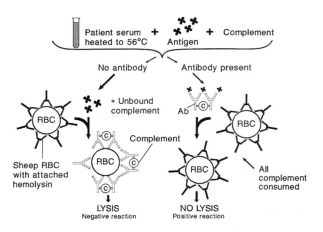

Complement Fixation

Figure 21.   Complement fixation.

amount of complement present in the reaction mixture is taken up by complexes of antigen and antibody. The consumption or binding of complement by antigen-antibody complexes. This serves as the basis for a serologic assay in which antigen is combined with a serum specimen suspected of containing the homologous antibody. Following the addition of a measured amount of complement, which is fixed or consumed only if antibody was present in the serum and has formed a complex with the antigen, sheep red blood cells sensitized (coated) with specific antibody are added to determine whether or not complement has been fixed in the first phase of the reaction. Failure of the sensitized sheep red blood cells to lyse constitutes a positive test since no complement is available. However, sheep red blood cell lysis indicates that complement was not consumed during the first phase of the reaction, implying that homologous antibody was not present in the serum, and complement remains free to lyse the sheep red blood cells sensitized with antibody. Hemolysis constitutes a negative reaction. The sensitivity of the complement fixation test falls between that of agglutination and precipitation. Complement fixation tests may be carried out in microtiter plates, which are designed for the use of relatively small volumes of reagents. The lysis of sheep red blood cells sensitized with rabbit antibody is measured either in a spectrophotometer at 413nm or by the release of ^{51}Cr from red cells that have been previously labeled with the isotope. Complement fixation can detect either soluble or insoluble antigen. Its ability to detect virus antigens in impure tissue preparations makes the test still useful in diagnosis of virus infections.

Complement deficiency conditions are rare inherited deficiencies. In healthy Japanese blood donors, only 1 in 100,000 persons had no C5, C6, C7 and C8. 3 of 1,000 individuals contained no C9. Most individuals with missing complement components do not manifest clinical symptoms. Additional

pathways provide complement-dependent functions that are necessary to preserve life. If C3, factor I or any segment of the alternative pathway is missing, the condition may be life-threatening with markedly decreased opsonization in phagocytosis. C3 is depleted when factor I is absent. C5, C6, C7 or C8 deficiencies are linked with infections, mainly meningococcal or gonococcal which usually succumb to complement's bactericidal action. Deficiencies in classical complement pathway activation are often associated with connective tissue or immune complex diseases. Systemic lupus erythematosus may be associated with C1qrs, C2 or C4 deficiencies. Hereditary angioedema (HANE) patients have a deficiency of C1 inactivator. A number of experimental animals with specific complement deficiencies has been described, such as C6 deficiency in rabbits and C5 deficiency in mice. Acquired complement deficiencies may be caused by either accelerated complement consumption in immune complex diseases with a type III mechanism or by diminished formation of complement proteins as in acute necrosis of the liver.

C1 deficiencies also are very rare. Only a few cases of C1q, C1r, or C1r and C1s deficiencies have been reported. These have an autosomal recessive mode of inheritance. Patients with these defects may manifest systemic lupus erythematosus, glomerulonephritis or pyogenic infections. They have an increased incidence of type III (immune complex) hypersensitivity diseases. Half of C1q deficient persons may contain physiologic levels of mutant C1q that is not functional.

C1 inhibitor (C1 INH) deficiencies are the most frequently found deficiency of the classic complement pathway and may be seen in patients with hereditary angioneurotic edema. This syndrome may be expressed as either a lack of the inhibitor substance or the C1 INH may be functionally inactive. The patient develops edema of the face, respiratory tract, including the glottis and bronchi, and the extremities. Severe abdominal pain may occur with intestinal involvement. Since C1 inhibitor can block Hagemann factor (Factor XII) in the blood clotting mechanism, its absence can lead to the liberation of kinin and fibrinolysis that results from the activation of plasmin. The disease is inherited as an autosomal dominant trait. When edema of the larynx occurs, the patient may die of asphyxiation. When abdominal attacks occur, there may be watery diarrhea and vomiting. These bouts usually span 48 hours followed by rapid recovery. During an attack of angioedema, C$\overline{1}$r is activated to produce C$\overline{1}$s, which depletes its substrates C4 and C2. The action of activated C1s on C4 and C2 leads to the production of a substance that increases vascular permeability, especially that of post capillary venules. C1 and C4 cooperate with plasmin to split this active peptide from C2. 85% of the families of patients with hereditary angioneurotic edema do not contain C1 inhibitor. Treatment is by preventive maintenance. Patients are given inhibitors of plasmin, such as aminocaproic acid and tranexamic acid. Methyl testosterone which causes synthesis of normal C1 inhibitor in angioneurotic edema patients is effective by an unknown mechanism.

Angioedema refers to the significant localized swelling of tissues as a consequence of complement activation that takes place when C1 esterase inhibitor is lacking.

Angiogenesis factor is a macrophage-derived protein that facilitates neovascularization through stimulation of vascular endothelial cell growth. Among the five angiogenesis factors known, basic fibroblast growth factor may facilitate neovascularization in type IV delayed hypersensitivity responses.

C1q deficiency may be found in association with lupus-like syndromes. C1r deficiency, which is inherited as an autosomal recessive trait, may be associated with respiratory tract infections, glomerulonephritis, and skin manifestations that resemble SLE-like disease. C1s deficiency is transmitted as an autosomal dominant trait and patients may again show SLE-like signs and symptoms. Their antigen-antibody complexes can persist without resolution.

C2 deficiency is rarely found in individuals. Although no symptoms are normally associated with this trait, which has an autosomal recessive mode of inheritance, autoimmune-like manifestations that resemble features of certain collagen-vascular diseases, such as systemic lupus erythematosus, may appear. Thus, many genetically determined complement deficiencies are not associated with signs and symptoms of disease. When they do occur, it is usually manifested as an increased incidence of infectious diseases that affect the kidneys, respiratory tract, skin and joints.

C3 deficiency is an extremely uncommon genetic disorder that may be associated with repeated serious pyogenic bacterial infections and may lead to death. The C3 deficient individuals are deprived of appropriate opsonization, prompt phagocytosis and the ability to kill infecting microorganisms. There is defective classical and alternative pathway activation. Besides infections, these individuals may also develop immune complex disease such as glomerulonephritis. C3 levels that are one-half normal in heterozygotes are apparently sufficient to avoid the clinical consequences induced by a lack of C3 in the serum.

C4 deficiency is an uncommon genetic defect with an autosomal recessive mode of inheritance. Affected individuals have defective classical complement pathway activation. Those who manifest clinical consequences of the defect may develop systemic lupus erythematosus or glomeruloneophritis. Half of the patients with C4 and C2 deficiencies develop SLE but deficiencies in these two complement components are not usually linked to increased infections.

C5 deficiency is a very uncommon genetic disorder that has an autosomal recessive mode of inheritance. Affected individuals have only trace amounts of C5 in their plasma. They have a defective ability to form the membrane attack complex (MAC) which is necessary for the efficient lysis of invading microorganisms. They have an increased susceptibility to disseminated infections by *Neisseria* microorganisms such as *Neisseria meningitidis* and *Neisseria gonorrhoeae*. Heterozygotes may manifest 13–65% of C5 activity in their plasma and usually show no clinical effects of their partial deficiency. C5 deficient mice have also been described.

C6 deficiency is a highly uncommon genetic defect with an autosomal recessive mode of inheritance in which affected individuals have only trace amounts of C6 in their plasma. They are defective in the ability to form a membrane attack complex (MAC) and have increased susceptibility to disseminated infections by *Neisseria* microorganisms, that include gonococci and meningococci. C6 deficient rabbits have been described.

C7 deficiency is a highly uncommon genetic disorder with an autosomal recessive mode of inheritance in which the serum of affected persons contains only trace amounts of C7 in the plasma. They have defective ability to form a membrane attack complex (MAC) and show an increased incidence of disseminated infections caused by *Neisseria* microorganisms. Some may manifest an increased propensity to develop immune complex (type III hypersensitivity) diseases such as glomerulonephritis or systemic lupus erythematosus.

C8 deficiency is a highly uncommon genetic disorder with an autosomal recessive mode of inheritance in which affected individuals are missing C8 α, γ or β-chains. This is associated with a defective ability to form a membrane attack complex (MAC). Individuals may have an increased propensity to develop disseminated infections caused by *Neisseria* microorganisms, such as meningococci.

C9 deficiency is a highly uncommon genetic disorder with an autosomal recessive mode of inheritance in which only trace amounts of C9 are present in the plasma of affected persons. There is defective ability to form the membrane attack complex (MAC). The serum of C9 deficient subjects retains its lytic and bactericidal activity even though the rate of lysis is decreased compared to that induced in the presence of C9. There are usually no clinical consequences associated with this condition. The disorder is more common in the Japanese than in most other populations.

Hereditary complement deficiencies and microbial infection are associated with defects in activation of the classical pathway that lead to increased susceptibility to pyogenic infections. A deficiency of C3 leads to a defect in activation of both the classical and alternative pathways that lead to an increased frequency of pyogenic infections that may prove fatal. Such individuals also have defective opsonization and phagocytosis. Defects of alternate pathway factors D and P lead to impaired activation of the alternative pathway with increased susceptibility to pyogenic infections. Deficiencies of C5 through C9 are associated with defective membrane attack complex (MAC) formation and lysis of cells, including bacteria. This produces increased susceptibility to disseminated *Neisseria* infection.

12
Types I, II, III, and IV Hypersensitivity

Hypersensitivity refers to an increased reactivity or increased sensitivity by the animal body to an antigen to which it has been previously exposed. The term is often used as a synonym for allergy which describes a state of altered reactivity to an antigen. Hypersensitivity has been divided into categories based upon whether it can be passively transferred by antibodies or by specifically immune lymphoid cells. The most widely adopted current classification is that of Coombs and Gell that designates immunoglobulin-mediated (immediate) hypersensitivity reactions as types I, II and III and lymphoid cell-mediated (delayed-type) hypersensitivity/cell-mediated immunity as a type IV reaction. *Hypersensitivity* generally represents the "dark side" signifying the undesirable aspects of an immune reaction whereas the term *immunity* implies a desirable effect.

Immediate hypersensitivity is an antibody-mediated hypersensitivity. In man, this homocytotropic antibody is IgE and in certain other species IgG1. The IgE antibodies are attached to mast cells through their Fc receptors. Once the Fab regions of the mast cell-bound IgE molecules interact with specific antigen, vasoactive amines are released from the cytoplasmic granules as described under type I hypersensitivity reactions. The term "immediate" is used to indicate that this type of reaction occurs within seconds to minutes following contact of a cell-fixed IgE antibody with antigen. Skin tests and RAST are useful to detect immediate hypersensitivity in humans and passive cutaneous anaphylaxis reveals immediate hypersensitivity in selected other species. Examples of immediate hypersensitivity in humans include the classic anaphylactic reaction to penicillin administration, hay fever, and environmental allergens such as tree and grass pollens, bee stings, etc.

The **triple response of Lewis** refers to skin changes in immediate hypersensitivity illustrated by striking the skin with a sharp object such as the side of a ruler. The first response termed the "stroke response" is caused by the production of histamine and related mediators at the point of contact with the skin. The second response is a flare produced by vasodilation and resembles a red halo. The third response is a wheal characterized by swelling and blanching induced by histamine from mast cell degranulation. The swelling is attributable to edema between the junctions of cells that become rich in protein and fluid.

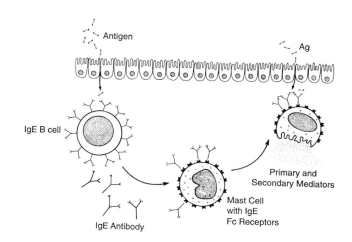

Figure 1. A type I hypersensitivity reaction in which antigen molecules cross-link IgE molecules on the surface of mast cells resulting in their degranulation with the release of both primary and secondary mediators of anaphylaxis.

Type I anaphylactic hypersensitivity (Figure 1) is a reaction mediated by IgE antibodies reactive with specific allergens (antigens that induce allergy) attached to basophil or mast cell Fc receptors. Cross-linking of the cell-bound IgE antibodies by antigen is followed by mast cell or basophil degranulation, with release of pharmacological mediators. These mediators include vasoactive amines such as histamine, which causes increased vascular permeability, vasodilation, bronchial spasm and mucous secretion (Figure 2). Secondary mediators of type I hypersensitivity include leukotrienes, prostaglandin D_2, platelet-activating factor and various cytokines. Systemic anaphylaxis is a serious clinical problem and can follow the injections of protein antigens, such as antitoxin or of drugs, such as penicillin.

Anaphylaxis is a shock reaction that occurs within seconds following the injection of an antigen or drug, or after a bee sting, to which the susceptible subject has IgE specific antibodies. There is embarrassed respiration due to laryngeal and bronchial constriction and shock associated with decreased blood pressure. Signs and symptoms differ among species based on the primary target organs or tissues. Type I hypersensitivity occurs following the crosslinking of IgE antibodies by specific antigen or allergen on the surfaces of basophils in the blood or mast cells in the tissues. This causes the release of the pharmacological mediators of immediate

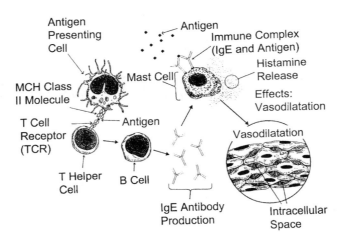

Figure 2.   Schematic representation of events that follow degranulation of mast cells in tissues resulting in vasodilatation of capillaries leading to the changes associated with type I hypersensitivity reactions in tissues.

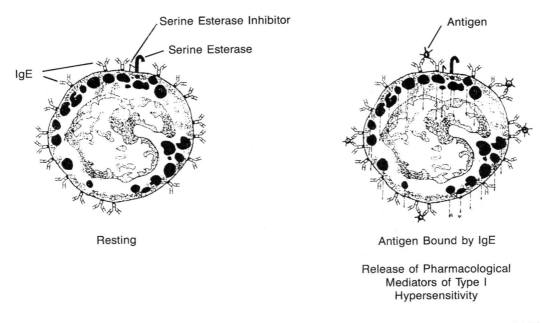

Figure 3.   Comparison of a resting basophil or mast cell in which serine esterase activity is blocked by serine esterase inhibitor with a mast cell or basophil undergoing degranulation as a consequence of antigen interaction with Fab regions of cell surface IgE molecules in which the serine esterase inhibitor activity is removed.

hypersensitivity with a reaction occurring within seconds of contact with antigen or allergen (Figure 3). Eosinophils, chemotactic factor, heparin, histamine, serotonin, together with selected other substances are released during the primary response. Acute phase reactants are formed and released in the secondary response. Secondary mediators include slow reacting substance of anaphylaxis (SRS-A), platelet activating factor and bradykinin. In addition to systemic anaphylaxis described below, local anaphylaxis may occur in the skin, gut or nasal mucosa following contact with antigen. The skin reaction, called urticaria, consists of a raised wheal surrounded by an area of erythema. Cytotoxic anaphylaxis follows the interaction of antibodies with cell surface antigens. **Active anaphylaxis** is an anaphylactic state induced by natural or experimental sensitization in atopic subjects or experimental animals. **Passive anaphylaxis** is an anaphylactic reaction in an animal which has been administered an antigen after it has been conditioned by an inoculation of antibodies derived from an animal immunized against the antigen of interest.

Antianaphylaxis is the inhibition of anaphylaxis through desensitization. This is accomplished by repeated injections of the sensitizing agent too minute to produce an anaphylactic reaction.

Desensitization is a method of treatment used by allergists to diminish the effects of IgE-mediated type I hypersensitivity (Figure 4). The allergen to which an individual has been sensitized is repeatedly injected in a form that favors the generation of IgG (blocking) antibodies rather than IgE antibodies that mediate type I hypersensitivity in humans. This method has been used for many years to diminish the symptoms of atopy, such as asthma and allergic rhinitis, and to prevent anaphylaxis produced by bee venom. IgG antibodies are believed to prevent antigen interaction with IgE antibodies anchored to mast cell surfaces by intercepting the antigen molecules before they reach the cell-bound IgE. Thus a type I hypersensitivity-reaction of the anaphylactic type is prevented.

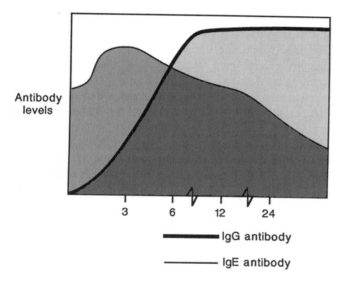

Antibody levels

3   6   12   24

■■■■ IgG antibody

——— IgE antibody

Figure 4.   Desensitization.

Bradykinin is a 9-amino acid peptide split by plasma kallikrein from plasma kininogens. It produces slow, sustained, smooth muscle contraction. Its action is slower than that of histamine (Figure 5). It is produced in experimental anaphylaxis in animal tissues. Its sequence is Arg Pro Pro Gly Phe Ser Pro Phe Arg. Besides anaphylaxis, bradykinin is also increased in endotoxin shock. Lysyl-bradyinin (kallidin), which is split from kininogens by tissue kallikreins, also has a lysine reside at the amino terminus.

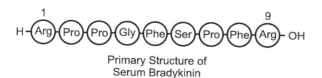

1   9
H—Arg—Pro—Pro—Gly—Phe—Ser—Pro—Phe—Arg— OH

Primary Structure of
Serum Bradykinin

Figure 5.   Active kinins.

Systemic anaphylaxis is a type I, immediate, anaphylactic type of hypersensitivity mediated by IgE antibodies anchored to mast cells that become cross-linked by homologous antigen (allergen) causing release of the pharmacological mediators of immediate hypersensitivity, producing lesions in multiple organs and tissue sites. This is in contrast to local anaphylaxis where the effects are produced in isolated anatomical location. The intravenous administration of a serum product, antibiotic or other substance against which the patient has anaphylactic IgE- type hypersensitivity may lead to the symptoms of systemic anaphylaxis within seconds and may prove lethal.

Passive systemic anaphylaxis renders a normal, previously unsensitized animal susceptible to anaphylaxis by a passive injection, often intravenoulsy, of homocytotrophic antibody derived from a sensitized animal, followed by antigen administration. Anaphylactic shock occurs soon after the passively transferred antibody and antigen interact *in vivo*, releasing the mediators of immediate hypersensitivity from mast cells of the host.

Generalized anaphylaxis occurs when the signs and symptoms of anaphylactic shock manifest within seconds to minutes following the administration of an antigen or allergen that interacts with specific IgE antibodies bound on mast cell or basophil surfaces, causing the release of pharmicologically active mediators that include vasoactive amines from their granules. Symptoms may vary from transient respiratory difficulties (due to contraction of the smooth muscle and terminal bronchioles) to even death.

Local anaphylaxis is a relatively common type I immediate hypersensitivity reaction. Local anaphylaxis is mediated by IgE cross-linked allergen molecules at the surface of mast cells which then release histamine and other pharmacological mediators that produce signs and symptoms. The reaction occurs in a particular target organ such as the gastrointestinal tract, skin or nasal mucosa. Hay fever and asthma represent examples.

Basophils are polymorphonuclear leukocytes of the myeloid lineage with distinctive basophilic secondary granules in the cytoplasm that frequently overlie the nucleus. These granules are storage depots for heparin, histamine, platelet activating factor and other pharmacological mediators of immediate hypersensitivity (Figure 6). Degranulation of the cells with release of these pharmacological mediators takes place following cross-linking by allergen or antigen of Fab regions of IgE receptor molecules bound through Fc receptors to the cell surface. They comprise less than 0.5% of peripheral blood leukocytes. Following cross-linking of surface bound IgE molecules by specific allergen or antigen, granules are released by exocytosis. Substances liberated from the granules are pharmacological mediators of immediate (Type I) anaphylactic hypersensitivity.

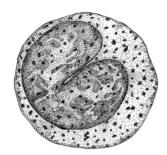

Figure 6. A peripheral blood basophil showing a bilobed nucleus and cytoplasmic granules that represent storage sites of pharmacological mediators of immediate type I hypersensitivity.

Degranulation is a mechanism whereby cytoplasmic granules in cells fuse with the cell membrane to discharge the contents from the cell. A classic example is degranulation of the mast cell or basophil in immediate (type I) hypersensitivity. In phagocytic cells, cytoplasmic granules combine with phagosomes and release their contents into the phagolysosome formed by their union.

Cromolyn (1,3-*bis*[2-carboxychromon-5-yloxy-2-hydroxypropane]) is a therapeutic agent that prevents mast cell degranulation (Figure 7). It has proven effective in the therapy of selected allergies that include allergic rhinitis and asthma.

Aggregate anaphylaxis is a form of anaphylaxis caused by aggregates of antigen and antibody in the fluid phase. The aggregates bind complement liberating complement fragments C3a, C5a, and C4a, also called toxins, which induce the release of mediators. Preformed aggregates of antigen-antibody complexes in the fluid phase fix complement. Frag-

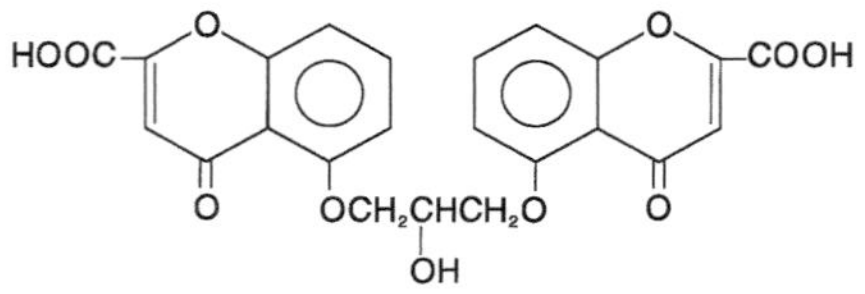

Figure 7. Structural formula for cromolyn.

ments of complement components, the anaphylatoxins, may induce experimentally the release of mediators from mast cells. There is no evidence that these components play a role in anaphylactic reactions *in vivo*. Aggregates of antigen-IgG antibody may, however, induce anaphylaxis, whose manifestations are different in the various species.

Histamine (Figure 8) is a biologically active amine, i.e., ß-aminoethylimidazole, of 111 molecular weight that induces contraction of the smooth muscle of human bronchioles and small blood vessels, increased capillary permeability and increased secretion by the mucous glands of the nose and bronchial tree. It is a principal pharmacological mediator of immediate (type I) hypersensitivity (anaphylaxis) in man and guinea pigs. Although found in many tissues, it is especially concentrated in mast cells of the tissues and basophils of the blood. It is stored in their cytoplasmic granules and is released following cross-linking of IgE antibodies by a specific antigen on their surfaces. It is produced by the decarboxylation of histidine through the action of histidine decarboxylase. When histamine combines with H_1 receptors, smooth muscle contraction and increased vascular permeability may result. Combination with H_2 receptors induces gastric secretion and blocks mediator release from mast cells and basophils. It may interfere with suppressor T cell function. Histamine

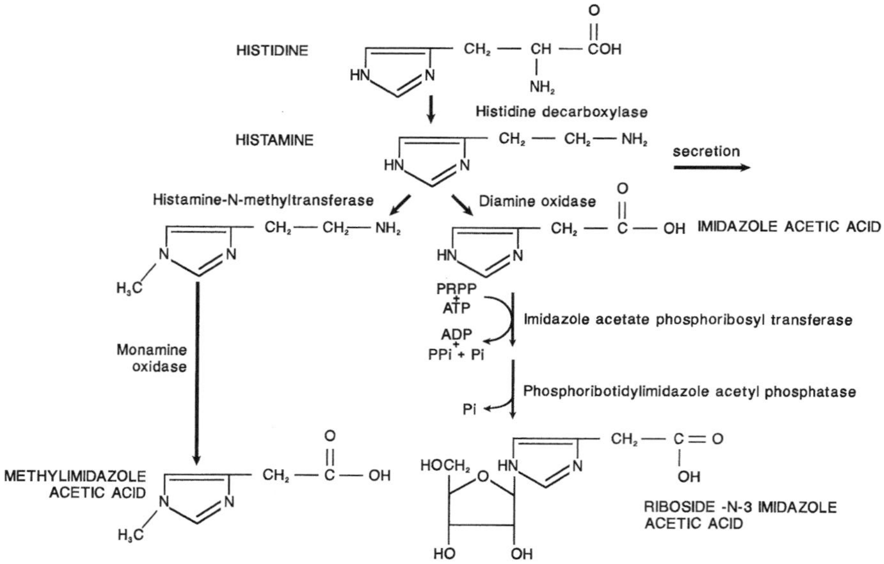

Figure 8. Schematic representation of the synthesis of histamine, a principal mediator of immediate (type I) hypersensitivity reactions.

attracts eosinophils that produce histaminase which degrades histamine.

Histaminase is a common tissue enzyme, termed diamine oxidase, that transforms histamine into imidazoleacetic acid, an inactive substance.

Histamine-releasing factor is a lymphokine produced from antigen-stimulated lymphocytes that induces the release of histamine from basophils.

Antihistamine is a substance that links to histamine receptors, therby inhibiting histamine action. Antihistamine drugs derived from ethylamine block H_1 histamine receptors, whereas those derived from thiourea block the H_2 variety.

Anaphylactoid reaction is a response resembling anaphylaxis except that it is not attributable to an allergic reaction mediated by IgE antibody. It is due to the nonimmunologic degranulation of mast cells such as that caused by drugs or chemical compounds such as aspirin, radiocontrast media, chymopapain, bee or snake venom and gum acacia which cause release of the pharmacological mediators of immediate hypersensitivity including histamine and other vasoactive molecules.

Serotonin (5-hydroxy tryptamine) [5HT] is a 176 mw catecholamine found in mouse and rat mast cells and in human platelets that participates in anaphylaxis in several species, such as the rabbit, but not in man (Figure 9). It induces contraction of smooth muscle, enhances vascular permeability of small blood vessels and induces large blood vessel vasoconstriction. 5-HT is derived from tryptophan by hydroxylation to 5-hydroxy tryptophan and decarboxylation to 5-hydroxy tryptamine. In man, gut enterochromaffin cells contain 90% of 5-HT with the remainder accruing in blood platelets and the brain. 5-HT is a potent biogenic amine with wide species distribution. 5-HT may stimulate phagocytosis by leukocytes and interfere with the clearance of particles by the mononuclear phagocyte system. Immunoperoxidase staining for 5-HT, which is synthesized by various neoplasms, especially carcinoid tumors, is a valuable aid in surgical pathologic diagnosis of tumors producing it.

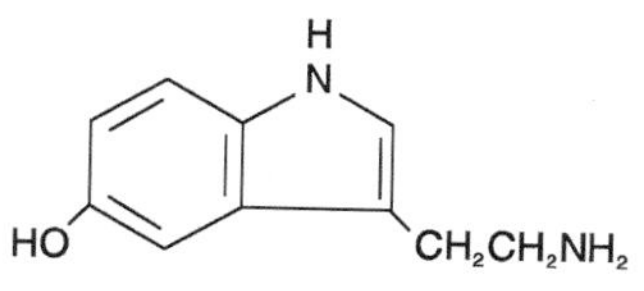

Figure 9. Structural formula of serotonin (5-hydroxytryptamine) that is released and participates in the mediation of anaphylactic reactions in some species and not others.

Vascular permeability factors are substances such as serotonins, histamines, kinins, and leukotrienes that increase the spaces between cells of capillaries and small vessels, facilitating the loss of protein and cells into the extravascular fluid.

An **eicosanoid** is an arachidonic acid-derived 20-carbon cyclic fatty acid (Figure10). It is produced from membrane phospholipids. Eicosanoids as well as other arachidonic acid metabolites are elevated during shock and following injury and are site-specific. They produce various effects, including bronchodilation, bronchoconstriction, vasoconstriction and vasodilation. Eicosanoids include: leukotrienes, prostaglandins, thromboxanes and prostacyclin.

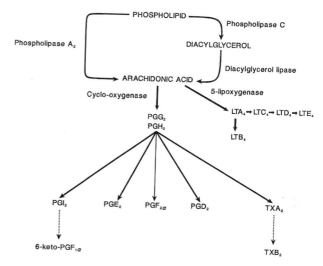

Figure 10. Schematic diagram of eicosanoids.

A **leukotriene** is a product of the enzymatic metabolism of arachidonic acid derived from the cell membrane. They are generated during an anaphylactic reaction by way of the lipoxygenase pathway (Figure 11).

Slow-reacting substance of anaphylaxis (SRS-A) is a 400 mol wt acidic lipoprotein derived from arachidonic acid that induces the slow contraction of bronchial smooth muscle and is produced following exposure to certain antigens. It is comprised of leukotrienes LTC_4, LTD_4, and LTE_4, which produce the effects observed in anaphylactic reactions. It is released, *in vitro*, in effleunts from synthesized lung tissue of guinea pig, rabbit, and rat profused with antigen. It has also been demonstrated in human lung tissue and nasal polyps. It contracts smooth muscle of guinea pig ileum. *In vitro*, it also increases vascular permeability upon intracutaneous injection and decreases pulmonary compliance by a mechanism independent of vagal reflexes. It also enhances some of the smooth muscle effects of histamine. the source of SRS-A is mast cells and certain other cells. It is found in immediate (type I) hypersensitivity reactions. SRS-A is not stored in a preformed state and is sequentially synthesized and released. The effects have a latent period before becoming manifest. Antihistamines do not neutralize the effects of SRS-A.

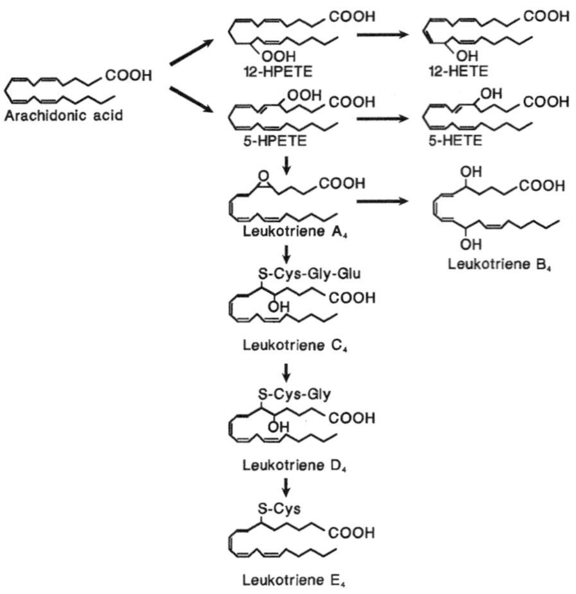

Figure 11. The lipoxygenase pathway of arachidonic acid metabolism that participates in the mediation of type I hypersensitivity reactions.

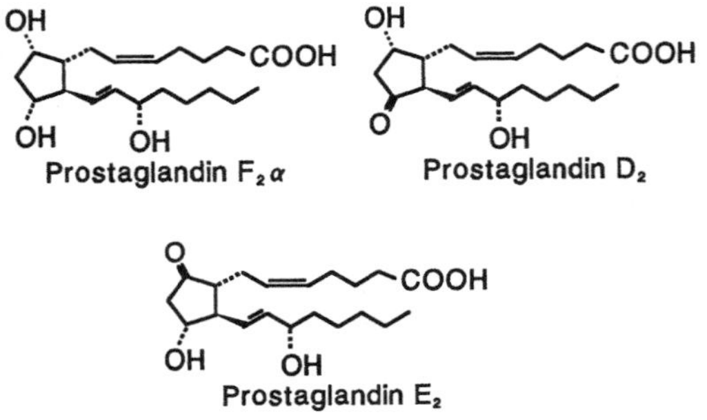

Figure 12. Structural formulae of prostaglandins, that are released and facilitate mediation of type I hypersensitivity reactions.

Prostaglandins (PG) are a family of biologically active lipids derived from arachidonic acid through the effects of the enzyme cyclooxygenase (Figures 12 and 13). Although first described in the prostate gland, they are now recognized in practically all tissues of mammals. The hormonal effects of prostaglandin include decreasing blood pressure, stimulating contraction of smooth muscle and regulation of inflammation, blood clotting and the immune response. Prostaglandins are grouped on the basis of their substituted five membered ring structure. During anaphylactic reactions mediated by IgE on mast cells, PGD_2 is released producing small blood vessel dilation and constriction of bronchial and pulmonary blood vessels. Mononuclear phagocytes may release PGE_2 after binding of immune complexes to Fcg receptors. Other effects of PGE_2 include blocking of MHC class II molecule expression in T cells and macrophages and inhibition of T cell growth. PGD_2 and PGE_2 both prevent

aggregation of platelets. Anti-inflammatory agents such as aspirin block prostaglandin synthesis.

Thromboxanes comprise a group of biologically active compounds with a physiological role in homeostasis and a pathophysiological role in thrombo-embolic disease and anaphylactic reactions. They are cyclopentane derivatives of polyunsaturated fatty acids and derived by isomerization from the prostaglandin endoperoxide PGH_2, the immediate precursor. The isomerizing enzyme is called thromboxane synthetase. The active compound, thromboxane A_2 is unstable (half life about 35 sec. at pH 7.4), being degraded to thromboxane B_2 which is stable but inactive on blood vessels; it has, however, polymorphonuclear cell chemotactic activity. The short notation is TXA_2 and TXB_2. TXA_2 and TXB_2 represent the major pathway of conversion of prostaglandin endoperoxide precursors. TXA_2 derived from prostaglandin G_2 generated from arachidonic acid by cyclooxygenase, increases following injury to vessels. It stimulates a primary hemostatic response. TXA_2 is a potent inducer of platelet aggregation, smooth muscle contraction and vasoconstriction. TXA was previously called rabbit aorta contacting substance (RACS) and is isolated from lung perfusates during anaphylaxis. It appears to be a peptide containing less than 10 amino acid residues. Thromboxane formation in platelets is associated with the dense tubular system. PMNs, spleen, brain and inflammatory granulomas have been demonstrated to produce thromboxanes.

Nonsteroidal anti-inflammatory drugs (NSAIDs) are used in the treatment of arthritis. A group of drugs used in the treatment of rheumatoid arthritis, gouty arthritis, ankylosing spondylitis, and osteoarthritis, the drugs are weak organic acids. They block prostaglandin synthesis by inhibiting cyclooxygenase and lipoxygenase. They also interrupt membrane-bound reactions such as NADPH oxidase in neutrophils, monocyte phospholipase C, and processes regulated by G protein. They also exert a number of other possible activities such as diminished generation of free redicals and superoxides which may alter intracellular cAMP levels, diminishing vasoactive mediator release from granulocytes, basophils, and mast cells.

Prostacyclin (PC) is a derivative of arachidonic acid that is related to prostaglandins. It has a second 5-membered ring (Figure 14). It inhibits aggregation of platelets and is a potent vasodilator. Prostacyclin's actions are the opposite of the actions of thromboxanes.

Anaphylatoxins are substances generated by the activation of complement that lead to increased vascular permeability as a consequence of the degranulation of mast cells with the release of pharmacologically active mediators of immediate hypersensitivity. These biologically active peptides of low molecular weight are derived from C3, C4, and C5. They are generated in serum during fixation of complement by Ag-Ab complexes, immunoglobulin aggregates, etc. Small

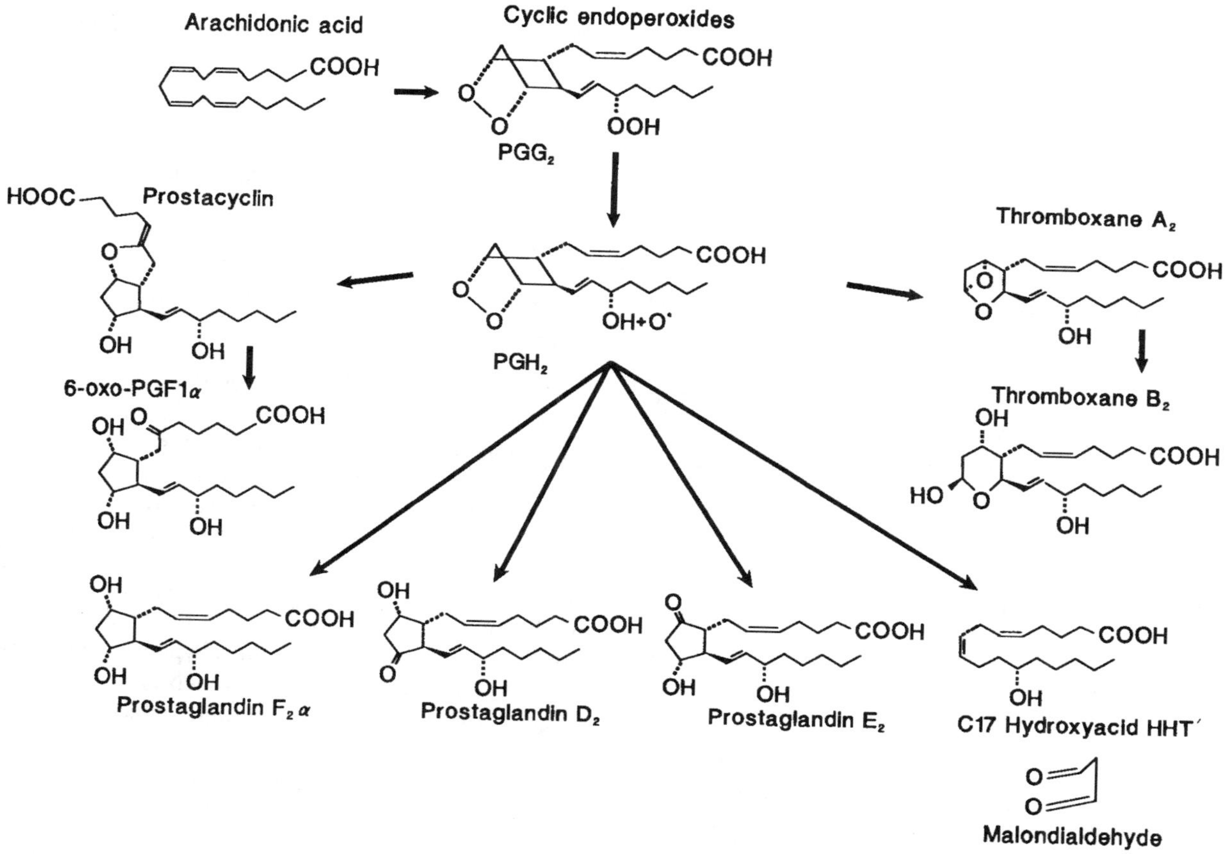

Figure 13.   Cyclooxygenase pathway of arachidonic acid metabolism that participates in the mediation of type I hypersensitivity reactions.

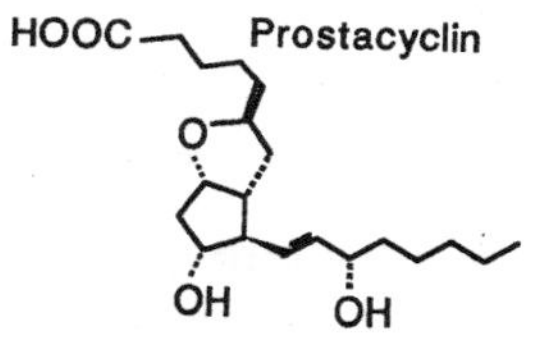

Figure 14.   Structural formula for prostacyclin which is released and participates in mediation of the effects on tissues of type I immediate hypersensitivity.

blood vessels, mast cells, smooth muscle, and leukocytes in peripheral blood are targets of their action. Much is known about their primary structure. These complement fragments are designated C3a, C4a and C5a. They cause smooth muscle contraction, mast cell degranulation with histamine release, increased vascular permeability and the triple response in skin. They induce anaphylactic-like symptoms upon parenteral inoculation.

Anaphylatoxin inactivator is a 300kD α globulin carboxy peptidase in serum that inactivates the anaphylatoxin activity of C5a, C3a and C4a by cleaving their carboxy-terminal arginine residues.

Atopy is a type of immediate (type I) hypersensitivity to common environmental allergens in man mediated by humoral antibodies of the IgE class formerly termed reagins, which are able to passively transfer the effect. Atopic hypersensitivity states include hay fever, asthma, eczema, urticaria and certain gastrointestinal disorders. There is a hereditary predisposition to atopic hypersensitivities, which affect more than 10 percent of the human population. Antigens which sensitize atopic individuals are termed allergens. They include: (1) grass and tree pollens, (2) dander, feathers, and hair (3) eggs, milk and chocolate, and (4) house dust, bacteria and fungi. IgE antibody is a skin-sensitizing homocytotropic antibody which occurs spontaneously in the sera of human subjects with atopic hypersensitivity. IgE antibodies are non-precipitating (*in vitro*), heat-sensitive (destroyed by heating to 60°C for 30 to 60 minutes), not able to pass across the placenta, remain attached to local skin sites for weeks after injection, and fail to induce passive cutaneous anaphylaxis (PCA) in guinea pigs.

Eczema is a skin lesion that is characterized as a weeping eruption consisting of erythema, pruritus with edema, papules, vesicles, pustules, scaling, and possible exudation. It occurs in individuals who are atopic, such as those with atopic dermatitis. Application to the skin or the ingestion of drugs that may themselves act as haptens may induce this type hypersensitivity. It may be seen in young children who subsequently develop asthma in later life.

An **allergen** is an antigen that induces an allergic or hypersensitivity response in contrast to a classic immune response produced by the recipient host in response to most immunogens. Allergens include such environmental substances as pollens, i.e., their globular proteins, from trees, grasses and ragweed as well as certain food substances, animal danders and insect venom. Selected subjects are predisposed to synthesizing IgE antibodies in response to allergens and are said to be atopic. The cross-linking of IgE molecules anchored to the surfaces of mast cells or basophils through their Fc regions result in the release of histamine and other pharmacological mediators of immediate hypersensitivity from mast cells/basophils. Allergen immunotherapy is desensitization treatment.

A **secondary allergen** is an agent that induces allergic symptoms because of crossreactivity with an allergen to which the individual is hypersensitive.

An **allergic response** is a response to an antigen (allergen) that leads to a state of increased reactivity or hypersensitivity rather than a protective immune response.

Allergoids are allergens that have been chemically altered to favor the induction of IgG rather than IgE antibodies in order to diminish allergic manifestations in the hypersensitive individual. These formaldehyde-modified allergens are analogous to toxoids prepared from bacterial exotoxins. Some of the physical and chemical characteristics of allergens are similar to those of other antigens. However, the MW of allergens is lower.

Allergy is a term that was coined by Clemens von Pirquet in 1906 to describe the altered reactivity of the animal body to antigen. Presently, the term allergy refers to altered immune reactivity to a spectrum of environmental antigens which includes pollen, insect venom, and food. Allergy is also referred to as hypersensitivity and usually describes type I immediate hypersensitvity of the atopic/anaphylactic type. Some allergies, especially the delayed T cell type, develop in subjects infected with certain microorganisms such as *Mycobacterium tuberculosis* or certain pathogenic fungi.

A **food allergy** is a type I (anaphylactic) or type III (antigen-antibody complex) hypersenstitivity mechanism response to allergens or antigens in foods that have been ingested and may lead to intestinal distress, producing nausea, vomiting, and diarrhea. There may be edema of the buccal mucosa, generalized urticaria, or eczema. Food categories associated with food allergy in some individuals include eggs, fish or nuts. Both skin tests and RAST tests using the appropriate allergen or antigen may identify individuals with a particular food allergy.

A **house dust allergy** is a type I immediate hypersensitivity reaction in atopic individuals exposed to house dust in which the principal allergen is *Dermatophagoides pteronyssinus*, the house dust mite. The condition is expressed as a respiratory allergy with the atopic subject manifesting either asthma or allergic rhinitis.

A **horse serum sensitivity** is an allergic or hypersensitivie reaction in a human or other animal receiving antitoxin or antithymocyte globulin generated by immunization of horses whose immune seurm is used for therapeutic purposes. Classic serum sickness is an example of this type of hypersensitivity which first appeared in children receiving diphtheria antitoxin early in the 20th century.

A **pollen hypersensitivity** is an immediate (type I) hypersensitivity which atopic individuals experience following inhalation of pollens such as ragweed in the U.S. This is an IgE-mediated reaction that results in respiratory symptoms expressed as hay fever or asthma. Sensitivity to certain pollens can be detected through skin tests with pollen extracts.

A **wheal and flare reaction** is an immediate hypersensitivity, IgE-mediated (in man) reaction to an antigen. Application of antigen by a scratch test in a hypersensitive individual may be followed by erythema, which is the red flare, and edema, which is the wheal. Atopic subjects who have a hereditary component to their allergy experience the effects of histamine and other vasoactive amine released from mast cell granules following crosslinking of surface IgE molecules by antigen or allergen.

Venom is a poisonous or toxic substance which selected species such as snakes, arthropods, and bees produce. The poison is transmitted to the recipient through a bite or sting.

Hypersensitivity angiitis is a small vessel inflammation most frequently induced by drugs.

Hypersensitivity pneumonitis is a lung inflammation induced by antibodies specific for substnces that have been inhaled. Within hours of inhaling the causative agent dypsnea, chills, fever, and coughing occur. Hisopathology of the lung reveals inflammation of alveoli in the interstitium with obliterating bronchiolitis. Immunofluorescence examination reveals deposits of C3. Hyperactivity of the lungs to air-borne immunogens or allergens may untimately lead to interstitial lung disease. An example is farmer's lung, which is characterized by malaise, coughing, fever, tightness in the chest, and myalgias. Of the numerous syndromes and associated antigens that may induce hypersensitivity pneumonitis, humidifier lung (thermophilic actinomycetes), bagassosis (*Thermoactinomyces vulgaris*), and bird fancier's lung (bird droppings) are well known.

Hypersensitivity vasculitis is an allergic response to drugs, microbial antigens, or antigens from other sources, leading to an inflammatory reaction involving small arterioles, venules, and capillaries.

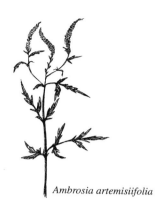

Ambrosia artemisiifolia

Figure 15. *Ambrosia artemisiifolia*, commonly termed ragweed.

Ragweed (*Ambrosia*) is distributed throughout the warmer parts of the western hemisphere but poses the greatest clinical problem in North America (Figure 15). Airborne ragweed pollen constitutes a troublesome respiratory allergen. Ragweed pollen appears in the air in northern states of the U.S.A. and adjacent eastern Canada in the latter days of July, when it reaches levels of up to thousands of grains per cubic meter by early September and then declines. Pure ragweed pollinosis has usually subsided by mid-October in the North. Short ragweed (*Ambrosia artemisiifolia*) and giant ragweed (*Ambrosia trifida*) are found widely from the Atlantic coast to the Midwest, Ozark plateau and Gulf states. Short ragweed reaches to northern Mexico and is only sparsely found in the Pacific Northwest. Giant ragweed is abundant in the Mississippi Delta and along the flood plains of Southeastern rivers. Pollen allergens of ragweed that have been characterized include:

Allergen source	Allergen
Ambrosiae artemisiifolia (ragweed)	Molecular weight (KD) SDS-page
AMB alph I (AGE)	38
AMB alpha II (AGK)	38
AMB alpha III (Ia3)	12
AMB alpha IV (Ra4)	23
AMB alpha V (Ra5)	5
AMB alpha VI (Ra6)	8
AMB alpha VII	—
Ambrosiae trifida (giant ragweed) AMB T V(Ra6)	4.4

Urticaria is a pruritic skin rash identified by localized elevated, edematous, erythematous, and itching wheals with a pale center encircled by a red flare. It is due to the release of histamine and other vasoactive substances from mast cell cytoplasmic granules based upon immunologic sensitization or due to physical or chemical substances. It is a form of type I immediate hypersensitivity. It is mediated by IgE antibodies in man. The action of allergen or antigen with

IgE antibodies anchored to mast cells can lead to this form of cutaneous anaphylaxis of hives. The wheal is due to leakage of plasma from venules, and the flare is caused by neurotransmitters.

Phacoanaphylaxis is a hypersensitivity to lens protein of the eye following an injury that introduces lens protein, normally a sequestered antigen, into the circulation. The immune system does not recognize it as self and responds to it as it would any other foreign antigen.

The Prausnitz-Küstner (PK) reaction (historical) is a skin test for hypersensitivity in which serum containing IgE antibodies specific for a particular allergen is transferred from an allergic individual to a nonallergic recipient by intradermal injection. This is followed by injection of the antigen or allergen in question into the same site as the serum injection. Fixation of the IgE antibodies in the "allergic" serum to mast cells in the recipient results in local release of the pharmacological mediators of immediate hypersensitivity including histamine. It results in a local anaphylactic reaction with a wheal and flare response.

Cutaneous anaphylaxis is a local reaction specifically elicited in the skin of an actively or passively sensitized animal. Causes of cutaneous anaphylaxis include immediate wheal and flare response following prick tests with drugs or other substances, insect stings or bites, contact urticaria in response to food substances such as nuts, fish, eggs or other substances such as rubber, dander or other environmental agents. The signs and symptoms of anaphylaxis are associated with the release of chemical mediators that include histamine and other substances from mast cell or basophil granules following cross-linking of surface IgE by antigen or by nonimmunological degranulation of these cells. The pharmacological mediators act principally on the blood vessels and smooth muscle. The skin may be the site where an anaphylytic reaction is induced or it can be the target of a systemic anaphylactic reaction resulting in itching (pruritus), urticaria, and angioedema.

Passive cutaneous anaphylaxis (PCA) is a skin test that involves the *in vivo* passive transfer of homocytotropic antibodies that mediate type I immediate hypersensitivity (e.g., IgE in man) from a sensitized to a previously nonsensitized individual by injecting the antibodies intradermally which become anchored to mast cells through their Fc receptors (Figure 16). This is followed hours or even days later by intravenous injection of antigen mixed with a dye such as Evans Blue. Crosslinking of the cell-fixed (e.g., IgE) antibody receptors by the injected antigen induces a type I immediate hypersensitivity reaction in which histamine and other pharmacological mediators of immediate hypersensitivity are released. Vascular permeability factors act on the vessels to permit plasma and dye to leak into the extravascular space forming a blue area which can be measured with

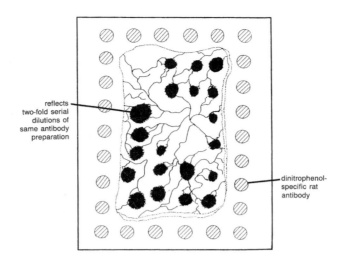

Figure 16. Passive cutaneous anaphylaxis in rats to dinitrophenol-specific rat reagin antibody. The diminished size of areas of increased capillary permeability is a consequence of two-fold serial dilutions of the antibody.

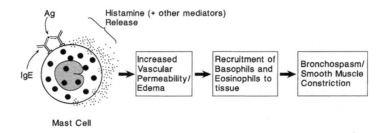

Figure 17. Events occurring in asthma.

calipers. In humans, this is called the Prausnitz-Küstner (P-K) reaction.

Reverse passive cutaneous anaphylaxis (RPCA) is a passive cutaneous anaphylaxis assay in which the order of antigen and antibody administration is reversed, i.e., the antigen is first injected followed by the antibody. In this case, the antigen must be an immunoglobulin that can fix to tissue cells.

Asthma is a disease of the lungs characterized by reversible airway obstruction (in most cases), inflammation of the airway with prominent eosinophil participation, and increased responsiveness by the airway to various stimuli (Figure 17). There is bronchospasm associated with recurrent paroxysmal dyspnea and wheezing. Some cases of asthma are allergic, i.e., bronchial allergy, mediated by IgE antibody to environmental allergens. Other cases are provoked by non-allergic factors that are not discussed here.

Type II antibody-mediated hypersensitivity is induced by antibodies and has three forms (Figure 18).

The classic type of hypersensitivity involves the interaction of antibody with cell membrane antigens followed by complement lysis (Figure 19). These antibodies are directed against antigens intrinsic to specific target tissues. Antibody-coated

cells also have increased susceptibility to phagocytosis. Examples of type II hypersensitivity include the anti-glomerular basement membrane antibody that develops in Goodpasture's syndrome and antibodies that develop against erythrocytes in Rh incompatibility leading to erythroblastosis fetalis or autoimmune hemolytic anemia.

A second variety of type II hypersensitivity is antibody-dependent cell-mediated cytotoxicity (ADCC). Killer (K) cells or NK cells, which have Fc receptors on their surfaces may bind to the Fc region of IgG molecules. They may react with surface antigens on target cells to produce lysis of the antibody-coated cell. Complement fixation is not required and does not participate in this reaction. In addition to K and NK cells, neutrophils, eosinophils and macrophages may participate in ADCC.

A third form of type II hypersensitivity is antibody against cell surface receptors that interfere with function, as in the case of antibodies against acetylcholine receptors in motor endplates of skeletal muscle in myasthenia gravis (Figure 20). This interference with neuromuscular transmission results in muscular weakness, ultimately affecting the muscles of respiration producing death. By contrast, stimulatory antibodies develop in hyperthyroidism (Graves' disease).

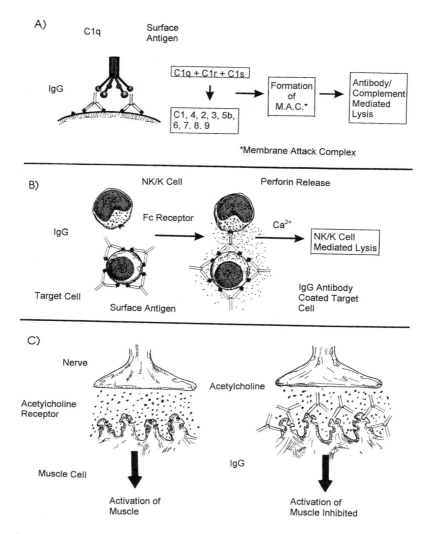

Figure 18.   Three separate forms of type II hypersensitivity. The uppermost diagram depicts antibody and complement-mediated lysis of a nucleated cell as a consequence of formation of the membrane attack complex. The middle diagram shows antibody-dependent cell-mediated cytotoxicity through the action of either an NK or a K cell with surface antibody specific for a target cell. The bottom figure illustrates inhibition of transmission of the nerve impulse by antibodies against acetylcholine receptors as occurs in myasthenia gravis.

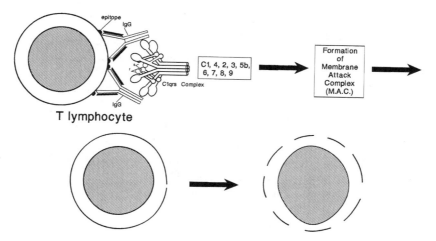

Figure 19.   Schematic representation of the action of specific IgG antibody on surface epitopes of a T lymphocyte leading to antibody-complement mediated-lysis of that cell.

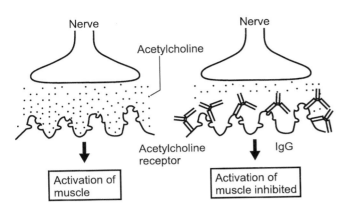

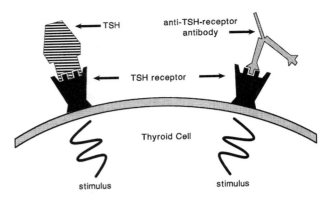

Figure 20. Schematic representation of the interference by acetylcholine receptor antibodies of chemical transmission of the nerve impulse. Acetylcholine receptor (AChR) antibodies are IgG autoantibodies that cause loss of function of acetylcholine receptors that are critical to chemical transmission of the nerve impulse at the neuromuscular junction. This represents a type II mechanism of hypersensitivity according to the Coombs and Gell classification. AChR antibodies are heterogeneous with some showing specificity for antigenic determinants other than those that serve as acetylcholine or alpha-bungarotoxin binding sites. As many as 85 to 95% of myasthenia gravis patients may manifest acetylcholine receptor antibodies.

They react with thyroid stimulating hormone receptors on thyroid epithelial cells to produce hyperthyroidism.

Long acting thyroid stimulator (LATS) is an IgG autoantibody that mimics the action of thyroid stimulating hormone in its effect on the thyroid (Figure 21). The majority of patients with Graves' disease, i.e., hyperthyroidism, produce LATS. This IgG autoantibody reacts with the receptors on thyroid cells that respond to thyroid stimulating hormone. Thus, the antibody-receptor interaction results in the same biological consequence as does hormone interaction with the receptor. This represents a stimulatory type of hypersensitivity and is classified in the Gell and Coombs classification as one of the forms of type II hypersensitivity.

Type III immune complex-mediated hypersensitivity is a type of hypersensitivity mediated by antigen-antibody-complement complexes (Figure 22). Antigen-antibody complexes can stimulate an acute inflammatory response that leads to complement activation and PMN leukocyte infiltration. The immune complexes are formed either by exogenous antigens such as those from microbes or by endogenous antigens such as DNA, a target for antibodies produced in systemic lupus erythematosus. Immune complex-mediated injury may be either systemic or localized. In the systemic variety, antigen-antibody complexes are produced in the circulation, deposited in the tissues and initiate inflammation. Acute serum sickness occurred in children treated with diphtheria antitoxin earlier in this century as a consequence of antibody produced against the horse serum protein. When immune complexes are deposited in tissues, complement is fixed, and PMNs are attracted to the site. Their lysosomal

Figure 21. Schematic representation of the third form of type II hypersensitivity in which long acting thyroid stimulator (LATS), an IgG antibody specific for the TSH receptor leads to continuous stimulation of thyroid parenchyma cells leading to hyperthyroidism. The IgG antibody mimics the action of TSH.

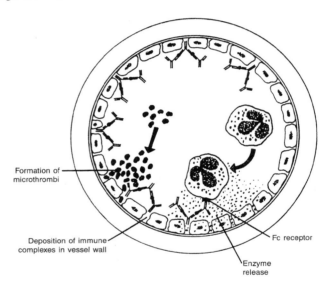

Figure 22. Schematic representation of the formation and deposition of immune complexes in vessel walls in type III hypersensitivity.

enzymes are released resulting in tissue injury. Localized immune complex disease, sometimes called the Arthus reaction, is characterized by an acute immune complex vasculitis with fibrinoid necrosis occurring in the walls of small vessels.

Serum sickness is a systemic reaction that follows the injection of a relatively large, single dose of serum (e.g., antitoxin) into humans or other animals. It is characterized by systemic vasculitis (arteritis), glomerulonephritis and arthritis. The lesions follow the deposition in tissues, such as the microvasculature, of immune complexes that form after antibody appears in the circulation between the fifth and 14th day following antigen administration. The antigen-antibody complexes fix complement and initiate a classic type III hypersensitivity reaction resulting in immune-mediated tissue injury. Patients may develop fever, lymphaden-

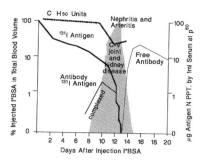

Figure 23.   Serum sickness.

opathy, urticaria and sometimes arthritis. The pathogenesis of serum sickness is that of a classic type III reaction. Antigen escaping into circulation from the site of injection forms immune complexes that damage the small vessels. The antibodies involved in the classic type of serum sickness are of the precipitating variety, usually IgG. They may be detected by passive hemagglutination. Pathologically, serum sickness is a systemic immune complex disease characterized by vasculitis, glomerulonephritis and arthritis due to the intravascular formation and deposition of immune complexes that subsequently fix complement and attract polymorphonuclear neutrophils to the site through the chemotactic effects of C5a, thereby initiating inflammation. The classic reaction which occurs 7–15 days after the triggering injection is called the primary form of serum sickness. Similar manifestations appearing only 1–3 days following the injection, represent the accelerated form of serum sickness and occur in subjects presumably already sensitized. A third form, called the anaphylactic form, develops immediately after injection. This latter form is apparently due to reaginic IgE antibodies and usually occurs in atopic subjects sensitized by horse dander or by previous exposure to serum treatment. The serum sickness-like syndromes seen in drug allergy have a similar clinical picture and similar pathogenesis (Figure 23).

Herxheimer reaction is a serum sickness (type III) form of hypersensitivity that occurs following the treatment of selected chronic infectious disease with an effective drug. When the microorganisms are destroyed in large numbers in the blood circulation, a significant amount of antigen is released from the disrupted microbes that tend to react with preformed antibodies in the circulation. This type of reaction has been described following the use of effective drugs to teat syphilis, trypanosomiasis, and brucellosis.

Arthus reaction is induced by repeated intradermal injections of antigen into the same skin site (Figure 24). It is dependent upon the development of humoral antibodies of the precipitation type which react *in vivo* with specific antigen at a local site. It may also be induced by the inoculation of antigen into a local skin site of an animal possessing performed IgG antibodies specific for the antigen. Immune complexes are com-

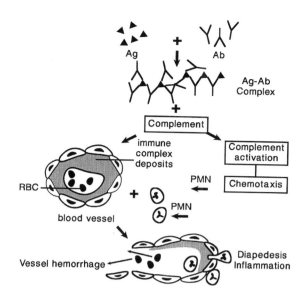

Figure 24.   Schematic representation of molecular, cellular and tissue interactions in the Arthus reaction.

prised of antigen, antibody and complement formed in vessels. The chemotactic complement fragment C5a and other chemotactic peptides produced attract neutrophils to antigen-antibody-complement complexes. This is followed by lysosomal enzyme release, which induces injury to vessel walls with the development of thrombi, hemorrhage, edema and necrosis. Events leading to vascular necrosis include: blood stasis, thrombosis, capillary compression in vascular injury which causes extravasation, venule rupture, hemorrhage and local ischemia. There is extensive infiltration of polymorphonuclear cells, especially neutrophils, into the connective tissue. Grossly, edema, erythema, central blanching, induration and petechiae appear. Petechiae develop within two hours, reach a maximum between four and six hours and then may diminish or persist for 24 hours or longer with associated central necrosis, depending on the severity of the reaction. If the reaction is more prolonged, macrophages replace neutrophils; histiocytes and plasma cells may also be demonstrated. The Arthus reaction is considered a form of immediate-type hypersensitivity but does not occur as rapidly as does anaphylaxis. It takes place during a four-hour period and diminishes after twelve hours. Thereafter, the area is cleared by mononuclear phagocytes. The passive cutaneous Arthus reaction consists of the inoculation of antibodies intravenously into a nonimmune host followed by local cutaneous injection of antigen. The reverse passive cutaneous Arthus reaction requires the intracutaneous injection of antibodies followed by the intravenous or incutaneous (at the same site) administration of antigen. The Authus reaction is a form of type III hypersensitivity since it is based upon the formation of immune complexes with complement fixation. Clinical situations for which it serves as an animal model include serum sickness, glomerulonephritis and farmer's lung.

Bagassosis is a hypersensitivity among sugar cane workers to a fungus, *Thermoactinomyces saccharic*, that thrives in the pressing from sugar cane. The condition is expressed as a hypersensitivity pneumonitis. Subjects develop type III (Arthus reaction) hypersensitivity following inhalation of dust from molding hot sugar cane bagasse.

Reverse passive Arthus reaction is a reaction that differs from a classic Arthus reaction only in that precipitating antibody is injected into an animal intracutaneously, and after an interval of one-half hour to two hours, the antigen is administered intravenously. In this situation, antigen, rather than antibody, diffuses from the blood into the tissues, and antibody, rather than antigen, diffuses into the tissue, where it encounters and interacts with antigen with the consequent typical changes in the microvasculature and tissues associated with the Arthus reaction.

The **Shwartzman** (or **Shwartzman-Sanarelli**) **reaction** is a nonimmunologic phenomenon in which endotoxin (lipopolysaccharides) induces local and systemic reactions. Following the initial or preparatory injection of endotoxin into the skin, polymorphonuclear leukocytes accumulate and are then thought to release lysosomal acid hydrolases that injure the walls of small vessels preparing them for the second provocative injection of endotoxin. The intradermal injection of endotoxin into the skin of a rabbit followed within 24 hours by the intravenous injection of the same or a different endotoxin leads to hemorrhage at the local site of the initial injection (Figures 25 and 26). Although the local Shwartzman reaction may resemble an Arthus reaction in appearance, the Arthus reaction is immunological whereas the Shwartzman reaction is not. In the Shwartzman reaction there is insufficient time between the first and second injections to induce an immune reaction in a previously unsensitized host. There is also a lack of specificity since even a different endotoxin may be used for first and second injections.

The generalized or systemic Shwartzman reaction again involves two injections of endotoxin. However, both are administered intravenously, one 24 hours following the first. The generalized Shwartzman reaction is the experimental equivalent of disseminated intravascular coagulation that occurs in a number of human diseases. Following the first injection, sparse fibrin thrombi (Figure 27) are formed in the vasculature of the lungs, kidney, liver and capillaries of the spleen. There is blockage of the reticuloendothelial system as its mononuclear phagocytes proceed to clear thromboplastin and fibrin. Administration of the second dose of endotoxin while the reticuloendothelial system is blocked leads to profound intravascular coagulation since the mononuclear phagocytes are unable to remove the thromboplastin and fibrin. There is bilateral cortical necrosis of the kidneys and splenic hemorrhage and necrosis. Neither platelets nor leukocytes are present in the fibrin thrombi that are formed.

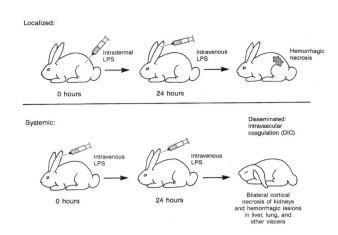

Figure 25. Schematic representation of the localized and systemic Shwartzman reaction.

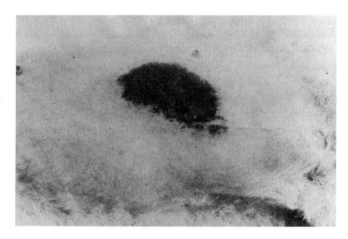

Figure 26. The ventral surface of a rabbit in which the localized Shwartzman reaction has been induced with endotoxin showing hemorrhage and necrosis.

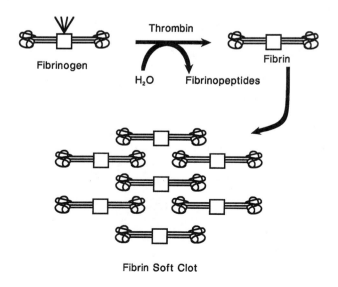

Figure 27. Fibrin.

Type IV cell-mediated hypersensitivity is a form of hypersensitivity mediated by specifically sensitized cells (Figure 28). Whereas antibodies participate in type I, II and III reactions, T lymphocytes mediate type IV hypersensitivity. Two types of reactions, mediated by separate T cell subsets are observed. Delayed-type hypersensitivity (DTH) is mediated by CD4+ T cells and cellular cytotoxicity is mediated principally by CD8+ T cells.

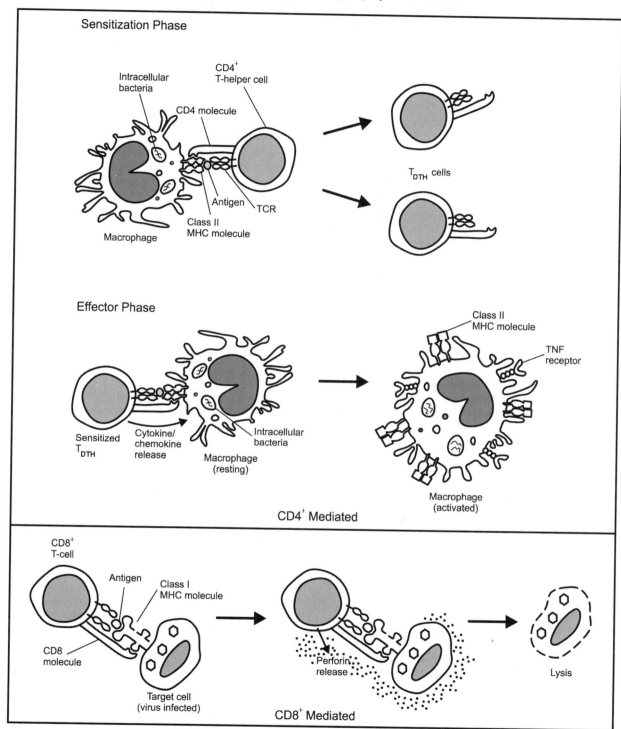

Figure 28. Schematic representation of type IV (cell-mediated) hypersensitivity. The upper frame illustrates tuberculin reactivity in the skin that is mediated by CD4+ helper/inducer T cells and represents a form of bacterial allergy. The lower frame illustrates the cytotoxic action of CD8+ T cells against a virus-infected target cell that presents antigen via class I MHC molecules to its TCR resulting in the release of perforin molecules that lead to target cell lysis.

A classic delayed hypersensitivity reaction is the tuberculin or Mantoux reaction. Following exposure to *Mycobacterium tuberculosis*, CD4+ lymphocytes recognize the microbe's antigens complexed with class II MHC molecules on the surface of antigen-presenting cells that process the mycobacterial antigens. Memory T cells develop and remain in the circulation for prolonged periods. When tuberculin antigen is injected intradermally, sensitized T cells react with the antigen on the antigen presenting cell's surface, undergo transformation and secrete lymphokines that lead to the manifestations of hypersensitivity. Unlike an antibody-mediated hypersensitivity, lymphokines are not antigen-specific.

In T cell-mediated cytotoxicity, CD8+ T lymphocytes kill antigen-bearing target cells. The cytotoxic T lymphocytes play a significant role in resistance to viral infections. Class I MHC molecules present viral antigens to CD8+ T lymphocytes as a viral peptide-class I molecular complex, which is transported to the infected cell's surface. Cytotoxic CD8+ cells recognize this and lyse the target before the virus can replicate, thereby stopping the infection.

Delayed-type hypersensitivity (DTH) is cell-mediated immunity, or hypersensitivity mediated by sensitized T lymphocytes (Figure 29). Although originally described as a skin reaction that requires 24–48 hours to develop following challenge with antigen, current usage emphasizes the mechanism, which is T cell-mediated, as opposed to emphasis on the temporal relationship of antigen injection and host response. The CD4+ T lymphocyte is the principal cell that mediates delayed-type hypersensitivity reactions. To induce a DTH reaction, antigen is injected intradermally in a primed individual. If the reaction is positive, an area of erythema and induration develops 24–48 hours following antigen challenge. Edema and infiltration by lymphocytes and macrophages occurs at the local site. The CD4+ T lymphocytes identify antigen on Ia positive macrophages and release lymphokines which entice more macrophages to enter the area where they become activated.

Skin tests are used clinically to reveal delayed-type hypersensitivity to infectious disease agents. Skin test antigens include such substances as tuberculin, histoplasmin, candidin, etc. Tuberculin or purified protein derivative (PPD), which are extracts of the tubercle bacillus, have long been used to determine whether or not a patient has had previous contact with the organism from which the test antigen was derived. Delayed-type hypersensitivity reactions are always cell-mediated. Thus, they have a mechanism strikingly different from anaphylaxis or the Arthus reaction, which occur within minutes to hours following exposure of the host to antigen and are examples of antibody-mediated reactions. DTH is classified as type IV hypersensitivity (Coombs and Gell classification). A T$_{DTH}$ lymphocyte is a delayed type hypersensitivity T lymphocyte

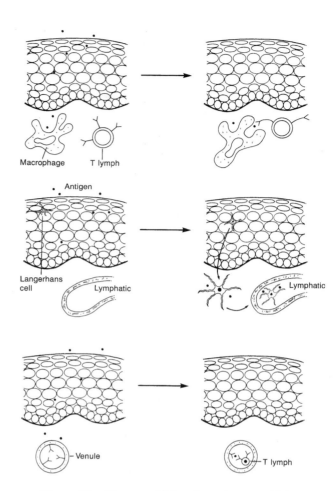

Figure 29.   Diagram of delayed type hypersensitivity.

Dhobi itch is contact hypersensitivity (type IV) induced by using a laundry marking ink made from Indian ral tree nuts. It occurs in subject sensitized by wearing garments marked with such ink. It induces a dermatitis at sites of contact with the laundry marking ink.

Infection or **bacterial allergy** is a hypersensitivity, especially of the delayed T cell type, that develops in subjects infected with certain microorganisms, such as *Mycobacterium tuberculosis* or certain pathogenic fungi.

An **infection allergy** is a T cell-mediated delayed-type hypersensitivity associated with infection by selected microorganisms such as *Mycobacterium tuberculosis*. This represents type IV hypersensitivity to antigenic products of microorganisms inducing a particular infection. It also develops in *Brucellosis, Lymphogranuloma venereum*, mumps, and vaccinia. Also called infection hypersensitivity.

An **infection hypersensitivity** is a tuberculin-type sensitivity that is more evident in some infections than others. It develops with great facility in tuberculosis, brucellosis, lymphogranuloma venereum, mumps, and vaccinia. The sensitizatng component of the antigen molecule is usually protein, although polysaccharides may induce delayed reactivity in cases of systemic fungal infections such as those caused by *Blastomyces*, *Histoplasma*, and *Coccidioides*.

The **Koch phenomenon** is a delayed hypersensitivity reaction in the skin of a guinea pig after it has been infected with *Mycobacterium tuberculosis* (Figure 30). Robert Koch described the phenomenon in 1891 following the injection of either living or dead *Mycobacterium tuberculosis* microorganisms into guinea pigs previously infected with the same microbes. He observed a severe necrotic reaction at the site of inoculation which occasionally became generalized and induced death. The injection of killed *Mycobacterium tuberculosis* microorganisms into healthy guinea pigs caused no ill effects. This is a demonstration of cell-mediated immunity and is the basis for the tuberculin test.

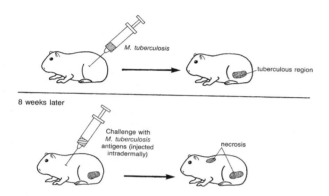

Figure 30. Illustration of the Koch phenomenon.

Tuberculid is a hypersensitivity skin reaction to mycobacteria. The lesion may be either a papulonecrotic tuberculid, with sterile papules ulcerated in the center and obliterative vasculitis, or crops of small red papules, with a sarcoid-like appearance that represent lichen scrofulosorum.

Tuberculin is a sterile solution containing a group of proteins derived from culture medium where *Mycobacterium tuberculosis* microorganisms have been grown. It has been used for almost a century as a skin test preparation to detect delayed-type (type IV) hypersensitivity to infection with *M. tuberculosis*. Many tuberculin preparations have been used in the past, but only old tuberculin (OT) and purified protein derivative (PPD) are still used. Whereas OT is a heat-concentrated filtrate of the culture medium in which *M. tuberculosis* was grown, PPD of tuberculin is a trichloroacetic acid precipitate of the growth medium. Tuberculin is a mitogen for murine B lymphocytes, as well as a T lymphocyte mitogen.

Tuberculin hypersensitivity is a form of bacterial allergy specific for a product in culture filtrates of *Mycobacterium tuberculosis which*, when injected into the skin, elicits a cell-mediated delayed-type hypersensitivity (type IV) response. Tuberculin-type hypersensitivity is mediated by CD4+ T

lymphocytes. Following the intracutaneous inoculation of tuberculin extract or purified protein derivative (PPD), an area of redness and induration develops at the site within 24 to 48 h in individuals who have present or past interaction with *M. tuberculosis*.

Tuberculin reaction is a test of *in vivo* cell-mediated immunity. Robert Koch observed a localized lesion in the skin of tuberculous guinea pigs inoculated intradermally with broth from a culture of tubercle bacilli. The body's immune response to infection with the tubercle bacillus is signaled by the appearance of agglutinins, precipitations, opsonins, and complement-fixing antibodies in the serum. This humoral response is, however, not marked, and such antibodies are present in low titer. The most striking response is the development of delayed-type hypersensitivity (DTHY), which has a protective role in preventing reinfection with the same organism. Subcutaneous inoculation of tubercle bacilli in a normal animal produces no immediate response, but in 10 to 14 days a nodule develops at the site of inoculation. The nodule then becomes a typical tuberculous ulcer. The regional lymph nodes become swollen and caseous. In contrast, a similar inoculation in a tuberculous animal induces an indurated area at the site of injection within 1 to 2 days. This becomes a shallow ulcer which heals promptly. No swelling of the adjacent lymphoatics is noted. The tubercle bacillus antigen which is responsible for DTH is wax D, a lipopolysaccharide-protein complex of the bacterial cellwall. The active peptide comprises diaminopimelic acid, glutamic acid, and alanine. Testing for DTH to the tubercle bacillus is done with tuberculin, a heat-inactivated culture extract containing a mixture of bacterial proteins, or with PPD, a purified protein derivative of culture in nonproteinaceous media. Both these compounds are capable of sensitizing the recipient themselves. The protective role of DTH is supported by the observation that in positive reactors living cells are usually free of tubercle bacilli and the bacteria are present in necrotic areas, separated by an avascular barrier. By contrast, in infected individuals giving a negative reaction, the tubercle bacilli are found in great numbers in living tissues. The reaction is permanently or transiently negative in individuals whose cell-mediated immune responses are transiently or permanently impaired.

A **tuberculin test** is the 24–48-hour response to intradermal injection of tuberculin. If positive, it signifies delayed-type hypersensitivity (type IV) to tuberculin and implies cell-mediated immunity to Mycobacterium tuberculosis. The intradermal inoculation of tuberculin or of purified protein derivative (PPD) leads to an area of erythema and induration within 24–48 h in positive individuals. A positive reaction signifies the presence of cell-mediated immunity to M. tuberculosis as a consequence of past or current exposure to this microorganism. However, it is not a test for the diagnosis of active tuberculosis.

A **tuberculin-type reaction** is a cell-mediated delayed-type hypersensitivity skin response to an extract such as candidin, brucellin, or histoplasmin. Individuals who have positive reactions have developed delayed-type hypersensitivity or cell-mediated immunity mediated by T lymphocytes following contact with the microorganism in question.

A **tuberculosis immunization** is the induction of protective immunity through injection of an attenuated vaccine containing Bacille-Calmette-Guerin (BCG). This vaccine was more widely used in Europe than in the U.S. in an attempt to provide protection against development of tuberculosis. A local papule develops several weeks after injection in individuals who were previously tuberculin negative, as it is not administered to positive individuals. It is claimed to protect against development of tuberculosis, although not all authorities agree on its efficacy for this purpose. In recent years, oncologists have used BCG vaccine to reactivate the cellular immune system of patients bearing neoplasms in the hope of facilitating antitumor immunity.

Anergy is a diminished or absent delayed-type hypersensitivity, i.e., type IV hypersensitivity, as revealed by lack of responsiveness to commonly used skin test antigens, including PPD, histoplasmin, candidin, etc. Decreased skin test reactivity may be associated with uncontrolled infection, tumor, Hodgkin's disease, sarcoidosis, etc. (Figure 31). There is decreased capacity of T lymphocytes to secrete lymphokines when their T cell receptors interact with specific antigen.

Contact hypersensitivity is a type IV delayed-type hypersensitivity reaction in the skin characterized by a delayed-type hypersensitivity (cell-mediated) immune reaction produced by T lymphocytes invading the epidermis (Figure 32). It is often

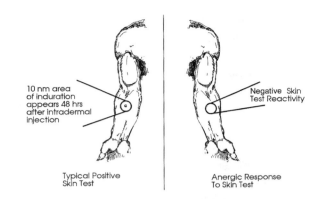

Figure 31. Representation of anergy.

induced by applying a skin-sensitizing simple chemical such as dinitrochlorobenzene (DNCB) that acts as a hapten uniting with proteins in the skin leading to the delayed-type hypersensitivity response mediated by CD4+ T cells. Although substances such as DNCB alone are not antigenic, they may combine with epidermal proteins which serve as carriers for these simple chemicals acting as haptens. Contact hypersensitivity may follow sensitization by topical drugs, cosmetics, or other types of contact chemicals. The causative agents, usually simple, low molecular weight compounds (mostly aromatic molecules) may also behave as haptens. The development of sensitization depends on the penetrability of the agent and its ability to form covalent bonds with protein. Part of the sensitizing antigen molecule is thus represented by protein, usually the fibrous protein of the skin. Local skin conditions that alter local proteins, such as inflammation, stasis, and others, facilitate the development of contact hypersensitivity, but some chemicals such as penicillin, picric acid or sulfonamides are

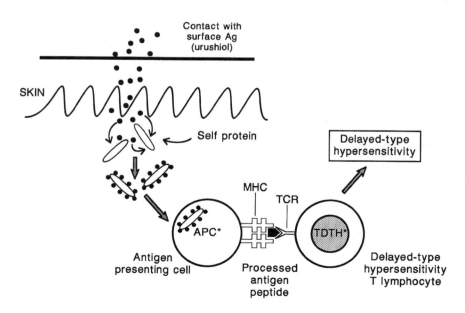

Figure 32. Contact sensitivity to poison ivy plants containing the chemical urushiol that induces delayed-type hypersensitivity mediated by CD4+ T cells with skin lesions.

unable to conjugate to proteins, but their degradation products may have this property.

Contact sensitivity (CS or allergic contact dermatitis) is a form of DTH reaction limited to the skin and consisting of eczematous changes. It follows sensitization by topical drugs, cosmetics, or other types of contatct chemicals. The causative agents, usually simple, low molecular weight compounds (mostly aromatic molecules), behave as haptens. The development of sensitization depends on the penetrability of the agent and its ability to form covalent bonds with protein. Part of the sensitizing antigen molecule is thus represented by protein, usually the fibrous protein of the skin. Local skin conditions that alter local proteins, usually the fibrous protein of the skin. Local skin conditions that alter local proteins, such as inflammation, stasis, and others, facilitate the development of CS, but some chemicals such as penicillin, picric acid, or sulfonamides are unable to conjugate to proteins. It is believed that in this case the degradation products of such chemicals have this property. CS may also be induced by hapten conjugates given by other routes in adjuvant. That actual immunogen in CS remains unidentified. CS may also have a toxic, nonimmunologic component, and frequently both toxic and sensitizing effects can be produced by the same compound. With exposure to industrial compounds, an initial period of increased sensitivity is followed by a gradual decrease in reactivity. This phenomenon is called hardening and could represent a process of spontaneous desensitization. The histologic changes in CS are characteristic.

An **id reaction** is a dermatophytid reaction. It is a sudden rash linked to, but anatomically separated from an inflammatory reaction of the skin in a sensitized individual with the same types of lesions elsewhere. The hands and arms are usual sites of id reactions that are expressed as sterile papulovesicular pustules. They may be linked with dermatophytosis such as tinea capitis or tenia pedis. They may also be associated with stasis dermatitie, contact dermatitis, and eczema.

Poison ivy is a plant containing the chemical urushiol which may induce severe contact hypersensitivity of the skin in individuals who have come into contact with it (Figure 33).

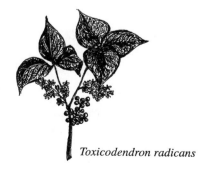

Toxicodendron radicans

Figure 33.   Poison ivy.

Urushiol is also found in mango trees, Japanese lacquer trees and cashew plants. Urushiol is present not only in *Toxicodendron radicans* (poison ivy) found in the Eastern United States but also in *T. diversilobium* (poison oak) found in the Western U.S. and *T. vernix* (poison sumac) found in the Southern U.S. Setting fire to these plants is also hazardous in that the smoke containing the chemical may induce tracheitis and pulmonary edema in allergic individuals. The chemical may remain impregnated in unwashed clothing and cause reactions in people who may come into contact with it for long periods of time.

Poison ivy hypersensitivity is principally type IV contact hypersensitivity induced by urushiols which are chemical constituents of poison ivy (*Rhus toxicodendron*), when poison ivy plants containing this chemical come into contact with the skin (Figure 34). The urushiol acts as a hapten by complexing with skin proteins to induce cellular (type IV) hypersensitivity on contact. This is a type of delayed-type hypersensitivity.

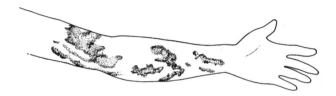

Figure 34.   Contact hypersensitivity induced by exposure to poison ivy.

Urushiols are catechols in poisonous (*Rhus toxicodendron*) plants that act as allergens to produce contact hypersensitivity, i.e., contact dermatitis at skin sites touched by the urushiol-bearing plant. The cutaneous lesion is T cell mediated and is classified as type IV hypersensitivity. There are four *Rhus* catechols that differ according to pentadecyl side chain saturation. They induce type IV delayed hypersensitivity. These substances are present in such plants as poison oak, poison sumac and poison ivy (Figure 35).

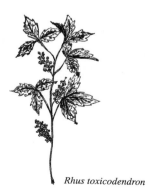

Rhus toxicodendron

Figure 35.   *Rhus toxicodendron* is now commonly called *Toxicodendron radicans*.

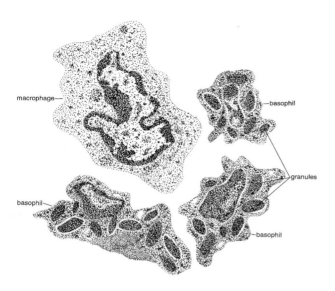

Figure 36. Cutaneous basophil hypersensitivity.

Cutaneous basophil hypersensitivity (Jones-Mote hypersensitivity) is a type of delayed (type IV) hypersensitivity in which there is prominent basophil infiltration of the skin immediately beneath the epidermis (Figure 36). It can be induced by the intradermal injection of a soluble antigen such as ovalbumin incorporated into Freund's incomplete adjuvant. Swelling of the skin reaches a maximum within 24 hours. The hypersensitivity reaction is maximal between seven and ten days following induction and vanishes when antibody is formed. Histologically, basophils predominate but lymphocytes and mononuclear cells are also present. Jones-Mote hypersensitivity is greatly influenced by lymphocytes that are sensitive to cyclophosphamide (suppressor lymphocytes).

Jones-Mote reaction is a delayed type hypersensitivity to protein antigens associated with basophil infiltration, which gives the reaction the additional name of cutaneous basophil hypersensitivity. Compared to the other forms of delayed-type hypersensitivity, it is relatively weak and appears on challenge several days following sensitization with minute quantities of protein antigens in aqueous medium or in incomplete Freund's adjuvant. No necrosis is produced. Jones-Mote hypersensitivity can be produced in laboratory animals such as guinea pigs appropriately exposed to protein antigens in aqueous media or in incomplete Freund's adjuvant. It can be passively transferred by T lymphocytes.

Penicillin hypersensitivity is an allergic reaction to penicillin or its degradation products such as penicillinic acid and may be either antibody-mediated or cell-mediated (Figure 37). Penicillin derivatives may act as haptens by conjugating to tissue proteins to yield penicilloyl derivatives. These conjugates may induce antibody-mediated hypersensitivity manifested as an anaphylactic reaction when the patient is subsequently exposed to penicillin, or it may be manifested as a serum sickness type reaction with fever, urticaria, and joint pains. Penicillin hyper-

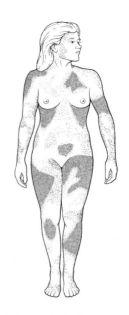

Figure 37. Penicillin hypersensitivity.

sensitivity may also be manifested as hemolytic anemia in which the penicillin derivatives have become conjugated to the patient's red blood cells, or as allergic contact dermatitis especially in pharmacists or nurses who come into contact with penicillin on a regular basis. Whereas the patch test using material impregnated with penicillin may be applied to the skin to detect cell-mediated (delayed-type, type IV, hypersensitivity), individuals who have developed anaphylactic hypersensitivity with IgE antibodies specific for penicilloyl-protein conjugates may be identified by injecting penicilloyl-polylysine into their skin. The development of a wheal and flare response signifies the presence of IgE antibodies which mediate anaphylactic reactivity in man.

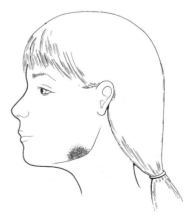

Figure 38. Fixed drug eruption.

Fixed drug eruption is a hypersensitivity reaction to a drug that appears at the same local site on the body surface regardless of the route by which the drug is administered. The lesion is a clearly circumscribed plaque that is reddish-brown or purple and edematous (Figure 38). It may be covered by a bulla. Common sites of occurrence include the extremities, hands, and glans penis. Drugs that may induce this reaction include sulfonamides, barbiturates, quinine and tetracycline, among other substances. There is hydropic degeneration of the basal layer.

13
Immunoregulation, Tolerance, and Autoimmunity

Immunoregulation refers to control of both humoral and cellular limbs of the immune response by mechanisms such as antibody feedback inhibition, the immunoglobulin idiotype-antiidiotype network, helper and suppressor T cells and cytokines. Results of these immunoregulatory interactions may lead to either suppression or potentiation of one or the other limbs of the immune response.

Tolerance is an active state of unresponsiveness by lymphoid cells to a particular antigen (tolerogen) as a result of the cells' interaction with that antigen. The immune response to all other immunogens is unaffected. Thus, this is an acquired nonresponsiveness to a specific antigen. When inoculated into a fetus or a newborn, an antigenic substance will be tolerated by the recipient in a manner that will prevent manifestations of immunity when the same individual is challenged with this antigen as an adult. This treatment has no suppressive effect on the response to other unrelated antigens. Immunologic tolerance is much more difficult to induce in an adult whose immune systems is fully developed. However, it can be accomplished by administering repetitive minute doses of protein antigens or by administering them in large quantities. Mechanisms of tolerance induction have been the subject of numerous investigations, and clonal deletion is one of these mechanisms. Either helper T or B lymphocytes may be inactivated or suppressor T lymphocytes may be activated in the process of tolerance induction. In addition to clonal deletion, clonal anergy and clonal balance are among the complex mechanisms proposed to account for self-tolerance in which the animal body accepts its own tissue antigens as self and does not reject them. Nevertheless, certain autoantibodies form under physiologic conditions and are not pathogenic. However, autoimmune phenomena may form under disease conditions and play a significant role in the pathogenesis of autoimmune disease.

An immunological adaptation to a specific antigen is distinct from unresponsiveness which is the genetic or pathologic inability to mount a measurable immune response. Tolerance involves lymphocytes as individual cells, whereas unresponsiveness is an attribute of the whole organism. The humoral or cell-mediated response may be affected individually or at the same time. The genetic form of unresponsiveness has been demonstrated with the immune response to synthetic antigens and has led to characterization of the immune response (Ir) locus of the major histocompatibility complex. The immune response of experimental animals which are classified as high, intermediate, or as nonresponders is not defective, but it is not reactive to the particular antigen. In some cases, suppressor cells prevent the development of an appropriate response. Unresponsiveness may also be the result of immunodeficiency states, some with clinical expression, or may be induced by immunosuppressive therapy such as that following X-irradiation, chemotherapeutic agents, or antilymphocyte sera. Tolerance, as the term is currently used, has a broader connotation and is intended to represent all instances in which an immune response to a given antigen is not demonstrable. Immunologic tolerance refers to a lack of response as a result of prior exposure to antigen.

Immunologic tolerance is an active but carefully regulated response of lymphocytes to self antigens. Autoantibodies are formed against a variety of self antigens. Maintenance of self tolerance is a quantitative process. When comparing the ease with which T cell and B cell tolerance may be induced, it was found that T cell tolerance is induced more rapidly and is longer lasting than is B cell tolerance. For example, T cell tolerance may be induced in a single day whereas B cells may require ten days for induction. In addition, one hundred times more tolerogen may be required for B cell tolerance than for T cell tolerance. The duration of tolerance is much greater in T cells, which is 150 days compared to that in B cells, which is only 50 to 60 days. T suppressor cells are also very important in maintaining natural tolerance to self antigens. For example, they may suppress T helper cell activity. Maintenance of tolerance is considered to require the continued presence of specific antigens. Low antigen doses may be effective in inducing tolerance in immature B cells leading to clonal abortion, whereas T cell tolerance does not depend upon the level of maturation. Another mechanism of B cell tolerance is cloning exhaustion in which the immunogen activates all of the B lymphocytes specific for it. This leads to maturation of cells and transient antibody synthesis thereby exhausting and diluting the B cell response. Antibody-forming cell blockade is another mechanism of B cell tolerance. Antibody-expressing B cells are coated with excess antigen rendering them unresponsive to the antigen.

Tolerogen is an antigen that is able to induce immunologic tolerance. The production of tolerance rather than immunity in response to antigen depends on such variables as physical state of the antigen, i.e., soluble or particulate, route of administration, level of maturation of the recipient's immune system, and immunologic competence. For example, soluble antigens administered intravenously will favor tolerance in many situations, as opposed to particulate antigens injected into the skin which might favor immunity. Immunologic tolerance with cells is easier to induce in the fetus or neonate than it is in adult animals, who would be more likely to develop immunity rather than tolerance.

Self-tolerance is a term used to describe the body's acceptance of its own epitopes as self antigens (Figure 1). The body is tolerant to these autoantigens which are exposed to the lymphoid cells of the host immune system. Tolerance to self antigens is developed during fetal life. Thus, the host is immunologically tolerant to self or autoantigens.

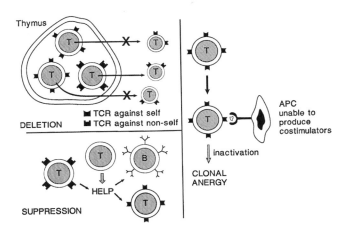

Figure 1. A schematic representation of the mechanism of self-tolerance.

Acquired tolerance is induced by the inoculation of a neonate or fetus *in utero* with allogeneic cells prior to maturation of the recipient's immune response (Figure 2). The inoculated antigens are accepted as self. Immunologic tolerance may be induced to some soluble antigens by low-dose injections of neonates with the antigen or to older animals by larger doses, the so-called low-dose and high-dose tolerance, respectively.

High-dose tolerance is a specific immunologic unresponsiveness induced in immunocompetent adult animals by the repeated administration of large doses of antigen (tolerogen) if the substance is a protein. A massive single dose is administered if the substance is a polysaccharide. Although no precise inducing dose of antigen can be defined, in high-dose

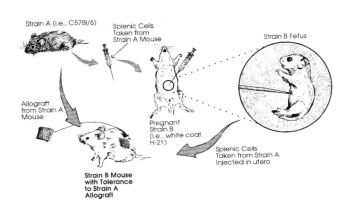

Figure 2. Acquired immunologic tolerance.

tolerance the antigen level usually exceeds 10^{-4} mol Ag per kilogram of body weight. This is also called high-zone tolerance.

Low-dose tolerance is an antigen-specific immunosuppression induced by the administration of antigen in a suboptimal dose. Low-dose tolerance is achieved easily in the neonatal period, in which the lymphoid cells of the animal are not sufficiently mature to mount an antibody or cell-mediated immune response. This renders helper T lymphocytes tolerant, thereby inhibiting them from signaling B lymphocytes to respond to immunogenic challenge. Although no precise inducing dose of antigen can be defined, in low-dose tolerance 10^{-8} mol Ag per kilogram of body weight is usually effective. Low-dose tolerance is relatively long lasting. This is also called low-zone tolerance. **Central tolerance** is the mechanism involved in the functional inactivation of cells requisite for initiation of an immune response. Central tolerance affects the afferent limb of the immune response, which is concerned with sensitization and cell proliferation.

Peripheral tolerance is involved in the inhibition of expression of the immune response. The cells delivering the actual response are functionally impaired but not defective. Peripheral tolerance affects the efferent limb of the immune response, which is concerned with the generation of effector cells.

Mechanisms that interfere with maturation or stimulation of lymphocytes with the potential for reacting with self include self-tolerance which is acquired and not inherited. Lymphocytes reactive with self may be either inhibited from responding to self or inactivated upon combination with self antigens. Self tolerance may involve both central and peripheral tolerance. In central tolerance, immature lymphocytes capable of reacting with self encounter self antigen producing tolerance instead of activation. By contrast, peripheral tolerance involves the interaction of mature self-reactive lymphocytes with self antigens in peripheral tissues if the interaction is under conditions that promote tolerance instead of activation. Clonal deletion and clonal anergy are also principal mechanisms of tolerance in clones of lymphocytes reactive with self antigens.

Clonal ignorance also may play a role that is yet ill-defined. Tolerance of T or B lymphocytes reactive with self antigen may also contribute to tolerance to self proteins. Properties of self antigens that render them tolerogenic and govern their ability to induce central or peripheral tolerance include self antigen concentration and persistence in the formative lymphoid organs, the type and strength of signals that self antigens activate in lymphocytes, and the ability to recognize antigens in the absence of costimulators.

T cell tolerance to self antigens involves the processing and presentation of self proteins complexed with major histocompatibility complex (MHC) molecules on antigen-presenting cells of the thymus. The interaction of immature T cells in the thymus with self peptide-MHC molecules leads to either clonal deletion or clonal anergy. Through this mechanism of negative selection, the T lymphocytes exiting the thymus are tolerant to self antigens. Tolerance of T cells to tissue antigens not represented in the thymus is maintained by peripheral tolerance. It is attributable to clonal anergy in which antigen-presenting cells recognize antigen in the absence of costimulation. Thus, cytokines are not activated to stimulate a T cell response. The activation of T lymphocytes by high antigen concentrations may lead to their death through Fas-mediated apoptosis. Regulatory T lymphocytes may also suppress the reactivity of T lymphocytes specific for self antigens. IL-10 or TGF-β or some other immunosuppressive cytokine produced by T lymphocytes reactive with self may facilitate tolerance. Clonal ignorance may also be important in preventing autoimmune reactivity to self.

B cell tolerance is manifested as a decreased number of antibody-secreting cells following antigenic stimulation, compared to a normal response. Hapten-specific tolerance can be induced by inoculation of deaggregated haptenated-gammaglobulins (Ig). Induction of tolerance requires membrane Ig cross-linking. Tolerance may have a duration of two months in B cells of the bone marrow and six to eight months in T cells. Whereas prostaglandin E enhances tolerance induction, IL-1, LPS or 8-bromoguanosine block tolerance instead of an immunogenic signal. Tolerant mice carry a normal complement of hapten-specific B cells. Tolerance is not attributable to a diminished number or isotype of antigen receptor. It has also been shown that the six normal activation events related to membrane Ig turnover and expression do not occur in tolerant B cells. Whereas tolerant B cells possess a limited capacity to proliferate, they fail to do so in response to antigen. Antigenic challenge of tolerant B cells induces them to enlarge and increase expression, yet they are apparently deficient in a physiologic signal requisite for progression into a proliferative stage.

Much of the understanding of **B cell tolerance to self** has been developed through models that permit the investigation

of B cell development and function following exposure to self antigen in the absence of T cell help. Both central and peripheral mechanisms may be involved in B lymphocyte tolerance to self antigens. The amount and valence of antigens in the bone marrow control the fate of immature B lymphocytes specific for these self antigens. Concentrated antigens that are multivalent may cause death of B lymphocytes. Other B cells specific for self antigens may survive to maturity following interaction with specific antigen but are permanently barred from migration to lymphoid follicles in the peripheral lymphoid tissues. Therefore, they do not respond to antigen in peripheral lymphoid sites. Soluble self antigens in lower concentrations may interact with B cells to produce anergy which could be attributable to diminished membrane Ig receptor expression on B lymphocytes or a failure in transmission of activation signals following interaction of antigen with its receptor. Thus, the power of the signal induced by antigen may determine the fate. In brief, larger concentrations of multivalent antigen may activate a powerful signal that results in cell death, whereas a weaker signal may lead to unresponsiveness.

If specific helper T lymphocytes are absent in peripheral lymphoid tissues, mature B cells may interact with self antigen there to become tolerant. Following interaction with antigen, some B lymphocytes may be unable to activate tyrosine kinases and others may diminish their antigen receptor expression after they have interacted with self antigen. Exposure to self antigen fails to cause self reactive B lymphocyte proliferation or increased expression of costimulators. These B cells also fail to become activated when aided by T cells. Other B cells may become blocked from terminal differentiation into antibody forming cells following reaction with self antigens. B cells capable of reacting with self may remain inactive in the absence of helper T cell activity.

Clonal deletion (negative selection) is the elimination of self-reactive T lymphocytes in the thymus during the development of natural self-tolerance. T cells recognize self antigens only in the context of major histocompatibility complex (MHC) molecules. Autoreactive thymocytes are eliminated following contact with self antigens expressed in the thymus before maturation is completed. The majority of CD4+ T lymphocytes in the blood circulation that survived clonal deletion in the thymus failed to respond to any stimulus. This reveals that clonal anergy participates in suppression of autoimmunity. Clonal deletion represents a critical mechanism to rid the body of autoreactive T lymphocytes. This is brought about by minor lymphocyte stimulation (mls) antigens that interact with the T cell receptor's V_β region of the T lymphocyte receptor thereby mimicking the action of bacterial super antigen. Intrathymic and peripheral tolerance in T lymphocyte can be accounted for by clonal deletion and functional inactivation of T cells reactive against self.

Clonal anergy is the interaction of immune system cells with antigen, without a second antigen signal, of the type usually needed for a response to an immunogen. This leads to functional inactivation of the immune system cells in contrast to the development of antibody formation or cell-mediated immunity. Clonal ignorance refers to lymphocytes that survive the principal mechanisms of self tolerance and remain functionally competent but are unresponsive to self antigens and do not cause autoimmune reactions.

It is convenient to describe **clonal balance** as an alteration in the helper/suppressor ratio with a slight predominance of helper activity. Factors that influence the balance of helper to suppressor cells include aging, steroid hormones, viruses and chemicals. The genetic constitution of the host and the mechanism of antigen presentation are the two most significant factors that govern clonal balance. Immune response genes associated with the MHC determine class II MHC antigen expression on cells presenting antigen to helper CD4+ lymphocytes. Thus the MHC class II genotype may affect susceptibility to autoimmune disease. Other genes may be active as well. Antigen presentation exerts a major influence on the generation of an autoimmune response. Whereas a soluble antigen administered intravenously with an appropriate immunologic adjuvant may induce an autoimmune response leading to immunopathologic injury, the same antigen injected intravenously without the adjuvant may induce no detectable response. Animals rendered tolerant to foreign antigens possess suppressor T lymphocytes associated with the induced unresponsiveness. Thus, self-tolerance could be due, in part, to the induction of suppressor T cells. This concept is called clonal balance rather than clonal deletion. Self antigens are considered to normally induce mostly suppressor rather than helper T cells leading to a negative suppressor balance in the animal body. Three factors with the potential to suppress immune reactivity against self include nonantigen-specific suppressor T cells, antigen-specific suppressor T cells and anti-idiotypic antibodies. Suppressor T lymphocytes may leave the thymus slightly before the corresponding helper T cells. Suppressor T cells specific for self antigens are postulated to be continously stimulated and usually in greater numbers than the corresponding helper T cells.

There is a bidirectional regulatory circuit between the **immune** and **neuroendocrine systems** (Figures 3 and 4). The neuroendocrine and immune systems affect each other. Receptors for neurally-active polypeptides, neurotransmitters and hormones are present on immune system cells, whereas receptors reactive with products of the immune system may be identified on nervous system cells. Neuroendocrine hormones have variable immunoregulatory effects mediated through specific receptors. Neurotransmitter influence on cell function is determined in part by the receptor-linked signal amplification associated with second messenger systems. Neuroimmunoregulation is mediated either

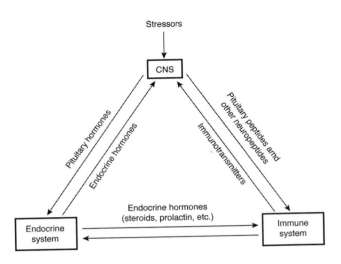

Figure 3. Interactions among the endocrine, central nervous, and immune system.

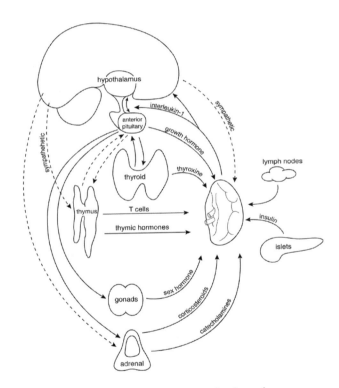

Figure 4. Immune-neuroendocrine axis.

through a neural pathway involving pituitary peptides and adrenal steroid hormones or through a second pathway that consists of direct innervation of immune system tissues. The thymus, spleen, bone marrow and perhaps other lymphoid organs contain afferent and efferent nerve fibers. ACTH, endorphins, enkephalins, and adrenal cortical steroids derived from the pituitary represent one direction for modulating the immune response. For example, prolactin (PRL) regulates lymphocyte function. Stimulated lymphocytes or nonstimulated macrophages may produce neuroendocrine hormone-related peptides, ACTH and endorphins. The participation of these substances in a stress response represents the opposite direction of regulation. Thymic hormones may also induce an endocrine response.

Neuroendocrine hormones may exert either a positive or negative regulatory effect on the macrophage, which plays a key role in both inflammation and immune responsiveness. Leukocyte mediators are known to alter both central nervous system and immune system functions. IL-1 acts on the hypothalamus to produce fever and participates in antigen-induced activation. IL-1 is synthesized by macrophages and has a major role in inflammation and immune responsiveness.

Substance P (SP) has been postulated to have an effect in hypersensitivity diseases including arthritis and asthma. The nervous system may release SP into joints in arthritis and into the respiratory tract in asthma perpetuating inflammation. SP has also been found to participate in immune system functions such as the induction of monocyte chemotaxis in *in vitro* experiments. Through their effect on mast cells, enkephalins influence hypersensitivity reactions. Enkephalins have been shown to diminish antibody formation against cellular and soluble immunogens and to diminish passive cutaneous anaphylaxis. Mast cells, which can be stimulated by either immunologic or nonimmunologic mechanisms, may be significant in immune regulation of neural function.

Oral tolerance is discussed in Chapter 14. **Split tolerance** includes several mechanisms. 1) Specific immunological unresponsiveness (tolerance) affecting either the B cell (antibody) limb or the T lymphocyte (cell-mediated) limb of the immune response. The unaffected limb is left intact to produce antibody or respond with cell-mediated immunity, depending on which limb has been rendered specifically unresponsive to the antigen in question. 2) The induction of immunologic tolerance to some epitopes of allogeneic cells while leaving the remaining epitopes capable of inducing an immune response characterized by antibody production and/or cell-mediated immunity.

In an **immune deviation**, antigen-mediated suppression of the immune response may selectively affect delayed-type hypersensitivity leaving certain types of immunoglobulin responses relatively intact and unaltered. This selective suppression of certain phases of the immune response to an antigen without alteration of others have been termed immune deviation. Thus, "split tolerance" or immune deviation offers an experimental model for dissection of the immune response into its component parts. It is necessary to use an antigen capable of inducing formation of humoral antibody and development of delayed-type hypersensitivity to induce immune deviation. Since it is essential that both humoral and cellular phases of the immune response be directed to the same antigenic determinant group, defined antigens are required. Immune deviation selectively suppresses delayed-type hypersensitivity and IgG_2 antibody production. By contrast, immunologic tolerance affects both IgG_1 and IgG_2 antibody production and delayed-type hypersensitivity. For example, prior administration of certain protein antigens to guinea pigs may lead to antibody production. However, the subsequent injection of antigen incorporated into Freund's complete adjuvant leads to deviation from the expected heightened delayed-type hypersensitivity and formation of IgG_2 antibodies to result in little of either, i.e., negligible delayed-type hypersensitivity and suppression of IgG_2 formation.

Immunological ignorance is a type of tolerance to self in which a target antigen and lymphocytes capable of reacting with it are both present simultaneously in an individual without an autoimmune reaction occurring. The abrogation of immunologic ignorance may lead to autoimmune disease.

Infectious tolerance was described in the 1970s. Animals rendered tolerant to foreign antigens were found to possess suppressor T lymphocytes associated with the induced unresponsiveness. Thus, self-tolerance was postulated to be based on the induction of suppressor T cells. Rose has referred to this concept as clonal balance rather than clonal deletion. Self antigens are considered to normally induce mostly suppressor rather than helper T cells leading to a negative suppressor balance in the animal body. Three factors with the potential to suppress immune reactivity against self include nonantigen-specific suppressor T cells, antigen-specific suppressor T cells and anti-idiotypic antibodies. Rose suggested that suppressor T lymphocytes leave the thymus slightly before the corresponding helper T cells. Suppressor T cells specific for self antigens are postulated to be continuously stimulated and usually in greater numbers than the corresponding helper T cells.

Immunologic paralysis is an immunologic unresponsiveness induced by the injection of large doses of pneumococcal polysaccharide into mice where it is metabolized slowly (Figure 5). Any antibody that is formed is consumed and not detectable. The pneumococcal polysaccharide antigen remained in tissues of the recipient for months during which time the animals produced no immune response to the antigen. Immunologic paralysis is much easier to induce with polysaccharide than with protein antigens. It is highly specific for the antigen used for its induction. Felton's first observation of immunologic paralysis preceded the demonstration of acquired immunologic tolerance by Medawar, et al.

Immunologic enhancement refers to the prolonged survival, conversely the delayed rejection, of a tumor allograft in a host as a consequence of contact with specific antibody. Both the peripheral and central mechanisms have been postulated. Coating of tumor cells with antibody was presumed, in the past, to interfere with the ability of specifically reactive

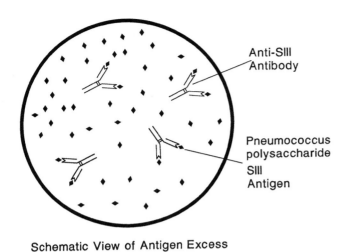

Schematic View of Antigen Excess

Figure 5.   Immunologic paralysis.

lymphocytes to destroy them, but a central effect in suppressing cell-mediated immunity, perhaps through suppressor T lymphocytes, is also possible.

In several forms of tolerance, the unresponsive state can be terminated by appropriate experimental manipulation. There are several methods for the **termination of tolerance**. (1) Injection of normal T cells. Tolerance to heterologous gammaglobulin can be terminated by normal thymus cells. It is, however, possible only in adoptive transfer experiments with cells of tolerant animals at 81 days after the induction of tolerance and after supplementation with normal thymus cells. By this time, B cell tolerance vanishes and only the T cells remain tolerant. Similar experiments at an earlier date do not terminate tolerance. (2) Injection of allogeneic cells. Allogeneic cells injected at the time when B cell tolerance has vanished or has not yet been induced, can also terminate or prevent tolerance. The mechanism is not specific and involves the allogeneic effect factor with activation of the unresponsive T cell population. (3) Injection of lipopolysaccharide (LPS). This polyclonal B cell activator is also capable of terminating tolerance if the B cells are competent. It has the ability to bypass the requirements for T cells in the response to the immunogen by providing the second (mitogenic) signal required for a response. The termination of tolerance by LPS does not involve T cells at all. LPS may also circumvent tolerance to self by a similar mechanism. (4) Crossreacting immunogens. Crossreacting immunogens (some heterologous protein in aggregated form or a different heterologous protein) also are capable of terminating tolerance to the soluble form of the protein. Termination also occurs by a mechanism which bypasses the unresponsive T cells and is obtainable at time intervals after tolerization when the responsiveness of B cells is restored. The antibody produced to the crossreacting antigen also reacts with the tolerogenic protein and is indistinguishable from the specificity produced by this protein in the absence of tolerance.

Autoimmunity is an immune reactivity involving either antibody-mediated (humoral) or cell-mediated limbs of the immune response against the body's own (self) constituents, i.e., autoantigens. When autoantibodies or autoreactive T lymphocytes interact with self-epitopes, tissue injury may occur e.g., in rheumatic fever the autoimmune reactivity against heart muscle sacrolemmal membranes occurs as a result of crossreactivity with antibodies against streptococcal antigens (molecular mimicry). Thus, the immune response can be a two-edged sword, producing both beneficial (protective effects) while also leading to severe injury to host tissues. Reactions of this deleterious nature are referred to as hypersensitivity reactions, which are subgrouped into four types.

Abrogation of tolerance to self antigens often leads to autoimmunity. This may result from altered regulation of lymphocytes reactive with self or in aberrations in self antigen presentation. Many factors participate in the generation of autoimmunity. Autoimmune reactants may be a consequence, and not a cause, of a disease process. Autoimmune diseases may be organ specific, such as autoimmune thyroiditis, or systemic, such as systemic lupus erythematosus. Different hypersensitivity mechanisms, classified from I–IV may represent mechanisms by which autoimmune diseases are produced. Thus, antibodies or T cells may be the effector mechanisms mediating tissue injury in autoimmune disease. The T or B cell abnormalities may contribute to the development of autoimmunity. Helper T cells control the immune response to protein antigens. Therefore, defects in this cell population may lead to high affinity autoantibody production specific for self antigens. MHC molecules, which are often linked genetically to the production of autoimmune disease, present peptide antigens to T lymphocytes. Various immunologic alterations may lead to autoimmunity. Experimental evidence supports the concept that autoimmunity may result from a failure of peripheral T lymphocyte tolerance, but little is known about whether or not loss of peripheral B cell tolerance is a contributory factor in autoimmunity. Processes that activate antigen presenting cells in tissues, thereby upregulating their expression of costimulators and leading to the formation of cytokines, may abrogate T lymphocyte anergy. The mouse model of human systemic lupus erythematosus involves *lpr/lpr* and *gld/gld* mice that succumb at six months of age from profound systemic autoimmune disease with nephritis and autoantibodies. The *lpr/lpr* is associated with a defect in the gene that encodes **Fas** which determines the molecule that induces cell death. The *gld/gld* is attributable to a point mutation in the **Fas ligand** which renders the molecule unable to signal. Thus, abnormalities in the Fas and Fas ligand prolong the survival of helper T cells specific for self antigens since they fail to undergo activation-induced cell death. Thus, this deletion failure mechanism involves peripheral tolerance rather than central tolerance. A decrease of regulatory T cells which synthesize lymphokines that mediate immunosuppression and maintain self tolerance might lead to autoimmunity even though no such condition has yet been described.

Autoantigens are normal body constituents recognized by autoantibodies specific for them. T cell receptors may also identify autoantigen (self antigen) when the immune reactivity has induced a cell-mediated T lymphocyte response.

An **autoantibody** recognizes and interacts with an antigen present as a natural component of the individual synthesizing the autoantibody (Figure 6). The ability of these autoantibodies to "crossreact" with corresponding antigens from other members of the same species provides a method for *in vitro* detection of such autoantibodies. **Autoallergy** is a tissue injury or disease induced by immune reactivity against self antigens.

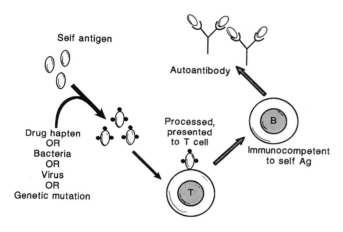

Figure 6.   Autoantibody formation.

Sequestered antigen is anatomically isolated and not in contact with the immunocompetent T and B lymphoid cells of the immune system (Figure 7). Examples include myelin basic protein, sperm antigens and lens protein antigens. When a sequestered antigen such as myelin basic protein is released by one or several mechanisms including viral inflammation, it can activate both immunocompetent T and B cells. An example of the sequestered antigen release mechanism of autoimmunity is found in experimental and post-infectious encephalomyelitis. Cell-mediated injury represents

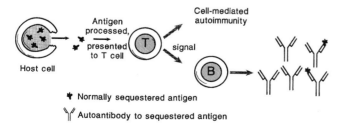

♠ Normally sequestered antigen

⅄ Autoantibody to sequestered antigen

Figure 7.   Release of sequestered antigen.

the principal mechanism in experimental and post-viral encephalitis. In vasectomized males, antisperm antibodies are known to develop when sperm antigens become exposed to immunocompetent lymphoid cells. Likewise, lens protein of the eye that enters the circulation as a consequence of either crushing injury to an eye or exposure of lens protein to immunocompetent cells inadvertently through surgical manipulation may lead to an anti-lens protein immune response. Autoimmunity induced by sequestered antigens is relatively infrequent and is a relatively rare cause of autoimmune disease.

Adjuvant is a substance that facilitates or enhances the immune response to an antigen with which it is combined (Figure 8). Various types of adjuvants have been described, including Freund's complete and incomplete adjuvants, aluminum compounds, and muramyl dipeptide. Some of these act by forming a depot in tissues from which an antigen is slowly released. In addition, Freund's adjuvant attracts a large number of cells to the area of antigen deposition to provide increased immune responsiveness to it. Modern adjuvants include such agents as muramyl dipeptide. The ideal adjuvant is one that is biodegradable with elimination from the tissues once it nonspecifically facilitates an immune response to antigen. An adjuvant usually combines with the immunogen, but is sometimes given prior to or following antigen administration. Adjuvants represent a heterogenous class of compounds capable of augmenting the humoral or cell-mediated immune response to a given antigen. They are widely used in experimental work and for therapeutic purposes in vaccines. Adjuvants comprise compounds of mineral nature, products of microbial origin, and synthetic compounds. The primary effect of some adjuvants is postulated to be the retention of antigen at the inoculation site so that the immunologic stimulus persists for a longer period of time. However, the mechanism by which adjuvants augment the immune response is poorly understood. The macrophage may be the target and mediator of action of some adjuvants, whereas others may require T cells for their response augmenting effect. Adjuvants such as lipopolysaccharide (LPS) may act directly on B lymphocytes.

Autoimmune complement fixation reaction refers to the ability of human blood serum from patients with certain autoimmune diseases, such as systemic lupus erythematosus, chronic active hepatitis, etc., to fix complement when combined with kidney, liver or other tissue suspensions in saline.

Viral infections may stimulate the production of **autoantibodies** in three ways: (1) by complexing with cell surface histocompatibility antigens to form new immunogenic units, (2) by nonspecifically stimulating the proliferation of lymphocytes, e.g., after infection with Epstein-Barr virus, (3) by inducing the expression of antigens normally repressed in the host cells. The nonspecific response includes clones

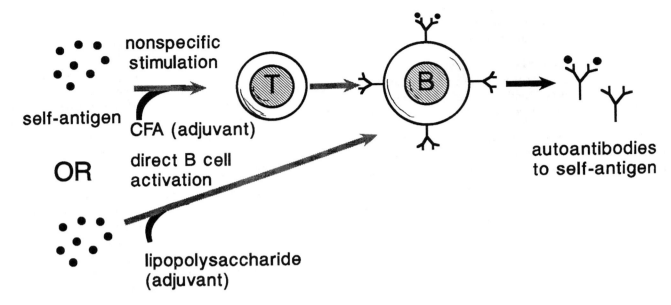

Figure 8. Adjuvant-induced autoimmunity.

of cells specific for autoantigens. In an **autoimmune disease**, pathogenic consequences, including tissue injury, produced by autoantibodies or autoreactive T lymphocytes interact with self epitopes, i.e., autoantigens. The mere presence of autoantibodies or autoreactive T lymphocytes does not prove that there is any cause and effect relationship between these components and a patient's disease. To show that autoimmune phenomena are involved in the etiology and pathogenesis of human disease, Witebsky suggested that certain criteria be fulfilled. In addition to autoimmune reactivity against self constituents, tissue injury in the presence of immunocompetent cells corresponding to the tissue distribution of the autoantigen, duplication of the disease features in experimental animals injected with the appropriate autoantigen, and passive transfer with either autoantibody or autoreactive T lymphocytes to normal animals offer evidence in support of an autoimmune pathogenesis of a disease.

Molecular mimicry is the sharing of antigenic determinants or epitopes between cells of an immunocompetent host and a microorganism. This may lead to pathologic sequelae if antibodies produced against the microorganism combine with antigens of self and lead to immunologic injury. Ankylosing spondylitis and rheumatic fever are examples. Immunologic cross-reactivity between a viral antigen and a self antigen or between a bacterial antigen such as streptococcal M protein and human myocardial sarcolemmal membranes may lead to tissue injury.

Genetics has long been recognized to play an important role in autoimmunity. Susceptibility genes increase probability but do not determine by themselves development of an autoimmune disease. MHC genes have been shown to have

a strong association with selected autoimmune diseases. This is especially true of the class II MHC genes. In addition, some non-MHC genes may also play a role in the development of autoimmunity. There is a higher frequency of certain HLA alleles in persons with selected autoimmune diseases than in members of the general population.

Relative risk (RR) is the association of a particular disease with a certain HLA antigen. This represents the chance a person with the disease-associated HLA antigen has of developing the disease compared with that of a person who does not possess that antigen. Relative risk is calculated as follows:

$$RR = (p^+ \times c^-)/(p^- \times c^+)$$

where

p^+ = number of patients possessing a particular HLA antigen
c^- = number of controls not possessing the particular HLA antigen
p^- = number of patients not possessing the particular HLA antigen
c^+ = number of controls possessing the particular HLA antigen

It is through the ability of MHC molecules to govern T lymphocyte selection and activation that they have an effect on the development of autoimmunity. Whereas some MHC genes may be predisposing factors in the development of autoimmune disease, others may be protective. HLA gene expression alone does not induce autoimmune disease, but it often serves as one of several determinants that lead to autoimmunity.

In addition to aberrations of immune responsiveness and susceptibility genes, autoimmunity may result from certain viral and bacterial infections. It may also result from tissue inflammation, injury or trauma leading to self antigen exposure to the immune system and hormonal influences. Estrogens have long been known to promote certain autoimmune diseases such as systemic lupus erythematosus that affects females 10 times more frequently than males.

In type I **MAD (multiple autoimmune disorders)**, a patient must manifest a minimum of two of the diseases designated Addison's disease, mucocutaneous candidiasis or hypoparathyroidism. Type II MAD is known as Schmidt syndrome, in which patients manifest at least two conditions from a category that includes autoimmune thyroid disease, Addison's disease, mucocutaneous candidiasis and insulin-dependent diabetes mellitus, with or without hypopituitarism.

Some mechanisms in **drug-induced autoimmunity** are similar to those induced by viruses (Figure 9). Autoantibodies may appear as a result of the helper determinant effect. With some drugs such as hydantoin, the mechanism resembles that of the Epstein-Barr virus (EBV). The generalized lymphoid hyperplasia also involves clones specific for autoantigens. Another form is that seen with α-methyldopa. This drug induces the production of specific antibodies. The drug attaches to cells *in vivo* without changing the surface antigenic makeup. The antibodies, which often have anti-e (Rh series) specificity, combine with the drug on cells, fix complement, and induce a bystander type of complement-mediated lysis. Another form of drug-induced autoimmunity is seen with nitrofurantoin, in which the autoimmunity involves cell-mediated phenomena without evidence of autoantibodies.

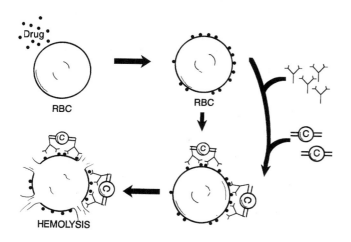

Figure 9. Drug-induced hemolysis.

Although both warm antibody and cold antibody types of **autoimmune hemolytic anemia** are known, the warm antibody type is the most common and is characterized by a positive direct antiglobulin (Coombs' test) associated with lymphoreticular cancer or autoimmune disease and splenomegaly. Patients may have anemia, hemolysis, lymphadenopathy, hepatosplenomegaly, or features of autoimmune disease. They commonly have a normochromic, normocytic

anemia with spherocytosis and nucleated red blood cells in the peripheral blood. Leukocytosis and thrombocytosis may also occur. There is a significant reticulocytosis and an elevated serum indirect (unconjugated) bilirubin. IgG and complement adhere to red blood cells. Antibodies are directed principally against Rh antigens. There is a positive indirect antiglobulin test in 50% of cases and agglutination of enzyme-treated red blood cells in 90% of cases. In the cold agglutinin syndrome, IgM antibodies with an anti-I specificity are involved. Warm-autoantibody autoimmune hemolytic anemia has a fairly good prognosis.

Autoimmune neutropenia can be either an isolated condition or secondary to autoimmune disease. Patients may either have recurrent infections or remain asymptomatic. Antigranulocyte antibodies may be demonstrated. There is normal bone marrow function with myeloid hyperplasia and a shift to the left as a result of increased granulocyte destruction. The autoantibody may suppress myeloid cell growth. The condition is treated by immunosuppressive drugs, corticosteroids or splenectomy. Patients with systemic lupus erythematosus, Felty's syndrome (rheumatoid arthritis, splenomegaly and severe neutropenia), and other autoimmune diseases may manifest autoimmune neutropenia.

Acetylcholine receptor (AChR) antibodies are IgG autoantibodies that cause loss of function of acetylcholine receptors that are critical to chemical transmission of the nerve impulse at the neuromuscular junction. This represents a type II mechanism of hypersensitivity according to the Coombs and Gell classification. AChR antibodies are heterogeneous with some showing specificity for antigenic determinants other than those that serve as acetylcholine or alpha-bungarotoxin binding sites. As many as 85 to 95% of myasthenia gravis patients may manifest acetylcholine receptor antibodies.

Spontaneous autoimmune thyroiditis (SAT) occurs in the obese strain (OS) of chickens. It is an animal model of Hashimoto's thyroiditis in man. Many mononuclear cells infiltrate the thyroid gland leading to disruption of the follicular architecture. Immunodysregulation is critical in the etiopathogenesis of SAT. Endocrine abnormalities play a role in the pathogenesis and disturbances in communication between the immune and endocrine systems in the disease. Dysregulation leads to hyperreactivity of the immune system which combined with a primary genetic defect-induced alteration of the thyroid gland leads to autoimmune thyroiditis. Both T and B lymphocytes are significant in the pathogenesis of SAT. T cell effector mechanisms have greater influence than do humoral factors in initiation of the disease and most lymphocytes infiltrating the autoimmune thyroid are mature cells. Not only do autoantibodies have a minor role in the pathogenesis but T cells, rather than B cells, of OS chickens are defective.

Experimental allergic thyroiditis is an autoimmune disease produced by injecting experimental animals with thyroid tissue or extract or thyroglobulin incorporated into Freund's complete adjuvant (Figure 10). It represents an animal model of Hashimoto's thyroiditis in humans, with mixed extensive lymphocytic infiltrate. Another animal model is the spontaneous occurrence of this disease in the obese strain of chickens as well as Buffalo rats.

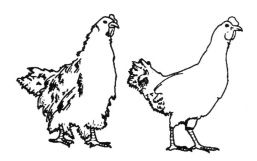

Figure 10. Experimental allergic thyroiditis (EAT).

Experimental autoimmune thyroiditis (EAT) includes a murine model for Hashimoto's thyroiditis. There is a strong MHC genetic component in susceptibility to Hashimoto's thyroiditis, which has been shown to reside in the *IA* subregion of the murine MHC (H-2), governing the immune response (*Ir*) genes to mouse thyroglobulin (MTg). Following induction of EAT with MTg, autoantibodies against MTg appear and mononuclear cells infiltrate the thyroid. Repeated administration of soluble, syngeneic MTg without adjuvant leads to thyroiditis only in the murine haplotype susceptible to EAT. Autoreactive T cells proliferate *in vitro* following stimulation with MTg. The disease can be passively transferred to naive recipients by adoptive immunization and differentiate into cytotoxic T lymphocytes (Tc) *in vitro*. Thus, lymphoid cells rather than antibodies represent the primary mediator of the disease. *In vitro* proliferation of murine-autoreactive T cells was found to show a good correlation with susceptibility to EAT and was dependent on the presence of Thy-1$^+$, Lyt-1$^+$, Ia$^+$ and L3T4$^+$ lymphocytes. Effector T lymphocytes (T$_E$) in EAT comprise various T cell subsets and Lyt-1 (L3T4) and Lyt-2 phenotypes. T lymphocytes cloned from thyroid infiltrates of Hashimoto's thyroiditis patients reveal numerous cytotoxic T lymphocytes and clones synthesizing IL-2 and IFN-γ. While the T cell subsets participate in the pathogenesis of Hashimoto's thyroiditis, autoantibody synthesis appears to aid perpetuation of the disease or result from it.

Myasthenia gravis (MG) is an autoantibody-mediated autoimmune disease. Experimental forms of myasthenia gravis (MG) were made possible through the ready availability of AChR from electric fish. Monoclonal antibodies were developed followed by molecular cloning techniques, that permitted definition of the AChR structure.

Experimental autoimmune myasthenia gravis (EAMG) can be induced in more than one species of animals by immunizing them with purified AChR from the electric ray (*Torpedo californica*). The autoantigen, nicotinic AChR, is T cell dependent. The *in vivo* synthesis of anti-AChR antibodies requires helper T cell activity. Antibodies specific for the nicotinic acetylcholine receptors (AChR) of skeletal muscle react with the postsynaptic membrane at the neuromuscular junction.

Experimental allergic encephalomyelitis is an autoimmune disease induced by immunization of experimental animals with preparations of brain or spinal cord incorporated into Freund's complete adjuvant. After ten to twelve days, perivascular accumulations of lymphocytes and mononuclear phagocytes surround the vasculature of the brain and spinal cord white matter. Demyelination may also be present, worsening as the disease becomes chronic. The animals often develop paralysis. The disease can be passively transferred from a sick animal to a healthy one of the same strain with T lymphocytes but not with antibodies. The mechanism involves T cell receptor interaction with an 18kD myelin basic protein molecule, which is an organ-specific antigen of nervous system tissue. The CD4$^+$ T lymphocyte represents the phenotype that is reactive with myelin basic protein. The immune reaction induces myelinolysis, wasting and paralysis. Peptides derived from myelin basic protein or MBP itself may be used to induce experimental allergic encephalomyelitis in animals. This experimental autoimmune disease is an animal model for multiple sclerosis and post-vaccination encephalitis in man.

A **NOD (nonobese diabetic) mouse** is one of a mutant mouse strain that spontaneously develops type I, insulin-dependent diabetes mellitus, an autoimmune disease. There is an autosomal recessive pattern of inheritance for the NOD mutation. Lymphocytes infiltrate NOD mouse islets of Langerhans in the pancreas and kill beta cells. There is a defect in HLA-DQ part of the MHC class II region in humans with insulin dependent diabetes mellitus and in the class II IA region of the mouse MHC class II. A major DNA segment is missing from the NOD mouse MHC IE region. When the IE segment is inserted or the IA defect is corrected in transgenic NOD mice, disease progression is halted.

A **NON mouse** the normal control mouse for use in studies involving the NOD mouse strain that spontaneously develops type I (insulin-dependent) diabetes mellitus. The two strains differ only in genes associated with the development of diabetes.

Polyclonal activation is the stimulation of multiple lymphocyte clones, thereby leading to a heterogeneous immune response. **Polyclonal activators** are substances that activate multiple lymphocyte clones including both T and B lymphocytes regardless of antigen specificity. Phytohemagglutinin activates mainly T lymphocytes, whereas staphylococcal protein A stimulates human B lymphocytes, and lipopolysaccharide derived from gram negative bacteria stimulates murine B lymphocytes. Con A stimulates T cells.

Bacterial lipopolysaccharide (LPS) acts as a **polyclonal lymphocyte activator** in murine B cells, but fails to stimulate human B lymphocytes. Among the B lymphocyte stimulated are self reactive ones that are anergic. LPS injection may result in the production of many autoantibodies in mice. Superantigens may cause polyclonal T cell stimulation which has been suggested to be a mechanism for autoimmunity but evidence is lacking. Graft vs. host reactivity also has many autoimmune-like features. Response of the human body to microbial antigens may lead to an immune response that cross-reacts with self antigens. For example, antibodies to streptococci in rheumatic fever may cross-react with antigens of the myocardium in man leading to myocarditis. If helper T cells are absent, autoreactive B cells may not produce autoantibodies. Antigens consisting of several determinants that include a self epitope reactive with B lymphocytes and a foreign epitope that activates helper T cells can result in stimulation of B lymphocytes with autoantibody synthesis.

A **MRL-*lpr/lpr* mouse** is from a strain genetically prone to develop lupus erythematosus-like disease spontaneously. Its congenic subline is MRL-+/+. The lymphoproliferation *(lpr)* gene in the former strain is associated with development of autoimmune disease, i.e., murine lupus. Although the MRL-+/+ mice are not normal immunologically, they develop autoimmune disease only late in life and without lymphadenopathy. MRL-lpr/lpr mice differ from New Zealand mice mainly in the development of striking lymphadenopathy in both males and females of the MRL-lpr/lpr strain between eight and 16 weeks of age with a 100-fold increase in lymph node weight. Numerous Thy-1+, Ly-1+, Ly-2−, L3T4− lymphocytes that express and rearrange α and β genes of the T cell receptor but fail to rearrange immunoglobulin genes are present in the lymph nodes. Multiple antinuclear antibodies including anti-Sm, are among serological features of murine lupus in the MRL-*lpr/lpr* mouse model. These are associated with the development of immune complexes which mediate glomerulonephritis. Although the *lpr* gene is clearly significant in the pathogenesis of autoimmunity, the development of anti-DNA and anti-Sm even in low titers and late in life in the MRL-+/+ congenic line points to the role of factors other than the lpr gene in the development of autoimmunity in this strain.

The ***gld/gld* mice** (generalized lymphoproliferation disease) are an experimental inbred strain. The mice develop progressive lymphadenopathy and lupus-like immunopathology. The ***gld*** gene is the murine mutant gene on chromosome 1. **New Zealand black (NZB) mice** are an inbred strain of mice that serves as an animal model of autoimmune hemolytic anemia. They develop antinuclear antibodies in low titer, have defective T lymphocytes, defects in DNA repair and have B cells that are spontaneously activated. **New Zealand white (NZW) mice** are an inbred strain of white mice which when mated with NZB strain that develop autoimmunity, produce an F_1 generation of NZB/NZW mice that represent an animal model of autoimmune disease and especially of a lupus erythematosus-like condition.

14

Mucosal Immunity

Local immunity refers to immunologic reactivity confined principally to a particular anatomic site such as the respiratory or gastrointestinal tract. Local antibodies, as well as lymphoid cells, present in the area may mediate a specific immunologic effect. For example, secretory IgA produced in the gut may react to food or other ingested antigens.

The **mucosal immune system** describes aggregates of lymphoid tissues or lymphocytes near mucosal surfaces of the respiratory, gastrointestinal and urogenital tracts (Figures 1–4). There is local synthesis of secretory IgA and T cell immunity at these sites. The mucosal epithelial layer serves as a mechanical barrier against foreign antigens and invading microorganisms. A specialized immune system, sometimes referred to as the common mucosal immune system (CMIS) located at epithelial surfaces represents a critical defense mechanism. The mucosal immune system consists of secretory IgA molecules produced by plasma cells in the lamina propria and subsequently transported across epithelial cells with the aid of the polyimmunoglobulin receptor. Both αβ and γδ T lymphocytes are present in the mucosal epithelial layer as intraepithelial lymphocytes. They are also found in the lamina propria of the mucosa where they serve as an integral component of the cellular immune system. These T lymphocytes function in the induction and regulation of responses by antigen-specific IgA B cells as well as effector T cells. The epithelial cells lining mucosal surfaces furnish signals that are significant for the initiation of the mucosal inflammatory response and critical communications between epithelial cells and mucosal lymphoid cells. The immune response to oral antigens differs from the response to parenterally administered immunogens. Oral tolerance may follow the ingestion of some protein antigens but a vigorous local mucosal immune response with the production of high concentrations of IgA may follow oral immunization with selected vaccines such as the Sabin oral polio vaccine.

Mucosa-associated lymphoid tissue (MALT) includes extranodal lymphoid tissue associated with the mucosa at various anatomical sites, including the skin (SALT), bronchus (BALT), gut (GALT), breast, and uterine cervix. The mucosa-associated lymphoid tissues provide localized or regional immune defense since they are in immediate contact with foreign antigenic substances, thereby differing from the lymphoid tissues associated with lymph nodes, spleen, and thymus. Secretory or exocrine IgA is associated with the MALT system of immunity.

Gut-associated lymphoid tissue (GALT) describes lymphoid tissue in the gastrointestinal mucosa and submucosa. It constitutes the gastrointestinal immune system (Figure 5). GALT is present in the appendix, in the tonsils, and in the Peyer's patches subjacent to the mucosa. GALT represents the counterpart of BALT and consists of radially arranged and closely packed lymphoid follicles which impinge upon the intestinal epithelium, forming dome-like structures. In GALT, specialized epithelial cells overlie the lymphoid follicles, forming a membrane between the lymphoid cells and the lumen. These cells are called M cells. They are believed to be "gatekeepers" for molecules passing across. Other GALT components include IgA-synthesizing B cells and intraepithelial lymphocytes such as CD8[+] T cells, as well as the lymphocytes in the lamina propria that include CD4[+] T lymphocytes, B lymphocytes which synthesize IgA and null cells.

The **lamina propria** is the thin connective tissue layer that supports the epithelium of the gastrointestinal, respiratory and genitourinary tracts (Figure 6). The epithelium and lamina propria form the mucous membrane. The lamina propria may be the site of immunologic reactivity in the gastrointestinal tract, representing an area where lymphocytes, plasma cells, and mast cells congregate.

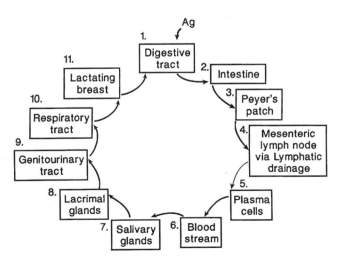

Figure 1. Secretory immune system.

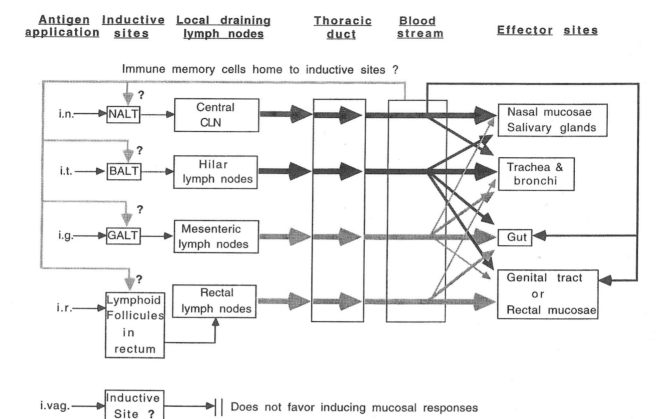

Figure 2. Compartmentalized common mucosal immune system.

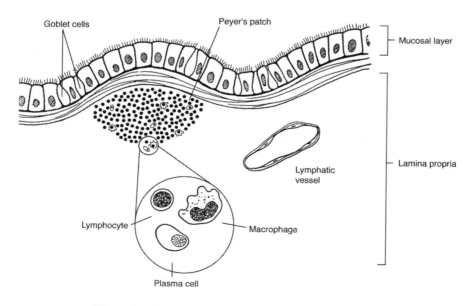

Figure 3. The mucosal system and its cellular components.

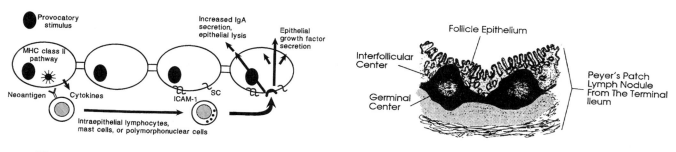

Figure 4. Common mucosal inflammatory pathway.

Figure 5. GALT (Gut-associated lymphoid tissue).

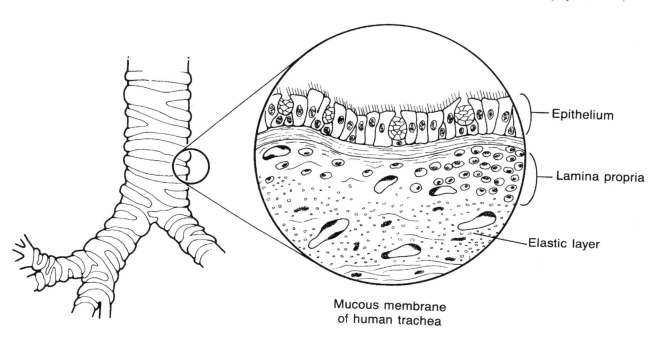

Figure 6. Lamina propria.

A **polyimmunoglobulin receptor** is an attachment site for polymeric immunoglobulins located on epithelial cell and hepatocyte surfaces that facilitate polymeric IgA and IgM transcytosis to the secretions. After binding, the receptor-immunoglobulin complex is endocytosed and enclosed within vesicles for transport. Exocytosis takes place at the cell surface where the immunoglobulin is discharged into the intestinal lumen. A similar mechanism in the liver facilitates IgA transport into the bile. The receptor-polymeric immunoglobulin complex is released from the cell following cleavage near the cell membrane. The receptor segment that is bound to the polymeric immunoglobulin is known as the secretory component which can only be used once in the transport process.

Lymphocytes in the gastrointestinal mucosa may be present in the lamina propria, Peyer's patches and the epithelial layer. In humans, the intraepithelial lymphocytes are mostly CD8+ T cells. γδ T cells make up these intraepithelial lymphocytes to varying degrees according to the species but

constitute approximately 10% in the human. The γδ as well as the αβ intraepithelial T cells have restricted specificities probably corresponding to antigens frequently found in the gut. Numerous activated B cells, plasma cells, activated CD4+ T cells, eosinophils, macrophages, and mast cells are present in the lamina propria of the intestine. T cells are believed to interact with antigen in regional mesenteric lymph nodes and then return to the intestinal lamina propria.

Mucosa homing is a selective return of immunologically reactive lymphoid cells, that originated in mucosal follicles and migrated to other anatomical locations, to return to their site of origin in mucosal areas. Receptors on lymphoid cells and ligands on endothelial cells are responsible for the cellular migration involving the mucosal immune system (Figure 7).

MadCAM-1 is a mucosal addressin cell adhesion molecule-1 which is an addressin in Peyer's patches of mice (Figure 8). This three Ig domain structure with a polypeptide backbone binds the α4β7 integrin. MadCAM-1 facilitates

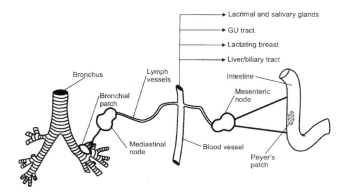

Figure 7.   Cell traffic.

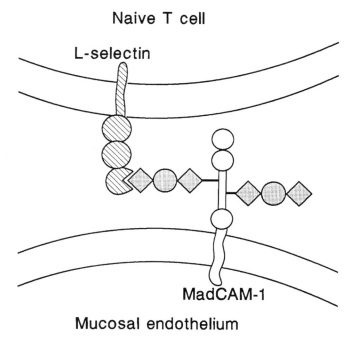

Figure 8.   MadCAM-1.

access of lymphocytes to the mucosal lymphoid tissues, as in the gastrointestinal tract. **Addressin** is a molecule such as a peptide or protein that serves as a homing device to direct a molecule to a specific location. Lymphocytes from Peyer's patches home to mucosal endothelial cells bearing ligands for the lymphocyte homing receptor.

L-selectin is a molecule found on lymphocytes that is responsible for the homing of lymphocytes to lymph node high endothelial venules. L-selectin is also found on neutrophils where it acts to bind the cells to activated endothelium early in the inflammatory process. L-selectin is also called CD62L.

Mucosal lymphoid follicles include such structures as Peyer's patches in the small intestine and pharyngeal tonsils. The appendix and other areas of the gastrointestinal tract and respiratory tract contain similar aggregates of lymphoid cells. Germinal centers at the center of lymphoid follicles have an abundance of B cells. CD4+ T cells are present in interfollicular regions of Peyer's patches. One-half to three-quarters of the lymphocytes in murine Peyer's patches are B cells, whereas 10 to 30% are T lymphocytes. M cells overlying Peyer's patches are membranous (M) cells devoid of microvilli, are pinocytic and convey macromolecules to subepithelial tissues from the lumen of the intestine. Although M cells are believed to transport antigens to Peyer's patches, they do not act as antigen-presenting cells. Lymphoid cells in the blood migrate to the gut mucosa. The integrin α_4 associated with β_7 is critical for endothelial binding of lymphocytes in the intestine and migration of cells into the mucosa.

The **M cell** is a gastrointestinal tract epithelial cell that conveys microorganisms and macromolecular substances from the gut lumen to Peyer's patches. The M cell cytoplasmic processes extend to CD4+ T cells underneath them. Materials attached to microvilli are conveyed to coated pits and moved to the basolateral surface, which has pronounced invaginations rich in leukocytes and mononuclear phagocytes. Thus, materials gaining access by way of M cells come into contact with lymphoid cells as they reach the basolateral surface. This is believed to facillitate induction of immune responsiveness.

Secretory IgA is a dimeric molecule comprised of two IgA monomers joined by a J polypeptide chain and a glycopeptide secretory component (Figure 9). This is the principal molecule of mucosal immunity. IgA is the only immunoglobulin isotype that can be selectively passed across mucosal walls to reach the lumens of organs lined with mucosal cells. Specific FαR that bind IgA molecular dimers are found on intestinal epithelial cells. The FcαR, also known as secretory (S protein) joins the antibody molecule to the epithelial cell's basal surface that is exposed to the blood. It is bound to the polyimmunoglobulin receptor on the epithelial cell's basolateral surface and facilitates vesicular transport of the anchored IgA across the cell to the surface of the mucosa. Once this complex reaches its

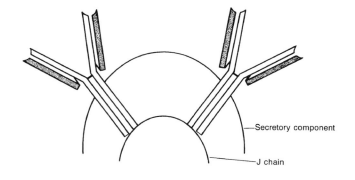

Figure 9.   Secretory IgA.

destination, FcαR (S protein) is split in a manner that permits the dimeric IgA molecule to retain an attached secretory piece which has a strong affinity for mucous, thereby facilitating the maintenance of IgA molecules on mucosal surfaces. Secretory or exocrine IgA appears in the colostrum, intestinal and respiratory secretions, saliva, tears and other secretions.

Secretory component (T piece) or **secretory piece** is a 75kD molecule synthesized by epithelial cells in the lamina propria of the gut that becomes associated with IgA molecules produced by plasma cells in the lamina propria of the gut (Figure 10). It can be found in three molecular forms: as an SIgM and SIgA stabilizing chain, as a transmembrane receptor protein, and as free secretory component in fluids. Secretory piece also has the important function of protecting the secreted IgA molecules from proteolytic digestion by enzymes of the gut. These latter two functions are in addition to its active role in transporting the IgA molecule through the epithelial cell.

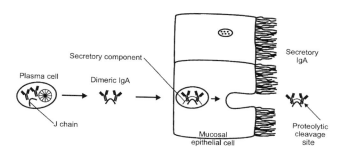

Figure 10. Secretory component.

Secretory component deficiency is a lack of IgA in secretions as a consequence of gastrointestinal tract epithelial cells' inability to produce secretory component to be linked to the IgA molecules synthesized in the lamina propria of the gut to prevent their destruction by the proteolytic enzymes in the gut lumen. The disorder is very infrequent but is characterized by protracted diarrhea associated with gut infection.

Bronchial-associated lymphoid tissue (BALT) is present in both mammals, including man and birds (Figure 11). In many areas it appears as a collar containing nodules located

deep around the bronchus and connected with the epithelium by patches of loosely arranged lymphoid cells. Germinal centers are absent (except in the chicken), although cells in the center of nodules stain lighter than do those at the periphery. Plasma cells are present occasionally beneath the epithelium. The cells in BALT have a high turnover rate and apparently do not produce IgG. BALT development is independent of that of the peripheral lymphoid tissues or antigen

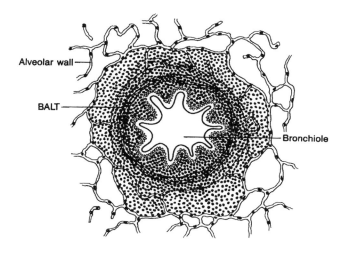

Figure 11. BALT (Bronchial-associated lymphoid tissue).

exposure. The cells of the BALT apparently migrate there from other lymphoid areas.

Oral unresponsiveness is the mucosal immune system's selective ability to not react immunologically against antigens or food and intestinal microorganisms even though it responds vigorously to pathogenic microorganisms.

Oral feeding of a protein antigen may lead to profound systemic immunosuppression involving both the B cell (antibody-mediated) and T cell (cell mediated) limbs of the immune response to that specific antigen (Figure 12). T cell clonal anergy is induced to some protein antigens administered by this route. Antigen presented by antigen-presenting

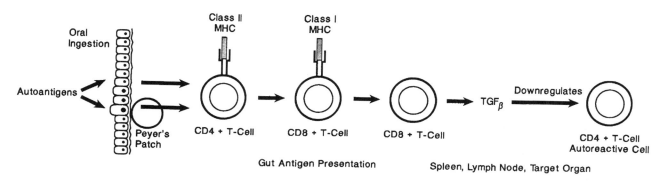

Figure 12. Antigen feeding.

cells deficient in costimulatory molecules may induce tolerance. Yet possible nonprofessional antigen-presenting cells involved in the induction of oral tolerance have not been identified.

It has also been postulated that the immunosuppressive cytokine TGF-β may be released during the induction of **oral tolerance** through its ability to block lymphocyte proliferation and to induce B lymphocyte switching to IgA production. Paradoxically it remains a mystery why large doses of soluble proteins induce systemic T lymphocyte tolerance, whereas the components of vaccines such as the Sabin polio vaccine induce an effective local immune response. Specific local immunity may be attributable to activation or infection of antigen-presenting cells in the intestinal epithelium. Nevertheless, oral tolerance is beneficial through its prevention of the body's reaction to oral antigens or food or gastrointestinal bacteria. Feeding of autoantigen to induce oral tolerance has potential therapeutic value for the treatment of autoimmune disease.

Antigen fed orally soon reaches the lymphatics of the intestine and is transported to the mesenteric lymph nodes, where it stimulates an immune response. Antigen may also reach Peyer's patches through M cells and lead to a T and B cell response. Activated lymphocytes in mesenteric lymph nodes may migrate to the lamina propria, whereas those in the Peyer's patches may reach either the lamina propria or mesenteric lymph nodes.

The epithelial layer is not only a mechanical barrier against pathogenic microorganisms but is the site in the gastrointestinal and respiratory tracts of secretory IgA antibodies. This class of immunoglobulin is also responsible for the passive transfer of immunity from mother to young through the milk and colostrum. Most of the antibodies produced in the normal adult are of the secretory IgA class. Antigens conveyed to Peyer's patches of the intestine activate T lymphocytes and follicular B cells. IgA-synthesizing lymphocytes enter the lamina propria. IL-5 and TGF-β facilitate IgA isotype switching. Antibody affinity maturation occurs in germinal centers of Peyer's patches where stimulated B lymphocytes have seeded and proliferated. IgA-synthesizing B lymphocytes populate the lamina propria or other mucosal tissues.

The relatively large quantity of secretory IgA synthesized in tissues of the mucosal immune system is attributable to the tendency of B cells that form IgA to populate the lamina propria and Peyer's patches. IgA-producing B lymphocytes in other parts of the body are responsible for serum IgA.

The **Sulzberger-Chase phenomenon** is the induction of immunological unresponsiveness to skin-sensitizing chemicals such as picryl chrloride by feeding an animal (e.g., guinea pig) the chemical in question prior to application to the skin. Intravenous administration of the chemical may also block the development of delayed-type hypersensitivity when the same chemical is later applied to the skin. Simple chemicals such as picryl chloride may induce contact hypersensitivity when applied to the skin of guinea pigs. The unresponsiveness may be abrogated by adoptive immunization of a tolerant guinea pig with lymphocytes from one that has been sensitized by application of the chemical to the skin without prior oral feeding.

SKIN IMMUNITY

The skin, the largest organ in the body, shields the body's interior environment from a hostile exterior (Figure 13). The skin defends the host through stimulation of inflammatory and local immune responses. Antigen applied to or injected into the skin drains to the regional lymph nodes through the skin's extensive lymphatic network. Cells of both the epidermis, papillary and reticular dermis have critical roles in the skin's immune function. Keratinocytes, which are epidermal epithelial cells, secrete various cytokines such as granulocyte-macrophage colony-stimulating factor, interleukin 1, interleukin 3, interleukin 6, and tumor necrosis factor. T lymphocytes in the skin may secrete IFN-γ or other cytokines that cause these epithelial cells to synthesize chemokines that lead to leukocyte chemotaxis and activation. Stimulation by IFN-γ may also lead to their expression of class II MHC molecules. Other epidermal cells include Langerhans cells which form an extensive network in the epidermis that permits their interaction with any antigen entering the skin. The few lymphocytes in the epidermis are principally CD8+ T cells often with restricted antigen receptors. In the mouse, these are mostly γδ T cells. Skin lymphocytes and macrophages are mostly in the dermis. The T cells are of CD4+ and CD8+ phenotypes and often perivascular.

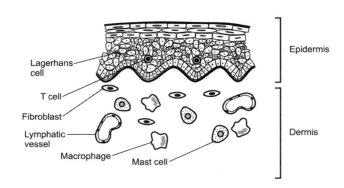

Figure 13. The cutaneous immune system and its cellular components.

Langerhans cells are the principal antigen-presenting cells in the skin. They encounter antigen entering through the skin and process it. Langerhans cells may reach the parafollicular cortical areas of the regional lymph nodes via lymphatic vessels of the skin. These Langerhans cells develop into effective antigen-presenting cells as a result of up-regulation of class II MHC molecules and of costimulatory molecules. In the lymph nodes they present antigen to CD4+ T lymphocytes after becoming interdigitating dendritic cells. Dermal macrophages may present protein antigens to previously activated T cells. Delayed type hypersensitivity reactions are mediated by T cells in the skin reacting to soluble protein antigens or to chemicals acting as haptens that combine with self proteins producing new epitopes. This cell-mediated immune reaction is accompanied by the release of cytokines from the activated T cells. With respect to the antibody response of the skin, secretory IgA is found in sweat which aids in defense against infection. IgE on the surface of mast cells in the dermis participates in the generation of immediate type I hypersensitivity reactions in the skin.

15

Immunohematology

An article in the *Berliner klinische Wochenschrift* in 1900 by Ehrlich and Morgenroth which described blood groups in goats based on antigens of their red cells led Karl Landsteiner, a Viennese pathologist, to successfully identify the human ABO blood groups. He took samples of his own blood from his colleagues Sturli and Ardhein, Dr. Pietschnig and his assistant Zaritsch. The small tables Landsteiner used to illustrate his reasoning bear the names of these colleagues. In 1902, Sturli and Alfred Descastello, under Landsteiner's direction, designated one more group which was actually not named "AB" until 10 years later when von Dungen and Hirszfeld studying the genetic inheritance of blood types, designated the fourth type and gave Landsteiner's "C" group the designated O. It was for this discovery, rather than his elegant studies on immunochemical specificity, that he won the Nobel Prize in Medicine 30 years later.

Among those who worked with him in the field of immunohematology were Alexander Weiner and Philip Levine. Landsteiner and Levine discovered the M and N blood group antigen by injecting human erythrocytes into rabbits. The antisera which they raised were able to divide human blood into three groups M, N and MN based on their antigenic content. They showed that these antigens were under the genetic control of codominant alleles. Landsteiner and Weiner described the Rh factor in 1940. At first thought to be a simple system involving a single antigen, it was shown to be genetically, immunologically and clinically complex. In studies of M-like factors on the erythrocytes of rhesus monkeys, antisera raised by injecting rabbits with rhesus red cells cross-reacted with human erythrocytes containing M antigen. It was subsequently demonstrated that the red cells of about 85% of the human population reacted with antisera against rhesus red cells. Thus, those individuals who shared an antigen with the rhesus monkeys red cells were termed Rh positive and those who did not were termed Rh negative. It was subsequently demonstrated that multiple pregnancies with Rh(D) positive fetuses in Rh negative mothers leads to stimulation of maternal anti-D antibodies of the IgG class which cross the placenta and cause lysis of fetal red cells. Unless the mother is treated with antibody against the D-antigen after parturition, hemolytic disease of the newborn (erythroblastosis fetalis) may result on subsequent births. Besides those mentioned above, other red blood cell antigens discovered in the intervening years included Kell, Diego, P, Duffy and I blood group systems and soluble antigens, such as the Lewis, Lutheran antigens that are in the secretions and are adsorbed to the red cell surface. Although most red cell groups are inherited as autosomal characteristics, the Xg blood group system is sex linked. Historically, new red blood cell antigens were discovered as a result of transfusion incompatibility reactions that could not be explained on the basis of existing or known antigens (Figure 1).

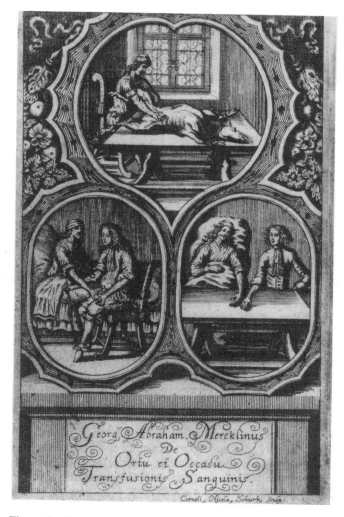

Figure 1. Engraved title page from G.A. Mercklin, *Tractatio med. curiosa de ortu et sdanguinis,* 1679. This is one of the best early pictures of blood transfusion. (From the Cruse Collection, Middleton Library, University of Wisconsin)

Blood grouping (Figures 2 and 3) is the classification of erythrocytes based on their surface isoantigens. Among the well known human blood groups are the ABO, Rh and MNS systems.

T a b e l l e I, betreffend das Blut sechs anscheinend gesunder Männer.

	Sera					
Dr. St.	—	+	+	+	+	—
Dr. Plecn.	—	—	+	+	—	—
Dr. Sturl.	—	+	—	—	+	—
Dr. Erdh.	—	+	—	+	+	—
Zar.	—	+	+	+	+	—
Landst.	+	+	+	+	+	—

Blutkörperchen von: Dr. St., Dr. Plecn., Dr.Sturl., Dr.Erdh., Zar., Landst.

T a b e l l e II, betreffend das Blut von sechs anscheinend gesunden Puerperae.

	Sera					
Seil.	—	—	+	—	—	+
Linsm.	+	—	+	+	+	+
Lust.	+	—	+	—	+	—
Mittelb.	—	—	+	—	—	+
Tomsch.	—	—	+	—	+	—
Graupn.	+	—	—	+	+	—

Blutkörperchen von: Seil., Linsm., Lust., Mittelb., Tomsch., Graupn.

Figure 2. Table illustrating ABO blood groups. *Wien. klin. Wschr.* *14:* 1132–1134, 1901.

Blood Type	RBC surface antigen	Antibody in Serum
A	A antigen	Anti-B
B	B antigen	Anti-A
AB	AB antigens	no antibody
O	no A or B antigens	Both Anti-A and Anti-B

Figure 3. ABO blood group antigens and antibodies.

ABO blood group substances are glycopeptides with oligosaccharide side chains manifesting ABO epitopes of the same specificity as those present on red blood cells of the individual in whom they are detected. Soluble ABO blood group substances may be found in mucous secretions of man such as saliva, gastric juice, ovarian cyst fluid, etc. Such persons are termed secretors whereas those without the blood group substances in their secretions are nonsecretors.

The **ABO blood group system** was the first of the human blood groups to be described based upon carbohydrate alloantigens present on red cell membranes. Anti-A or anti-B isoagglutinins (alloantibodies) are present only in the blood sera of individuals not possessing that specificity, i.e.,

anti-A is found in the serum of group B individuals and anti-B is found in the serum of group A individuals. This serves as the basis for grouping humans into phenotypes designated A, B, AB and O. Type AB subjects possess neither anti-A nor anti-B antibodies, whereas group O persons have both anti-A and anti-B antibodies in their serum. Blood group methodology to determine the ABO blood type makes use of the agglutination reaction. The ABO system remains the most important in the transfusion of blood and is also critical in organ transplantation. Epitopes of the ABO system are found on oligosaccharide terminal sugars. The genes designated as *A/B*, *Se*, *H*, and *Le* govern the formation of these epitopes and of the Lewis (Le) antigens (Figure 4). The two precursor substances, type I and type II, differ only in that the terminal galactose is joined to the penultimate N-acetyl-glucosamine in, β 1-3 linkage in type α chains but in β 1-4 linkage in type II chain.

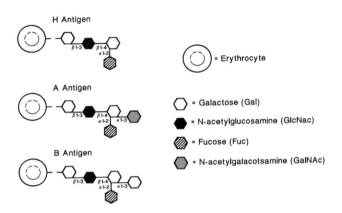

Figure 4. Chemical structure of AB and H antigens of the ABO blood group system.

In the **ABO blood group system**, O antigen is an oligosaccharide precursor form of A and B antigens; a fucose-galactose-N-acetylglucosamine-glucose. The O blood group is one of those described by Landsteiner (Figures 5–7).

The **Bombay phenotype (O$_h$)** is an ABO blood group antigen variant on human erythrocytes in rare subjects. These red blood cells do not possess A, B or H antigens on their surfaces, even though the subject does not have anit-A, anti-B, and anti-H antibodies in the serum. The Bombay phenotype may cause difficulties in crossmatching for transfusion.

Front typing (Figure 8) refers to blood typing for transfusion, antibodies of known specificity are used to identify erythrocyte ABO antigens. Differences between front and back typing might be attributable to acquired group B or B subtypes, cold agglutinins, diminished immunoglobulins, anti-B and anti-A$_1$ antibody polyagglutination, rouleaux formation, Wharton's jelly or two separate cell populations.

Back typing detects antibodies in an individual's serum that react with known antigens of an erythrocyte panel. It is

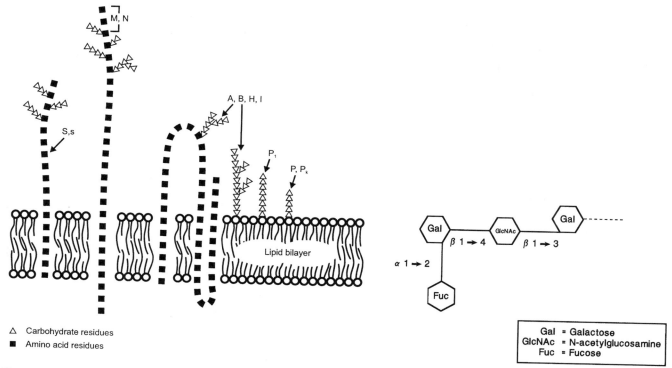

Figure 5.   Schematic representation of membrane glycoproteins and glycosphingolipids that carry blood group antigens.

Figure 6.   Chemical structure of H antigen, which is a specificity of the ABO blood group system.

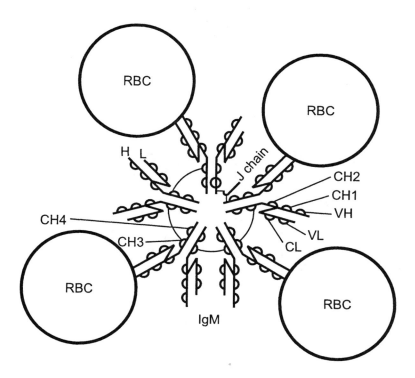

Figure 7.   Schematic representation of the agglutination of human red cells by the natural isohemagglutinins, which are antibodies of the IgM class that constitute the natural isohemagglutinins in serum.

Front Typing		Back Typing			
Reaction of Cells Tested with		Reaction of Serum Tested Against			Interpretation
Anti-A	Anti-B	A Cells	B Cells	O Cells	ABO Group
O	O	+	+	O	O
+	O	O	+	O	A
O	+	+	O	O	B
+	+	O	O	O	AB

+ = agglutination
O = no agglutination

Figure 8.   ABO blood grouping by front and back typing.

designed to ascertain whether or not the person's serum contains antierythrocyte antibodies. It is also called reversed typing.

A **secretor** (Figure 9) is an individual who secretes ABH blood group substances into body fluids such as saliva, gastric juice, tears, ovarian cyst fluid, etc. At least 80% of the human population are secretors. The property is genetically determined and requires that the individual be either homozygous dominant (*Se/Se*) or heterozygous (*Se/se*) for the *Se* gene.

The **Rhesus blood group system** (Figure 10) is comprised of Rhesus monkey erythrocyte antigens such as the D antigen that are found on the red cells of most humans, who are said to be Rh positive. This blood group system was discovered by Landsteiner *et al.* in the 1940s when they injected Rhesus monkey erythrocytes into rabbits and guinea pigs. Subsequent studies showed the system to be quite complex, and the rare Rh alloantigens are still not characterized biochemically (Figure 11). Three closely linked pairs of alleles designated

Secretors in ABO Blood Group	Antigens in Saliva
O	A, H
A	B, H
B	A, B, H
AB	H

Figure 9.   The secretor phenomenon in which AB and H substances are detectable in the saliva of individuals with ABO blood groups.

Haplotype	Fisher-Race	Wiener	Frequency (%)	
			Whites	Arican Am.
R¹	CDe	Rh₁	42	17
r	cde	rh	37	26
R²	cDE	Rh₂	14	11
R⁰	cDe	Rh₀	4	44
r′	Cde	rh′	2	2
r″	cdE	rh″	1	<1
Rᶻ	CDE	Rhᵤ	Very rare	Very rare
Rʸ	CdE	rhʸ	Very rare	Very rare

Figure 10. Principal *Rh* genes and their frequencies of occurance among Whites and African Americans.

Dd, Cc, and *Ee* are postulated to be at the Rh locus, which is located on chromosome 1. There are several alloantigenic determinants within the Rh system. Clinically, the D antigen is the one of greatest concern since RhD negative individuals who receive RhD positive erythrocytes by transfusion can develop alloantibodies that may lead to severe reactions with further transfusions of RhD positive blood. The D antigen also poses a problem in RhD negative mothers who bear a

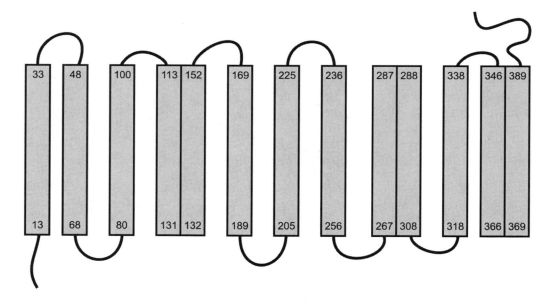

Figure 11.   Schematic representation of the suggested molecular structure of the Rh polypeptide.

child with RhD positive red cells inherited from the father. The entrance of fetal erythrocytes into the maternal circulation at parturition or trauma during the pregnancy (such as in amniocentesis) can lead to alloimmunization against the RhD antigen which may cause hemolytic disease of the newborn in subsequent pregnancies. This is now prevented by the administration of $Rh_o(D)$ immune globulin to these women within 72 hours of parturition. Further confusion concerning this system has been caused by the use of separate designations by the Wiener and Fisher systems. Rh antigens are a group of 7–10 kD erythrocyte membrane-bound antigens that are independent of phosphatides and proteolipids. Antibodies against Rh antigens do not occur naturally in the serum.

Rhesus antigen refers to an erythrocyte antigen of man that shares epitopes in common with rhesus monkey red blood cells. Rhesus antigens are encoded by allelic genes. D antigen has the greatest clinical significance as it may stimulate antibodies in subjects not possessing the antigen and induce hemolytic disease of the newborn or cause transfusion incompatibility reactions. Rhesus antibody reacts with rhesus antigen, especially RhD (Figure 12).

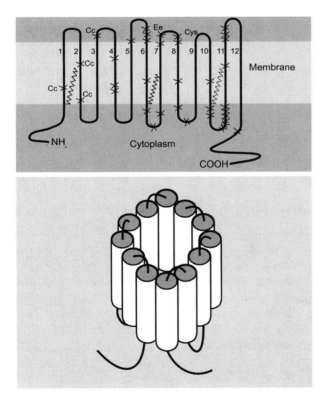

Figure 12. Schematic representation of CcEe and D polypeptide topology within the erythrocyte membrane. There are 12 membrane-spanning domains and cytoplasmic N- and C-termini. The linear diagram depicts probable sites of palmitoylation (Cys-Leu-Pro Motifs).

Anti-D (Figure 13) is an antibody against the Rh blood group D antigen. This antibody is stimulated in RhD negative mothers by fetal RhD positive red blood cells that enter her circulation at parturition. Anti-D antibodies become a problem usually with the third pregnancy resulting from the booster immune response against the D antigen to which the mother was previously exposed. IgG antibodies pass across the placenta leading to hemolytic disease of the newborn (erythroblastosis fetalis). Anti-D antibody (Rhogam®) administered up to 72 hours following parturition may combine with the RhD positive red blood cells in the mother's circulation, thereby facilitating their removal by the reticuloendothelial system. This prevents maternal immunization against the RhD antigen.

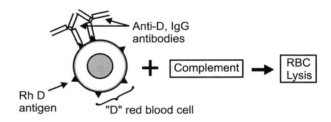

Figure 13. Complement-mediated lysis of RhD antigen positive red blood cells through doublets of anti-D, IgG antibodies on the red cell surface.

Rhesus incompatibility refers to the stimulation of anti-RhD antibodies in a Rh negative mother when challenged by RhD positive red cells of her baby (especially at parturition) that may lead to hemolytic disease of the newborn. The term also refers to the transfusion of RhD positive blood to an Rh negative individual who may form anti-D antibodies against the donor blood leading to subsequent incompatibility reactions if given future RhD positive blood.

Dextrans (Figure 14) of relatively low molecular weight have been used as plasma expanders.

The **Coombs' test** (Figure 15) is an antiglobulin assay that detects immunoglobulin on the surface of a patient's red blood cells. The test was developed by Robin Coombs to demonstrate autoantibodies on the surface of red blood cells that fail to cause agglutination of these red cells. In the direct Coombs' test, rabbit antihuman immunoglobulin is added to a suspension of patient's red cells and if they are coated with autoantibody, agglutination results. In the indirect Coombs' test, the patient's serum can be used to coat erythrocytes which are then washed and the antiimmunoglobulin reagent added to produce agglutination if the antibodies in question had been present in the serum sample. The Coombs' test has long been a part of an autoimmune disease evaluation of patients. An incomplete antibody is nonagglutinating and must have a linking agent such as anti-IgG to reveal its presence in an agglutination reaction.

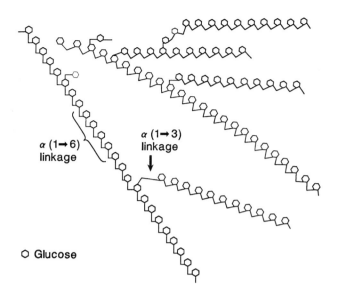

Figure 14. α (1-6) linkages and β (1-3) linkages are shown in the dextran molecule.

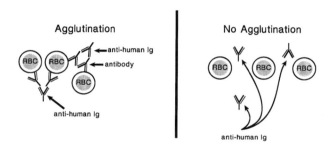

Figure 15. Schematic representation of the mechanism of the Coombs' test.

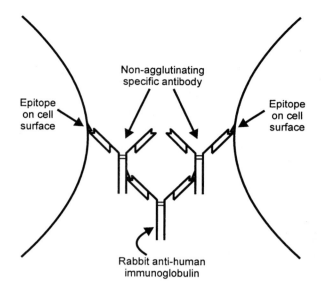

Figure 16. Schematic representation of the mechanism of the antiglobulin test to demonstrate nonagglutinating antibodies on red cell surfaces in autoimmune hemolytic anemia.

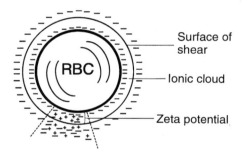

Figure 17. Schematic representation of the zeta potential surrounding red blood cells.

The **antiglobulin test** (Figure 16) is an antibody raised by immunization of one species, such as a rabbit, with immunoglobulin from another species, such as man. Rabbit anti-human globulin has been used for many years in an antiglobulin test to detect incomplete antibodies coating red blood cells as in erythroblastosis fetalis or autoimmune hemolytic anemia. Antiglobulin antibodies are specific for epitopes in the Fc region of immunoglobulin molecules used as immunogen, rendering them capable of agglutinating cells whose surface antigens are combined with the Fab regions of IgG molecules whose Fc regions are exposed.

The **zeta potential** (Figures 17 and 18) is a collective negative charge on erythrocyte surfaces that causes them to repulse one another in cationic medium. Some cations are red cell surface bound whereas others are free in the medium. The boundary of shear is between the two cation planes where the zeta potential may be determined as –mV. IgM antibodies have an optimal zeta potential of –22 to –17mV, and IgG antibodies have an optimum of –11 to –4.5mV. The less the absolute mV, the less the space between cells in

suspension. The addition of certain proteins, such as albumin, to the medium diminishes the zeta potential.

Hemolytic disease of the newborn (HDN) (Figure 19) is a condition in which a fetus with RhD positive red blood cells can stimulate an RhD negative mother to produce anti-RhD IgG antibodies that cross the placenta and destroy the fetal red blood cells when a sufficient titer is obtained. This is usually not until the third pregnancy with an Rh positive fetus. At parturition, the RhD positive red blood cells enter the maternal circulation and subsequent pregnancies provide a booster to this response. With the third pregnancy, a sufficient quantity of high titer antibody crosses the placenta to produce considerable lysis of fetal red blood cells. This may lead to erythroblastosis fetalis (hemolytic disease of the newborn). 70% of HDN cases are due to RhD incompatibility between mother and fetus. Exchange transfusions may be required for treatment. Two other antibodies against erythrocytes that may likewise be a cause for transfusion exchange

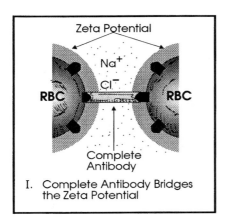

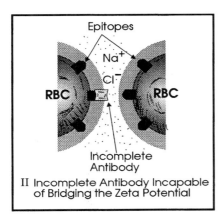

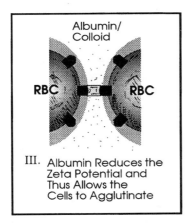

Figure 18. Comparison of the ability of complete antibody to bridge the zeta potential with the inability of incomplete antibody to do so.

include anti-Fy^a and Kell. As bilirubin levels rise, the immature blood-brain barrier permits bilirubin to penetrate and deposit on the basal ganglia. Injection of the mother with anti-D antibody following parturition unites with the RhD+ red cells leading to their elimination by the mononuclear phagocyte system.

P antigen (Figure 20) is an ABH blood group-related antigen found on erythrocyte surfaces that is comprised of the three sugars galactose, N-isoacetyl-galactosamine and N-acetyl-glucosamine. The P antigens are designated P$_1$, P$_2$, P^k and p. P$_2$ subjects rarely produce anti-P$_1$ antibody which may lead to hemolysis in clinical situations. Paroxysmal cold hemagglutinuria patients develop a biphasic autoanti-P antibody that fixes complement in the cold and lyses red blood cells at 37°C.

The **MNSs blood group system** (Figure 21) refers to human erythrocyte glycophorin epitopes. There are four distinct sialoglycoproteins (SGP) on red cell membranes. These include α-SGP (glycophorin A, MN), β-SGP (glycophorin C), γ-SGP (glycophorin D) and δ-SGP (glycophorin B). MN antigens are present on α-SGP and δ-SGP. M and N antigens are present on α-SGP, with approximately one half million copies detectable on each erythrocyte. This is a 31kD structure that is comprised of 131 amino acids with about 60% of the total weight attributable to carbohydrate. This transmembrane molecule has a carboxyl terminus that stretches into the cytoplasm of the erythrocyte with a 23-amino-acid hydrophobic segment embedded in the lipid bilayer. The amino terminal segment extends to the extracellular compartment. Blood group antigen activity is in the external segment. In α-SGP with M antigen activity, the first amino acid is serine and the fifth is glycine. When it carries N antigen activity, leucine and glutamic acid replace serine and glycine at positions 1 and 5, respectively. The Ss antigens are encoded by allelic genes at a locus closely linked to the MN locus. The U antigen is also considered a part of the MNSs system. Whereas anti-M and anti-N antibodies may occur without red cell stimulation, antibodies against Ss and U antigens generally follow erythrocyte stimulation. The MN and Ss alleles positioned on chromosome 4 are linked. Antigens of the MNSs system may provoke the formation of antibodies that can mediate hemolytic disease of the newborn (Figure 22).

The **Lewis blood group system** (Figures 23 and 24) is an erythrocyte antigen system that differs from other red cell groups in that the antigen is present in soluble form in the blood and saliva. Lewis antigens are adsorbed from the plasma onto the red cell membrane. The Lewis phenotype expressed is based on whether the individual is a secretor or a nonsecretor of the Lewis gene product. Expression of the Lewis phenotype is dependent also on the ABO phenotype. Lewis antigens are carbohydrates. Lewis blood secretors have an increased likelihood of urinary tract infections induced by *Escherichia coli* or other microbes because of the linkage of carbohydrate residues of glycolipids and glycoproteins on urothelial cells.

Kell blood group system (Figure 25) was named for an antibody that induces hemolytic disease of the newborn, described in 1946, was specific for the K(KEL1) antigen. 9% of Caucasian and 2% of African Americans have the *K* gene that encodes this antigen. Subsequently, the *K* allele

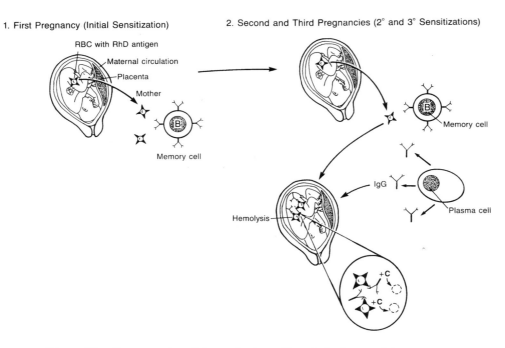

1. First Pregnancy (Initial Sensitization)

2. Second and Third Pregnancies (2° and 3° Sensitizations)

Figure 19.   Representation of the mechanism of hemolytic disease of the newborn.

Phenotype	Reactions with Anti-				Phenotype Frequency	
	P_1	P	P^k	$PP_1 P^k$	Whites	African Am.
P_1	+	+	0	+	79	94
P_2	0	+	0	+	21	6
p	0	0	0	0	Very rare	
P_1^k	+	0	+	+	Very rare	
P_2^k	0	0	+	+	Very rare	

Figure 20.   P antigen.

Reactions		Phenotype	Phenotype Frequency	
Anti-M	Anti-N		Whites	African Am.
+	0	M+N−	28	26
+	+	M+N+	50	45
0	+	M−N+	22	30
Anti-s	Anti-s			
+	0	S+s−	11	3
+	+	S+s+	43	28
0	+	S−s+	45	69
0	0	S−s−	0	<1

Figure 21.   MNSs blood group system.

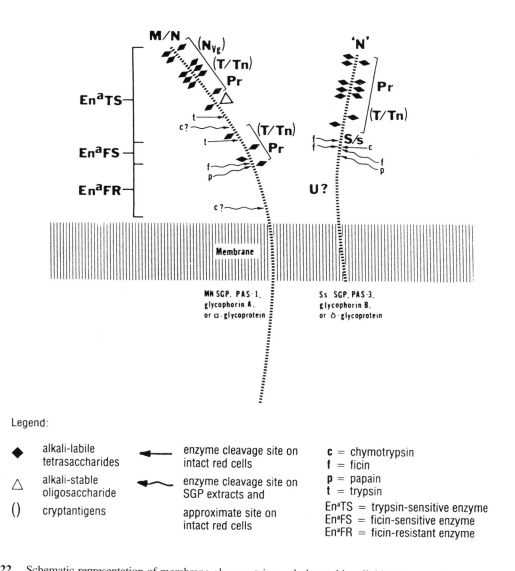

Legend:

◆	alkali-labile tetrasaccharides	←	enzyme cleavage site on intact red cells	**c** = chymotrypsin
△	alkali-stable oligosaccharide	↜	enzyme cleavage site on SGP extracts and	**f** = ficin
()	cryptantigens		approximate site on intact red cells	**p** = papain

c = chymotrypsin
f = ficin
p = papain
t = trypsin
En^{a}TS = trypsin-sensitive enzyme
En^{a}FS = ficin-sensitive enzyme
En^{a}FR = ficin-resistant enzyme

Figure 22. Schematic representation of membrane glycoproteins and glycosphingolipids that carry blood group antigens.

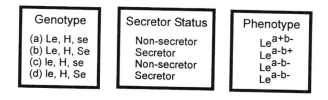

Figure 23. Lewis blood group system.

was identified. Anti-k(KEL2) antibodies reacted with the erythrocytes of more than 99% of the random population. Kell system antigens are present only in relatively low density on the erythrocyte membrane. The strong immunogenicity of the K antigen leads to the presence of anti-K antibodies in sera of transfused patients. Anti-K antibodies cause hemolytic transfusion reactions of both immediate and delayed varieties. 90% of donors are K⁻, which considerably simplifies the task of finding compatible blood for patients with anti-K.

The **Duffy blood group** (Figure 26) is comprised of human erythrocyte epitopes encoded by *Fya* and *Fyb* genes, located on chromosome 1. Since these epitopes are receptors for *Plasmodium vivax*, African-Americans who often express the Fy(a⁻b⁻) phenotype are not susceptible to the type of malaria induced by this species. Mothers immunized through exposure to fetal red cells bearing the Duffy antigens which she does not possess may synthesize antibodies that cross the placenta and induce hemolytic disease of the newborn (Figure 27).

Kidd blood group system (Figure 28) was named fo anti-Jkª antibodies which were originally detected in the blood serum of a woman giving birth to a baby with hemolytic disease of the newborn. Anti-Jkᵇ antibodies were discovered in the serum of a patient following a transfusion reaction.

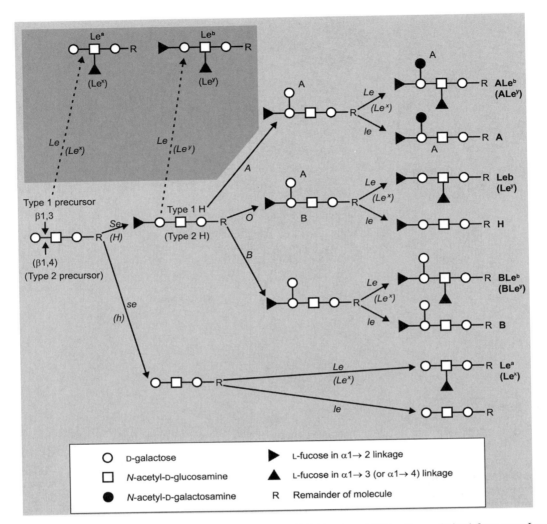

Figure 24.   Schematic representation of the biosynthetic pathways of ABH, Lewis and XY antigens derived from type I and type II core chains. Genes controlling steps in the pathway are shown in italics. Type I and type II precursors differ in the nature of the linkage between the non-reducing terminal galactolose and N-acetylglucosamine: Beta 1–3 in type I and Beta 1–4 in type II. Type II structures and the genes acting on them are shown in parenthesis. Dash lines show how Le^a and (Le^x) Le^d (Le^y), produced from the precursor and H structures, respectively are not substrate for the H–, Se–, or ABO-transferases and remain unconverted.

Phenotype	Reactions with Anti-						Phenotype Frequency	
	K	K	Kp^a	Kp^b	Js^a	Js^b	Whites	African Am.
K+k-	+	0					0.2	Rare
K+k+	+	+					8.8	2
K-k+	0	+					91	98
Kp (a+b-)			+	0			Rare	0
Kp (a+b+)			+	+			2.3	Rare
Kp (a-b+)			0	+			97.7	100
Js (a+b-)					+	0	0	1
Js (a+b+)					+	+	Rare	19
Js (a-b+)					0	+	100	80
K$_0$	0	0	0	0	0	0	Very rare	Very rare

Figure 25.   Kell blood group system.

Phenotype	Reactions with Anti-		Phenotype Frequency	
	Fy^a	Fy^b	Whites	African Am.
Fy (a+b-)	+	0	17	9
Fy (a+b+)	+	+	49	1
Fy (a-b+)	0	+	34	22
Fy (a-b-)	0	0	Very rare	68

Figure 26.   Duffy blood group.

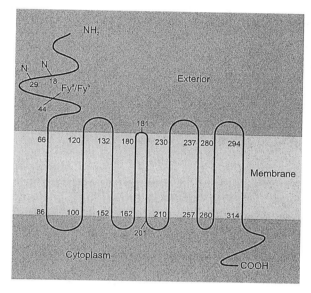

Figure 27.   Schematic representation of the proposed topography of the Duffy glycoprotein within the red cell membrane. Numbers represent amino acid residues with the transcription-initiating methionine residue as 1. An extracellular N-terminal domain of 65 amino acids containing two N-glycosylation sites (N) and the site of the Fy^a/Fy^b polymorphism is followed by nonmembrane-spanning domains, or alternatively seven membrane spanning domains in common with other chemokine receptors.

Phenotype	Reactions with Anti-		Phenotype Frequency	
	Jk^a	Jk^b	Whites	African Am.
Jk (a+b-)	+	0	28	57
Jk (a+b+)	0	+	49	34
Jk (a-b+)	+	+	23	9
Jk (a-b-)	0	0	Very rare	Very rare

Figure 28.   Kidd blood group system.

Although Kidd system antibodies sometimes lead to HDN, it is not usually severe. However, the antibodies are problematic and cause severe hemolytic transfusion reactions, especially of the delayed type. These occur when antibodies developing quickly in a booster response to antigens on transfused erythrocytes destroy red cells in the circulation. As shown in the table, four phenotypes are revealed by the reactions of anti-Jk^a and anti-Jk^b antibodies. A dominant inhibitor gene (*In[Jk]*) may encode a null phenotype. Jk3 is believed to be present on both Jk(a+) and Jk(b+) red cells. Anti-Jk3 is frequently induced by red blood cells stimulation.

Ii antigens (Figure 29) are two nonallelic carbohydrate epitopes on the surface membrane of human erythrocytes. They may also occur on some nonhematopoietic cells. The

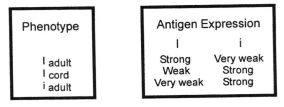

Figure 29.   Ii antigens.

| Phenotype | Reactions with Anti- | | Phenotype Frequency |
	Lu^a	Lu^b	
Lu (a+b-)	+	0	0.15
Lu (a+b+)	+	+	7.5
Lu (a-b+)	0	+	92.35
Lu (a-b-)	0	0	Very rare

Figure 30.   Lutheran blood group.

Phenotype	C4d Component Present	Frequency (%) Whites
Ch(a+), Rg(a+)	C4dS, C4df	95
Ch(a-), Rg(a+)	C4df	2
Ch(a+), Rg(a-)	C4dS	3
Ch(a-), Rg(a-)	None	Very rare

Figure 31.   Chido (Ch) and Rodgers (Rg) antigens.

i epitope is found on fetal erythrocytes and red cell blood precursors. The I antigen is formed when aliphatic galactose-N-acetyl-glucosamine is converted to a complex branched structure. I represents the mature form and i the immature form. Mature erythrocytes express I. Antibodies against i antigen are hemolytic in cases of infectious mononucleosis.

The **Lutheran blood group** (Figure 30) consists of human erythrocyte epitopes recognized by alloantibodies against Lu^a and Lu^b products. Antibodies developed against Lutheran antigens during pregnancy may induce hemolytic disease of the newborn.

The **Chido (Ch) and Rodgers (Rg) antigens** (Figure 31) are epitopes of C4d fragments of human complement component C4. They are not intrinsic to the erythrocyte membrane. The Chido epitope is found on C4d from C4B, whereas the Rodgers epitope is found on C4A derived from C4d. The Rodgers epitope is Val-Asp-Leu-Leu, and the Chido epitope is Ala-Asp-Leu-Arg. They are situated at residue positions 1188–1191 in the C4 α chain's C4d region. Antibodies against Ch and Rg antigenic determinants agglutinate saline suspensions of red blood cells coated with C4d.

Since C4 is found in human serum, anti-Ch and anti-Rg are neutralized by sera of most individuals which contain the relevant antigens. Ficin and papain destroy these antigens.

C4A is a very polymorpholic molecule expressing the Rodgers epitope that is encoded by the *C4A* gene. The equivalent murine gene encodes sex-limited protein (SLP). It has less hemolytic activity than does C4B. C4A and C4B differ in only 4 amino acid residues in the α chain's C4d region. C4A is Pro-Cys-Pro-Bal-Leu-Asp, whereas C4B is Leu-Ser-Pro-Bal-Ile-His.

C4B is a polymorpholic molecule that usually expresses the Chido epitope and is encoded by the *C4B* gene. The murine equivalent gene encodes Ss protein. It shows greater hemolytic activity than does C4A.

Xg^a, the sex-linked blood antigen (Figure 32) is an antibody more common in women than in men. It is specific for the Xg^a antigen, in recognition of its X-born pattern of inheritance. This table gives phenotype frequencies in Caucasian males and females. The antibody is relatively uncommon and has not been implicated in hemolytic disease of the

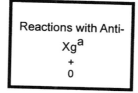

Figure 32. Xgᵃ, the sex-linked blood antigen.

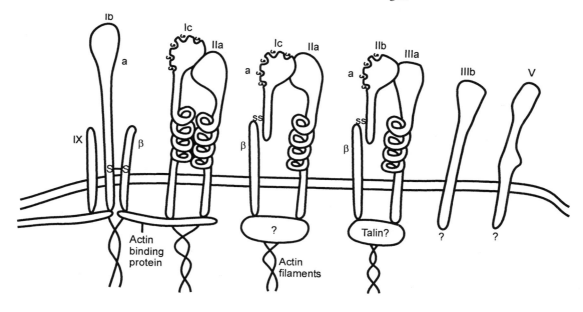

Figure 33. Schematic representation of the principal platelet membrane glycoproteins indicating known or suspected complexes, disulfide bonds between chains, calcium-bonding domains and interactions with cytoskeletal components.

newborn or in hemolytic transfusion reactions even though it can bind complement and may occasionally be an autoantibody. Anti-Xgᵃ antibodies might be of value in identifying genetic traits transmitted in association with the X chromosome.

Platelet antigens are surface epitopes on thrombocytes that may be immunogenic leading to platelet antibody formation leading to such conditions as neonatal alloimmune thrombocytopenia and post-transfusion purpura. The Plᴬ¹ antigen may induce platelet antibody formation in Plᴬ¹ antigen-negative individuals. Additional platelet antigens associated with purpura include Plᴬ², Bakᵃ, and HLA-A2. Bakᵃ is a normal human platelet (thrombocyte) antigen. Anti-Bakᵃ IgG antibody synthesized by a Bakᵃ negative pregnant female may be passively transferred across the placenta to induce immune thrombocytopenia in the neonate.

Platelets possess surface FcγRII that combine to IgG or immune complexes (Figures 33 and 34). The platelet surfaces can become saturated with immune complexes as in autoimmune (or idiopathic) thrombocytopenic purpura (ITP) or AITP. Fab-mediated antibody binding to platelet antigens

may be difficult to distinguish from Fc-mediated binding of immune complexes to the surface.

The administration of platelet concentrates prepared by centrifuging a unit of whole blood at low speed to provide 40 to 70 ml of plasma that contains 3 to 4 × 10¹¹ platelets for platelet transfusion. This amount can increase an adult's platelet concentration by 10,000/mm³ blood. It is best to store platelets at 20 to 24°C, subjecting them to mild agitation. They must be used within five days of collection.

Transfusion reaction(s) may be either immune or nonimmune and follow the administration of blood. Transfusion reactions with immune causes are considered serious and occur in 1 in 3,000 transfusions. Patients may develop urticaria, itching, fever, chills or even collapse, chest pains, cyanosis and hemorrhage. The appearance of these symptoms together with an increase in temperature by 1°C signals the need to halt the transfusion. Immune, noninfectious transfusion reactions include allergic urticaria (immediate hypersensitivity), anaphylaxis, as in the administration of blood to IgA deficient subjects, some of whom develop anti-IgA antibodies of the IgE class, and serum sickness, in which

Antigen System	Glycoprotein (GP) Location	Other Names	Antigens	Other Names	Phenotype Frequency (%)	
					White	Japanese
HPA-1	GPIIIa	Zw, Pl^A	HPA-1a	Zw^a, Pl^{A1}	97.9	99.9
			HPA-1b	Zw^b, Pl^{A2}	26.5	3.7
HPA-2	GPIb	Ko, Sib	HPA-2a	Ko^b	99.3	NT
			HPA-2b	Ko^a, Sib^a	14.6	25.4
HPA-3	GPIIb	Bak, Lek	HPA-3a	Bak^a, Lek^a	87.7	78.9
			HPA-3b	Bak^b	64.1	NT
HPA-4	GPIIIa	Pen, Yuk	HPA-4a	Pen^a, Yuk^b	99.9	99.9
			HPA-4b	Pen^b, Yuk^a	0.2	1.7
HPA-5	GPIa	Br, Hc, Zav	HPA-5a	Br^b, Zav	99.2	NT
			HPA-5b	Br^a, Zav^a, Hc^a	20.6	NT

Figure 34.   Nomenclature and phenotype frequency of human platelet antigens.

the serum proteins such as immunoglobulins induce the formation of precipitating antibodies that lead to immune complex formation.

TRALI (transfusion-related acute lung injury) (Figure 35) is a form of acute respiratory distress that often occurs within four hours following a blood transfusion. It is attributable to leukocyte antibodies and is an acute pulmonary reaction leading to noncardiac pulmonary edema. It is a form of ARDS with a reasonably good prognosis. Mortality is 10% as opposed to 50% to 60% for other forms of ARDS. 80% of TRALI patients experience rapid resolution of pulmonary infiltrates and restoration of arterial blood gas values to normal within 96 hours. 17% of TRALI patients retain pulmonary infiltrates for a week following the transfusion reactions. TRALI reactions have been reported in 1 in 5000 units of blood transfused. Leukoagglutinating antibodies as well as some lymphocytotoxins have been implicated. The offending antibody is passively transfused in donor plasma rather than the donor's leukocytes reacting with recipient antibody. Both donor granulocyte antibodies and donor lymphocyte antibodies have been implicated in TRALI reactions. 65% of cases revealed the presence of HLA-specific antibodies. However, HLA antibodies may be present in the plasma of donors but not cause TRALI reactions. Donor plasma implicated in TRALI reactions are often from multiparous females and individuals who have received multiple blood transfusions. There is difficulty in explaining the pathophysiology of a mechanism whereby such a small amount of antibody could induce a severe clinical reaction unless it initiates an amplification mechanism such as activation of complement. Such a mechanism could cause the formation of C5a that attaches to granulocytes altering their membrane in such a way that they adhere nonspecifically to various surfaces. Once these cells are sequestered in the pulmonary vascular bed they may become activated and release proteolytic enzymes in toxic oxygen metabolites leading to acute lung injury. Pulmonary sequestration of granulocytes could lead to further endothelial injury and microvascular occlusion. The activation of complement, generation of C5a and pulmonary sequestration of granulocytes that occurs when blood comes into contact with hemodialysis membranes further supports a role for complement activation. In summary, TRALI depends on the simultaneous presence of antibody, complement and antigen positive cells leading to extensive capillary leakage.

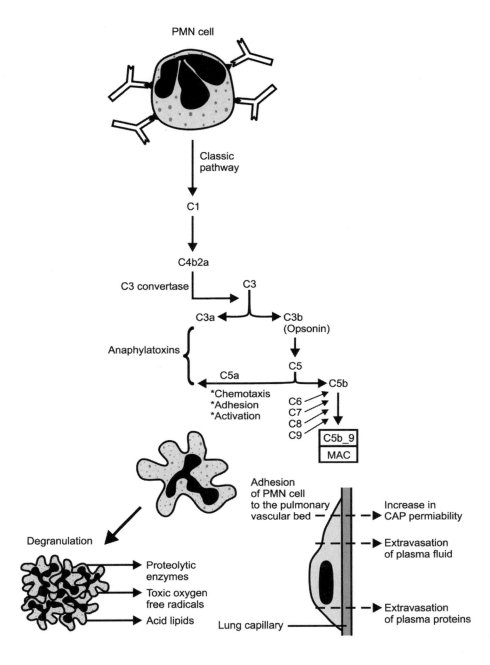

Figure 35. Schematic representation of molecular and cellular events that lead to the production of transfusion-related acute lung injury (TRALI), believed to be a form of adult respiratory distress syndrome (ARDS).

16

Immunological Diseases and Immunopathology

Immunological diseases include those conditions in which there is either an abberation in the immune response or the immune response to the disease agent leads to pathological changes. This category includes diseases with an immunological etiology or pathogenesis, immunodeficiency, hyperactivity of the immune response, or autoimmunity that leads to pathological sequelae.

BLOOD

Autoimmune neutropenia can be either an isolated condition or secondary to autoimmune disease. Patients may either have recurrent infections or remain asymptomatic. Antigranulocyte antibodies may be demonstrated. There is normal bone marrow function with myeloid hyperplasia and a shift to the left as a result of increased granulocyte destruction. The autoantibody may suppress myeloid cell growth. The condition is treated by immunosuppressive drugs, corticosteroids or splenectomy. Patients with systemic lupus erythematosus, Felty's syndrome (rheumatoid arthritis, splenomegaly and severe neutropenia) as well as other autoimmune diseases may manifest autoimmune neutropenia.

Idiopathic thrombocytopenic purpura is an autoimmune disease in which antiplatelet autoantibodies destroy platelets. Splenic macrophages remove circulating platelets coated with IgG autoantibodies at an accelerated rate. Thrombocytopenia occurs even though the bone marrow increases platelet production. This can lead to purpura and bleeding. The platelet count may fall below 20,000 to 30,000/μL. Antiplatelet antibodies are detectable in the serum and on platelets. Platelet survival is decreased. Splenectomy is recommended in adults. Corticosteroids facilitate a temporary elevation in the platelet count. This disease is characterized by decreased blood platelets, hemorrhage and extensive thrombotic lesions.

Acute lymphoblastic leukemia (ALL) (Figures 1–4) consist of a heterogeneous group of lymphopoietic stem cell disorders in which lymphoblasts accumulate in the bone marrow and suppress normal hemopoietic cells. Eighty percent of ALL cases are of the B cell type whereas the remainder are T cell with rare cases of null cell origin. Ten percent of leukemias as ALL and 60% of ALL cases are in children. Chromosomal abnormalities have been found in most cases of ALL. B-ALL (L3) is characterized by one of three chromosomal translocations. Most B-ALL cases have a translo-

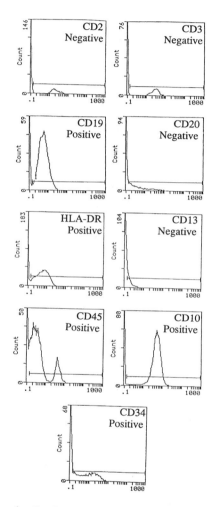

Figure 1. Pre-B cell acute lymphoblastic leukemia.

cation of *c-myc* protooncogene on chromosome 8 to the immunoglobulin coding gene region on chromosome 14. Lymphoblasts that are unable to differentiate and mature continue to accumulate in the bone marrow. ALL patients develop anemia, granulocytopenia and thrombocytopenia. L1, L2 and L3 lymphoblast cytologic subtypes are recognized. ALL is diagnosed by the demonstration of lymphoblasts in the bone marrow. The total leukocyte count is normal or decreased in half the cases with or without lymphoblast in the peripheral blood. An elevated leukocyte count is usually accompanied by lymphoblast in the peripheral blood. Patients develop a normal chromic, normocytic ane-

283

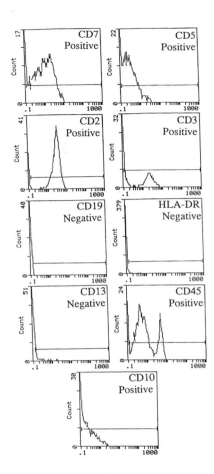

Figure 2.   T cell acute lymphocytic leukemia (T-ALL).

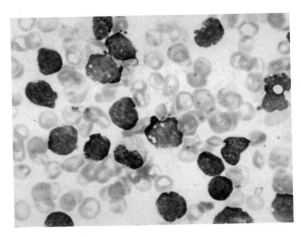

Figure 3.   Acute lymphoblastic leukemia (ALL).

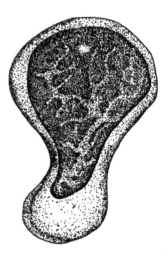

Figure 4.   Hand mirror cell.

mia with thrombocytopenia and neutropenia. They may develop weakness, malaise, and pallor, secondary to anemia. Half the individuals develop bleeding secondary to thrombocytopenia and many develop bacterial infections secondary to neutropenia. Patients also experience bone pain. There is generalized lymphadenopathy especially affecting the cervical lymph nodes. Frequently, there is hepatosplenomegaly and leukemic meningitis. Age at onset and initial total blood leukocyte count are valuable prognostic features. Ninety percent of children with L1 morphology cells experience complete clinical remission with chemotherapy.

B-cell chronic lymphocytic leukemia (B-CLL) (Figure 5) is a lymphoproliferative disorder characterized by sustained lymphocytosis of lymphocytes that are light chain-restricted. There is splenomegaly, lymphadenopathy and hepatomegaly with lymphocytosis ranging from 4×10^9/L to lymphocyte counts exceeding 400×10^9/L. The lymphocytes are relatively small with condensed nuclear chromatin and sparse cytoplasm. They have a uniform appearance and injured cells are often present. Injured cells are often present. Nucleoli are not usually visible. The mixed cell type may reveal both large and small lymphocytes. The more diffuse the pattern of involvement, the more aggressive the disease. B cell CLL

lymphocytes express pan-B cell antigens and meager quantities of light chain-restricted immunoglobulins on the cell surface. The lymphocytes usually express CD5, a pan T cell antigen and rosette spontaneously with mouse red blood cells. One half to three-fourths of B-CLL patients are hypogammaglobulinemic. Autoimmune hemolytic anemia, neutropenia or thrombocytopenia develop in 15 to 30% of cases. Those cases of B cell CLL that become aggress-ive with pyrexic, weight loss and fatigue and large cell lymphoma are referred to as having undergone Richter transformation, usually leading to death.

CD10 (CALLA) is an antigen, also referred to as common acute lymphoblastic leukemia antigen (CALLA), that has a MW of 100 kD. CD10 is now known to be a neutral endopeptidase (enkephalinase). It is present on many cell types, including stem cells, lymphoid progenitors of B and T cells, renal epithelium, fibroblasts, and bile canaliculi.

Acute myelogenous leukemias (AML) (Figure 6) consist of a heterogeneous group of disorders characterized by neo-

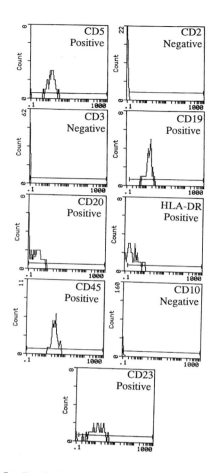

Figure 5. B cell chronic lymphocytic leukemia (B-CLL).

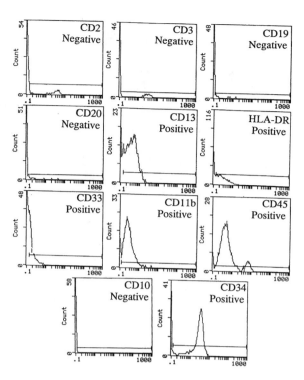

Figure 6. Acute myeloid leukemia (AML).

plastic transformation in a multipotential hematopoietic stem cell or in one of restricted lineage potential. Since multipotential hematopoietic stem cells of the precursors of granulocytes, monocytes, erythrocytes and megakaryocytes, one or all of these cell types may be affected. Differentiation usually ends at the blast cell stage causing myeloblasts to accumulate in the bone marrow. AML is diagnosed by the discovery of 30% myelogenous blasts in the bone marrow, whether or not they are present in the peripheral blood. The total peripheral blood leukocyte count may be normal, low or elevated. There may be thrombocytopenia, neutropenia and anemia. The presenting symptoms and signs are non-specific and may be secondary to anemia. Patients may experience fatigue, weakness, and pallor. One-third of AML patients are found to have hepatosplenomegaly. One-third of patients may have bleeding secondary to thrombocytopenia. GI tract or CNS hemorrhage may occur when platelet counts decrease below 20,000/µL. Decreased neutrophil counts may increase secondary infections.

Unfavorable prognostic findings include (1) an age of diagnosis greater than 60 years, (2) 5q- and 7q- chromosomal abnormalities, (3) a history of myelodysplastic syndrome, (4) a history of radiation or chemotherapy for cancer, and

(5) a leukocytosis exceeding 100,000/µL. If untreated, AML leads to death in less than two months through hemorrhage or infection. Both chemotherapy and bone marrow transplantation are modes of therapy.

Philadelphia chromosome (Figures 7 and 8) is the translocation of one arm of chromosome 22 to chromosome 9 or 6 in chronic granulocytic leukemia cells in humans.

Angioimmunoblastic lymphadenopathy (AILA) (Figure 9) is the proliferation of hyperimmune B lymphocytes. Immunoblasts, both large and small, form a pleomorphic infiltrate together with plasma cells in lymph nodes revealing architectural effacement. There is arborization of newly formed vessels and proliferating vessels with hyperplasia of endothelial cells. In the interstitium amorphous eosinophilic PAS-positive deposits, possibly representing debris from cells, is found. Fever, night sweats, weight loss, generalized lymphadenopathy, hepatosplenomegaly, hemolytic anemia, polyclonal gammopathy and skin rashes may characterize the disease in middle aged to older subjects. Patients live approximately 15 months with some developing immunoblastic lymphomas or monoclonal gammopathy. AILA must be differentiated from AIDS, Hodgkin's disease, immunoblastic lymphoma, histocytosis X and a variety of other conditions affecting the lymphoid tissues.

Plasmacytoma (Figure 10) is a plasma cell neoplasm. Also termed myeloma or multiple myeloma. To induce an experimental plasmacytoma in laboratory mice or rats, paraffin oil is injected into the peritoneum. Plasmacytomas may

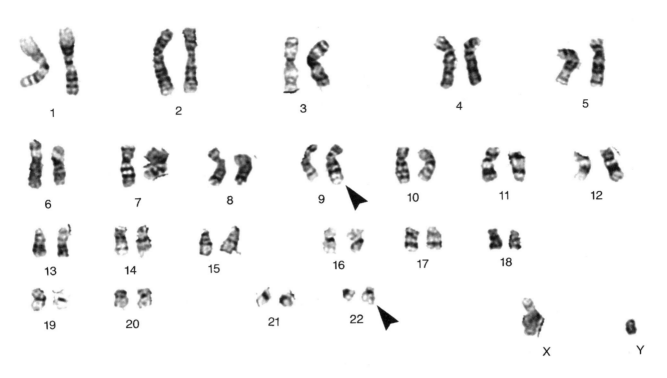

Figure 7.   Philadelphia chromosome.

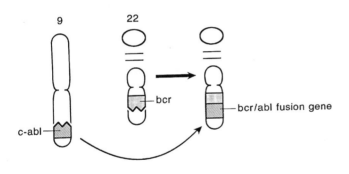

Figure 8.   Philadelphia chromosome.

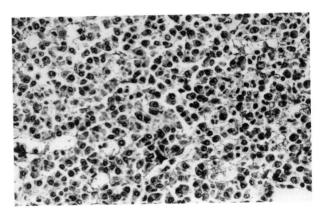

Figure 10.   Bone marrow plasmacytoma with pure plasma cell infiltrate.

occur spontaneously. These tumors, comprised of neoplastic plasma cells, synthesize and secrete monoclonal immunoglobulins yielding a homogeneous product that forms a spike in electrophoretic analysis of the serum. Plasmacytomas were used extensively to generate monoclonal immunoglobulins prior to the development of B cell hybridoma technology to induce monoclonal antibody synthesis at will to multiple antigens.

Hodgkin's disease (Figure 11) is a type of lymphoma that involves the lymph nodes and spleen causing a replacement of the lymph node architecture with binucleated giant cells

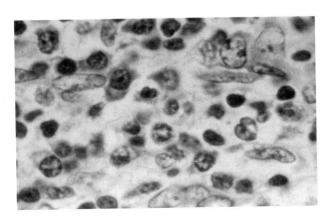

Figure 9.   Angioimmunoblastic lymphadenopathy

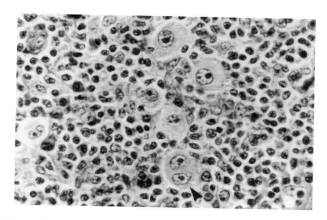

Figure 11. Hodgkin's disease. Hodgkin cell and Reed-Sternberg cell.

known as Reed Sternberg cells, reticular cells, neutrophils, eosinophils, and lymphocytes. There is both lymphadenopathy and splenomegaly. Patients manifest a deficiency of cell-mediated immunity which causes skin tests of the tuberculin type to be negative. By contrast, there is no alteration in their B cell function. They may have an increase in suppressor cell activity. There is also increased susceptibility to opportunistic infections.

Reed-Sternberg cells (Figures 12 and 13) are binucleated giant cells that contain prominent nucleoli. They are classically associated with Hodgkin's disease.

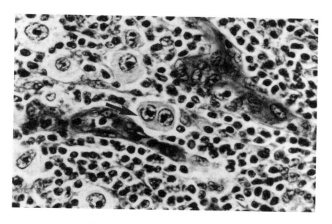

Figure 12. Reed-Sternberg cell.

SKIN

Allergic contact dermatitis is delayed-type hypersensitivity mediated by specifically sensitized T lymphocytes (type IV hypersensitivity) in response to the covalent linkage of low molecular weight chemicals, often of less than 1,000 M_r to proteins in the skin. The inflammation induced by these agents is manifested as erythema and swelling at approximately 12 hours after contact and is maximal at 24 to 48 hours. Blisters form that are filled with serum, neutrophils and mononuclear cells. There is perivascular cuffing with

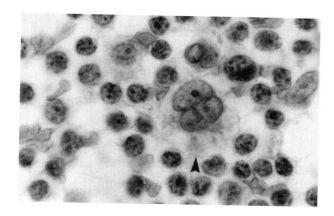

Figure 13. Touch preparation. Reed-Sternberg cell.

lymphocytes, vesiculation and necrosis of epidermal cells. Basophils, eosinophils and fibrin deposition appear together with edema of the epidermis and dermis. Langerhans cells in the skin serve as antigen processing cells where the allergen has penetrated. Sensitization lasts for many years and becomes generalized in the skin. Chemicals become conjugated to skin proteins and serve as haptens. Therefore, the hapten alone can elicit the hypersensitivity once sensitization is established. After blistering, there is crust formation and weeping of the lesion. It is intensely pruritic and painful. Metal dermatitis, such as that caused by nickel, occurs as a patch which corresponds to the area of contact with the metal or jewelry. Dyes in clothing may produce skin lesions at points of contact with the skin. The patch test is used to detect sensitivity to contact allergens. Rhus dermatitis represents a reaction to urushiols in poison oak or ivy which elicit vesicles and bullae on affected areas. Treatment is with systemic corticosteroids or the application of topical steroid cream to localized areas. Dinitrochlorobenzene (DNCB) and dinitrofluorobenzene (DNFB) are chemicals that have been used to induce allergic contact dermatitis in both experimental animals and in man.

Atopic dermatitis (Figure 14) is a chronic eczematous skin reaction marked by hyperkeratosis and spongiosis especially in children with a genetic predisposition to allergy. These are often accompanied by elevated serum IgE levels, which are not proved to produce the skin lesions.

Bullous pemphigoid (Figures 15 and 16) is a blistering skin disease with fluid filled bullae developing at flexor surfaces of extremities, groin, axillae and inferior abdomen. IgG is deposited in a linear pattern at the lamina lucida of the dermal-epidermal junction in most (50–90%) patients and linear C3 in nearly all cases. The blisters are subepidermal bullae filled with fluid containing fibrin, neutrophils, eosinophils and lymphocytes. Antigen-antibody-complement interaction and mast cell degranulation release mediators that attract inflammatory cells and facilitate dermal-epidermal separation.

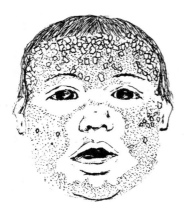

Figure 14. Atopic dermatitis.

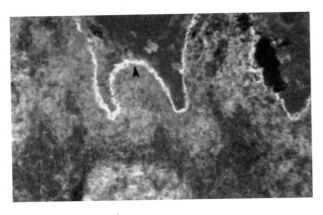

▲ bulla formation
▲ linear IgG and C3
   at dermal-epidermal junction

Figure 15. Bullous pemphigoid.

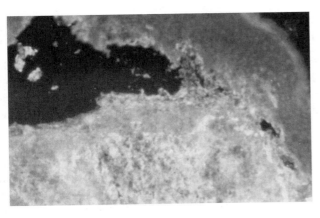

Figure 16. Bullous pemphigoid.

Pemphigus vulgaris (Figures 17–19) is a blistering lesion of the skin and mucous membranes. The bullae develop on normal appearing skin and rupture easily. The blisters are prominent on both oral and anal genital mucous membranes. The disorder may have an insidious onset appearing in middle aged individuals and tends to be chronic. It may be associated with autoimmune diseases, thymoma and myasthenia gravis. Certain drugs may induce a pemphigus-like condition. By light microscopy, intraepidermal bullae are present. There is suprabasal epidermal acantholysis with only mild inflammatory reactivity in early pemphigus. Suprabasal unilocular bullae develop and there are autoantibodies to intercellular substance with activation of classic pathway- mediated immunologic injury. Acantholysis results as the epidermal cells become disengaged from one another as the bulla develops. Epidermal proteases activated by autoantibodies may actually cause the loss of intercellular bridges. Immunofluorescence staining reveals IgG, Clq and C3 in the intercellular substance between epidermal cells. 80 to 90% of pemphigus vulgaris patients have circulating pemphigus antibodies. Their titer usually correlates positively with clinical manifestations. Corticosteroids and immunosuppressive therapy as well as plasmapheresis have been used with some success.

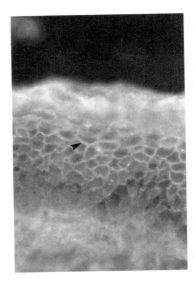

Figure 17. Pemphigus vulgaris. "Chickenwire staining" antibody to intercellular antigen.

Erythema multiforme (Figure 20) is a skin lesion resulting from subcutaneous vasculitis produced by immune complexes, that are frequently linked to drug reactions. The lesions are identified by a red center encircled by an area of pale edema which is encircled by a red or erythematous ring. This gives it a target appearance. Erythema multiforme usually signifies drug allergy or may be linked to systemic infection. Lymphocytes and macrophages infiltrate the lesions. When there is involvement and sloughing of the

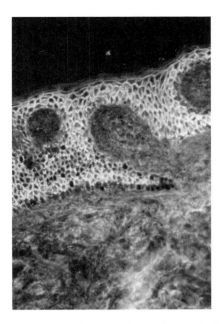

Figure 18. Pemphigus vulgaris. "Chickenwire staining" antibody to intercellular antigen.

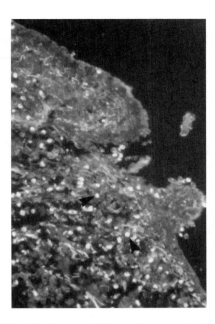

Figure 20. Erythema multiforme. Immunocytes in dermis.

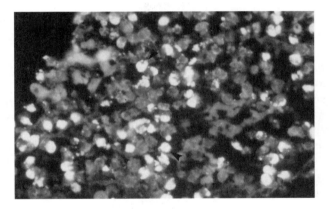

Figure 21. Immunocytes in reticular dermis.

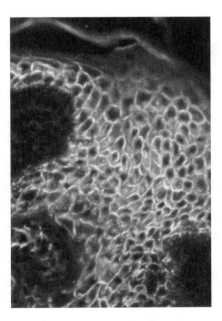

Figure 19. Pemphigus vulgaris. "Chickenwire staining" antibody to intercellular antigen at higher magnification.

mucous membranes, the lesion is considered quite severe and even life-threatening. This form is called the Stevens-Johnson syndrome.

Immunocyte (Figures 21 and 22) literally means "immune cell". A term sometimes used by pathologists to describe plasma cells in stained tissue sections, e.g., in the papillary or reticular dermis in erythema multiforme.

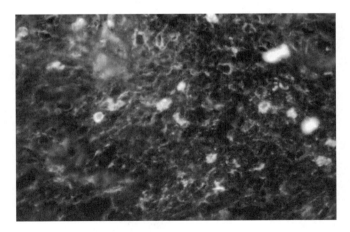

Figure 22. Immunocytes in dermis.

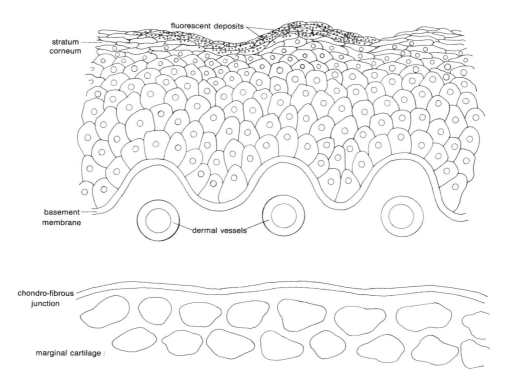

stratum
corneum

fluorescent deposits

basement
membrane

dermal vessels

chondro-fibrous
junction

marginal cartilage

Figure 23. Psoriasis vulgaris.

Psoriasis vulgaris (Figure 23) is a chronic, recurrent papulosquamous disease. Clinical features include the appearance of a discrete, papulosquamous plaque on areas of
trauma such as the elbow, knee or scalp, although it may
appear elsewhere on the skin. There is a relatively high
instance of HLA-B13 and B17 antigen and decreased T
suppressor cell function in psoriasis patients. It may coexist
with lupus erythematosus in some individuals. Peripheral
blood helper/inducer CD4+ T lymphocytes are significantly
decreased in psoriasis patients. It may be treated with pso-
ralens and long-wave ultraviolet radiation. Psoriasis patients
develop Monro microabscesses, hyperkeratosis, parakerato-
sis, irregular acanthosis, papillary edema and mild chronic
inflammation of the dermis. By immunofluorescence, there
are focal granular or globular deposits of immunoglobulins
and C3 in the stratum corneum. The finely granular deposits
principally contain IgG, IgA and C3. They are deposited in
areas where stratum corneum antigens are located. C3 and
properdin deposits suggest activation of the alternate complement pathway.

VASCULATURE

Leukocytoclastic vasculitis (Figure 24) is a type of vasculitis in which there is karyorrhexis of inflammatory cell
nuclei. Fragments of neutrophil nuclei immune complexes
are deposited in vessels. Direct immunofluorescence reveals
IgM, C3 and fibrin in vessel walls. There is nuclear dust,
necrotic debris and fibrin staining of the post capillary

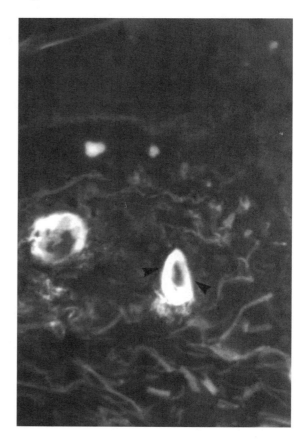

Figure 24. Leukocytoclastic vasculitis.

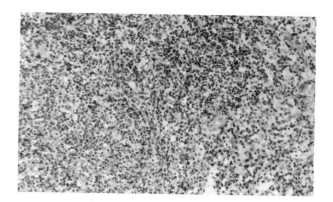

Figure 25.   Inflammation of ethmoid and maxillary sinuses.

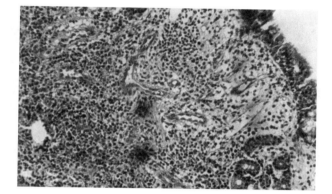

Figure 26.   Necrosis in respiratory epithelium.

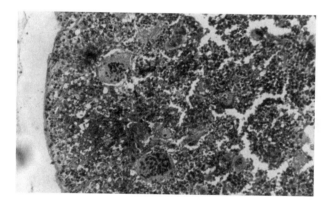

Figure 27.   Giant cells in the respiratory epithelium.

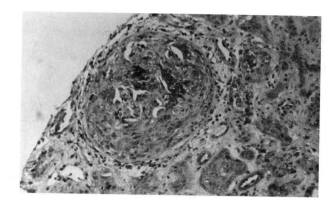

Figure 28.   Obsolescent renal glomerulus in Wegener's granulomatosis.

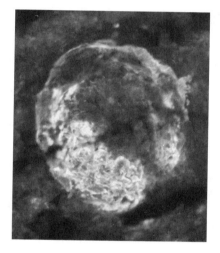

Figure 29.   Immunofluorescence of renalglomerulis in Wegener's granulomatosis.

antineutrophil cytoplasmic antibodies (ANCA). It may be treated successfully in many subjects by cyclophosphamide therapy (Figures 28 and 29).

Anti-neutrophil cytoplasmic antibodies (ANCA) (Figure 30) are antibodies detected in 84–100% of generalized active Wegener's granulomatosis patients. These antibodies react with the cytoplasm of fixed neutrophils. They may also be detected in patients with microscopic polyarteritis. ANCA may be quantified by flow cytometry in conjunction with indirect immunofluorescence microscopy which permits observation of antibody reactivity with the cytoplasm. There is a positive correlation between antibody levels and disease activity, with a decrease following therapy. The staining pattern is to be distinguished from that produced by anti-myeloperoxidase antibodies that display perinuclear staining. One of the antibodies producing diffuse cytoplasmic fluorescence is against proteinase 3. Sera from some HIV positive subjects may prove false-positive for ANCA.

venules. Leukocytoclastic vasculitis represents a type of allergic cutaneous arteriolitis or necrotizing angiitis. It is seen in a variety of diseases including Henoch-Schonlein purpura, rheumatoid arthritis, polyarteritis nodosa and Wegener's granulomatosis, as well as other diseases.

Wegener's granulomatosis (Figures 25–27) refers to necrotizing sinusitis with necrosis of both the upper and lower respiratory tract. The disease is characterized by granulomas, vasculitis, granulomatous arteritis and glomerulonephritis. The condition is believed to have an immunological etiology although this remains to be proven. Patients develop

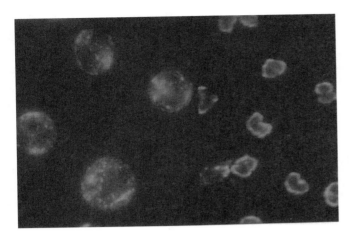

Figure 30.   Anti-neutrophil cytoplasmic antibodies (ANCA).

Polyarteritis nodosa is a necrotizing vasculitis of small and medium sized muscular arteries. It often involves renal and visceral arteries and spares the pulmonary circulation. The disease is often characterized by immune complex deposition in arteries, often associated with chronic hepatitis B virus infection. Early lesions of the vessels often reveal hepatitis B surface antigen, IgM and complement components. This uncommon disease has a male/female ratio of 2.5 to 1. Forty-five years of age is the mean age at onset. Characteristically the kidneys, heart, abdominal organs and both peripheral and central nervous systems are involved. Lesions of vessels are segmental and show preference for branching and bifurcation in small and medium sized muscular arteries. Usually the venules and veins are unaffected and only rarely are granulomas formed. Characteristically aneurysms form following destruction of the media and internal elastic lamina. There is proliferation of the endothelium with degeneration of the vessel wall and fibrinoid necrosis, thrombosis, ischemia and infarction developing. Other than hepatitis B, polyarteritis nodosa is also associated with tuberculosis, streptococcal infections and otitis media. Presenting signs and symptoms include weakness, abdominal pain, leg pain, fever, cough and neurologic symptoms. There may be kidney involvement, arthritis, arthralgia or myalgia as well as hypertension. 40% of patients may have skin involvement manifested as a maculopapular rash. Laboratory findings include elevated erythrocyte sedimentation rate, leukocytosis, anemia, thrombocytosis and cellular casts in the urinary sediment signifying renal glomerular disease. Angiography is important in revealing the presence of aneurysm and changes in vessel caliber. There is no diagnostic immunologic test but immune complexes, cryoglobulins, rheumatoid factor and diminished complement component levels are often found. Biopsies may be taken from skeletal muscle or nerves for diagnostic purposes. Corticosteroids may be used but cyclophosphamide is the treatment of choice in the severe progressive form. Hypersensitivity angiitis is a type of small vessel inflammation most frequently induced by drugs.

Henoch-Schoenlein purpura is a systemic form of small vessel vasculitis that is characterized by arthralgias, nonthromocytopenic purpuric skin lesions, abdominal pain with bleeding and renal disease. Immunologically, immune complexes containing IgA activate the alternate pathway of complement. Patients may present with upper respiratory infections preceding onset of the disease. Certain drugs, food and immunizations have also been suspected as etiologic agents. The disease usually occurs in children 4 to 7 years of age although it can occur in adults. Histopathologically, there is a diffuse leukocytoclastic vasculitis involving small vessels. The submucosa or subserosa of the bowel may be sites of hemorrhage. There may be focal or diffuse glomerulonephritis in the kidneys. Children may manifest lesions associated with the skin, gastrointestinal tract or joints, whereas in adults the disease is usually associated with skin findings. The skin lesions begin as a pleuritic urticarial lesion that develops into a pink maculopapular spot which matures into a raised and darkened lesion. The maculopapular lesion may ultimately resolve in two weeks without leaving a scar. Patients may also have arthralgias associated with the large joints of the lower extremities. Skin biopsy reveals the vasculitis and immunofluorescence examination shows IgA deposits in vessel walls which is in accord with a diagnosis of Henoch-Schoenlein purpura.

MUSCLE

Inflammatory myopathy (Figure 31) occurs when there is a necrosis and phagocytosis of muscle fibers with inflammatory cells.

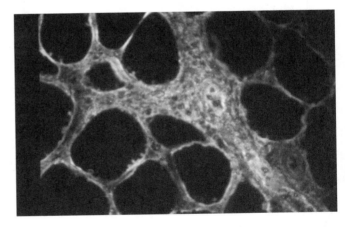

Figure 31.   Inflammatory myopathy. Both regenerating and atrophic fibers are present with fibrosis.

Dermatoysitis (Figures 32–34) is a connective tissue or collagen disease characterized by skin rash and muscle inflammation. It is a type of polymyositis presenting with a purple-tinged skin rash that is prominent on the superior

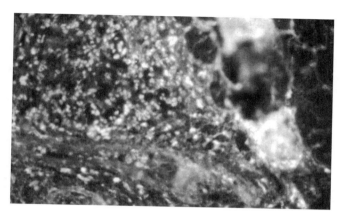

Figure 32.   Dermatomyositis. Anti IgG staining.

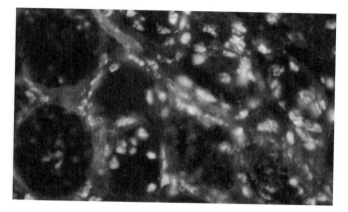

Figure 33.   Dermatomyositis. Anti IgG staining.

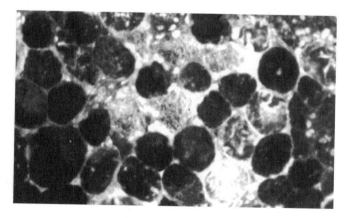

Figure 34.   Dermatomyositis. Anti IgG staining.

eyelids, extensor joint surfaces, and base of the neck. There is weakness, muscle pain, edema, and calcium deposits in the subcutaneous tissue, especially prominent late in the disease. Blood vessels reveal lymphocyte cuffing, and autoantibodies against tRNA synthetases appear in the serum.

Polymyositis is a acute or chronic inflammatory disease of muscle that occurs in women twice as commonly as in men.

Lymphocytes in polymyositis subjects produce a cytotoxin when incubated with autologous muscle. Biopsies of involved muscle reveal infiltration by lymphocytes and plasma cells. Antibodies can be demonstrated against the nuclear antigens Jo-1, PM-Scl, and RNP. Patients may develop polyclonal hypergammaglobulinemia. One-fifth of patients may develop rheumatoid factors and antinuclear antibodies. Cellular immunity appears important in the pathogenesis. This is exemplified by lymphocytes of patients with polymyositis responding to their own muscle antigens as if they were alien. Patients often complain of muscle weakness especially in the proximal muscles of extremities. To diagnose polymyositis, a minimum of three of the following must be present: (1) shoulder or pelvic girdle weakness, (2) myositis as revealed by biopsy, (3) increased levels of muscle enzymes, and (4) electromyographic findings of myopathy. Corticosteroids have been used to decrease muscle inflammation and increase strength. Methotrexate or other cytotoxic agents may be used when steroids prove ineffective.

NEURO-MUSCULAR

Myasthenia gravis (MG) (Figure 35) is an autoantibody-mediated autoimmune disease. Antibodies specific for the nicotinic acetylcholine receptor (AChR) of skeletal muscle react with the postsynaptic membrane at the neuromuscular junction and diminish the number of functional receptors. Patients develop muscular weakness and some voluntary muscle fatigue. Thus, MG represents a receptor disease mediated by antibodies. The nicotinic AChR is the autoantigen. Contemporary research hopes to identify epitopes on the autoantigen(s) that interact with B and T cells in an autoimmune response. AChR is a four subunit transmembrane protein. Most autoantibodies in humans are against the main immunogenic regions (MIR). Antibodies against the MIR cross-link AChR molecules, leading to their internalization and lysosomal degradation. This leads to a decreased number of postsynaptic membrane AChRs. Humans with MG and animals immunized against AChR

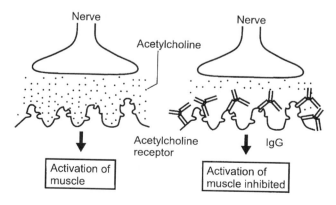

Figure 35.   Myasthenia gravis.

develop circulating antibodies and clinical manifestations of MG. A subgroup of patients are seronegative MG, resemble classic MG patients clinically, but have no anti-AChR antibodies in their circulation. Since the IgG anti-acetylcholine receptor autoantibodies cross the placenta from mother to fetus, newborns of mothers with this disease may also manifest signs and symptoms of the disease. Neonatal MG establishes the antibody-mediated autoimmune nature of the disease. The thymus of an MG patient may reveal either lymphofollicular hyperplasia (70%) or thymoma (10%). Anti-AChR synthesizing B cells and T helper lymphocytes may be found in hyperplastic follicles. These are often encircled by myoid cells that express AChR. Interdigitating follicular dendritic cells closely associated with myoid cells have been suggested to present AChR autoantigen to autoreactive T helper lymphocytes. Anti-idiotypic antibodies have been used to suppress or enhance experimental autoimmune myasthenia gravis (EAMG) depending on the antibody concentration employed. Conjugate immunotoxins to anti-Id antibodies have been able to suppress autoimmunity to AChR. Thymectomy and anti-cholinesterase drugs have both proven useful in treatment.

Acetylcholine receptor (AChR) antibodies are IgG autoantibodies that cause loss of function of acetylcholine receptors that are critical to chemical transmission of the nerve impulse at the neuromuscular junction. This represents a type II mechanism of hypersensitivity according to the Coombs and Gell classification. AChR antibodies are heterogeneous with some showing specificity for antigenic determinants other than those that serve as acetylcholine or alpha-bungarotoxin binding sites. As many as 85 to 95% of myasthenia gravis patients may manifest acetylcholine receptor antibodies.

THYROID

Hashimoto's disease (chronic thyroiditis) is an inflammatory disease of the thyroid (Figure 36) found most frequently in middle age to older women. There is extensive infiltration of the thyroid by lymphocytes which completely replace the normal glandular structure of the organ. There are numerous plasma cells and macrophages and germinal centers which give the appearance of node structure within the thyroid gland. Both B cells and CD4+ T lymphocytes comprise the principal infiltrating lymphocytes. Thyroid function is first increased as inflammatory reaction injures thyroid follicles causing them to release thyroid hormones. However, this is soon replaced by hypothyroidism in the later stages of Hashimoto's thyroiditis. Patients with this disease have an enlarged thyroid gland. There are circulating autoantibodies against thyroglobulin and thyroid microsomal antigen (thyroid peroxidase). Cellular sensitization to thyroid antigens may also be detected. Thyroid hormone replacement therapy is given for the hypothyroidism that develops (Figures 37–38).

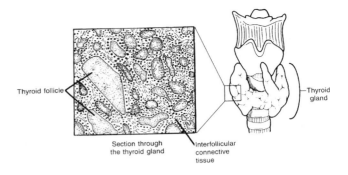

Figure 36. Thyroid gland.

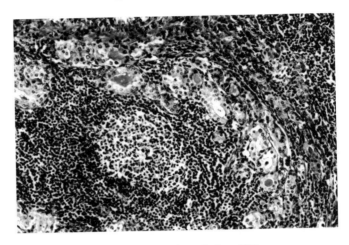

Figure 37. Hashimoto's thyroiditis.

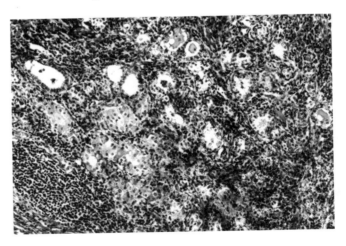

Figure 38. Hashimoto's thyroiditis.

Thyroid autoantibodies are found in patients with Hashimoto's thyroiditis or those with thyrotoxicosis (Graves' disease) that are organ-specific for the thyroid. Antibodies against thyroglobulin and antibodies against the microsomal antigen of thyroid acinar cells may appear in patients with autoimmune thyroiditis. Antibodies against TSH receptors appear in Graves' disease patients and cause stimulatory hypersensitivity. They mimic the action of TSH. This is an

IgG molecule termed long acting thyroid stimulator (LATS). LATS levels are increased in many patients with thyrotoxicosis or Graves' disease.

Graves' disease (hyperthyroidism) is a thyroid gland hyperplasia with increased thyroid hormone secretion produces signs and symptoms of hyperthyroidism in the patient. Patients may develop IgG autoantibodies against thyroid stimulating hormone (TSH) receptors. This autoantibody is termed long-acting thyroid stimulator (LATS). When the LATS IgG antibody binds to the TSH receptor, it has a stimulatory effect on the thyroid promoting hyperactivity. This IgG autoantibody can cross the placenta and produce transient hyperthyroidism in a newborn infant. The disease has a female predominance.

Thyrotoxicosis is a disease of the thyroid in which there is hyperthyroidism with elevated levels of thyroid hormones in the blood and thyroid gland hyperplasia or hypertrophy. Thyrotoxicosis may be autoimmune as in Graves' disease in which there may be diffuse goiter. Autoantibodies specific for thyroid antigens mimic thyroid stimulating hormones (TSH) by stimulating thyroid cell function. In addition, patients with Graves' disease develop ophthalmopathy and proliferative dermopathy. It occurs predominantly in females (70 females to 1 male) and appears usually in the 30 to 40 year old age group. In Caucasians, it is a disease associated with DR3. Patients may develop nervousness, tachycardia and numerous other symptoms of hyperthyroidism. They also have increased levels of total and free T3 and T4. There is a diffuse and homogenous uptake of radioactive iodine in these patients. Three types of antithyroid antibodies occur: (1) thyroid stimulating immunoglobulin, (2) thyroid growth-stimulating immunoglobulin and (3) thyroid binding-inhibitory immunoglobulin. Their presence confirms a diagnosis of Graves' disease. The thyroid gland may be infiltrated with lymphocytes. Long-acting thyroid stimulator (LATS) is classically associated with thyrotoxicosis. It is an IgG antibody specific for thyroid hormone receptors. It induces thyroid hyperactivity by combining with TSH receptors.

Long acting thyroid stimulator (LATS) is an IgG autoantibody that mimics the action of thyroid stimulating hormone in its effect on the thyroid. The majority of patients with Graves disease, i.e., hyperthyroidism, produce LATS. This IgG autoantibody reacts with the receptors on thyroid cells that respond to thyroid stimulating hormone. Thus, the antibody-receptor interaction results in the same biological consequence as does hormone interaction with the receptor. This represents a stimulatory type of hypersensitivity and is classified in the Gell and Coombs classification as one of the forms of Type II hypersensitivity.

LUNG

Usual interstitial pneumonia (UIP) (Figures 39–41) is a lung disease associated with interstitial inflammation and

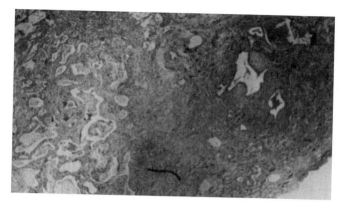

Figure 39. Usual interstitial pneumonitis. Biopsy revealed idiopathic pulmonary fibrosis. Histopathology reveals a bronchus that has divided chronic lymphocytic infiltrate, interstitial inflammation, and fibrosis edema. Only a few air spaces are irregularly located.

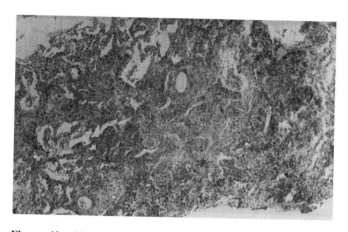

Figure 40. Usual interstitial pneumonitis. Histopathology reveals fibrosis and inflammation, numerous plasma cells, fibroblasts, histiocytes, and vascular destruction.

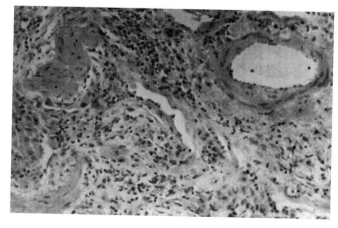

Figure 41. Usual interstitial pneumonitis.

fibrosis that lead to progressive respiratory insufficiency. It is the most frequent type of idiopathic interstitial pneumonitis and has been referred to by various names including Hamman-Rich syndrome. It is believed to have an immunologic basis with 20% of cases associated with collagen vascular diseases such as rheumatoid arthritis, progressive systemic sclerosis and systemic lupus erythematosus. Autoantibodies in these patients include anti-nuclear antibodies and rheumatoid factor. Immune complexes may be found in the blood, alveolar walls and bronchoalveolar lavage fluid yet the antigen remains unknown. Alveolar macrophages are believed to become activated after phagocytizing immune complexes. This might be followed by the release of cytokines that attract neutrophils that cause injury of alveolar walls leading to interstitial fibrosis. Pathologically, this is chronic inflammation in the interstitial space and extensive fibrosis of alveolar cepta. There are intermittent areas of extensive alveolar damage and of normal lung parenchyma. Areas of diffuse alveolar damage contain infiltrates of lymphocytes and plasma cells in alveolar walls and hypoplasia of type II pneumocytes. Fibrosis varies from mild to severe leading even to honeycomb lung in string cases. The distal acinus shrinks and proximal bronchioles dilate as fibrosis follows alveolitis. Multiple cystic spaces separated by scars occur in the end-stage of severe cases. The inflammation fibrosis may be accompanied by pulmonary hypertension. UIP may occur over a five to 10 year period with development of dyspnea on exertion and dry cough. The disease may follow acute viral infection of the respiratory tract in one-third of patients or in rare cases may have acute fulminating interstitial inflammation and fibrosis leading to Hamman-Rich syndrome that may lead to death without delay. Treatment modalities include corticosteroids or cytophosphamide in lung transplantation.

Lymphocytic interstitial pneumonia (LIP) (Figure 42) is a diffuse pulmonary disease of middle-aged females who may also have Sjögren's disease, hypergammaglobulinemia or hypogammaglobulinemia. They develop shortness of breath, and reticulonodular infiltrates appear on chest films. Mature lymphocytes and plasma cells appear in the nodular interstitial changes in alveolar and interlobular septae with perivascular accumulation of round cells. LIP may resemble lymphoma based on the monotonous accumulation of small lymphocytes, and patients may ultimately develop end-stage lung disease or lymphoma.

Farmer's lung (Figure 43) is a pulmonary disease of farm workers who have been exposed repeatedly to organic dust and fungi such as *Aspergillus* species. It occurs as an extrinsic allergic alveolitis or hypersensitivity pneumonitis in nonatopic subjects. It is mediated by IgG1. 90% of individuals manifest antibodies specific for moldy hay in which a number of fungi grow readily. These include *Microspora vulgaris* and *Micropolyspora faeni*. The pathogenesis is believed to involve a type III hypersensitivity mechanism

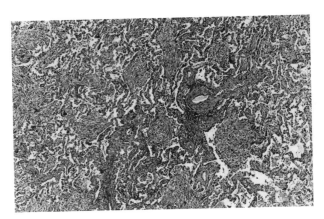

Figure 42.   Lymphocytic interstitial pneumonia (LIP) with organization.

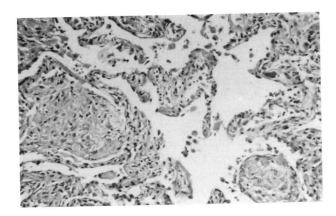

Figure 43.   Farmer's lung.

with the deposition of immune complexes in the lung. Patients become breathless within hours after inhaling the dust and may develop interstitial pneumonitis with cellular infiltration of the alveolar walls where monocytes and lymphocytes are prominent. This may lead to pulmonary fibrosis following chronic inflammation, peribronchiolar granulomatous reaction and foreign body-type giant cell reactions. Corticosteroids are used for treatment.

Sarcoidosis (Figures 44 and 45) is a systemic granulomatous disease that involves lymph nodes, lungs, eyes and skin. There is a granulomatous hypersensitivity reaction that resembles that of tuberculosis and fungus infections. Sarcoidosis has a higher incidence in African Americans than in Caucasians and is prominent geographically in the Southeastern United States. It is of unknown etiology. Immunologically, there is a decrease in circulating T cells. There is decreased delayed-type hypersensitivity as manifested by anergy to common skin test antigens. Increased antibody formation leads to polyclonal hypergammaglobulinemia. There is a marked cellular immune response in local areas of disease activity. Tissue lesions consist of inflammatory cells and granulomas, comprised of activated mononuclear phagocytes such as epithelioid cells, multinucleated giant

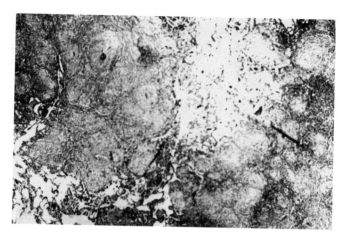

Figure 44.   Open lung biopsy showing sarcoidosis.

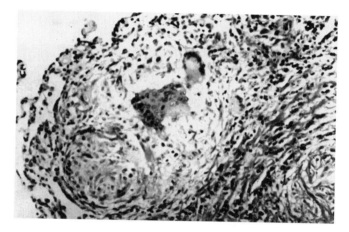

Figure 45.   Open lung biopsy showing sarcoidosis.

cells and macrophages. Activated T cells are present at the periphery of the granuloma. CD4[+] T cells appear to be the immunoregulatory cells governing granuloma formation. Mediators released from T cells nonspecifically stimulate B cells resulting in the polyclonal hypogammaglobulinemia. The granulomas are typically non-caseating, distinguishing them from those produced in tuberculosis. Patients may develop fever, polyarthritis, erythema nodosum, and iritis. They also may experience loss of weight, anorexia, weakness, fever, sweats, nonproductive cough and increasing dyspnea on exertion. Pulmonary symptoms occur in greater than 90% of patients. Angiotensin-converting enzyme is increased in the serum of sarcoid patients. Disease activity is monitored by measuring the level of this enzyme in the serum. The subcutaneous inoculation of sarcoidosis lymph node extracts into patients diagnosed with sarcoidosis leads to a granulomatous reaction in the skin three to four weeks after inoculation. This was used in the past as a diagnostic test, of questionable value, termed the Kveim reaction. Sarcoidosis syptoms can be treated with corticosteroids but only in patients where disease progression occurs. It is a relatively

mild disease with 80% resolving spontaneously and only 5% dying of complications.

Asthma is a disease of the lumgs characterized by reversible airway obstruction (in most cases), inflammation of the airway with prominent eosinophil participation, and increased responsiveness by the airway to various stimuli. There is bronchospasm associated with recurrent paroxysmal dyspnea and wheezing. Some cases of asthma are allergic, i.e., bronchial allergy, mediated by IgE antibody to environmental allergens. Other cases are provoked by nonallergic factors that are not discussed here.

Bird fancier's lung (Figures 46 and 47) is a respiratory disease in which subjects are hypersensitive to plasma protein antigens of birds following exposure of the subject to bird feces or skin and feather dust. Hypersensitive subjects have an Arthus type of reactivity or type III hypersensitivity to the plasma albumin and globulin components. Precipitates may be demonstrated in the blood sera of hypersensitivity subjects.

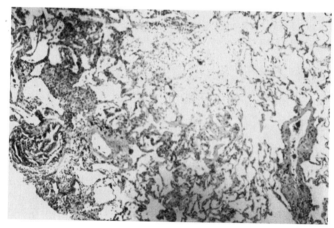

Figure 46.   Bird fancier's lung. Lung biopsy showing an interstitial granulomatous pneumonitis consistent with bird fancier's lung.

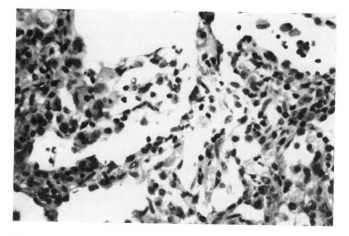

Figure 47.   Bird fancier's lung. Lung biopsy showing an interstitial granulomatous pneumonitis consistent with bird fancier's lung.

Pulmonary vasculitis (Figures 48–51) is a vasculitis characterized by chronic inflammation, necrotizing and non-necrotizing granulomatous inflammation, fibrinoid necrosis, arterial wall medial thickening and intimal proliferation.

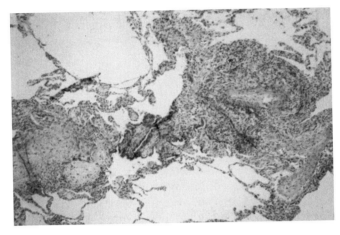

Figure 48. Pulmonary vasculitis. There is necrosis of endothelial cells and supporting stromal structures with acute and chronic inflammation. There is exudation of polymorphonuclear leukocytes, eosinophils and extravasated erythrocytes. Magnification: 35X.

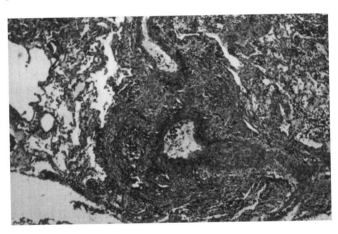

Figure 49. Pulmonary vasculitis. There is necrosis of endothelial cells and supporting stromal structures with acute and chronic inflammation. There is exudation of polymorphonuclear leukocytes, eosinophils and extravasated erythrocytes. Magnification: 50X.

MULTISYSTEM

Rheumatic fever (RF) is an acute, nonsuppurative, inflammatory disease that is immune-mediated and occurs mainly in children a few weeks following an infection of the pharynx with Group A β hemolytic streptococci. M protein, a principal virulence factor associated with specific strains of the streptococci, induces antibodies that cross-react with epitopes of human cardiac muscle. These antibodies may not produce direct tissue injury but together with other immune mechanisms evoke acute systemic disease characterized mainly by polyarthritis, skin lesions and carditis.

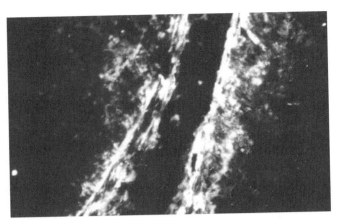

Figure 50. Pulmonary vasculitis. Direct immunoflorescence reveals coalescent and granular deposits of IgM and C3 in the walls of some muscular arteries and occasional large veins consistent with immune complex vasculitis involving large vessels. Magnification: 200X.

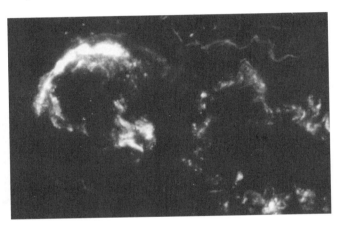

Figure 51. Pulmonary vasculitis. Direct immunoflorescence reveals coalescent and granular deposits of IgM and C3 in the walls of some muscular arteries and occasional large veins consistent with immune complexes vasculitis involving large vessels. Magnification: 500X.

Whereas the arthritis and skin lesions resolve, the cardiac involvement may lead to permanent injury to the valves producing fibrocalcific deformity. Foci of necrosis of collagen with fibrin deposition surrounded by lymphocytes, macrophages and plump modified histiocytes are termed Aschoff bodies, which are ultimately replaced years later by fibrous scars. Aschoff bodies may be found in any of the three layers of the heart. In the pericardium they are accompanied by serofibrinous (bread and butter) pericarditis. In the myocardium they are scattered in the interstitial connective tissue often near blood vessels. There may be dilatation of the heart and mitral valve ring. There may be inflammation of the endocardium mainly affecting the left-sided valves. Small vegetations may form along the lines of closure. Other tissues may be affected with the production of acute nonspecific arthritis affecting the larger joints. Fewer than half of the patients develop skin lesions such as subcutaneous nodules or erythema marginatum. Subcutaneous nodules that appear at pressure points overlying extensor tendons of extremities at the wrist, elbows, ankles and knees consist of central fibrinoid necrosis enclosed by a palisade of fibroblasts and mononuclear inflammatory cells. Rheumatic arteritis has been described in coronary, renal, mesenteric and cerebral arteries as well as in the aorta and pulmonary vessels. Rheumatic interstitial pneumonitis is a rare complication of the disease. Antistreptolysin O (ASO) and antistreptokinase (ASK) antibodies are found in the serum of affected individuals. Myocarditis that develops during an acute attack may induce arrhythmias such as atrial fibrillation, or cardiac dilatation with potential mitral valve insufficiency. Long-term antistreptococcal therapy must be given to any patient with a history of rheumatic fever as subsequent streptococcal infections may worsen the carditis.

Aschoff bodies (Figure 52) are areas of fibrinoid necrosis encircled first by lymphocytes and macrophages with a rare plasma cell. The mature Aschoff body reveals prominent modified histiocytes termed Anitschkow cells or Aschoff cells in the inflammatory infiltrate. These cells have round to oval nuclei with wavy ribbon-like chromatin and amphophilic cytoplasm. Aschoff bodies are pathognomonic of rheumatic fever. They may be found in any of the heart's three layers, i.e., pericardium, myocardium or endocardium.

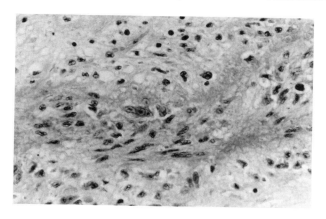

Figure 52. Aschoff body.

DIGESTIVE SYSTEM

Crohn's disease is a condition usually expressed as ileocolitis but can affect any segment of the gastrointestinal tract. Crohn's disease is associated with transmural granulomatous inflammation of the bowel wall characterized by lymphocyte, plasma cell and eosinophil infiltration. Goblet cells and gland architecture are not usually affected. Granuloma formation is classically seen in Crohn's disease, appearing in 70% of patients. The etiology is unknown. *Mycobacterium paratuberculosis* has been found in a few patients with Crohn's disease although no causal relationship has been established. An immune effector mechanism is believed to be responsible for maintaining chronic disease in these

patients. Their serum immunoglobulins and peripheral blood lymphocyte counts are usually normal except for a few diminished T cell counts in selected Crohn's disease patients. Helper/suppressor ratio are also normal. Active disease has been associated with reduced suppressor T cell activity which returns to normal during remission. Patients have complexes in their blood that are relatively small and contain IgG, although no antigen has been identified. The complexes may be merely aggregates of IgG. Complexes in Crohn's disease patients are associated with involvement of the colon and are seen less often in those with disease confined to the ileum. During active disease, serum concentrations of C3, Factor B, C1 inhibitor and C3b inactivator are elevated but return to normal during remission. Patients with long standing disease often develop high titers of immunoconglutinins which are antibodies to activated C3. High titer antibodies against bacterial antigens such as those of *E. coli* and *Bacteroides* crossreact with colonic globlet cell lipopolysaccharides. Patients' peripheral blood lymphocytes can kill colonic epithelial cells *in vitro*. Colonic mucosa lymphocytes in these patients are also cytotoxic for colonic epithelial cells.

Ulcerative colitis (immunologic colitis) (Figure 53) is an ulcerative condition that may involve the entire colon but does not significantly affect the small intestine. There is neutrophil, plasma cell and eosinophil infiltration of the colonic mucosa. This is followed by ulceration of the surface epithelium, loss of globlet cells and formation of crypt abscess. The etiology is unknown. An immune effector mechanism is believed to maintain chronic disease in these patients. Their serum immunoglobulins and peripheral blood lymphocyte counts usually are normal. Complexes present in the blood are relatively small and contain IgG although no antigen has been identified. The complexes could be merely aggregates of IgG. These patients have diarrhea with blood and mucus in the stool. The signs and symptoms are intermittent, and there is variation in the severity of colon lesions. The patient's lymphocytes are cytotoxic for colon epithelial cells. Antibodies against *E. coli* may crossreact

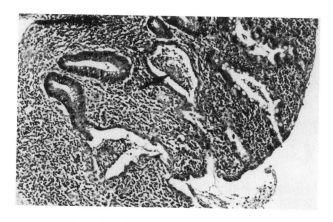

Figure 53. Ulcerative colitis. Crypt abcess.

with colonic epithelium in these patients. However, whether or not such antibodies have a role in etiology and pathogenesis remains to be proven.

Pernicious anemia (PA) (Figures 54 and 55) is an autoimmune disease characterized by the development of atrophic gastritis, achlorhydria, decreased synthesis of intrinsic factor and mild absorption of vitamin B_{12}. Patients present with megaloblastic anemia caused by the vitamin B_{12} deficiency that develops. The majority of pernicious anemia patients develop anti-parietal cell antibodies and at least half of them also develop antibodies against intrinsic factor, which is necessary for the absorption of B_{12}. The anti-parietal cell antibodies are against a microsomal antigen found in gastric parietal cells. Intrinsic factor is a 60kD substance that links to vitamin B_{12} and aids its uptake in the small intestine. PA may be a complication of common variable immunodeficiency or may be associated with autoimmune thyroiditis. Pernicious anemia is caused principally by injury to the stomach mediated by T lymphocytes. Patients may manifest megaloblastic anemia, deficiency of vitamin B_{12} and increased gastrin in serum.

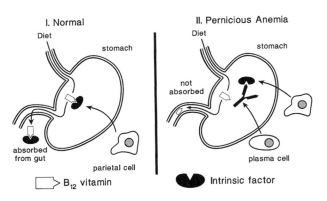

Figure 54. Pernicious anemia.

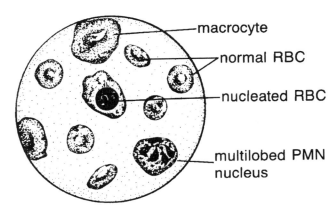

Figure 55. Macrocytic anemia.

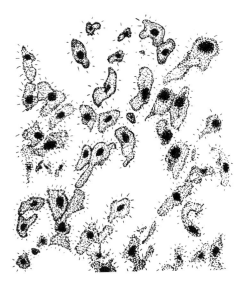

Figure 56. Pernicious anemia. Parietal cell antibody. (FITC-labelled).

Parietal cell antibodies (Figure 56) are antibodies present in 50 to 100% of pernicious anemia (PA) patients. They are also found in 2% of normal individuals. Their frequency increases with aging and in subjects with insulin-dependent diabetes mellitus. The frequency of parietal cell antibodies diminishes with disease duration in pernicious anemia. Parietal cell autoantibodies in pernicious anemia and in autoimmune gastritis recognize the α and β-subunits of the gastric protein proton pump (H+/K+ ATPase) which are the principal target antigens. Parietal cell antibodies react with α and β subunits of the gastric proton pump and inhibits the gastric mucosa's acid-producing H+/K+ adenosine triphosphatase. Parietal cell antibodies relate to type A gastritis in which there is fundal mucosal atrophy, achlorhydria, development of pernicious anemia and autoimmune endocrine disease.

LIVER

Chronic active hepatitis (autoimmune) (Figure 57) is a disease that occurs in young females who may develop fever, arthralgias and skin rashes. They may be of the HLA-B8, -DR3 haplotype and suffer other autoimmune disorders. Most develop antibodies to smooth muscle, principally against actin, and autoantibodies to liver membranes. They also have other organ- and non-organ-specific autoantibodies. A polyclonal hypergammaglobulinemia may be present. Lymphocytes infiltrating portal areas destroy hepatocytes. Injury to liver cells produced by these infiltrating lymphocytes produces piecemeal necrosis. The inflammation and necrosis are followed by fibrosis and cirrhosis. The T cells infiltrating the liver are CD4+. Plasma cells are also present and immunoglobulins may be deposited on hepatocytes. The autoantibodies against liver cells do not play a pathogenetic role in liver injury. There are no serologic findings that are diagnostic. Corticosteroids are useful in treatment. The

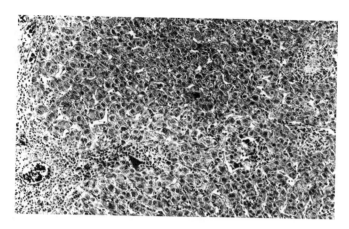

Figure 57. Chronic active hepatitis piecemeal necrosis.

immunopathogenesis of autoimmune chronic active hepatitis involves antibody, K cell cytotoxicity and T cell reactivity against liver membrane antigens. Antibodies and specific T suppressor cells reactive with LSP are found in chronic active hepatitis patients, all of whom develop T cell sensitization against asialo-glycoprotein (AGR) antigen. Chronic active hepatitis has a familial predisposition.

Smooth muscle antibodies are autoantibodies belonging to the IgM or IgG class that are found in the blood sera of 60% of chronic active hepatitis patients. 30% of biliary cirrhosis patients may also be positive for these antibodies. Low titers of smooth muscle antibodies may be found in certain viral infections of the liver.

Primary biliary cirrhosis is a chronic liver disease of unknown cause that affects middle aged women in 90% of cases. There is chronic intrahepatic cholestasis caused by chronic inflammation and necrosis of intrahepatic bile ducts with progression to biliary cirrhosis. It is believed to be an autoimmune disease based on its association with autoimmune conditions and the presence of autoantibodies. Patients develop pruritis, fatigue, steatorrhea, renal tubular acidosis, hepatic osteodystrophy and increased incidence of hepatocellular carcinoma and breast carcinoma. Four-fifths of patients also have a connective tissue or autoimmune disease such as rheumatoid arthritis, autoimmune thyroiditis, scleroderma and Sjogren's syndrome. Most patients manifest a high titer of antimitochondrial antibodies. There is elevated IgM in the serum. Lymphocytic infiltration occurs together with intrahepatic bile duct destruction. Alkaline phosphatase is greatly increased in addition to the elevation of IgM and anti-mitochondrial antibodies. The M2 antimitochondrial antibody is most frequently associated with PBC. In addition to hepatosplenomegaly and skin hyperpigmentation, patients may develop severe jaundice, petechiae and purpura as the disease progresses. Liver transplantation is the only treatment for end-stage disease.

Hepatitis (immunopathology panel) is a profile of assays that are very useful to establish the clinical and immune status of a patient believed to have hepatitis. The panel for acute hepatitis may include hepatitis B surface antigen (HBsAg), antibody to hepatitis B core antigen (anti-HBc), anti-hepatitis B surface antigen (anti-ABs), anti-hepatitis A (IgM), anti-HBe and anti-hepatitis C. The panel for chronic hepatitis (carrier) includes all of these except for the anti-hepatitis A test.

Hepatitis B (Figure 58) is a DNA virus that is relatively small and has four open reading frames. The S gene codes for HBsAg. The P gene codes for a DNA polymerase. There is an X gene and core gene that code for HBcAg and the pre-core area that codes for HBeAg.

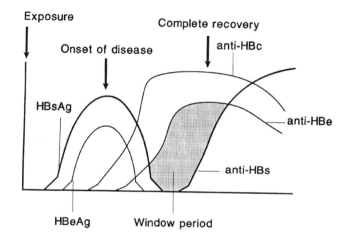

Figure 58. Hepatitis B.

Delta agent [hepatitis D virus (HDV)] is a viral etiologic agent of hepatitis that is a circular single-stranded incomplete RNA virus without an envelope. It is a 1.7 kilobase virus and consists of a small, highly conserved domain and a larger domain manifesting epitopes. HDV is a subviral satellite of the hepatitis B virus (HBV), on which it depends to fit its genome into viral particles. Thus the patient must first be infected with HBV to have HDV. Individuals with the delta agent in their blood are positive for HBsAg, anti-HBC and often HBe. This agent is frequently present in IV drug abusers and may appear in hemophiliacs and AIDS patients.

Hepatitis non-A, non-B (C) (NANBH) is the principal cause of hepatitis that is transfusion-related. Risk factors include intravenous drug abuse (42%), unknown risk factors (40%), sexual contact (6%), blood transfusion (6%), household contact (3%) and health professionals (2%). There are 150,000 cases per year in the United States. 30–50% of these become chronic carriers and one-fifth develop cirrhosis. Parenteral NANBH is usually hepatitis C and enteric NANBH is usually hepatitis E.

Hepatitis serology refers to hepatitis B antigens and antibodies against them. Core antigen is designated HBc. The HBc particle is comprised of double-stranded DNA and DNA polymerase. It has an association with HBe antigens. Core antigen signifies persistence of replicating hepatitis B virus. Anti-HBc antibody is a serologic indicator of hepatitis B. It is an IgM antibody that increases early and is still detectable 20 years post infection. The IgM anti-HBc antibody assay is the one best antibody assay for acute hepatitis B. The HBe antigen (HBe) follows the same pattern as HBsAg antigen. When found, it signifies a carrier state. The anti-HBe increases as HBe decreases. It appears in patients who are recovering and may last for years after the hepatitis has been resolved. The first antigen that is detectable following hepatitis B infection is surface antigen (HBs). It is detectable a few weeks before clinical disease and is highest with the first appearance of symptoms. This antigen disappears six months from infection. Antibody to HBs increases as the HBsAg levels diminish. Anti-HBs often is detectable for the lifetime of the individual.

PANCREAS

Insulin dependent diabetes mellitus, type I (Figures 59 and 60) is a disease in which autoantibodies against islet cells (and insulin) may be identified. Among the three to six

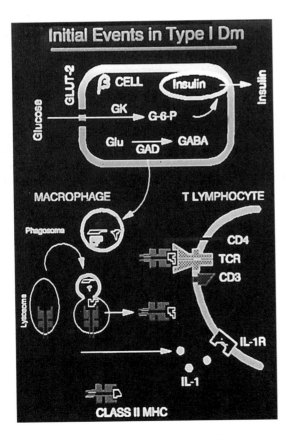

Figure 59.   Diabetes mellitus, Type I.

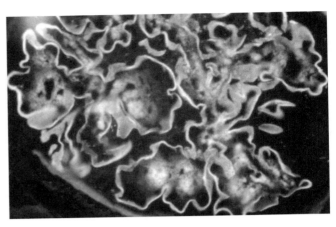

Figure 60.   Diabetic glomerulopathy. Discontinuous linear fluorescence-anti IgG.

genes governing susceptibility to type I diabetes are those encoding the MHC. Understanding human diabetes has been greatly facilitated by both immunological and genetic studies in experimental animal models including nonobese diabetic mice (NOD mice) and biobreeding rats (BB rats). Human type I diabetes mellitus results from autoimmune injury of pancreatic β cells. Specific autoantibodies signal pancreatic β cell destruction. The autoantibodies are against islet cell cytoplamic or surface antigens or insulin. Antiidiotypic antibodies may also develop against antiinsulin antibodies, possibly leading to antibody blockade of insulin receptors and thereby inducing insulin resistance and β cell exhaustion. Autoantibodies have also been demonstrated against a 64-kD third islet cell antigen which could represent a primary target of autoimmune reactivity in type I diabetes and have been found in the sera of diabetic before clinical onset of the disease. HLA typing is also useful. DNA sequence analysis has revealed that alleles of HLA-DQ β chain govern diabetes susceptibility and resistance. The amino acid at position 57 has a critical role in disease susceptibility and resistance. Although pancreatic β cells fail to express MHC class II antigens under normal circumstances, they become Ia MHC class II antigen positive following stimulation by INF-α and TNF or lymphotoxin. Class II postive pancreatic β cells may present islet cell autoantigens to T lymphocytes inaugurating an immune response.

Patients at risk for diabetes or prediabetes might benefit from immunosuppresive therapy, such as cyclosporine, although most are still treated with insulin. Transplantation of pancreatic islet cells remain a bright possibility in future treatment strategies.

Acanthosis nigricans (Figure 61) is a condition in which the afflicted subject develops insulin receptor autoantibodies associated with insulin-resistant diabetes mellitus, as well as thickened and pigmented skin.

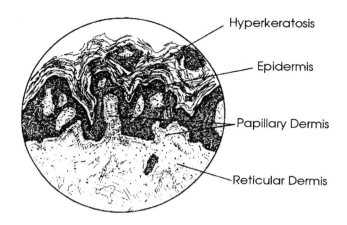

Figure 61.   Acanthosis Nigricans.

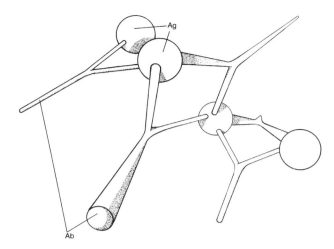

Figure 62.   Immune complex.

KIDNEY

Immune complex disease (ICD) (Figures 62–64) is described under type III hypersensitivity reaction, antigen-antibody complexes have a fate that depends in part on the size. The larger insoluble immune complexes are removed by the mononuclear phagocyte system. The smaller immune complexes become lodged in the microvasculature such as the renal glomeruli. They may activate the complement system, and attract polymorphonuclear neutrophils, initiating an inflammatory reaction. The antigen of an immune complex may be from microorganisms such as streptococci leading to subepithelial deposits in renal glomeruli in post-streptococcal glomerulonephritis, or endogenous such as DNA or nuclear antigens in systemic lupus erythematosus. Diphtheria antitoxin prepared in horses induced serum sickness when the foreign horse serum proteins stimulated antibodies in human recipients. Immune complex disease is characterized clinically by fever, joint pain, lymphadenopathy, eosinophilia, hypocomplementemia, proteinuria, purpura and urticaria among other features. Laboratory techniques to detect immune complexes include the solid phase Clq assay, the Clq binding assay, the Raji cell technique and the staphylococcal protein assay among other methods. Most autoimmune diseases have a type III (antigen-antibody complex)-mediated mechanism. The connective tissue diseases such as systemic lupus erythematosus, polyarteritis nodosa, progressive systemic sclerosis, dermatomyositis, rheumatoid arthritis and others fall within this category. Viral infections such as hepatitis B, cytomegalovirus, infectious mononucleosis and Dengue as well as neoplasia such as carcinomas and melanomas may be associated with immune complex formation.

Membranous glomerulonephritis (Figures 65–67) is a disease induced by deposition of electron-dense, immune (Ag-Ab) deposits in the glomerular basement membrane in a subepithelial location. This leads to progressive thickening of glomerular membranes. Most cases are idiopathic, but

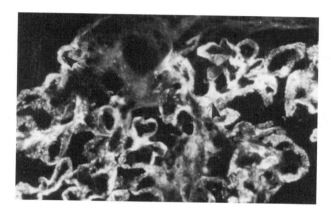

Figure 63.   Immune complexes in renal glomerulus.

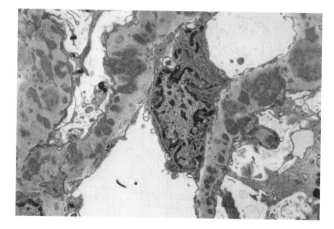

Figure 64.   Electron dense deposits. Immune complex disease (ICD).

membranous glomerulonephritis may follow development of other diseases such as systemic lupus erythematosus, lung or colon carcinoma, exposure to gold, mercury, penicillamine or captopril. It can also be a sequela of certain infections, e.g., hepatitis B, or metabolic disorders, e.g., diabetes

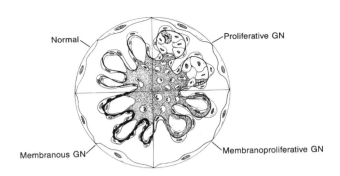

Figure 65.   Types of glomerulonephritis.

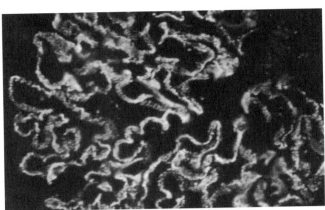

Figure 67.   Membranous glomerulonephritis.

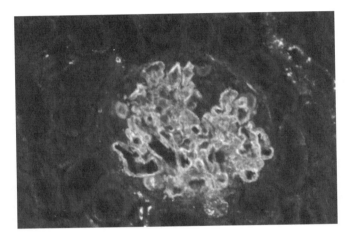

Figure 66.   Glomerulonephritis.

Masugi nephritis (Figure 68) is an experimental model of human anti-glomerular basement membrane (anti-GBM) nephritis. The disease is induced by the injection of rabbit anti-rat glomerular basement membrane antibody into rats. The antiserum for passive transfer is raised in rabbits immunized with rat kidney basement membranes. The passively administered antibodies become bound to the glomerular basement membrane, fix complement and induce glomerular basement membrane injury with increased permeability. Neutrophils and monocytes may infiltrate the area. Masugi nephritis is an experimental model of Goodpasture's syndrome in man. This also is called nephrotoxic nephritis.

mellitus. Clinically it is a principal cause of nephrotic syndrome in adults. The subepithelial immune deposits are shown by immunofluorescence to contain both immunoglobulins and complement. Proteinuria persists in 70–90% of cases, and half of the patients develop renal insufficiency over a period of years. 10–30% have a less severe course.

Heymann glomerulonephritis (Figure 69) is an experimental model of membranous glomerulonephritis induced by immunizing rats with proximal tubule brush border preparations containing subepithelial antigen or Heymann factor, a 330kD protein incorporated in Freund's adjuvant. The rats produce antibodies against brush border antigens and membranous glomerulonephritis is induced. Autoantibodies combine with shed epithelial cell antigen. The union of antibody

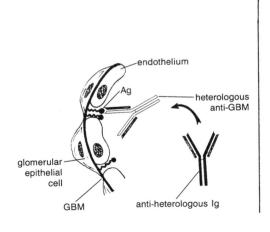

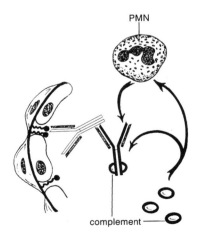

Figure 68.   Masugi Nephritis.

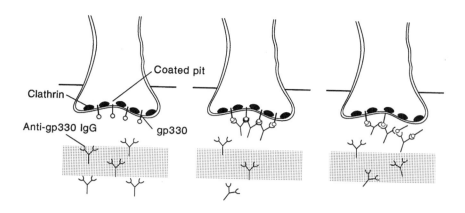

Figure 69.   Heymann glomerulonephritis.

with Heymann antigen, distributed in an interrupted manner along visceral epithelial cell surfaces leads to subepithelial electron-dense, granular deposits. Immunoglobulins and complement are deposited in a granular rather than linear pattern along the glomerular basement membrane, as revealed by immunofluorescence. The glomerulonephritis results from interaction of anti-brush border antibody with the 330kD glycoprotein that is fixed but discontinuously distributed on the base of visceral epithelial cells and is cross reactive with brush border antigens. Heymann nephritis closely resembles human membranous glomerulonephritis.

Post-streptococcal glomerulonephritis is an acute proliferative glomerulonephritis that may follow a streptococcal infection of the throat or skin by one to two weeks. It is usually seen in 6- to 10-year-old children but may occur in adults as well. The onset is heralded by evidence of acute nephritis. 90% of patients have been infected with Group A β hemolytic streptococci that are nephritogenic, specifically types 12, 4 and 1, which are revealed by their cell wall M protein. Post-streptococcal glomerulonephritis is mediated by antibodies induced by the streptococcal infection. Most patients show elevated anti-streptolysin-O (ASO) titers. Serum complement levels are decreased. Immunofluorescence of renal biopsies demonstrates granular immune deposits that contain immunoglobulin and complement in the glomeruli. This is confirmed by electron microscopy. The precise streptococcal antigen has never been identified, however, a cytoplasmic antigen termed endostreptosin together with some cationic streptococcal antigens are found in glomeruli. Subepithelial immune deposits appear as "humps". They are antigen-antibody complexes that may also appear in the mesangium or occasionally in a subendothelial or intramembranous position. These immune deposits stain positively for IgG and complement by immunofluorescence. Affected children develop fever, nausea, oliguria and hematuria within two weeks following a streptococcal sore throat or skin infection. Erythrocyte casts and mild proteinuria may be identified. There may be periorbital edema and hypertension upon examination. The BUN and ASO titer may also

be elevated. More than 95% of children with post-streptococcal glomerulonephritis recover although a few, less than 1%, develop rapidly progressive glomerulonephritis and a few others develop chronic glomerulonephritis.

Humps (Figure 70) are immune deposits containing IgG and C3 as well as the alternate complement pathway components, properdin and Factor B that occur in post infectious glomerulonephritis on the subepithelial side of peripheral capillary basement membranes. They resolve within 4 to 8 weeks of the infection in most individuals. They may also occur in selected other nonstreptococcal post infectious glomerulonephritides.

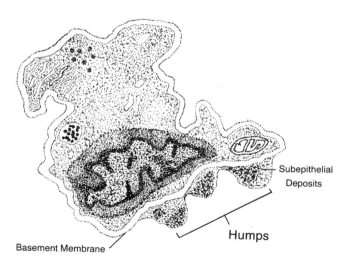

Figure 70.   Hump.

IgA nephropathy (Berger's disease) (Figures 71–73) is a type of glomerulonephritis in which prominent IgA-containing immune deposits are present in mesangial areas. Patients usually present with gross or microscopic hematuria and often mild proteinuria. By light microscopy, mesangial widening or proliferation may be observed. However, immunofluorescence microscopy demonstrating IgA and

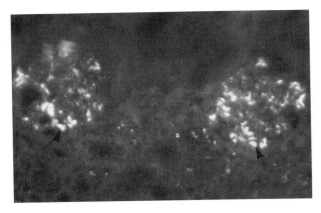

Figure 71. IgA nephropathy. Granular immune deposits in mesangial areas.

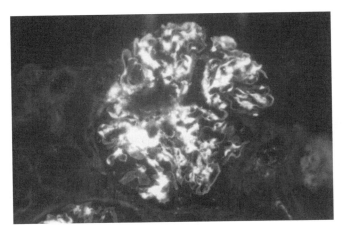

Figure 72. Berger's disease. Granular immune deposits containing IgG, IgA, and C3 in mesangial areas.

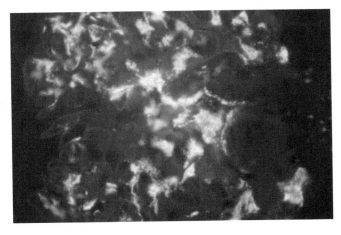

Figure 73. Berger's disease. Granular immune deposits containing IgG, IgA, and C3 in mesangial areas.

C3, fixed by the alternative pathway, is requisite for diagnosis. Electron microscopy confirms the presence of electron-dense deposits in mesangial areas. Half of the cases progress to chronic renal failure over a 20-year course.

Dense-deposit disease (Figure 74) is a type II membranoproliferative glomerulonephritis characterized by the deposition of electron-dense material, often containing C3, in the peripheral capillary basement membrane of the glomerulus. C3 is decreased in the serum as a consequence of alternate complement pathway activation. C4 is normal. There is an increase in sialic acid-rich glomerular basement membrane glycoproteins. Patients may possess a serum factor termed nephritic factor that activates the alternate complement pathway. This factor is an immunoglobulin molecule that reacts with alternate complement pathway-activated components such as the bimolecular C3b and activated factor B complex. Nephritic factor stabilizes alternate pathway C3 convertase.

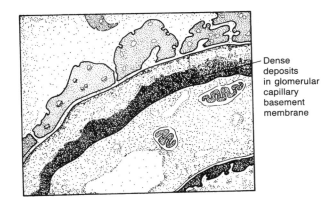

Figure 74. Dense deposit disease.

Goodpasture's syndrome (Figures 75–77) is a disease with pulmonary hemorrhage (with coughing up blood) and glomerulonephritis (with blood in the urine), induced by anti-glomerular basement membrane autoantibodies that also interact with alveolar basement membrane antigens. A linear pattern of immunofluorescent staining confirms interaction of the IgG antibodies with basement membrane antigens in the kidney and lung leading to membrane injury with pulmonary hemorrhage and acute (rapidly progressive or crescentic) proliferative glomerulonephritis. Pulmonary hemorrhage may precede hematuria. In addition to linear IgG, membranes may reveal linear staining for C3 (Figure 78).

Goodpasture's antigen is an antigen found in the noncollagenous part of type IV collagen. It is present in human glomerular and alveolar basement membranes, making them a target for injury-inducing anti-GBM antibodies in blood sera of Goodpasture's syndrome patients. Interestingly, individuals with Alport's (hereditary) nephritis do not have the Goodpasture antigen in their basement membranes. Thus, renal transplants stimulate anti-GBM antibodies in Alport's patients.

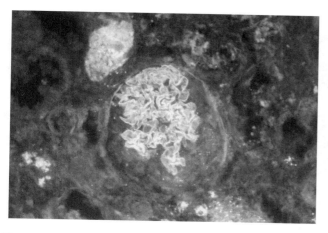

Figure 75.   Goodpasture's syndrome. Stained with anti-GBM antibody.

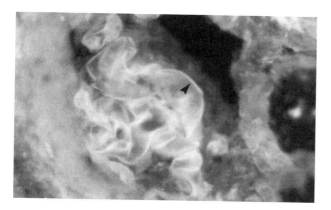

Figure 76.   Goodpasture's syndrome. Stained with anti-GBM antibody.

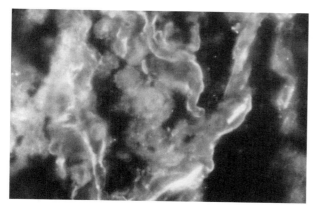

Figure 77.   Goodpasture's syndrome. Stained with anti-lung basement membrane antibody.

NERVOUS SYSTEM

Multiple sclerosis (MS) (Figure 79) is a demyelinating nervous system disease of unknown cause. It is most frequent in young adult females and has an incidence of 1 in 2500 individuals in the U.S.A. MS shows a disease association

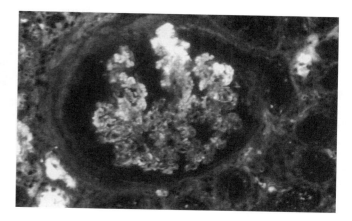

Figure 78.   Focal segmental glomerulosclerosis.

Zone electrophoresis patterns of cerebrospinal fluid

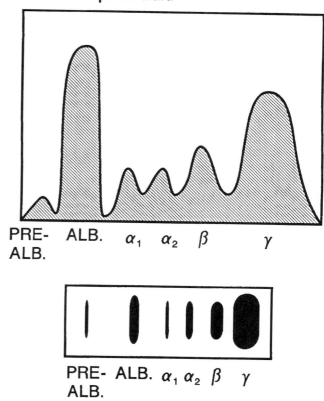

Figure 79.   Multiple sclerosis (100X concentrate).

with HLA-A3, B7, Dw2 haplotypes. Patients express multiple neurological symptoms that are worse at some times than others. They have paresthesias, muscle weakness, visual and gait disturbances, ataxia, and hyperactive tendon reflexes. There is infiltration of lymphocytes and macrophages in the nervous system which facilitates demyelination. Autoimmune mechanisms mediated by T cells, which constitute the majority of

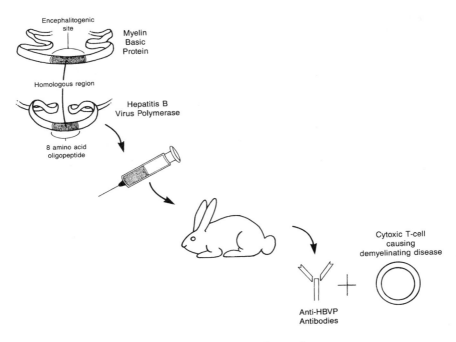

Figure 80. Myelin basic protein.

infiltrating lymphocytes, are involved. At least 20 viruses have been suggested to play a role in the etiology of MS. Infected oligodendrocytes are destroyed by the immune mechanism, and there may be also "innocent bystander" demyelination. Antibodies against HTLV-I GAG (p24) protein have been identified in the cerebrospinal fluid of MS patients. HTLV-I gene sequences have been identified in monocytes of MS patients. 90% of MS patients have an oligoclonal increase in CSF IgG. There is inflammation, demyelination and glial scarring. Paraventricular, frontal and temporal areas of the brain are first involved, followed by regions of the brainstem, optic tracts and white matter of the cortex with patchy lesions of the spinal cord. Attempts at treatment have included cop-1, a polypeptide mixture that resembles myelin basic protein and numerous other agents.

Myelin basic protein (MBP) (Figure 80) is a principal constituent of the lipoprotein myelin that first appears during late embryogenesis. It is a 19kD protein that is increased in multiple sclerosis patients who may generate T lymphocyte reactivity against MBP. T lymphocytes with the V-β 17 variant of the T cell receptor are especially prone to react to MBP.

When cerebrospinal fluid of some multiple sclerosis patients is electrophoresed in agarose gel, immunoglobulins with restricted electrophoretic mobility may appear as multiple distinct oligoclonal bands in the gamma region (Figure 81). Although nonspecific, 90–95% of multiple sclerosis patients show this. They may appear in selected other central nervous system diseases such as herpetic encephalitis, bacterial or viral meningitis, carcinomatosis, toxoplasmosis, neurosyphilis,

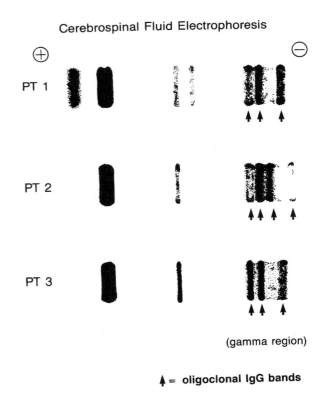

Cerebrospinal Fluid Electrophoresis

(gamma region)

↟ = oligoclonal IgG bands

Figure 81. Oligoclonal bands.

progressive multifocal leukoencephalopathy, subacute sclerosing pan-encephalitis and may appear briefly during the course of Guillian-Barre disease, lupus erythematosus vasculitis, spinal cord compression, diabetes, and amyotrophic lateral sclerosis.

Experimental allergic encephalomyelitis is an autoimmune disease induced by immunization of experimental animals with preparations of brain or spinal cord incorporated into Freund's complete adjuvant. After 10–12 days, perivascular accumulations of lymphocytes and mononuclear phagocytes surround the vasculature of the brain and spinal cord white matter. Demyelination may also be present, worsening as the disease becomes chronic. The animals often develop paralysis. The disease can be passively transferred from a sick animal to a healthy one of the same strain with T lymphocytes but not with antibodies. The mechanism involves T cell receptor interaction with an 18kD myelin basic protein molecule, which is an organ-specific antigen of nervous system tissue. The CD4+ T lymphocyte represents the phenotype that is reactive with myelin basic protein. The immune reaction induces myelinolysis, wasting and paralysis. Peptides derived from myelin basic protein or MBP itself may be used to induce experimental allergic encephalomyelitis in animals. This experimental autoimmune disease is an animal model for multiple sclerosis and post-vaccination encephalitis in man.

Postinfectious encephalomyelitis is a demyelinating disease following a virus infection that is mediated by autoimmune delayed-type (type IV) hypersensitivity to myelin.

EYE

Sympathetic ophthalmia is uveal inflammation of a healthy uninjured eye in an individual who has sustained a perforating injury to the other eye. The uveal tract reveals an infiltrate of lymphocytes and epithelioid cells, and there is granuloma formation. The mechanism has been suggested to be autoimmunity expressed as T lymphocyte-mediated immune reactivity against previously sequestered antigens released from the patient's other injured eye.

Vogt-Koyanagi-Harada (VKH) syndrome (Figures 82 and 83) is a uveal inflammation of the eye(s) with acute iridocyclitis, choroiditis, and retinal detachment. Initial manifestations include headache, dysacusis and sometimes vertigo. Scalp hair may show patchy loss or whitening. Vitiligo and poliosis occur often. The development of delayed-type hypersensitivity to melanin-containing tissue has been postulated. Apparently, pigmented constituents of the eye, hair and skin are altered by some type of insult in a manner that leads to a delayed-type hypersensitivity response to them. Possible autoantigens are soluble substances from the retinal photoreceptor layer. There is a predisposition to VKH in Asians. Uveal tissue extracts have been used in delayed-hypersensitivity skin tests. Antibodies to uveal antigens may

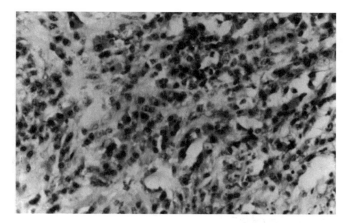

Figure 82. Hematoxylin and eosin (H & E) stained eye section showing extensive mononuclear cellular infiltrate of lymphocytes and plasma cells.

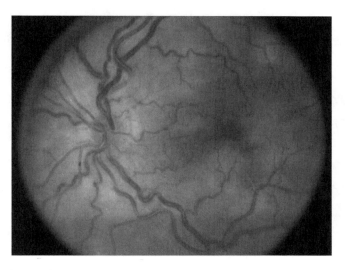

Figure 83. VKH funduscopic examination reveals venous engorgement and serous retinal detachment.

be present but are not specific for VKH. Corticosteroids, as well as chlorambucil, cyclophosphamide or cyclosporin A have been used for treatment.

Cicatricial ocular pemphigoid (Figures 84 and 85) is a rare blistering disorder of the conjunctival mucous membrane. This may lead to scarring that can result in blindness if untreated with corticosteroids. Histopathologically, the subepithelial unilocular bulla is accompanied by a mild inflammatory reaction. Direct immunoflorescence reveals a diffuse, linear deposition of immunoglobulins and complement components, mainly IgG and C3 at the epithelial-subepithelial junction.

SPERMATOZOA

Anti-sperm antibody (Figure 86) is specific for any one of several sperm constituents. Anti-sperm agglutinating antibodies are detected in blood serum by the Kibrick sperm

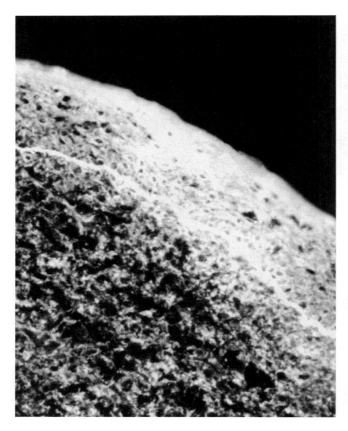

Figure 84. Cicatricial ocular pemphigoid. Stained with anti-IgGγ antibody.

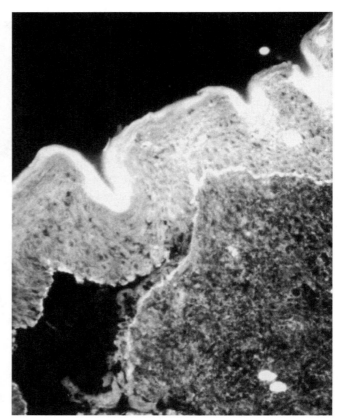

Figure 85. Cicatricial ocular pemphigoid. Stained with anti-IgGγ antibody.

agglutination test that uses donor sperm. Sperm-immobilizing antibodies are detected by the Isojima test. The subject's serum is incubated with donor sperm and motility examined. Testing for antibodies is of interest to couples with infertility problems. Treatment with relatively small doses of prednisone is sometimes useful in improving the situation by diminishing anti-sperm antibody titers. One-half of infertile females manifest IgG or IgA sperm immobilizing antibodies which affect the tail of the spermatozoa. By contrast, IgM anti-sperm head agglutinating antibodies may occur in homosexual males.

CARTILAGE

Relapsing polychondritis (Figures 87 and 88) is inflammation of the cartilage, especially that of the external pinnae of the ears, causing them to lose their structural integrity. It appears to have an immunological etiology, and anticollagen antibodies may be demonstrated in the serum of patients.

SYSTEMIC AUTOIMMUNE DISEASES

Systemic lupus erythematosus (SLE) (Figures 89–94) is a prototype of connective tissue diseases that involves multiple systems and has an autoimmune etiology. It is a disease with an acute or insidious onset. Patients may experience fever,

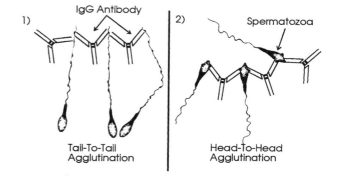

Figure 86. Antisperm Antibody.

malaise, loss of weight and lethargy. All organ systems may be involved. Patients form a plethora of autoantibodies, especially antinuclear autoantibodies. SLE is characterized by exacerbations and remissions. Patients often have injury to the skin, kidneys, joints, and serosal membranes. SLE occurs in one in 2,500 people in certain populations. It has a 9:1 female to male predominance. Its cause remains unknown. Antinuclear antibodies produced in SLE fall into four categories that include (1) antibodies against DNA, (2) antibodies against histones, (3) antibodies to nonhistone proteins bound to RNA, and (4) antibodies against nucleolar antigens.

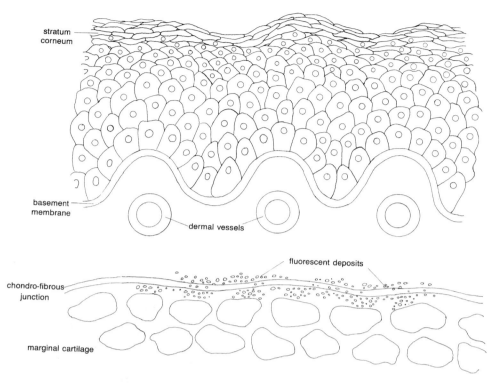

Figure 87.   Relapsing polychondritis.

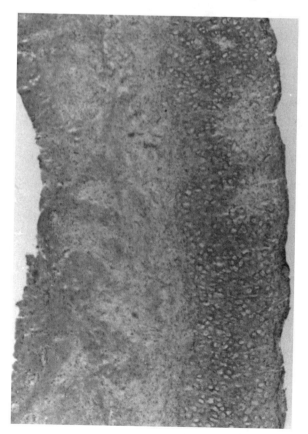

Figure 88.   Relapsing polychondritis.

Indirect immunofluorescence is used to detect nuclear fluorescence patterns that are characteristic for certain antibodies. These include homogeneous or diffuse staining, which reveals antibodies to histones and deoxyribonucleoprotein, rim or peripheral staining which signifies antibodies against double-stranded DNA, speckled pattern, which indicates antibodies to non-DNA nuclear components including histones and ribonucleoproteins, and the nucleolar pattern in which fluorescent spots are observed in the nucleus and reveal antibodies to nucleolar RNA. Antinuclear antibodies most closely associated with SLE are anti-double-stranded DNA and anti-Sm (Smith) antibodies.

There appears to be genetic predisposition to the disease which is associated with DR2 and DR3 genes of the major histocompatibility complex (MHC) in Caucasians of North America. Genes other than HLA genes are also important. In addition to the anti-double-stranded DNA and anti-Sm antibodies, other immunologic features of the disease include depressed serum complement levels, immune deposits in glomerular basement membranes and at the dermal-epidermal junction, and the presence of multiple other autoantibodies. Of all the immunologic abnormalities, the hyperactivity of B cells is critical to the pathogenesis of SLE. B cell activation is polyclonal leading to the formation of antibodies against self and nonself antigens. In SLE there is a loss of tolerance to self constituents leading to the formation of antinuclear antibodies. The polyclonal activation leads to antibodies of essentially all classes in immune

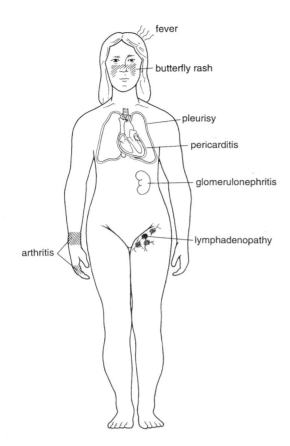

Figure 89. Systemic lupus erythematosus.

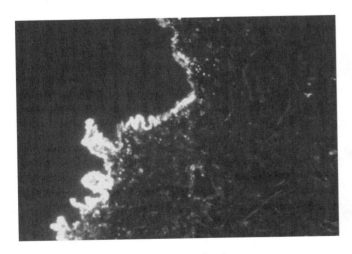

Figure 90. Lupus band test.

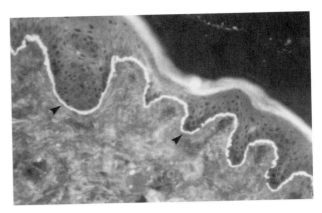

Figure 91. Lupus erythematosus. Immune deposits at dermal-epidermal junction.

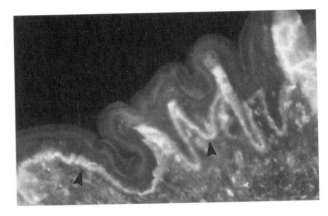

Figure 92. Systemic lupus erythematosus. Immune deposits at dermal-epidermal junction.

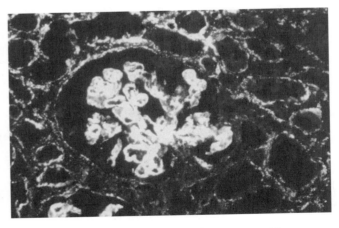

Figure 93. Diffuse proliferative lupus nephritis.

deposits found in renal biopsy specimens by immunofluorescence. In addition to genetic factors, hormonal and environmental factors are important in producing the B cell activation. Nuclei of injured cells react with antinuclear antibodies forming a homogeneous structure called an LE body or a hematoxylin body which is usually found in a neutrophil that has phagocytized the injured cell's denatured nucleus.

Tissue injury in lupus is mediated mostly by immune complex (type III hypersensitivity). There are also autoantibodies specific for erythrocytes, leukocytes, and platelets that induce injury through a type II hypersensitivity mechanism. There is an acute necrotizing vasculitis involving small arteries and arterioles present in tissues in lupus. Fibrinoid necrosis is classically produced. Most SLE patients have renal

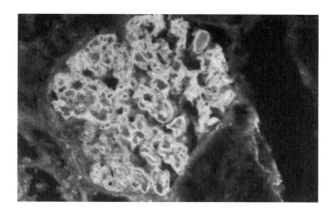

Figure 94.   Systemic lupus erythematosus. Diffuse immune deposits on peripheral capillary loops.

involvement which may take several forms with diffuse proliferative glomerulonephritis being the most serious. Subendothelial immune deposits in the kidneys of lupus patients are typical and may give a "wire loop" appearance to a thickened basement membrane.

In the skin, immunofluorescence can demonstrate deposition of immune complexes and complement at the dermal-epidermal junction. Immune deposits in the skin are especially prominent in sun-exposed areas of the skin. Joints may be involved but the synovitis is nonerosive. Typical female patients with lupus have a butterfly rash over the bridge of the nose in addition to fever and pain in the peripheral joints. However, the presenting complaints in SLE vary widely. Patients may have central nervous system involvement, pericarditis or other serosal cavity inflammation. There may be pericarditis as well as involvement of the myocardium or of the cardiac valves to produce Libman-Sacks endocarditis. There may be splenic enlargement, pleuritis and pleural effusion or interstitial pneumonitis as well as other organ or system involvement. Patients may also develop anti-phospholipid antibodies called lupus anticoagulants. They may be associated with a false positive VDRL test for syphilis. A drug such as hydrazaline may induce a lupus-like syndrome. However, the antinuclear antibodies produced in drug-induced lupus are often specific for histones, a finding not commonly found in classic SLE. Lupus erythematosus induced by drugs remits when the drug is removed. Discoid lupus refers to a form of the disease limited to the skin. Corticosteroids have proven very effective in suppressing immune reactivity in SLE. In more severe cases, cytotoxic agents such as cyclophosphamide, chlorambucil and azathioprine have been used.

A **butterfly rash** (Figure 95) is a facial rash in the shape of a butterfly across the bridge of the nose. It is seen especially in patients with lupus erythematosus. These areas are photosensitive and consist of erythematous and scaly patches that may become bulbous or secondarily infected. The rash is not specific for lupus erythematosus, since butterfly-type

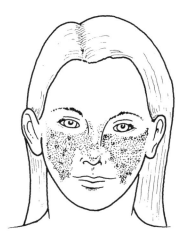

Figure 95.   Butterfly rash.

rashes may also occur in various other conditions including AIDS, dermatomyositis, ataxia-telangiectasia, erysipelas, pemphigus erythematosus, pemphigus foliaceous, etc.

An **LE cell** (Figures 96 and 97) is a neutrophil (PMN) in the peripheral blood or synovium of lupus erythematosus patients produced when the PMN phagocytizes a reddish-purple staining homogeneous lymphocyte nucleus that has

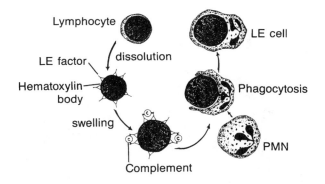

Figure 96.   Formation of an LE cell.

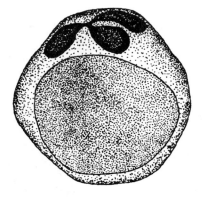

Figure 97.   Lupus erythematosus cell.

been coated with antinuclear antibody. In addition to lupus erythematosus, LE cells are seen also in scleroderma, drug-induced lupus erythematosus and lupoid hepatitis.

Antinuclear antibodies (ANA) (Figures 98–104) are antibodies found in the circulation of patients with various connective tissue disorders. They may show specificity for various nuclear antigens including single and double stranded DNA, histones and ribonucleoprotein. To detect

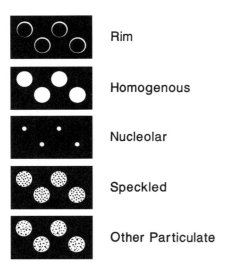

Figure 98.   Antinuclear antibody.

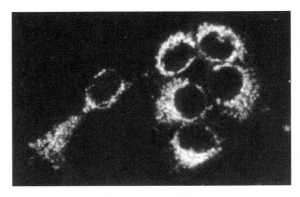

Figure 101.   AMA positive pattern.

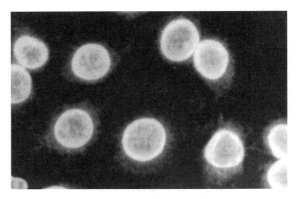

Figure 102.   ANA peripheral pattern.

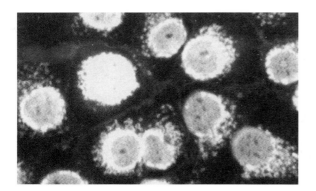

Figure 99.   ANA/AMA Mixed Pattern.

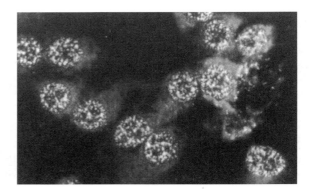

Figure 103.   ANA speckled pattern.

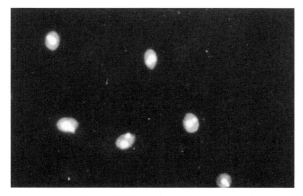

Figure 100.   nDNA antibody. Positive reaction.

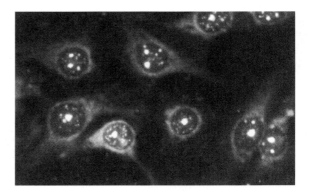

Figure 104.   ANA nucleolar pattern.

anti-nuclear antibodies, the patient's serum is incubated with Hep-2 cells and the pattern of nuclear staining determined by fluorescence microscopy. The homogeneous pattern of staining represents the morphologic expression of antinuclear antibodies specific for ribonucleoprotein which is positive in systemic lupus erythematosus, progressive systemic sclerosis, rheumatoid arthritis and other connective tissue disorders. Peripheral nuclear staining represents the morphologic expression of DNA antibodies associated with systemic lupus erythematosus. Nucleolar fluorescence signifies anti-RNA antibodies of the type that occurs in progressive systemic sclerosis (scleroderma). The speckled pattern of staining is seen in several connective tissue diseases.

Anti-double-stranded DNA (anti-dsDNA) (Figure 105) are antibodies present in the blood sera of systemic lupus erythematosus (SLE) patients. Among the detection methods is an immunofluorescence technique (IFT) using *Crithidia luciliae* as the substrate. In this method, fluorescence of the kinetoplast which contains mitochondrial DNA, signals the presence of anti-dsDNA antibodies. This technique is useful for assaying SLE serum which is usually positive in patients with active disease. A rim or peripheral pattern of nuclear staining of cells interacting with anti-nuclear antibody represents morphologic expression of anti-double-stranded DNA antibody.

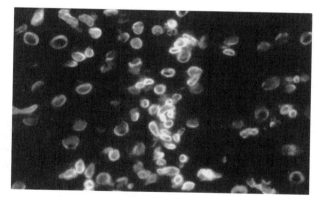

Figure 105. Anti-double stranded DNA.

Alopecia areata (Figure 106) describes hair loss in subjects who demonstrate autoantibodies against hair follicle capillaries.

Lupus anticoagulant is an IgG or IgM antibody that develops in lupus erythematosus patients as well as in certain individuals with neoplasia or drug reactions, in some normal persons and recently reported in AIDS patients who have active opportunistic infections. These antibodies are specific for phospholipoproteins or phospholipid constituents of coagulation factors. *In vitro*, these antibodies inhibit coagulation dependent upon phospholipids. If there are no other platelet or coagulation defects, they do not cause coagulopathy.

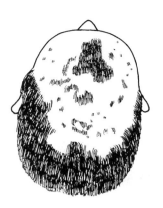

Figure 106. Alopecia areata.

Discoid lupus erythematosus (Figures 107 and 108) is a type of lupus erythematosus that involves only the skin which manifests a characteristic rash. The viscera are not involved, but the skin manifests erythematous plaques and telangiectasis with plugging of the follicles. Also called cutaneous lupus erythematosus.

Rheumatoid arthritis (Figure 109) is an autoimmune inflammatory disease of the joints which is defined according to special criteria designated 1 through 7. Criteria 1 through 4 must be present for more than six weeks. The "revised criteria" for rheumatoid arthritis are as follows: (1) morning stiffness in and around joints lasting at least 1 hour before maximum improvement; (2) soft tissue swelling (arthritis) of three or more joints observed by a physician; (3) swelling (arthritis) of the proximal interphalangeal, metacarpal phalangeal, or wrist joints; (4) symmetric swelling (arthritis); (5) rheumatoid nodules; (6) presence of rheumatoid factors; (7) roentgenographic erosions.

Pannus (Figure 110) refers to a granulation tissue reaction that is chronic and progressive and produces joint erosion in patients with rheumatiod arthritis. It is a structure that deveops in synovial membranes during the chronic proliferative and destructive phase of rheumatoid arthritis. It is a

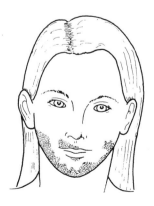

Figure 107. Discoid lupus erythematosus.

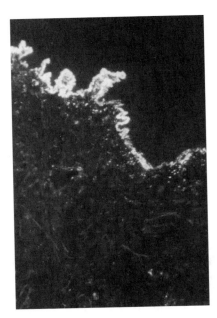

Figure 108.   Discoid lupus erythematosus. Immune deposits at dermal-epidermal junction.

Rheumatoid Arthritis

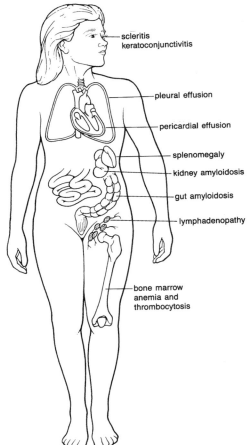

Figure 109.   Rheumatoid arthritis.

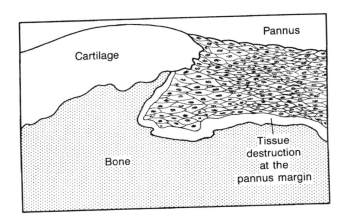

Figure 110.   Pannus.

membrane of granulation tissue induced by immune complexes that are deposited in the synovial membrane. They stimulate macrophages to release interleukin-1, fibroblast-activating factor, prostaglandins, substance P, and platelet-derived growth factor. This leads to extensive injury to chrondroosseous tissues. The articular surface of the joint is covered by the synovitis. There is edema, swelling, and erythema in the joints. Palisades of histiocytes are present. This entire process can fill the joint space, leading to demineralization and cystic resorption.

Rheumatoid factors is an autoantibody present in the serum of patients with rheumatoid arthritis but also found with varying frequency in other diseases such as subacute bacterial endocarditis, tuberculosis, syphilis, sarcoidosis, hepatic diseases and others, as well as in the sera of some human allograft recipients and apparently healthy persons. RF are immunoglobulins, usually of the IgM class and to a lesser degree of the IgG or IgA classes, with reactive specificity for the Fc region of IgG. This anti-immunoglobulin antibody, which may be either monoclonal or polyclonal, reacts with the Fc region epitopes of denatured IgG, including the Gm markers. Most RF are isotype-specific, manifesting reactivity mainly for IgG1, IgG2 and IgG4 but only weakly reactive with IgG3. Antigenic determinants of IgG that are potentially reactive with RF include (1) subclass specific or genetically defined determinants of native IgG (IgG1, IgG2, IgG4 and Gm determinants); (2) determinants present on complexed IgG but absent on native IgG; (3) determinants exposed after enzymatic cleavage of IgG. The Gm determinants are allotypic markers of the human IgG subclasses. They are located in the IgG molecule as follows: in the C_H1 domain in IgG1; in the C_H2 domain in IgG2; in C_H2 and C_H3 domains in IgG4.

Although rheumatoid factor titers may not be clearly correlated with disease activity, they may help perpetuate chronic inflammatory synovitis. When IgM rheumatoid factors and IgG target molecules react to form immune complexes, complement is activated leading to inflammation and immune injury. IgG rheumatoid factors may self-associate to form IgG-IgG immune complexes that help perpetuate chronic synovitis and vasculitis. IgG RF synthesized by plasma cells in the rheumatoid synovium fix complement and perpetuate inflammation. IgG RF has been shown in microbial infections, B lymphocyte proliferative disorders and malignancies, non-RA patients and aging individuals. RF might have a physiologic role in removal of immune complexes from the circulation. Rheumatoid factors (RF) were demonstrated earlier by the Rose-Waaler test but are now detected by the latex agglutination (or RA) test, which employs latex particles coated with IgG.

A **rheumatoid nodule** (Figure 111) is a granulomatous lesion characterized by central necrosis encircled by a palisade of mononuclear cells and an exterior mantle of lymphocytic infiltrate. The lesions occur as subcutaneous nodules, especially at pressure points such as the elbow, in individuals with rheumatoid arthritis or other rheumatoid diseases.

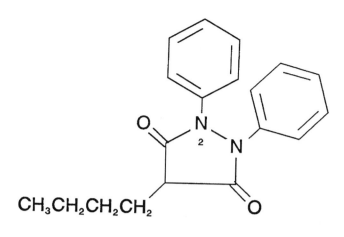

Figure 112. Phenylbutazone.

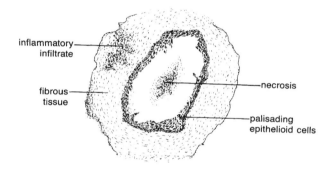

Figure 111. Rheumatoid nodule.

A **rheumatoid arthritis cell (RA cell)** is an irregular neutrophil that contains a variable number of black-staining cytoplasmic inclusions that are 0.2 to 2.0 μ in diameter. These cells contain IgM rheumatoid factor, complement, IgG and fibrin. They are found in synovial fluid of RA patients. Although RA cells may constitute 5 to 100% of an RA patient's neutrophils, they may also be present in patients with other connective tissue diseases.

Phenylbutazone (Figure 112) is a drug that prevents synthesis of prostaglandins and serves as a powerful antiinflammatory drug. It is used in therapy of rheumatoid arthritis and ankylosing spondylitis.

Ankylosing spondylitis (Figure 113) is a chronic inflammatory disease affecting the spine, sacroiliac joints and large peripheral joints. There is a strong male predominance with onset in early adult life. The erythrocyte sedimentation rate is elevated but subjects are negative for rheumatoid factor and antinuclear antibodies. Pathologically, there is chronic proliferative synovitis that resembles that seen in rheumatoid

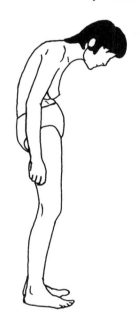

Figure 113. A patient with severe ankylosing spondylitis.

arthritis. The sacroiliac joints and interspinous and capsular ligaments ossify when the disease advances. There is a major genetic predisposition as revealed by increased incidence in selected families. Ninety percent of ankylosing spondylitis patients are positive for HLA-B27 compared to 8% among Caucasians in the U.S.A. The HLA-B27 genes may be linked to genes that govern pathogenic autoimmunity. There may be increased susceptibility to infectious agents, or molecular mimicry between HLA-B27 and an infectious agent such as *Klebsiella pneumoniae* leading to the synthesis of a cross reacting antibody. Treatment is aimed at diminishing inflammation and pain and providing physical therapy.

Adjuvant disease (Figure 114) may follow the injection of rats with Freund's complete adjuvant, a water-in-oil emulsion containing killed, dried mycobacteria, e.g., *Mycobacterium*

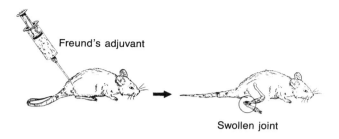

Figure 114. Adjuvant disease.

tuberculosis. This leads to the production of aseptic synovitis that closely resembles rheumatoid arthritis in man. Sterile inflammation occurs in the joints and lesions of the skin. In addition to swollen joints, inflammatory lesions of the tail may also result in animals developing adjuvant arthritis, which represents an animal model for RA.

Sjögren's syndrome (Figures 115 and 116) is a condition in which immunologic injury to the lacrimal and salivary glands leads to dry eyes (keratoconjunctivitis sicca) and dry mouth (xerostomia). It may occur alone as sicca syndrome (primary form) or together with an autoimmune disease such as rheumatoid arthritis (secondary form). The lacrimal and salivary glands show extensive lymphocytic infiltration and fibrosis. Most of the infiltrating cells are CD4+ T cells but there are some B cells (plasma cells) that form antibody. Approximately 75% of patients form rheumatoid factor. The LE cell test is positive in 25% of patients. Numerous antibodies are produced including autoantibodies against salivary duct cells, gastric parietal cells, thyroid antigens, and smooth muscle mitochondria. Antibodies against ribonucleoprotein antigens are termed SS-A (Ro) and SS-B (La). 90% of patients have these antibodies. Anti-SS-B shows greater specificity for Sjögren's syndrome than do anti-SS-A antibodies which also occur in SLE. Sjögren's syndrome patients who also have rheumatoid arthritis may have antibodies to

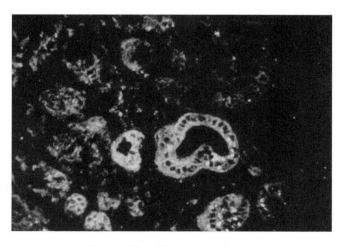

Figure 115. Sjörgren's syndrome.

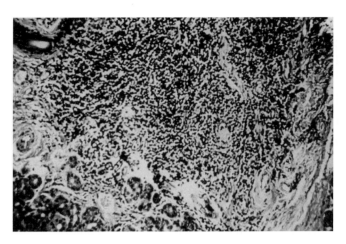

Figure 116. Sjögren's syndrome.

rheumatoid-associated nuclear antigen (RANA). There is a positive correlation between HLA-DR3 and primary Sjögren's syndrome and between HLA-DR4 and secondary Sjögren's syndrome associated with rheumatoid arthritis. Genetic predisposition, viruses and disordered immunoregulation may play a role in the pathogenesis. 90% of patients are 40–60 year-old females. In addition to dry eyes and dry mouth, with associated visual or swallowing difficulties, 50% of patients show parotid gland enlargement. There is drying of the nasal mucosa with bleeding, pneumonitis and bronchitis. A lip biopsy to examine minor salivary glands is needed to diagnose Sjögren's syndrome. Inflammation of the salivary and lacrimal glands was previously called Mikulicz's disease. Mikulicz's syndrome refers to enlargement of the salivary and lacrimal glands due to any cause. Enlarged lymph nodes that reveal a pleomorphic cellular infiltrate with many mitoses are typical of Sjögren's syndrome and have been referred to as "pseudolymphoma". These patients have a 40-fold greater risk of lymphoid neoplasms than do others.

SS-A is anti-RNA antibody that occurs in Sjögren's syndrome patients. The antibody may pass across the placenta in pregnant females and be associated with heart block in these infants. SS-A Ro is an antigen in the cytoplasm to which one-quarter of lupus erythematosus patients and 40% of Sjögren's syndrome patients synthesize antibodies.

Sixty percent of **Sjögren's syndrome (SS)** and 35% of **systemic lupus erythematosus (SLE)** patients have been shown by immunodiffusion to develop antibodies against SS-A/Ro antigen, (60 kD and 52 kD polypeptides complex with Ro RNAs). Ninety six percent of primary Sjögren's syndrome patients and in most individuals with SS secondary to rheumatoid arthritis or SLE have been shown by EIA to have SS-A antibodies. SS-A antibody levels are significantly higher in primary than in secondary (RA or SLE) Sjögren's syndrome. Cryostat sections of solid tissue and Hep-2 cell lines are used to detect SS-A/Ro and SS-B/La antibodies. There is a 5% risk of congenital heart block in babies born to mothers with SS-A/Ro antibodies. Passage of maternal SS-A antibodies across the placenta signifies neonatal lupus erythematosus. These antibodies from the mother may mediate congenital heart block. Mothers of babies with neonatal lupus erythematosus may range from asymptomatic to sicca syndrome or SLE. SS-A/Ro antibodies are demonstrable in cases of C2 and C4 deficiency, in subacute cutaneous lupus and in vasculitis with Sjögren's syndrome. Fewer than 1% of normal subjects have low levels of SS/A/Ro antibodies, detectable by EIA. The 2 to 5% of lupus patients who are ANA negative may manifest subacute cutaneous lupus, positive IgM-RF and SS-A antibodies. Approximately half of patients with Sjögren's syndrome and those with SLE, react with the 60 kD as well as the 52 kD components of the SS-A/Ro particle that is comprised of these proteins and RNA. Forty percent of patients with Sjögren's syndrome react with the 52 kD protein along, whereas 20% of SLE patients react only with the 60 kD component. Most patients with neonatal lupus erythematosus and complete heart block reveal antibodies against both 52 kD SS-A/Ro protein and 48 kD SS-B/La protein. Fetal cardiac tissue of 18 to 24 week gestation contains these antigens in significant quantities. The synthesis of SS-A, but not SS-B, antibodies within the blood-brain-barrier has been reported in cerebral vasculopathy.

SS-B is an anti-RNA antibody detectable in patients with Sjögren's syndrome as well as other connective tissue (rheumatic) diseases. SS-B La is an antigen in the cytoplasm to which Sjögren's syndrome and lupus erythematosus patients form antibodies. Anti-SS-B antibodies may portend a better prognosis in patients with lupus erythematosus.

Progressive systemic sclerosis (sclerederma) (Figure 117) is a connective tissue or collagen-vascular disease in which the skin and submucosal connective tissue become thickened and scarred. There is increased collagen deposition in the skin. It is slowly progressive and chronic and may involve internal organs. The female to male ratio is 2 to 1. Although the etiology is unknown, patients demonstrate anti-nuclear antibodies, rheumatoid factor and polyclonal hypergammaglobulinemia. There is no demonstrable immunoglobulin at the dermal-epidermal junction. These patients may have altered cellular immunity. The epidermis is thin, dermal appendages atrophy and rete pegs are lost. There is also a marked increase in collagen deposition in the reticular dermis together with fibrosis and hyalinization of arterioles. The GI tract may also reveal increased collagen deposition in the lamina propria, submucosa and muscularis layers. 90% of affected individuals experience Raynaud's phenomenon at the onset. Skin changes are usually the initial manifestation with involvement of the hands, feet, forearms and face or possibly diffuse involvement of the trunk. A variation of the disease is called CREST syndrome which consists of calcinosis, Raynaud's, esophageal dysmotility, sclerodactyly and telangiectasia. This form of the disease may become stabilized for a number of years. The skin may exhibit a bound, smooth, waxy appearance in the sclerotic phase with no wrinkles or folds apparent. Ulcers may develop on the fingertips in many patients with a mask-like appearance of the face with thin lips. The skin may either become atrophic or return to a normal soft structure. The lungs may be involved leading to dyspnea on exertion. Pulmonary fibrosis may lead to cor pulmonale. The principal immunologic findings include antinuclear antibodies with a speckled or nucleolar pattern, anti-centromere antibodies that are found in individuals with known CREST syndrome and the development of antibodies specific for acid-extractable nuclear antigen. Approximately one-third of individuals with diffuse involvement of the trunk reveal antibodies specific for topoisomerase (anti-Scl-70 antibodies).

Scl-70 antibody is an antinuclear antibody found in as many as 70% of diffuse-type scleroderma (progressive systemic sclerosis) patients, who experience extensive and rapid skin involvement as well as early visceral manifestations.

CREST complex includes calcinosis, Raynaud's phenomenon, esophageal dysmotility, sclerodactyly and telangiectasia associated with mixed connective tissue disease. The prognosis of CREST is slightly better than that of other connective tissue diseases but biliary cirrhosis and pulmonary hypertension are complications. CREST patients may develop anticentromere antibodies which may also occur in progressive systemic sclerosis patients, in aged females or in individuals with HLA-DR1. CREST represents a mild form of systemic sclerosis. CREST syndrome is a relatively mild clinical form of scleroderma (progressive systemic sclerosis). CREST is an acrynym for calcinosis, Raynaud's phenomenon, esophageal dysmotility, sclerodactyly and telangiectasis. Skin lesions are usually limited to the face and fingers, with only later visceral manifestations. Most (80–90%) of CREST patients have anti-centromere antibodies.

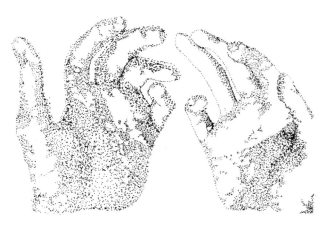

Figure 117.   Systemic sclerosis.

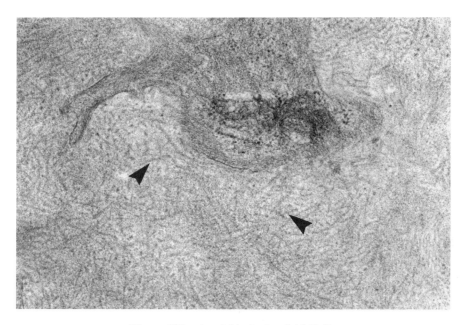

Figure 118. Amyloidosis. Amyloid fibrils.

GAMMAPATHIES

Amyloidosis (Figures 118–120) is a constellation of diseases characterized by the extracellular deposition of fibrillar material that has a homogeneous and eosinophilic appearance in conventional staining methods. It may compromise the function of vital organs. Diseases with which it is associated may be inflammatory, hereditary or neoplastic. All types of amyloid link to Congo red and manifest an apple-green birefrigence when viewed by polarizing light microscopy after first staining with Congo red. By electron microscopy, amyloid has a major fibrillar component and a minor rod-like structure which is shaped like a pentagon with a hollow core when observed on end, i.e., the P component. All forms of amyloid share the P component in common. It is found as a soluble serum protein in the circulation (SAP). Amyloid has a β-pleated sheet structure; it is insoluble in physiologic saline but is soluble in distilled water.

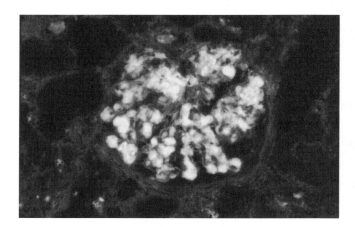

Figure 119. Amyloidosis.

The classification of amyloidosis depends upon the clinical presentation, anatomic distribution and chemical content of the amyloid. In the United States, AL amyloid is the most common type of amyloidosis which occurs in association with multiple myeloma and Waldenström's macroglobulinemia. These patients have free light chain production in association with the development of Bence-Jones proteins in myeloma. The light chain quality and degradation mechanism are critical in determining whether or not Bence Jones proteins will be deposited as amyloid. Chronic inflammation leads to increased levels of SAA, which are produced by the liver following IL-6 and IL-1 stimulation. Normally, SSA is degraded by the enzymes of monocytes. Thus, individuals

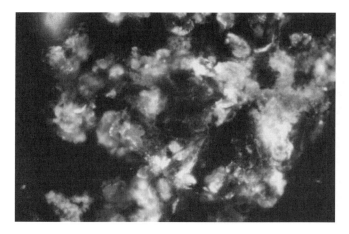

Figure 120. Amyloidosis.

with a defect in the degradation process could generate insoluble AA molecules. Likewise, there could be a defect in the degradation of immunoglobulin light chains in subjects who develop AL amyloidosis.

Amyloidosis secondary to chronic inflammation is severe with kidney, liver, spleen, lymph node, adrenal and thyroid involvement. These secondary amyloidosis deposits consist of amyloid A protein (AA) which makes up 85 to 90% of the deposits and serum amyloid P component which accounts for the remainder of the deposit. The AL type of amyloidosis more often involves the heart, gastrointestinal tract and respiratory tract, peripheral nerves and tongue. Amyloidosis may also be heredofamilial or associated with aging.

Amyloid (Figures 121 and 122) is an extracellular, homogenous eosinophilic material deposited in various tissues in disease states, designated primary and secondary amyloidosis. It is composed chiefly of protein and shows a green birefringence when stained with Congo red and observed by polarizing light microscopy. By electron microscopy, the fibrillar appearance is characteristic. By X-ray crystallography, it shows a β-pleated sheet structure, arranged in an antiparallel fashion. The amino termini of the individual chains face opposite directions and the chains are bound by hydroxyl bonds.

Amyloid consists of two principal and several minor biochemical varieties. Pathogenetic mechanisms for its deposition differ although the deposited protein appears similar from one form to another. Amyloid consists of nonbranching fibrils 7.5 to 10nm wide and are of indefinite length. X-ray crystallography reveals a β-pleated sheet configuration which gives the protein its optical and staining properties. It also has a P component that is nonfibrillary, is pentagonal in structure and constitutes a minor component of amyloid. Chemically amyloid falls into two principal classes, i.e., AL, consisting of amyloid light chains and AA (amyloid-associated) that is comprised of a nonimmunoglobulin protein called AA. These molecules are antigenically different and have dissimilar deposition patterns based on the clinical situation. AL amyloid is comprised of whole immunoglobulin light chains, their N-terminal fragments, or a combination of the two. λ light chains rather than κ are the ones usually found in AL. Proliferating immunoglobulin producing B cells, as in B cell dyscrasias, produce AL amyloid protein. AA amyloid fibroprotein is not an immunoglobulin and has a molecular wight of 8.5kD. Serum amyloid-associated protein (SAA) is the serum precursor of AA amyloid. It constitutes the protein constituent of high density lipoprotein and acts as an acute phase reactant. Thus, its level rises remarkably within hours of an acute inflammatory response. AA protein is the principal type of amyloid deposited in the tissues during chronic inflammatory diseases. Several other distinct amyloid proteins exist also.

AA amyloid is a nonimmunoglobulin amyloid fibril of the type seen following chronic inflammatory diseases, such as tuberculosis and osteomyelitis or more recently chronic noninfectious inflammatory disorders. Kidneys, liver and spleen are the most significant areas of AA deposition. The precursor for AA protein is apo-SAA with a monomer molecular weight of 12.5kD that is found in the circulation as a 220kD to 235kD molecular complex because it is linked to high density lipoprotein. IL-6 stimulates its synthesis. AA deposition is associated with either an amyloidogenic isotypical form of SAA or results from the inability to completely degrade SAA.

Amyloid consists of nonbranching fibrils 7.5 to 10nm in width and of indefinite length. Chemically, amyloid occurs in two classes. The AL (amyloid light chain) type consists of immunoglobulin light chains or parts of them. The AA (amyloid associated) type is derived from the SAA (serum amyloid-associated) protein in the serum. SAA acts like an acute phase reactant increasing greatly during inflammation. Thus, AA protein is the principal type of amyloid deposited in chronic inflammatory diseases. AL amyloid consists of either whole immunoglobulin light chains or their N-terminal fragments or combination of the two. λ light chain especially gives

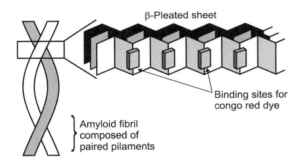

Figure 121.   Amyloid.

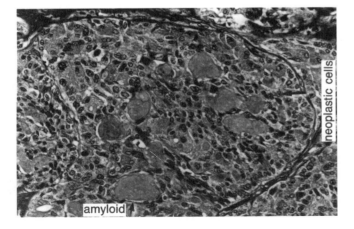

Figure 122.   Medullary carcinoma of thyroid with amyloid deposition.

rise to AL. AL amyloid protein is often deposited following or during B cell disorders. Other biochemical forms of amyloid include transthyretin, β_2 microglobulin, β_2 amyloid protein or additional forms. Amyloid filaments stained with Congo red exhibit green birefringence with polarized light.

Amyloid P component has a molecular weight of 180kD. It migrates in electrophoresis with the α globulin fraction and by electron microscopy has a pentagonal shape suggesting that it consists of subunits linked by hydrogen bonds. It is a minor component of all amyloid deposits and is nonfibrillar. It is a normal α_1 glycoprotein and has close structural homology with C-reactive protein. It has an affinity for amyloid fibrils and accounts for their PAS positive staining quality.

Multiple myeloma (Figures 123–125) is a clinical condition in which a plasmacytoma or plasma cell neoplasm is associated with the production of a paraprotein that appears in the serum. The neoplastic plasma cells usually synthesize and secrete monoclonal, highly homogenous, immunoglobulins. Serum electrophoresis reveals a narrow monoclonal band in 98 to 99% of patients. Eighty percent of myeloma patients manifest IgG paraimmunoglobulin, while 15% have monoclonal IgA. A few

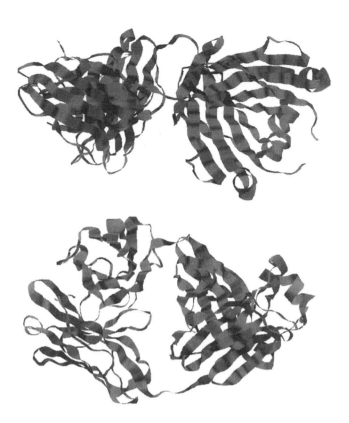

Figure 125.   From a patient with multiple myeloma and amyloidosis.

cases of the IgD and IgE types have been described. Homogeneous light chain dimers, which are identical to the corresponding light chain portion of immunoglobulin in the individual's blood, appear in the urine. These light chain dimers in the urine are called Bence-Jones proteins. These segments of light polypeptide chains do not represent degradation products of immunoglobulin, since they are synthesized separately from it. The disease affects three in 100,000 persons, usually men over 50 years of age. Patients develop anemia, anorexia and weakness. The tumor infiltrates the bone marrow cavities, ultimately leading to erosion of the bone cortex. This may take years. Osteolytic lesions are the hallmark of multiple myeloma. The long bones, ribs, vertebrae and skull manifest diffuse osteoporosis which leads to the appearance of punched-out areas and pathologic fractions. Tumor invasion of the marrow and erosion of the cortex as well as osteoclast-activating substances produce the bone lesions. Lung or renal infections may also occur. Hypogammagloblinemia results from decreased functioning of normal plasma cells that leads to diminished antibody to combat infections. The malignant plasma cells produce an excess of nonsense paraimmunoglobulin which does not protect against infection. There is also defective phagocytic activity. Patients may have altered B cell function and increased susceptibility to pyogenic infections. Some patients may develop myeloma kidney, signified by proteinuria followed by oliguria, kidney failure and possibly death.

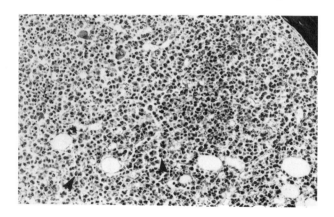

Figure 123.   Multiple myeloma. Bone marrow plasma cell myeloma.

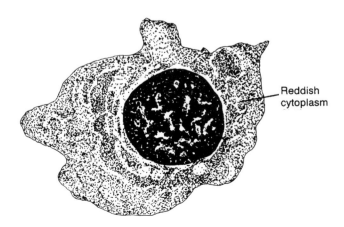

Reddish cytoplasm

Figure 124.   Flame cell.

Bence-Jones proteins (Figures 126 and 127) represent the light chains of either λ or κ variant excreted in the urine of patients with a paraproteinemia as a result of excess synthesis of such chains or from mutant cells which make only such chains. Both mechanisms appear operative and over 50% of patients with multiple myeloma, a plasma cell neoplasm, have B-J proteinuria. The highest frequency of B-J excretion is seen in IgD myeloma; the lowest in IgG myeloma. The daily amount excreted parallels the severity of the disease. The B-J proteins are secreted mostly as dimers and show unusual heat solubility properties. They precipitate at temperatures between 40°C to 60°C and redissolve again near 100°C. With proper pH control and salt concentration, precipitation may detect as low as 30 mg per 100 ml of urine. Better identification is by protein electrophoresis.

Waldenström's macroglobulinemia (Figure 128) is a paraproteinemia that is second in frequency only to multiple myeloma occurring mostly in people more than 50 years of age. It may be manifested in various clinical forms. Most of the features of the disease are related to the over-synthesis of monoclonal IgM. Relatively mild cases may be characterized by anemia and weakness or pain in the abdomen resulting from enlargement of the spleen and liver. A major difference from multiple myeloma is a lack of osteolytic lesions of the skeleton although patients may have peripheral lymphadenopathy. On bone marrow examination many kinds of cells are found with characteristics of plasma cells and lymphocytes constituting so-called lymphocytoid plasma cells. Many are transitional or intermediate between one type or another. Patients may develop bleeding disorders of some type due to the paraproteins in their circulation. The more severe forms of the disease are characterized by features that resemble chronic lymphocytic leukemia or even lymphosarcoma with a rapidly fatal course. Many individuals may develop anemia. The large molecules of IgM with a molecular weight approaching one million lead to increased viscosity of the blood. Central nervous system and visual difficulties may also be manifested.

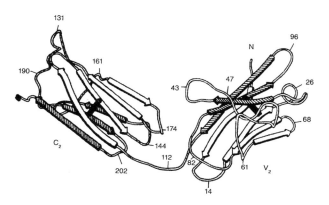

Figure 126. Bence-Jones protein.

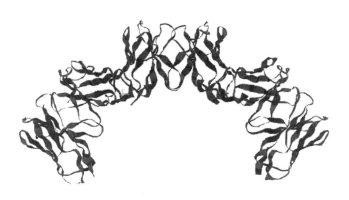

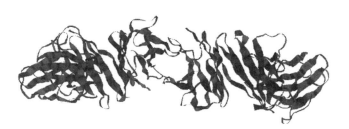

Figure 127. Bence-Jones protein.

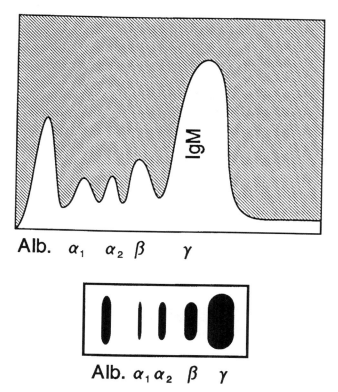

Figure 128. Waldenström's macroglobulinemia with IgM spike.

Macroglobulinemia of Waldenström is a condition usually of older men in which monoclonal IgM is detected in the serum, and elevated numbers of lymphoid cells and plasmacytoid lymphocytes expressing cytoplasmic IgM are found in the bone marrow. However, these subjects do not have the osteolytic lesions observed in multiple myeloma. Due to the high molecular weight of the IgM and increased levels of this immunoglobulin, blood viscosity increases, leading to circulatory embarassment. Patients often develop skin hemorrhages and anemia as well as neurological problems. This condition is considered less severe than multiple myeloma.

β-pleated sheet describes a protein configuration in which the β sheet polypeptide chains are extended and have a 35nm axial distance. Hydrogen bonding between NH and CO groups of separate polypeptide chains stabilize the molecules. Adjacent molecules may be either parallel or antiparallel. The β-pleated sheet configuration is characteristic of amyloidosis and is revealed by Congo red staining followed by polarizing light microscopy that yields an apple-green birefringence and ultrastructurally consists of non-branching fibrils.

In **amyloid β fibrillosis**, all amyloids have a β-pleated sheet structure which accounts for the ability of Congo red to stain them and the ability of proteolytic enzymes to digest them.

Burkitt's lymphoma (Figure 129) is an Epstein-Barr virus-induced neoplasm of B lymphocytes. It affects the jaws and abdominal viscera. It is seen especially in African children. The Epstein-Barr virus is present in tumor cells which may reveal rearrangement between the c-*myc* bearing chromosome and the immunoglobulin heavy chain gene-bearing chromosome. Burkitt's lymphoma patients have antibodies to the Epstein-Barr virus in their blood sera. The disease occurs in geographic regions that are hot and humid and where malaria is endemic. It occurs in subjects with acquired immuno-deficiency and in other immunosuppressed individuals. There is an effective immune response against the lymphoma that may lead to remission.

Sezary syndrome (Figure 130) is a disease that occurs in middle age affecting males more commonly than females. It is a neoplasm, i.e., a malignant lymphoma of CD4+ T helper lymphocytes with prominent skin involvement. There is a generalized erythroderma, hyperpigmentation and exfoliation. Fissuring and scaling of the skin on the palms of the hands and soles of the feet may occur. The peripheral blood and lymph nodes contain the typical cerebriform cells that have a nucleus that resembles brain. There is extensive infiltration of the skin by leukocytes with prominent clustering in the epidermis forming Pautrier's evidence. Late in the disease, T immunoblasts may appear. The so-called Sezary cells are T lymphocytes.

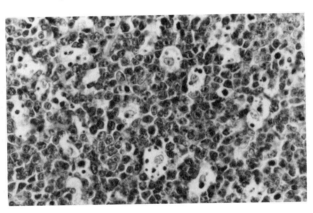

Figure 129.   Burkitt's lymphoma.

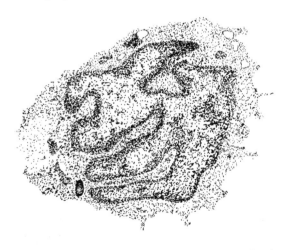

Figure 130.   Lymphocyte from a patient with Sezary Syndrome.

17
Immunodeficiencies: Congenital and Acquired

Immunodeficiencies are classified as either primary diseases with a genetic origin or those that are secondary to an underlying disorder. X-linked (congenital) agammaglobulinemia results from a failure of pre-B cells to differentiate into mature B cells. The defect in Bruton's disease is in rearrangement of immunoglobulin heavy chain genes. It occurs almost entirely in males and is apparent after 6 months of age following disappearance of the passively transferred maternal immunoglobulins. Patients have recurrent sinopulmonary infections caused by *Haemophilus influenzae, Streptococcus pyogenes, Staphlococcus aureus,* and *Streptococcus pneumoniae.* These patients have absent or decreased B cells and decreased serum levels of all immunoglobulin classes. The T-cell system and cell-mediated immunity appear normal.

Thymic hypoplasia (DiGeorge's syndrome) occurs when the immune system in infants is deprived of thymic influence. T cells are absent or deficient in the blood and thymus-dependent areas of lymph nodes and spleen. Infants with this condition are highly susceptible to infection by viruses, fungi, protozoa, or intracellular bacteria due to defective intracellular microbial killing by phagocytic cells with interferon. By contrast, B cells and immunoglobulins are not affected.

Severe combined immunodeficiency (Swiss-type agammaglobulinemia) comprises a group of conditions manifesting variable defects in both B and T cell immunity. In general, there is a lymphopenia with deficiency of T and B cell numbers and function. The thymus is hypoplastic or absent. Lymph nodes and other peripheral lymphoid tissues reveal depleted B- and T-cell regions. Infants with severe combined immunodeficiency show increased susceptibility to infections by viruses, fungi, and bacteria, and often succumb during the first year.

Secondary immunodeficiencies are more common than the primary forms. The best known is aquired immunodeficiency disease (e.g., AIDS), which results from destruction of the helper/inducer (CD4+) lymphocyte. Most of these individuals develop opportunistic infections caused by viruses, fungi, protozoa, and bacteria that are not commonly pathogenic (Figure 1).

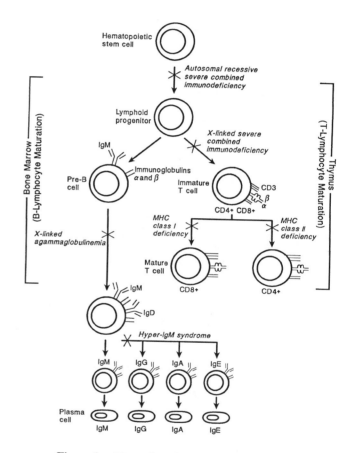

Figure 1. Maturation of T and B lymphocytes.

Immunodeficiency is a failure in humoral antibody or cell-mediated limbs of the immune response. If attributable to intrinsic defects in T and/or B lymphocytes, the condition is termed a primary immunodeficiency. If the defect results from loss of antibody and/or lymphocytes, the condition is termed a secondary immunodeficiency.

Congenital immunodeficiency refers to a varied group of unusual disorders with associated autoimmune manifestations, increased incidence of malignancy, allergy, and gastrointestinal abnormalities. These include defects in stem cells, B cells, T cells, phagocytic defects and complement defects. An example is severe combined immunodeficiency due to various causes. The congenital immunodeficiencies are described under the separate disease categories.

Agammaglobulinemia (hypogammaglobulinemia) (Figure 2) was used in earlier years before the development of methods sufficiently sensitive to detect relatively small quantities of gammaglobulin in the blood. Primary agammaglobulinemia was attributed to defective immunoglobulin formation, whereas secondary agammaglobulinemia referred to immunoglobulin depletion, as in loss through inflammatory bowel disease or through the skin in burn cases.

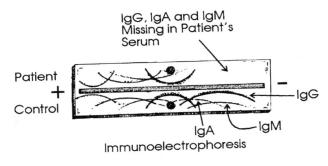

Figure 2.   Agammaglobuilinemia.

X-linked agammaglobulinemia (Bruton's X-linked agammaglobulinemia) affects males who develop recurrent sinopulmonary or other pyogenic infections at 5 to 6 months of age after disappearance of maternal IgG. There is defective B lymphocyte gene (chromosome Xq21.3-22). Whereas B cells and immunoglobulins are diminished, there is normal T cell function. Supportive therapy includes gammaglobulin injections and antibiotics. Repeated infections may lead to death in childhood. Their bone marrow contains pre-B cells with constant regions of immunoglobulin μ chains in the cytoplasm. There may be defective V_H-D-J_H gene rearrangement.

Swiss type agammaglobulinemia is a severe combined immunodeficiency disease. Refer to Swiss type of severe combined immunodeficiency.

Immunodeficiency with thymoma is an abnormality in B cell development with a striking decrease in B cell numbers and in immunoglobulins in selected patients with thymoma. There is a progressive decrease in their cell-mediated immunity as the disease continues. Most patients develop chronic sinopulmonary infections. Approximately 20% develop thrombocytopenia and about 25% have splenomegaly. Immunoglobulin class alterations are variable. Skin test reactivity and responsiveness to skin allografts are decreased. Patients have few or no lymphocytes expressing surface immunoglobulin. The disease is due to a stem cell defect. The preferred treatment is gammaglobulin administration.

B cell leukemias can be classified as **pre-B cell**, **B cell** or as **plasma cell neoplasms**. They include Burkitt's lymphoma,

Hodgkin's disease and chronic lymphocytic leukemia. Neoplasms of plasma cells are associated with multiple myeloma and Waldenström's macroglobulinemia. Many of these conditions are associated with hypogammaglobulinemia and a diminished capacity to form antibodies in response to the administration of an immunogen. In chronic lymphocytic leukemia, more than 95% of individuals have malignant leukemic cells that are identifiable as B lymphocytes expressing surface immunoglobulin. These patients frequently develop infections and have autoimmune manifestations such as autoimmune hemolytic anemia. CLL patients may have secondary immunodeficiency which affects both B and T limbs of the immune response. Diminished immunoglobulin levels are due primarily to diminished synthesis (Figure 3).

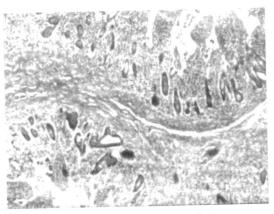

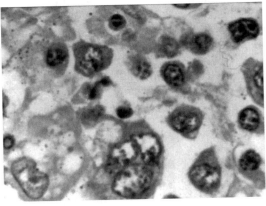

Figure 3.   B cell lymphoma of the gut.

Selective IgA deficiency is the most frequent immunodeficiency disorder. It occurs in approximately 1 in 600 individuals in the population. It is characterized by nearly absent serum and secretory IgA. The IgA level is less than 5mg/dL, whereas the remaining immunoglobulin class levels are normal or elevated. The disorder is either familial, or it may be acquired in association with measles, other types of virus infection, or toxoplasmosis. The patients may appear normal and asymptomatic, or they may have some form of an associated disease. IgA is the principal immunoglobulin in secretions and is an important part of the defense of mucosal surfaces. Thus IgA deficient individuals have an increased incidence of respiratory, gastrointestinal and urogenital infections. They may manifest sinopulmonary infections and diarrhea. Selective IgA deficiency is diagnosed by the demonstration of less than 5 mg/dL of IgA in serum. The etiology is unknown but is believed to be arrested B cell development. The B lymphocytes are normal with surface IgA and IgM or surface IgA and IgD.

Some patients also have an IgG2 and IgG4 subclass deficiency. They are especially likely to develop infections. IgA deficient patients have an increased incidence of respiratory allergy and autoimmune disease such as systemic lupus erythematosus, and rheumatoid arthritis. The principal defect is in IgA B lymphocyte differentiation. The 12- week-old fetus contains the first IgA B lymphocytes that bear IgM and IgD as well as IgA on their surface. At birth, the formation of mature IgA B lymphocytes begins. Most IgA B cells express IgA exclusively on their surface with only 10% expressing surface IgM and IgD in the adult. Patients with selective IgA deficiency usually express the immature phenotype, only a few of which can transform into IgA synthesizing plasma cells. Patients have an increased incidence of HLA-A1, -B8 and -Dw3. Their IgA cells form but do not secrete IgA. There is an increased incidence of the disorder in certain atopic individuals. Some selective IgA deficiency patients form significant titers of antibody against IgA. They may develop anaphylactic reactions upon receiving IgA-containing blood transfusions. The patients have an increased incidence of celiac disease and of several autoimmune diseases as indicated above. They synthesize normal levels of IgG and IgM antibodies. Autosomal recessive and autosomal dominant patterns of inheritance have been described. It has been associated with several cancers including thymoma, reticulum cell sarcoma, and squamous cell carcinoma of the esophagus and lungs. Certain cases may be linked to drugs such as phenytoin or other anticonvulsants. Some individuals develop antibodies against IgG, IgM and IgA. Gamma globulin should not be administered to selective IgA deficient patients.

Selective IgM deficiency occurs when IgM is absent from the serum. Although IgM may be demonstrable on plasma cell surfaces, it is not secreted. This could be related to an alteration in secretory peptide or due to the action of suppressor T lymphocytes specifically on IgM-synthesizing and secreting cells. Gram negative microorganisms may induce septicemia in affected individuals since IgM's major role in protection against infection is in the intravascular compartment rather than in extravascular spaces where other immunoglobulin classes may be active.

IgG subclass deficiency refers to decreased or absent IgG2, IgG3 or IgG4 subclasses. Total serum IgG is unaffected because it is 65 to 70% IgG1. Deletion of constant heavy chain genes or defects in isotype switching may lead to IgG subclass deficiency. IgG1 and IgG3 subclasses mature quicker than do IgG2 or IgG4. Patients have recurrent respiratory infections and recurring pyogenic sinopulmonary infections with *Hemophilus influenzae*, *Staphylococcus aureus*, and *Streptococcus pneumoniae*. Some patients may manifest features of autoimmune disease such as systemic lupus erythematosus. IgG2–IgG4 deficiency is often associated with recurrent infections or autoimmune disease. IgG2 deficiency is reflected as recurrent sinopulmonary infections and nonresponsiveness to polysaccharide antigens such as those of the pneumococcus. A few individuals have IgG3 deficiency and develop recurrent infections. In the IgG4 deficient patients, recurrent respiratory infections as well as autoimmune manifestations also occur. The diagnosis is established by the demonstration of significantly lower levels of at least one IgG subclass in the patient compared with IgG subclass levels in normal age-matched controls. Gammaglobulin is the treatment choice. Very infrequently, C-gene segment deletions may lead to IgG subclass deficiency.

Selective IgA and IgG deficiency affects both males and females, is either X-linked, autosomal recessive, or can be acquired later in life. There may be a genetic defect in the switch mechanism for immunoglobulin producing cells to change from IgM to IgG or IgA synthesis. Respiratory infections with pyogenic microorganisms or autoimmune states that include hemolytic anemia, thrombocytopenia, and neutropenia may occur. Numerous IgM-synthesizing plasma cells are demonstrable in both lymph nodes and spleen of affected individuals.

Selective IgA and IgM deficiency is a concomitant reduction in both IgA and IgM concentrations with normal IgG levels. The IgG produced in many individuals may not be protective and recurrent infections may result. There is an inadequate response to many immunogens in this disease which occurs in 4 males to every female affected.

Selective immunoglobulin deficiency is an insufficient quantity of one of the three major immunoglobulins or a subclass of IgG or IgA.

Common variable immunodeficiency (CVID) is a relatively common congenital or acquired immunodeficiency that may be either familial or sporadic. The familial form may have a variable mode of inheritance. Hypogammaglobulinemia is common to all of these patients and usually affects all classes of immunoglobulin but in some cases only IgG is affected. The World Health Organization (WHO) classifies three forms of the disorder: (1) an intrinsic B lymphocyte defect, (2) a disorder of T lymphocyte regulation that includes deficient T helper lymphocytes or activated T suppressor lymphocytes, and (3) autoantibodies against T and B lymphocytes. The majority of patients have an intrinsic B cell defect with normal numbers of B cells in the circulation that can identify antigens and proliferate but cannot differentiate into plasma cells. The ability of B cells to proliferate when stimulated by antigen is evidenced by hyperplasia of B cell regions of lymph nodes, spleen and other lymphoid tissues. Yet, differentiation of B cells into plasma cells is blocked. The deficiency of antibody that results leads to recurrent bacterial infections as well as intestinal infestation by *Giardia lamblia*, which produces a syndrome that resembles sprue. Noncaseating granulomas occur in many organs. There is an increased incidence of autoimmune diseases such as pernicious anemia, rheumatoid arthritis and hemolytic anemia. Lymphomas also occur in these immunologically deficient individuals.

DiGeorge syndrome (Figure 4) is a T cell immunodeficiency in which there is failure of T cell development but normal maturation of stem cells and B lymphocytes. This is attributable to failure in development of the thymus, depriving the individual of the mechanism for T lymphocyte development. Maldevelopment of the thymus gland is associated with thymic hypoplasia. Anatomical structures derived from the third and fourth pharyngeal pouches during embryogenesis fail to develop. This leads to a defect in function of both the thymus and parathyroid glands. DiGeorge syndrome is believed to be a consequence of intrauterine malfunction. It is not familial. Tetany and hypocalcemia, both characteristics of hypoparathyroidism, are observed in DiGeorge syndrome in addition to the defects in T cell immunity. Peripheral lymphoid tissues exhibit a deficiency of lymphocytes in thymic-dependent areas. By

contrast, the B or bursa equivalent-dependent areas, such as lymphoid follicles, show normal numbers of B lymphocytes and plasma cells. Serum immunoglobulin levels are within normal limits, and there is a normal immune response following immunization with commonly employed immunogens. A defect in delayed-type hypersensitivity is demonstrated by the failure of affected patients to develop positive skin tests to commonly employed antigens such as candidin or streptokinase and the inability to develop an allograft response. Defective cell-mediated immunity may increase susceptibility to opportunistic infections and render the individual vulnerable to a graft-versus-host reaction in blood transfusion recipients. There is also minimal or absent *in vitro* responsiveness to T cell antigens or mitogens. Considerable success in treatment has been achieved with fetal thymic transplants and by the passive administration of thymic humoral factors.

Thymic hypoplasia is an immunodeficiency that selectively affects the T cell limb of the immune response. Early symptoms soon after birth may stem from associated parathyroid abnormalities leading to hypocalcemia and heart defects which may lead to congestive heart failure. There is lymphopenia with diminished T cell numbers. T lymphocyte function cannot be detected in peripheral blood T cells. There is variation in antibody levels and function. The condition has been successfully treated by thymic transplantation. Some DiGeorge patients may have normal B cell immunity. All the others may have diminished immunoglobulin levels and may not form specific antibody following immunization. Clinically, DiGeorge patients may have a fish-shaped mouth, abnormal faces with low-set ears, hypertelorism, antimongoloid eyes in addition to the other features mentioned above.

Nezelof's syndrome is a hypoplasia of the thymus leading to a failure of the T lymphocyte compartment with no T cells and no T cell function. By contrast, B lymphocyte function remains intact. Thus, this is classified as a T lymphocyte immunodeficiency.

T cell immunodeficiency syndromes (TCIS) causes a decreased immune function as a consequence of complete or partial defects in the function of T lymphocytes. HUETER patients develop recurrent opportunistic infections; may manifest cutaneous anergy, wasting, diminished life expectancy, retardation in growth, increased likelihood of developing graft-versus-host disease and have very serious or even fatal reactions following immunization with BCG or live virus vaccines. They also have an increased likelihood of malignancy. T cell immunodeficiencies are usually more profound than are B cell immunodeficiencies. There is no effective treatment. This group of disorders includes thymic hypoplasia known as DiGeorge syndrome, cellular immunodeficiency with immunoglobulins termed Header syndrome and defects of T lymphocytes caused by deficiency

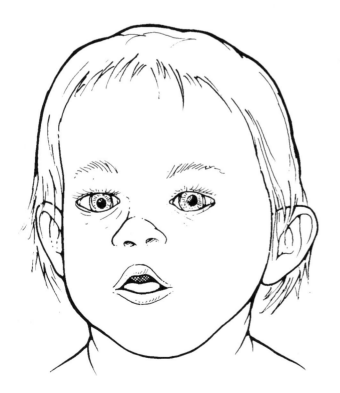

Figure 4. DiGeorge syndrome.

of purine nucleoside phosphorylase and lack of inosine phosphorylase.

Immunodeficiency with T cell neoplasms occurs in almost one-third of patients with acute lymphocytic leukemia (ALL), individuals with Sezary syndrome and a very few chronic lymphocytic leukemia (CLL) patients develop a malignant type proliferation of lymphoid cells. Sezary cells are poor mediators of T cell cytotoxicity but can produce migration inhibitory factor (MIF)-like lymphokine. They produce neither immunoglobulin nor suppressor substances but do have a helper effect for immunogloublin synthesis by B cell. In mycosis fungoides, skin lesions contain T lymphocytes and there is an increased number of null cells in the blood with a simultaneous decrease in the numbers of B and T cells. T cell immunity is decreased in this condition but IgA and IgE may be elevated. Whereas, acute lymphocytic leukemia (ALL) patients show major defects in cell-mediated or in humoral (antibody) immunity, a few of them manifest profound reduction in their serum immunoglobulin concentration. This has been suggested to be due to malignant expansion of their T suppressor lymphocytes.

Reticular dysgenesis is the most severe form of all combined immunodeficiency disorders. It is believed to be caused by a cellular defect at the level of hematopoietic stem cells. This leads to a failure in development of B cells, T cells and granulocytes. This condition is incompatible with life and leads to early death of affected infants. The only possibility for treatment is bone marrow transplantation. This condition has an autosomal recessive mode of inheritance.

Chronic mucocutaneous candidiasis is an infection of the skin, mucous membranes and nails by *Candida albicans* associated with defective T cell-mediated immunity that is specific to Candida. Skin tests for delayed-hypersensitivity to Candida antigen are negative. There may also be an associated endocrinopathy. The selective deficiency in T lymphocyte immunity leads to increased susceptibility to chronic Candida infection. T cell immunity to non-Candida antigens is intact. B cell immunity is normal which leads to an intact antibody response to Candida antigens. T lymphocytes form migration inhibitor factor (MIF) to most all antigens except for those of Candida microorganisms. The most common endocrinopathy that develops in these patients is hypoparathyroidism. Clinical forms of the disease may be either granulomatous or non-granulomatous. Candida infection of the skin may be associated with the production of granulomatous lesions. The second most frequent endocrinopathy associated with this condition is Addison's disease. The disease is difficult to treat. The antifungal drug ketoconazole has proven effective. Intravenous amphotericin B has led to improvement. Transfer factor has been administered with variable success in selected cases.

A **nude mouse** strain is hairless and has a congenital absence of the thymus and of T lymphocyte function. They serve as highly effective animal models to investigate immunologic consequences of not having a thymus. They fail to develop cell-mediated (T lymphocyte-mediated) immunity, are unable to reject allografts and are unable to synthesize antibodies against the majority of antigens. Their B lymphocytes and natural killer cells are normal even though T lymphocytes are missing. Also called *nu/nu* mice. Valuable in the investigation of graft vs. host disease.

Severe combined immunodeficiency syndrome (SCID) (Figure 5) is a profound immunodeficiency characterized by functional impairment of both B and T lymphocyte limbs of the immune response. It is inherited as an X-linked or autosomal recessive disease. The thymus has only sparse lymphocytes and Hassall's corpuscles or is bereft of them. Several congenital immunodeficiencies are characterized as SCID. There is T and B cell lymphopenia and decreased production of IL-2. There is an absence of delayed-type hypersensitivity, cellular immunity and of normal antibody synthesis following immunogenic challenge. SCID is a disease of infancy with failure to thrive. Affected individuals

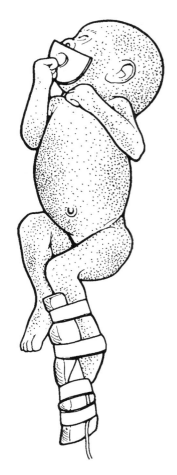

Figure 5. Severe combined immunodeficiency syndrome (SCID).

frequently die during the first two years of life. Clinically they may develop a measles-like rash, show hyperpigmentation and develop severe recurrent (especially pulmonary) infections. These subjects have heightened susceptibility to infectious disease agents such as *Pneumocystis carinii, Candida albicans,* and others. Even attenuated microorganisms, such as those used for immunization, e.g., attenuated poliomyelitis viruses, may induce infection in SCID patients. Graft-versus-host disease is a problem in SCID patients receiving unirradiated blood transfusions. Maternal-fetal transfusions during gestation or at parturition, or blood transfusions at a later date provide sufficient immunologically competent cells entering the SCID patient's circulation to induce graft-versus-host disease. SCID may be manifested in one of several forms. SCID is classified as a defect in adenosine deaminase (ADA) and purine nucleoside phosphorylase (PNP) enzymes and in a DNA-binding protein needed for HLA gene expression. Treatment is by bone marrow transplantation or gene therapy and enzyme reconstitution in those cases caused by a missing gene, such as adenosine deaminase deficiency.

Swiss type of severe combined immunodeficiency is a condition that results from a defect at the lymphocytic stem cell level. It results in cellular abnormalities that affect both T and B cell limbs of the immune response. This culminates in impaired cell-mediated immunity and humoral antibody responsiveness following challenge by appropriate immunogens. The mode of inheritance is autosomal recessive.

SCID mouse is a mouse with an autosomal recessive mutation expressed as severe combined immune deficiency in the CB-17Icr mouse strain. These mice do not have serum immunoglobulins yet their adenosine deaminase (ADA) levels are normal. They lack of T and B lymphocytes. Thus, they fail to respond to either T cell-dependent or to T cell-independent antigens when challenged. Likewise, their lymph node or spleen cells fail to proliferate following challenge by T or B lymphocyte mitogens. The lymphoid stroma in their lymph nodes and spleen is normal. Even though there is no evidence of T cell-mediated immunity, they do have natural killer cells and mononuclear phagocytes that are normal in number and function. The mutation likewise does not affect myeloid and erythroid lineage cells. B cell development is arrested at the pro-B cell stage before cytoplasmic or surface immunoglobulins are present. There are also normal numbers of macrophages in the spleen, peritoneum and liver. The SCID mutation is associated with an intrinsic defect in lymphoid stem cells. The main characteristic of SCID mice is the failure of their lymphocytes to express antigen-specific receptors. This is due to disordered rearrangements of T cell receptors or of immunoglobulin genes. The defect in recombination of antigen-specific receptor genes may be associated with the absence of a DNA recombinase specific for lymphocytes in these mice. This mouse model may be used to investigate the effects of anti-

HIV drugs as well as of immunostimulants as a substitute for human experimentation. This model is also useful for investigations of neoplasms in hosts lacking an effective immune response.

Adenosine deaminase (ADA) deficiency (Figure 6) is a form of severe combined immunodeficiency (SCID) in which affected individuals lack an enzyme, adenosine deaminase (ADA), which catalyses the deamination of adeosine as well as deoxyadenosine to produce inosine and deoxyinosine, respectively. Cells of the thymus, spleen, and lymph node as well as red blood cells contain free ADA enzyme. In contrast to the other forms of SCID, children with ADA deficiency possess Hassall's corpuscles in the thymus. The accumulation of deoxyribonucleotides in various tissues, especially thymic cells, is toxic and is believed to be a cause of immunodeficiency. As deoxyadenosine and deoxy-ATP accumulate, the latter substance inhibits ribonucleotide reductase activity which inhibits formation of the substrate needed for synthesis of DNA. These toxic substances are especially injurious to T lymphocytes. The autosomal recessive ADA deficiency leads to death. Two-fifths of severe combined immunodeficiency cases are of this type. The patient's signs and symptoms reflect defective cellular immunity with oral candidiasis, persistent diarrhea, failure to thrive and other disorders, with death occurring prior to two years of age. T lymphocytes are significantly diminished. There is eosinophilia and elevated serum and urine adenosine and deoxyadenosine levels. As bone marrow transplantation is relatively ineffective, gene therapy is the treatment of choice (Figure 7).

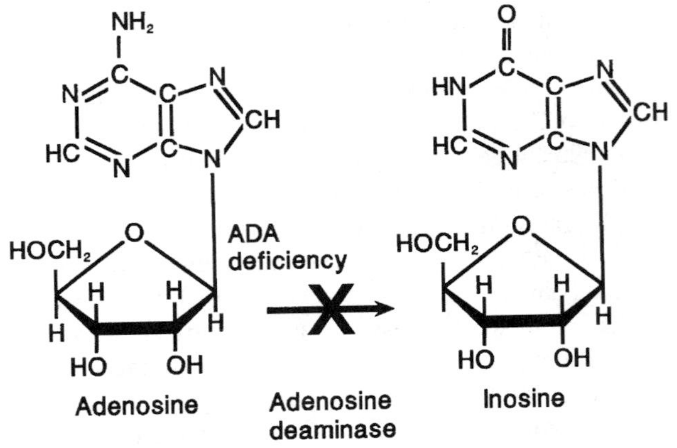

Figure 6.   ADA deficiency.

Purine nucleoside phosphorylase (PNP) deficiency is a type of severe combined immunodeficiency caused by mutant types of purine nucleoside phosphorylase. This results in the retention of metabolites that have a toxic effect on T cells. B lymphocytes appear unaffected and their numbers are normal. All cells of mammals contain PNP which

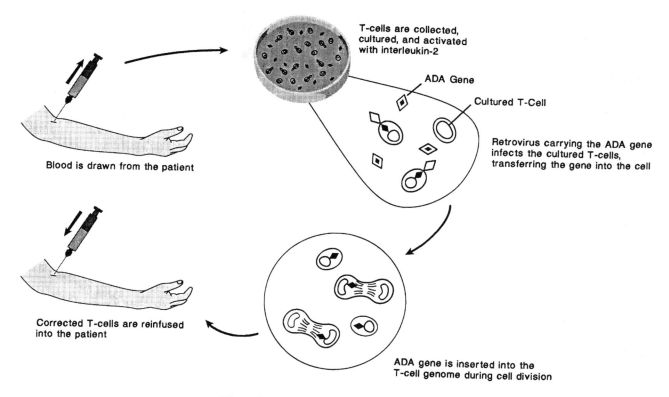

Figure 7. Gene Therapy for ADA deficiency.

acts as a catalyst in the phosphorolysis of guanosine, deoxyguanosine and inosine. Insufficient PNP leads to an elevation in the concentration within cells of deoxyguanosine, guanosine, deoxyguanosine triphosphate (dGTP) and guanosine triphosphate (GTP). dGTP blocks the enzyme ribonucleoside-diphosphate reductase which participates in DNA synthesis. T cell precursors are especially sensitive to death induced by these compounds. PNP is comprised of three 32kD subunits. Its gene, located on chromosome 14q13.1, codes for a 289-amino-acid-residue polypeptide chain. Immunologic defects associated with this disorder are characterized by anergy, lymphocytopenia and diminished T lymphocytes in the blood. By contrast, serum immunoglobulin levels and the response following deliberate immunization with various types of immunogens are within normal limits. There is an autosomal recessive mode of inheritance. Treatment is by bone marrow transplantation.

The term **bubble boy** refers to the 12 year-old male child who was maintained in a germ-free (gnotobiotic) environment in a plastic bubble from birth because of his severe combined immunodeficiency. A bone marrow transplant from a histocompatible sister was treated with monoclonal antibodies and complement to diminish alloreactive T lymphocytes. He died of a B cell lymphoma as a consequence of Epstein-Barr virus induced polyclonal gammopathy that transformed into monoclonal proliferation leading to lymphoma.

Bare lymphocyte syndrome causes a failure to express class I HLA-A, -B, or -C major histocompatibility antigens due to defective β_2 microglobulin expression on the cell surface. This immune deficiency is inherited as an autosomal recessive trait. In some individuals, the class II HLA-DR molecules are likewise not expressed. Patients may be asymptomatic or manifest respiratory tract infections, mucocutaneous candidiasis, opportunistic infections, chronic diarrhea and malabsorption, inadequate responsiveness to antigen, aplastic anemia, leukopenia, decreased T lymphocytes and normal or elevated B lymphocytes. The mechanism appears to be related to either defective gene activation or inaccessibility of promoter protein. DNA techniques are required for tissue typing.

Wiscott-Aldrich syndrome (Figure 8) is an X-linked recessive immunodeficiency disease of infants characterized by thrombocytopenia, increased IgA and IgE levels. There is decreased cell-mediated immunity (and delayed hypersensitivity), and the antibody response to polysaccharide antigens is defective with only minute quantities of IgM appearing in the serum. There may be an inability to recognize processed antigen. Male patients may have small platelets with absent surface glycoprotein Ib. Whereas IgA and IgE are increased, IgM is diminished although IgG serum concentrations are usually normal. By electron microscopy, T lymphocytes appear to be bereft of the markedly fimbriated surface of normal T cells. T lymphocytes have abnormal

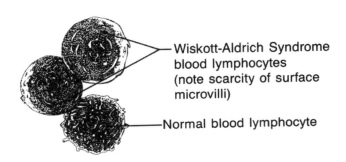

Figure 8.   Wiscott-Aldrich syndrome.

sialophorin. Patients may have an increased incidence of malignant lymphomas. Bone marrow transplantation corrects the deficiency.

Thymic alymphoplasia is a severe combined immune deficiency transmitted as an X-linked recessive trait.

Immunodeficiency with partial albinism is a type of combined immunodeficiency characterized by decreased cell-mediated immunity and deficient natural killer cells. Patients develop cerebral atrophy and aggregation of pigment in melanocytes. This disease, which leads to death, has an autosomal recessive mode of inheritance.

Ataxia-telangiectasia is a disorder characterized by cerebellar ataxia, oculocutaneous telangiectasis, variable immunodeficiency that affects both T and B cell limbs of the immune response, the development of lymphoid malignancies, and recurrent sinopulmonary infections. Clinical features may appear by two years of age. Forty percent of patients have selective IgA deficiency. The disease has an autosomal recessive mode of inheritance. There may be lymphopenia, normal or decreased T lymphocyte numbers and a normal or diminished lymphocyte response to PHA and allogeneic cells. The delayed-type hypersensitivity skin test may not stimulate any response. Some individuals may have an IgG2, IgG4 or IgA2 subclass deficiency. Other patients may reveal no IgE antibody level. There is diminished antibody responsiveness to selected antigens. B cell numbers are usually normal and NK cell function is within physiologic limits. The level of T cell deficiency varies. Defects in DNA repair mechanisms lead to multiple breaks, inversions and translocations within chromosomes rendering them highly susceptible to the injurious action of ionizing radiation and radiomimetic chemicals. The chromosomal breaks are especially apparent on chromosome 7 and 14 in the regions that encode immunoglobulin genes and T cell receptor genes. The multiple chromosomal breaks are believed to be linked to the high incidence of lymphomas in these patients. α-fetoprotein is also elevated. Endocrine abnormalities associated with the disease include glucose intolerance associated with anti-insulin receptor antibodies and hypogonadism in males. Patients may experience retarded growth, hepatic dysfunction and death may occur in many of the patients related to recurrent respiratory tract infections or lymphoid malignancies.

LFA-1 deficiency is an immunodeficiency that is caused by a defect in lymphocyte function-associated antigen, a 95kD β chain linked to CD11a which aids NK-binding T helper cell reactivity and cytotoxic T cell-mediated killing. This deficiency is associated with pyogenic mucocutaneous infections, pneumonia, diminished respiratory burst and abnormal cell adherence in chemotaxis causing poor wound healing among other features.

Chronic granulomatous disease (CGD) is a disorder that is inherited as an X-linked trait in two-thirds of cases and as an autosomal recessive trait in the remaining one-third. Clinical features are usually apparent before the end of the second year of life. There is an enzyme defect associated with NADPH oxidase. This enzyme deficiency causes neutrophils and monocytes to have decreased consumption of oxygen and diminished glucose utilization by the hexose monophosphate shunt. Although neutrophils phagocytize microorganisms, they do not form superoxide and other oxygen intermediates that usually constitute the respiratory burst. Neutrophils and monocytes also form a smaller amount of hydrogen peroxide, have decreased iodination of bacteria and diminished production of superoxide anions. All of this leads to decreased intracellular killing of bacteria and fungi. Thus these individuals have an increased susceptibility to infection with microorganisms that normally are of relatively low virulence. These include Aspergillus, *Serratia marcescens*, and *Staphylococcus epidermidis*. Patients may have hepatosplenomegaly, pneumonia, osteomyelitis, abscesses and draining lymph nodes. The quantitative nitroblue tetrazolium test (NBT) (Figure 9) and the quantitative killing curve are both employed to confirm the diagnosis. Most microorganisms that cause difficulty in CGD individuals are catalase positive. Therapy includes interferon-γ, antibiotics and surgical drainage of abscesses (Figure 10).

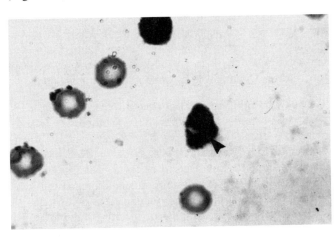

Figure 9.   NBT test.

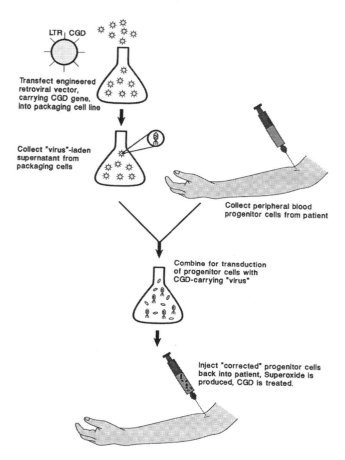

Figure 10. Strategy for gene therapy for CGD with peripheral blood progenitor cells.

Lazy leukocyte syndrome is a disease of unknown cause in which patients experience an increased incidence of pyogenic infections such as abscess formation, pneumonia and gingivitis which is linked to defective neutrophil chemotaxis in combination with neutropenia. Random locomotion of neutrophils is also diminished and abnormal. This is demonstrated by the vertical migration of leukocytes in capillary tubes. There is also impaired exodus of neutrophils from the bone marrow.

Leukocyte adhesion deficiency (LAD) is a recurrent bacteremia with staphylococci or *Pseudomonas* linked to defects in the leukocyte adhesion molecules known as integrins. These include the CD11/CD18 family of molecules. CD18 β chain gene mutations lead to a lack of complement receptors CR3 and CR4 to produce a congenital disease marked by recurring pyogenic infections. Deficiency of p150,95, LFA-1 and complement receptor 3 (CR3) membrane proteins leads to diminished adhesion properties and mobility of phagocytes and lymphocytes. There is a flaw in synthesis of the 95kD β chain subunit which all three of these molecules share. The defect in mobility is manifested as altered chemotaxis, defective random migration and

faulty spreading. Particles coated with C3 are not phagocytized and therefore fail to activate a respiratory burst. The CR3 and p150,95 deficiency account for the defective phagocytic activity. LAD patients' T cells fail to respond normally to antigen or mitogen stimulation and are also unable to provide helper function for B cells producing immunoglobulin. They are ineffective in fatally injuring target cells, and they do not produce the lymphokine, γ interferon. LFA-1 deficiency accounts for the defective response of these T lymphocytes as well as all natural killer cells, which also have impaired ability to fatally injure target cells. Clinically, the principal manifestations are a consequence of defective phagocyte function rather than of defective T lymphocyte function. Patients may have recurrent severe infections, a defective inflammatory response, abscesses, gingivitis and periodontitis. There are two forms of leukocyte adhesion deficiency. Those with the severe deficiency do not express the three α and 4 β chain complexes, whereas those with moderate deficiency express 2.5% to 6% of these complexes. There is an autosomal recessive mode of inheritance for leukocyte adhesion deficiency.

Job's syndrome (Figure 11) refers to cold staphylococcal abscesses or infections by other agents that recur. There is associated eczema, elevated levels of IgE in the serum and phagocytic dysfunction associated with glutathione reductase and glucose-6-phosphatase deficiencies. The syndrome has an autosomal recessive mode of inheritance.

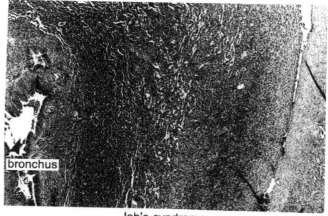

Job's syndrome
with bronchogenic abscess

Figure 11. Job's syndrome with bronchogenic abscess.

Hyperimmunoglobulin E syndrome (HIE) is a condition characterized by markedly elevated IgE levels, i.e., greater than 5000 IU/ml. The patients have early eczema and repeated abscesses of the skin, sinuses, lungs, eyes, and ears. *Staphylococcus aureus, Candida albicans, Hemophilus influenae, Streptococcus pneuomoniae,* and group A hemolytic streptococci are among the more common infectious agents. The principal infection produced by *Staphlococcus aureus* and

C. albicans is a "cold abscess" in the skin. The failure of IgE to fiz complement and therefore cause inflammation at the infection site is characteristic. IgG antibodies against IgE form complexes that bind to mononuclear phagocytes, resulting in monokine release that induces calcium resorption from bone. As calcium is lost from the bone, osteoporosis results, leading to bone fractures. Patients with HIE have diminished antibody responses to vaccines and to major histocompatibility antigens. They may be anergic, and *in vitro* challenge of their lymphocytes with mitogens or antigens leads to diminished responsiveness. There is also a decrease in the CD8+ T lymphocyte population in the peripheral blood. The disease becomes manifest in young infants, shows no predilection for males vs. females, and is not hereditary.

Myeloperoxidase is an enzyme present in the azurophil granules of neutrophilic leukocytes that catalyzes peroxidation of many microorganisms. Myeloperoxidase in conjunction with hydrogen peroxidase and halide has a bactericidal effect.

Myeloperoxidase (MPO) deficiency is a lack of 116kD myeloperoxidase in both neutrophils and monocytes. This enzyme is located in the primary granules of neutrophils. It possesses a heme ring which imparts a dark green tint to the molecule. MPO deficiency has an autosomal recessive mode of inheritance. Clinically, affected patients have a mild version of chronic granulomatous disease. *Candida albicans* infections are frequent in this condition.

Chediak-Higashi syndrome (Figure 12) is a childhood disorder with an autosomal recessive mode of inheritance and is identified by the presence of large lysosomal granules in leukocytes that are very stable and undergo slow degranulation. Multiple systems may be involved. Repeated bacterial infections with various micororganisms, partial albinism, central nervous system disorders, hepatosplenomegaly and an inordinate incidence of malignancies of the lymphoreticular tissues may occur. The large cytoplasmic granular inclusions that appear in white blood cells may also be observed in blood platelets and can be seen by regular light microscopy in peripheral blood smears. There is defective neutrophil chemotaxis and altered ability of the cells to kill ingested microorganisms. There is a delay in the killing time even though hydrogen peroxide formation, oxygen consumption and hexose monophosphate shunt are all within normal limits. There is also defective microtubule function leading to defective phagolysosome formation. Cyclic AMP levels may increase. This causes decreased neutrophil degranulation and mobility. High doses of ascorbic acid have been shown to restore normal chemotaxis, bactericidal activity, and degranulation. Natural killer cell numbers and function are decreased. There is an increased incidence of lymphomas in Chediak-Higashi patients. There is no effective therapy other than administration of antibiotics for the infecting microorganisms. The disease carries a poor prognosis because of the infections and the neurolgoical complications. The majority of affected individuals die during childhood although occasional subjects may live longer.

Beige mice are a mutant strain of mice that develops abnormalities in pigment, defects in natural killer cell function, and heightened tumor incidence. This serves as a model for Chediak-Higashi disease in man.

Complement deficiency conditions are rare. In healthy Japanese blood donors, only one in 100,000 persons had no C5, C6, C7 and C8. 3 of 1,000 individuals contained no C9. Most individuals with missing complement components do not manifest clinical symptoms. Additional pathways provide complement-dependent functions that are necessary to preserve life. If C3, factor I or any segment of the alternative pathway is missing, the condition may be life-threatening with markedly decreased opsonization in phagocytosis. C3 is depleted when factor I is absent. C5, C6, C7 or C8 deficiencies are linked with infections, mainly meningococcal or gonococcal which usually succumb to complement's bactericidal action. Deficiencies in classical complement pathway activation are often associated with connective tissue or immune complex diseases. Systemic lupus erythematosus may be associated with C1qrs, C2 or C4 deficiencies. Hereditary angioedemia (HAE) patients have a deficiency of C1 inactivator. A number of experimental animals with specific complement deficiencies has been described, such as C6 deficiency in rabbits and C5 deficiency in mice. Acquired complement deficiencies may be caused by either accelerated complement consumption in immune complex diseases with a type III mechanism or by diminished formation of complement proteins as in acute necrosis of the liver.

Hereditary angioedema (HAE) is a disorder in which recurrent attacks of edema, persisting for 48 to 72 hours occur in the skin, gastrointestinal and respiratory tracts. It is nonpitting and can threaten death if laryngeal edema becomes severe enough to obstruct the airway. Edema in the

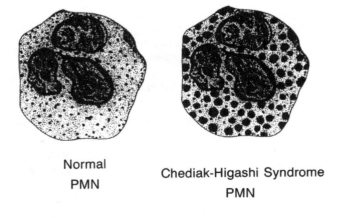

Normal
PMN

Chediak-Higashi Syndrome
PMN

Figure 12. Chediak-Higashi Syndrome.

jejunum may be associated with abdominal cramps and bilious vomiting. Edema of the colon may lead to watery diarrhea. There is no redness or itching associated with edema of the skin. Tissue trauma or no apparent initiating cause may induce an attack. It is due to decreased or absent C1 inhibitor (C1-INH). It is inherited in an autosomal dominant fashion. Heterozygotes for the defect develop the disorder. Greatly diminished C1-INH levels (5 to 30% of normal) are found in affected individuals. Activation of C1 leads to increased cleavage of C4 and C2, decreasing their serum levels during an attack. C1-INH is also a kinin system inactivator. The C1-INH deficiency in HAE permits a kinin-like peptide produced from C2b to increase vascular permeability leading to manifestations of HAE. Some have proposed that bradykinin may represent the vasopermeability factor. Hereditary angioedema has been treated with aminocaproic acid and transexamic acid but they do not elevate C1-INH or C4 levels. Anabolic steroids such as danazol and stanozolol, which activate C1-INH synthesis in affected individuals, represent the treatment of choice.

Secondary immunodeficiency is an immunodeficiency that is not due to a failure or intrinsic defect in the T and B lymphocytes of the immune system. It is a consequence of some other disease process and may be either transient or permanent. The transient variety may disappear following adequate treatment whereas the more permanent type persists. Secondary immunodeficiencies are commonly produced by many effects. For example, those that appear in patients with neoplasms may result from effects of the tumor. Secondary immunodeficiencies may cause an individual to become susceptible to microorganisms that would otherwise cause no problem. They may occur following immunoglobulin or T lymphocyte loss, the administration of drugs, infections, cancer, effects of ionizing radiation on immune system cells and other causes.

Immunodeficiency from hypercatabolism of immunoglobulin occurs when serum levels of immunoglobulins fluctuate according to their rates of synthesis and catabolism. Although many immunological deficiencies result from defective synthesis of immunoglobulins and lymphocytes, immunoglobulin levels in serum can decline as a consequence of either increased catabolism or loss into the gastrointestinal tract or other areas. Defective catabolism may affect one to several immunoglobulin classes. For example, in myotonic dystrophy, only IgG is hypercatabolized. In contrast to the normal levels of IgM, IgA, IgD, IgE, and albumin in the serum, the IgG concentration is markedly diminished. Synthesis of IgG in these individuals is normal, but the half-life of IgG molecules is reduced as a consequence of increased catabolism. Patients with ataxia telangiectasia and those with selective IgA deficiency have antibodies directed against IgA which remove this class of immunoglobulin. Patients with the rare condition known as

familial hypercatabolic hypoproteinemia demonstrate reduced IgG and albumin levels in the serum and slightly lower IgM levels, but the IgA and IgE concentrations are either normal or barely increased. Although synthesis of IgG and albumin in such patients is within normal limits, the catabolism of these two proteins is greatly accelerated.

Immunodeficiency from severe loss of immunoglobulins and lymphocytes occurs when the gastrointestinal and urinary tracts are two sources of serious protein loss in disease processes. The loss of integrity of the renal glomerular basement membrane, renal tubular disease or both may result in loss of immunoglobulin molecules into the urine. Since the small IgG molecules would pass through in many situations leaving larger IgA molecules in the intravascular space, all immunoglobulins are not lost from the serum at the same rate. More than 90 diseases that affect the gastrointestinal tract have been associated with protein-losing gastroenteropathy. This may be secondary to inflammatory or allergic disorders, or disease processes involving the lymphatics. In intestinal lymphangiectasia associated with lymphatic blockage, lymphocytes as well as protein are lost. Lymphatics in the small intestine are dilated.

Intestinal lymphangiectasia patients show defects in both humoral and cellular immune mechanisms. The major immunoglobulins are diminished to less than half normal. IgG is affected more than IgA and IgM, which are more affected than is IgE.

An **immunodeficiency associated with hereditary defective response to Epstein-Barr virus** is an immunodeficiency that develops in previously healthy subjects with a normal immune system who have developed a primary Epstein-Barr virus infection. They develop elevated numbers of natural killer cells in the presence of a lymphopenia. The condition is serious and its acute stage may lead to B cell lymphoma or failure of the bone marrow or agammaglobulinemia. The disease may be fatal. The condition was first considered to have an X-linked recessive mode of inheritance recurring only in males; it has now been found in occasional females. The term Duncan's syndrome is often used to describe the X-linked variety of this condition.

An **acquired immunodeficiency** is a decrease in the immune response to immunogenic (antigenic) challenge as a consequence of numerous diseases or conditions that include acquired immune deficiency syndrome (AIDS), chemotherapy, immunosuppressive drugs such as corticosteroids, psychological depression, burns, nonsteroidal antiinflammatory drugs, radiation, Alzheimer's disease, coeliac disease, sarcoidosis, lymphoproliferative disease, Waldenström's macroglobulinemia, multiple myeloma, aplastic anemia, sickle cell disease, malnutrition, aging, neoplasia, diabetes mellitus and numerous other conditions.

18

Acquired Immune Deficiency Syndrome (AIDS)

AIDS (acquired immune deficiency syndrome) is a disease induced by the human immunodeficiency retrovirus designated HIV-1. Although first observed in homosexual men, the disease affects both males and females equally in central Africa and is beginning to affect an increasing number of heterosexuals with cases in both males and females in the Western countries including North America and Europe. Following exposure to the AIDS virus, the incubation period is variable and may extend to 11 years before clinical AIDS occurs in HIV positive males in high risk groups. It is transmitted by blood and body fluids but is not transmitted through casual contact, or through air, food or other means. Besides homosexual and bisexual males, others at high risk include intravenous drug abusers, hemophiliacs, the offspring of HIV infected mothers, and sexual partners of any HIV infected individuals in the above groups.

AIDS belt (Figure 1) refers to the geographic area across central Africa that describes a region where multiple cases of heterosexual AIDS, related to sexual promiscuity, was reported. Nations in this belt include Burundi, Central African Republic, Kenya, the Congo, Malawi, Rwanda, Tanzania, Uganda and Zambia.

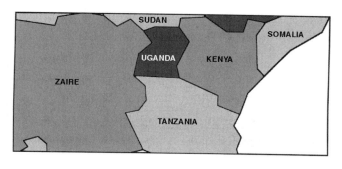

Figure 1. AIDS belt.

Retrovirus (Figures 2 and 3) is a reverse transcriptase-containing virus such as human immunodeficiency virus and human T cell leukemia virus. An RNA virus that can insert and efficiently express its own genetic information in the host cell genome through transcription of its RNA into DNA which is then integrated into the genome of host cells. Retroviruses are employed in research to deliberately insert foreign DNA into a cell. Thus, they have the potential for use in gene therapy when a host cell gene is either missing

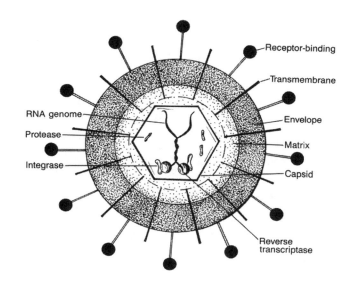

Figure 2. Retrovirus.

or defective. Retroviruses have been used to tag tumor-infiltrating lymphocytes in experimental cancer treatment.

Human immunodeficiency virus (HIV) (Figure 4) is the retrovirus that induces acquired immune deficiency syndrome (AIDS) and associated disorders. It was previously designated HTLV-III, LAV, or ARV. It infects CD4[+] T lymphocytes, mononuclear phagocytes carrying CD4 molecules on their surface, follicular dendritic cells and Langerhan's cells. It produces profound immunodeficiency affecting both humoral and cell-mediated immunity. There is a progressive decrease in CD4[+] helper/inducer T lymphocytes until they are finally depleted in many patients. There may be polyclonal activation of B lymphocytes with elevated synthesis of immunoglobulins. The immune response to the virus is not protective and does not improve the patient's condition. The virus is comprised of an envelope glycoprotein (gp160) which is its principal antigen. It has a gp120 external segment and a gp41 transmembrane segment. CD4 molecules on CD4[+] lymphocytes and macrophages serve as receptors for gp120 of HIV. It has an inner core that contains RNA and is encircled by a lipid envelope. It contains structural genes designated *env, gag* and *pol* that encode the envelope protein, core protein and reverse transcriptase, respectively. HIV also possesses at least six additional genes, i.e., *tat* that regulates HIV replication. It can increase production

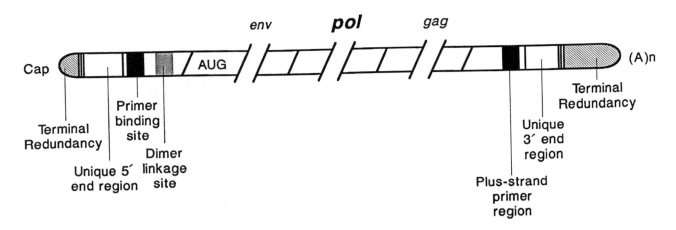

Figure 3. Retroviral genome.

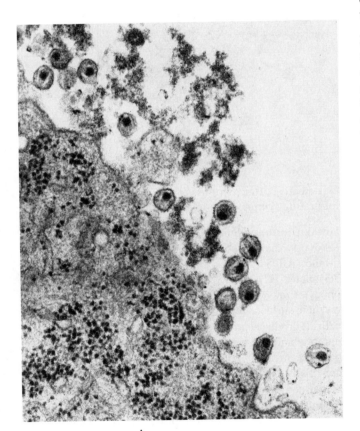

Figure 4. HIV. Electron microscopy. (Courtesy of Dr. Tom Folks, CDC, Atlanta, GA)

of viral protein several thousand-fold. *rev* encodes proteins that block transcription of regulatory genes. *vif (sor)* is the virus infectivity gene whose product increases viral infectivity and may promote cell to cell transmission. *nef* is a negative regulatory factor that encodes a product that blocks replication of the virus. *vpr* (viral protein R) gene and *vpu* (viral protein U) genes have also been described. No suc-

cessful vaccine has yet been developed although several types are under investigation.

HIV infection (Figure 5) is the recognition of infection by the human immunodeficiency virus (HIV) is through sero-conversion. Following conversion to positive reactivity in an antibody screening test, a Western blot analysis is performed to confirm the result of positive testing for HIV. HIV mainly affects the immune system and the brain. It affects primarily the CD4+ lymphocytes which are necessary to initiate an immune response by interaction with antigen-presenting cells. This also deprives other cells of the immune system from receiving a supply of interleukin-2 through CD4+ lymphocyte stimulation leading to a progressive decline in immune system function. HIV transmission is by either sexual contact, through blood products or horizontally from mother to young. Although first observed in male homosexuals, it later became a major problem of intravenous drug abusers and ultimately has become more serious in the heterosexual population affecting an increasing number of

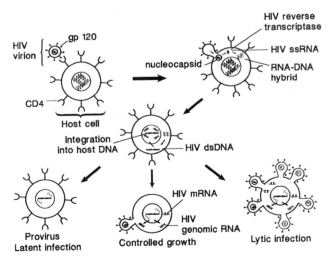

Figure 5. HIV infection.

women as well as men. Clinically individuals may develop acute HIV mononucleosis that usually occurs two to six weeks following infection although it may occur later. The main symptoms include headache, fever, malaise, sore throat and rash. Patients may develop pharyngitis, generalized lymphadenopathy, a macular or urticarial rash on the face, trunk and limbs and hepatosplenomegaly.

The severity of the symptoms may vary from one individual to another. Acute HIV infection may also induce neurologic disease including meningitis, encephalitis, and other neurologic manifestations. Some individuals may not develop symptoms or illness for years. Other individuals develop AIDS-related complex (ARC) which represents progressive immune dysfunction. Symptoms include fever, night sweats, weight loss, chronic diarrhea, generalized lymphadenopathy, herpes zoster and oral lesions. Individuals with ARC may progress to AIDS or death may occur in the ARC stage. ARC patients do not revert to an asymptomatic condition. Other individuals may develop persistent generalized lymphadenopathy (PGL) characterized by enlarged lymph nodes in the neck, axilla and groin. The Centers for Disease Control (CDC) has set up criteria for the diagnosis of AIDS. These include the individuals who develop certain opportunistic infections and neoplasms, HIV-related encephalopathy and HIV-induced wasting syndrome. The most frequent opportunistic infections in AIDS patients include *Pneumocystis carinii* which produces pneumonia and *Mycobacterium avium-intracellulare* among other microorganisms. The most frequent tumor in AIDS patients is Kaposi's sarcoma. The definition of AIDS by the CDC now includes HIV-related encephalopathy and HIV wasting syndrome. At the present time, AIDS is 100% fatal.

AIDS embryopathy is a condition in children born to HIV infected mothers, who are intravenous drug abusers. Affected children have craniofacial region defects that include microcephaly, hypertelorism, cube-shaped head, saddle nose, widened palpebral fissures with bluish sclera, triangular philtrum and widely spreading lips.

HIV-1 virus structure (Figure 6) is comprised of two identical RNA strands which constitute the viral genome. These are associated with reverse transcriptase and p17 and p24 which are core polypeptides. These components are all enclosed in a phospholipid membrane envelope that is derived from the host cell. Proteins gp120 and gp41 encoded by the virus are anchored to the envelope.

HIV-1 genes (Figures 7 and 8) include the *gag* gene which encodes the structural core proteins p17, p24, p15 and p55 precursor. *pol* encodes a protease (Figure 9) that cleaves *gag* precursors. It also encodes reverse transcriptase (Figure 10) that produces proviral DNA from RNA and encodes an integrase that is necessary for proviral insertion. *env* encodes gp160 precursor, gp120 and gp41 in mature proteins. gp120 binds CD4 molecules, and gp41 is needed for fusion of the

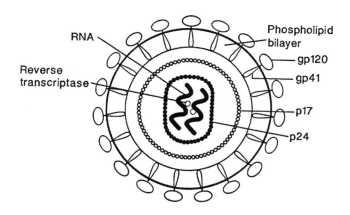

Figure 6. HIV-1 virus structure.

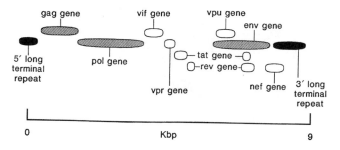

Figure 7. HIV-1 genes.

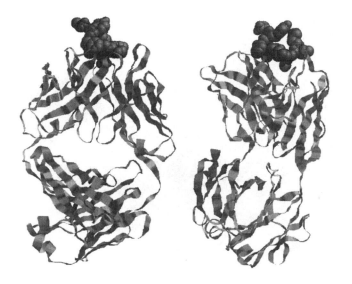

Figure 8. IgG/gp120 complex.

virus with the cell. *vpr's* function is unknown. *vif* encodes a 23kD product that is necessary for infection of cells by free virus and is not needed for infection from cell to cell. *tat* encodes a p14 product that binds to viral long terminal repeat (LTR) sequence and activates viral gene transcription. *rev* encodes a 20kD protein product that is needed for post-transcriptional expression of *gag* and *env* genes. *nef* encodes a 27kD protein that inhibits HIV transcription and slows viral

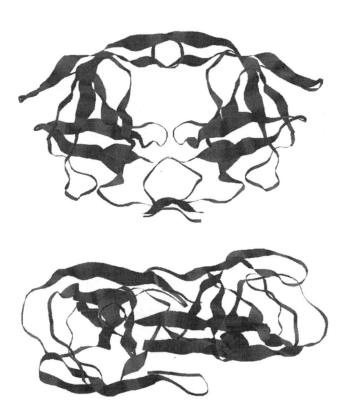

Figure 9.   HIV-1 protease. NMR.

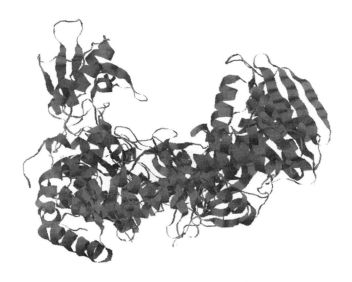

Figure 10.   HIV-1 reverse transcriptase.

replication. *vpu* encodes a 16kD protein product that may be required for assembly and packaging of new virus particles.

HIV-2 is an abbreviation for human immunodeficiency virus-2. Previously referred to as HTLV-IV, LAV-2 and SIV/AGM. This virus was first discovered in West African individuals who showed aberrant reactions to HIV-1 and simian immunodeficiency virus (SIV). It shows greater

sequence homology (70%) with SIV/MAC than with HIV-1 (40% sequence homology). It has only 50% conservation for *gag* and *pol*. The remaining HIV genes are even less conserved than this. It has p24, gp36 and gp140 structural antigens. Its clinical course resembles that of AIDS produced by HIV-1 but it is confined principally to Western Africa and is transmitted principally through heterosexual promiscuity.

The subject recently infected with HIV may develop either no symptoms or an acute infectious mononucleosis-like condition. The principal symptoms include headache, sore throat, fever, rash and malaise. This illness is apparent 2 to 6 weeks following infection but may occur between five days and three months. On examination, there is a macular or urticarial rash on the limbs, face and trunk, hepatosplenomegaly, generalized lymphadenopathy and pharyngitis. The illness ranges from mild to severe possibly requiring hospitalization. Acute HIV infection may also involve the nervous system and be associated with encephalitis, meningitis, carinal nerve palsies, peripheral neuropathy and myopathy.

Three to six weeks after infection with HIV-I there are high levels of HIV p24 antigen in the plasma (Figure 11). One week to three months following infection there is an HIV-specific immune response resulting in the formation of antibodies against HIV envelope protein gp-120 and HIV core protein p24. HIV-specific cytotoxic T lymphocytes are also formed. The result of this adoptive immune response is a dramatic decline in viremia and a clinically asymptomatic phase lasting from 2 to 12 years. As CD4+ T cell numbers decrease, the patient becomes clinically symptomatic. HIV-specific antibodies and cytotoxic T lymphocytes decline, and p24 antigen increases.

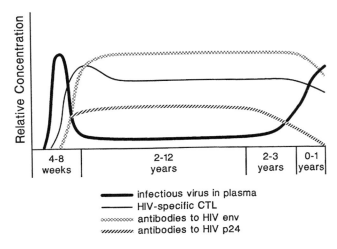

Figure 11.   AIDS serology.

AIDS-related complex (ARC) is the former term for the preamble to AIDS which consisted of a constellation of symptoms and signs that included a temperature of greater than 38°C, a greater than 10% loss of body weight, lymphadenopathy, diarrhea and night sweats of greater than three month duration and fatigue. Laboratory findings included CD4⁺ T lymphocyte levels of less than 0.4×10^9, a CD4:CD8 T lymphocyte ratio of less than 1.0, leukopenia, anemia and thrombocytopenia. There may be a decreased response to PHA, principally a T cell mitogen, and anergy, manifested as failure to respond to skin tests. In contrast, there may be a polyclonal gammopathy. A diagnosis of ARC required at least two of the clinical manifestations and two of the laboratory findings listed above.

Changes in the nomenclature for diseases associated with HIV caused AIDS-related complex (ARC) to be termed symptomatic HIV infection without an AIDS-defining condition. Progressive immune dysfunction is defined by manifestations of HIV-related symptoms. Patients experience persistent fever, night sweats, some weight loss, psoriasis, exemia, seborrheic dermatitis, diarrhea, herpes zoster, oral candidiasis and oral hairy leukoplakia. The latter two indicate the development of AIDS. A few developed blood platelet counts less than 50,000/μL.

The CDC criteria for diagnosing AIDS include the development of selected opportunistic infections and tumors, HIV-induced wasting syndrome, HIV-related encephalopathy and various other diseases indicative of AIDS based on laboratory findings. Subjects with a CD4 lymphocyte count below 200 cells/μL blood or a CD4 T lymphocyte level below 14% irrespective of clinical symptoms are considered to have AIDS. AIDS-defining illnesses also include recurrent bacterial pneumonia, pulmonary tuberculosis and invasive cervical cancer. Opportunistic infections common in these individuals include *Pneumocystitis carinii* pneumonia, disseminated toxoplasmosis, cryptococcus and Mycobacterial disease (include mycobacterium avium complex) and tuberculosis, the current herpes simplex infection, disseminated cytomegalovirus infection and histoplasmosis. AIDS patients are also prone to develop staphylococcal and pneumococcal infections as well as *Salmonella bacteriemia*. Lymphocytic interstitial pneumonitis and recurrent bacterial infections may have a higher incidence in children with AIDS than in adults. Kaposi's sarcoma is the most frequently associated tumor with AIDS. It involves the endothelium and mesenchyma stroma but is a less frequent presenting illness than in the past. HHV-8 herpes virus may be the causative agent of Kaposi's sarcoma. B cell lymphomas may also occur.

Up to two-thirds of AIDS patients may develop CNS signs and symptoms such as sustained cognitive behavior and motor impairment refered to as the AIDS dementia complex. This is believed to be associated with infection of microglial cells with the HIV-1 virus. This could be due to the structural similarity of gp120 of HIV-1 to neuroleukin. Patients have memory loss, are unable to concentrate, have poor coordi-

nation of gait, altered psychomotor function, among other symptoms. The subcortical white matter and deep gray matter degenerate; lateral and posterior spinal cord columns show white matter vacuolization; the gp120 of HIV serves as a calcium channel inhibitor causing toxic levels of calcium within neurons.

AIDS enteropathy is a condition which may be seen in AIDS related complex patients marked by diarrhea, especially nocturnal, wasting, possibly fever and defective D-xylose absorption leading to malnutrition. The small intestine may demonstrate atrophy of villi and hyperplasia of crypts. Both small and large intestines may reveal diminished plasma cells, elevated intraepithelial lymphocytes and viral inclusions.

***Pneumocystis cnarinii* (PCP)** (Figure 12) is a protozoan parasite that infects immunocompromised subjects such as AIDS patients, transplant recipients, lymphoma and leukemia patients, and others immunosuppresed for one reason or the other. It is diagnosed in tissue sections stained with the Gomori-methenamine silver stain. A mannose receptor facilitates the organism's uptake by macrophages. Approximately one-half of those hospitalized with a first infection by PCP die.

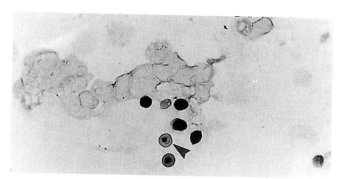

Figure 12. *Pneumocystis carinii.*

Cytomegalovirus (CMV) (Figure 13) is a herpes (DNA) virus group that is distributed worldwide and is not often a problem except in individuals who are immunocompromised, such as the recipients of organ or bone marrow transplants or individuals with acquired immunodeficiency syndrome (AIDS). Histopathologically, typical inclusion bodies that resemble an owl's eye are found in multiple tissues. CMV is transmitted in the blood.

Two classes of antiviral drugs are used to treat HIV infection and AIDS. Nucleotide analogues inhibit reverse transcriptase activity. They include azidothymidine (AZT) dideoxyinosine and dideoxycytidine. They may diminish plasma HIV RNA levels for considerable periods but often fail to stop disease progression because of development of mutated forms of reverse transcriptase that resist these drugs. Viral protease inhibitors are now used to block the

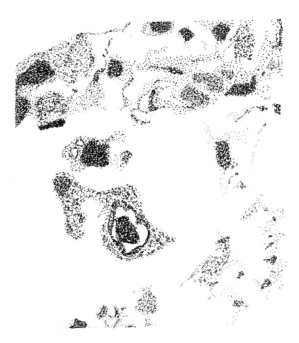

Figure 13.   CMV nuclear and cytoplasmic inclusions in the lung.

processing of precursor proteins into mature viral capsid and core proteins. Currently, a triple-drug therapy consisting of protease inhibitors (Figures 14–16) together with two separate reverse transcriptase inhibitors are used to reduce plasma viral RNA to very low levels in patients treated for more than one year. It remains to be determined whether or not resistance to this therapy will develop. Disadvantages include their great expense and the complexity of their administration. Antibiotics are used to treat the many infections to which AIDS patients are susceptible. Whereas, viral resistance to protease inhibitors may develop after only a few days, resistance to the reverse transcriptase inhibitor zidovudine may occur only after months of administration. Three of four mutations in the viral reverse transcriptase are necessary for resistance to zidovudine, yet only one mutation can lead to resistance to protease inhibitors.

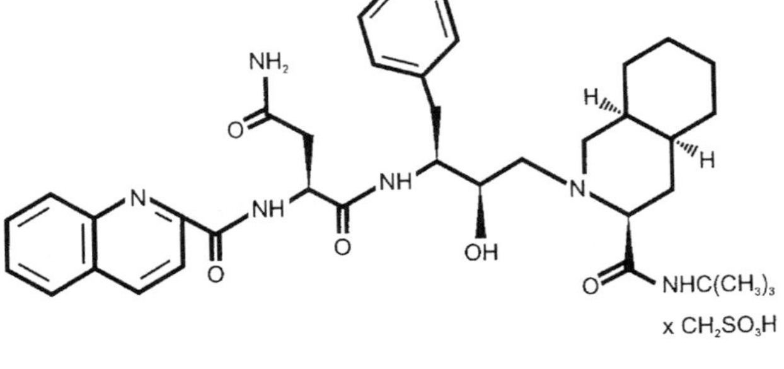

Figure 14.   Saquinavir mesylate.

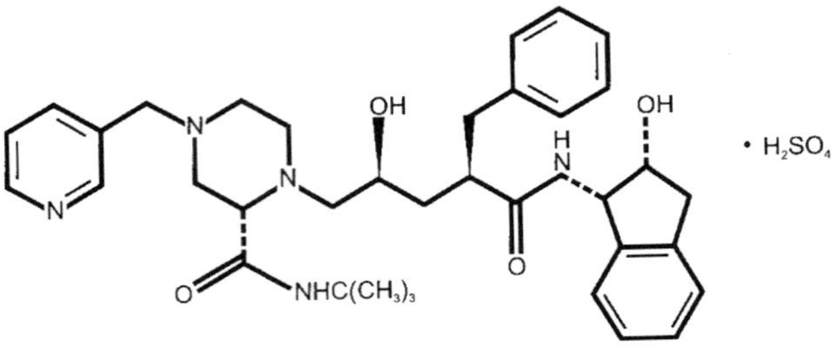

Figure 15.   Indinavir sulfate.

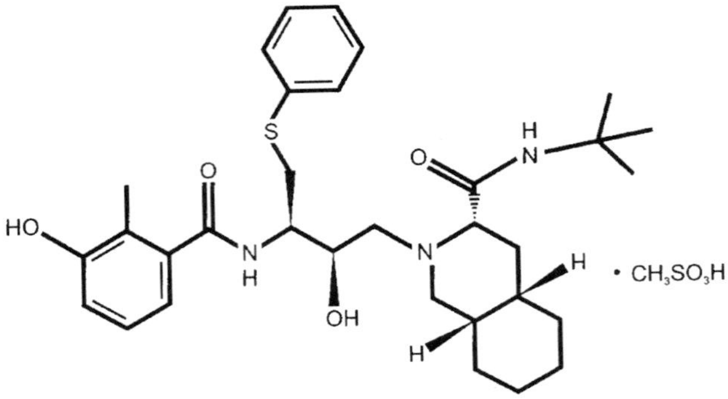

Figure 16.   Nelfinavir mesylate.

Many advances have been made in **AIDS treatment**. Although no drug is curative, zidovudine (azidothymidine-AZT), ddC (dideoxycytidine) and ddI (dideoxyinosine) are effective in delaying progression of the disease. Many experimental preparations are under investigation such as DAB/486 IL-2 which is cytotoxic for high affinity IL-2 receptors expressed on HIV-infected T lymphocytes.

Zidovudine (3′-azido-3′-deoxythymidine) or AZT (Figure 17) is a reverse transcriptase inhibitor that is a thymidine analogue. It is FDA approved for the treatment of acquired immune deficiency syndrome (AIDS). The mechanism of action includes phosphorylation of the drug *in vivo* to 3′-azido-3′deoxythymidine triphosphate. This combines with human immunodeficiency virus (HIV reverse transcriptase), which leads to cessation of DNA elongation.

Ribavarin (1-8-5-D-ribofuranosyl-1,2,4-triazole-3-carboxamide) (Figure 18) is a substance that interferes with mRNA capping of certain viruses thereby restricting the synthesis of viral proteins. It is used as an aerosol to treat severe respiratory syncytial virus infection in children.

Foscarnet (Figure 19) is an investigational drug used to combat cytomegalovirus-induced pneumonia, hepatitis, colitis and retinitis in AIDS patients rendered nonresponsive to gancyclovir, which is a frequently used treatment for cytomegalovirus infection.

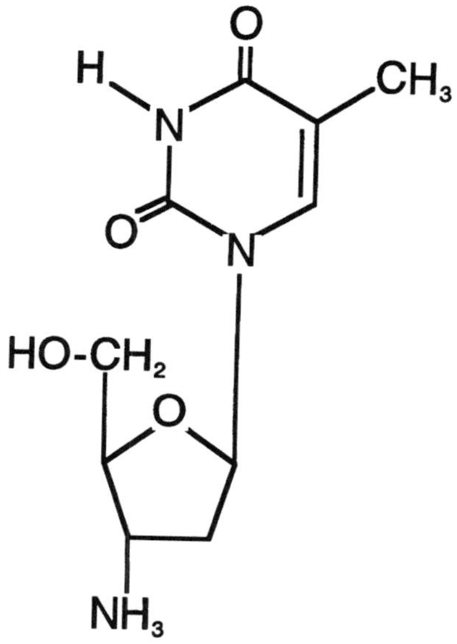

Figure 17. Zidovudine.

Figure 18. Ribavirin.

Development of an **AIDS vaccine** always has been made difficult by the genetic potential of HIV for extensive antigenic variations. Whereas, many of the viral gene products capable of inducing humoral immunity are known, humoral immunity is insufficient to prevent HIV disease. By contrast, viral products that can induce effective cell-mediated immunity require investigations to determine whether or not they can effectively prevent disease.

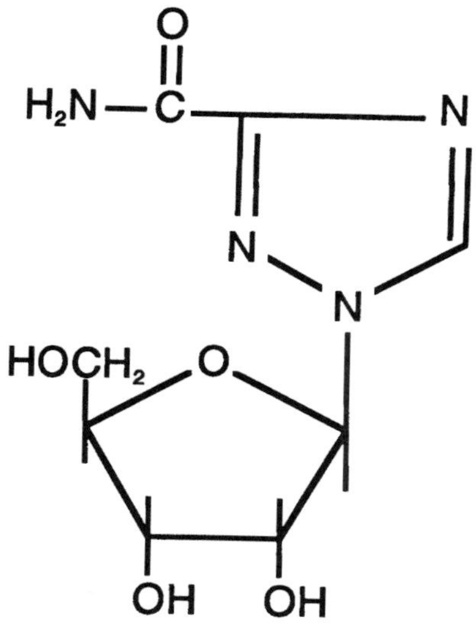

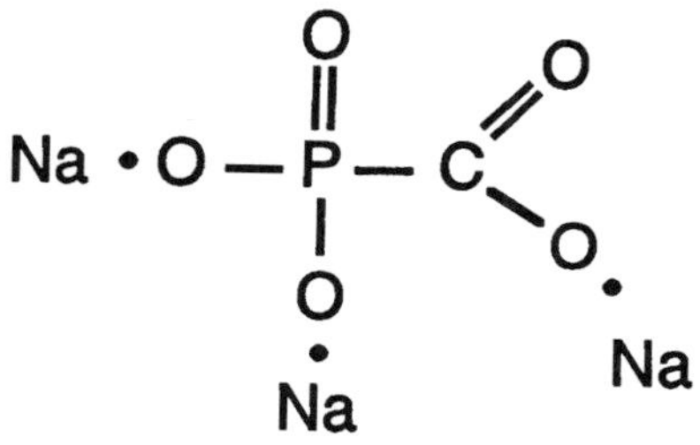

Figure 19. Foscarnet.

19

Immunosuppression

Clinical immunosuppression has been used to treat immunological diseases, including autoimmune reactions, as well as to condition recipients of solid organ allografts or of bone marrow transplants.

Immune suppression refers to decreased immune responsiveness as a consequence of therapeutic intervention with drugs or irradiation or as a consequence of a disease process that adversely affects the immune response.

Immunosuppression describes either the deliberate administration of drugs such as cyclosporine, azathioprine, corticosteroids, FK506 or rapamycin; the administration of specific antibody; the use of irradiation to depress immune reactivity in recipients of organ or bone marrow allotransplants; and the profound depression of the immune response that occurs in patients with certain diseases such as acquired immune deficiency syndrome in which the helper-inducer (CD4+) T lymphocytes are destroyed by the HIV-1 virus.

Immunosuppressive agents include drugs such as cyclosporine, FK506, rapamycin, azathioprine or corticosteroids; antibodies such as antilymphocyte globulin; and irradiation. These produce mild to profound depression of a host's ability to respond to an immunogen (antigen), as in the conditioning of an organ allotransplant recipient.

NONSPECIFIC IMMUNOSUPPRESSION

Corticosteroids (Figures 1–5) are lympholytic steroid hormones, such as cortisone, derived from the adrenal cortex. Glucocorticoids such as prednisone or dexamethasone can diminish the size and lymphocyte content of lymph nodes and spleen while sparing proliferating myeloid or erythroid stem cells of the bone marrow. Glucocorticoids may interfere with the activated lymphocyte's cell cycle. Glucocorticoids are cytotoxic for selected T lymphocyte subpopulations and are also able to suppress cell-mediated immunity and antibody synthesis as well as the formation of prostaglandin and leukotrienes. Corticosteroids may lyse either suppressor or helper T lymphocytes, but plasma cells may be more resistant to their effects. However, precursor lymphoid cells are sensitive to the drug which may lead in this way to decreased antibody responsiveness. The repeated administration of prednisone diminishes the concentration of specific antibodies in the IgG class whose fractional catabolic rate is increased by prednisone. Corticosteroids interfere with the phagocytosis of antibody-coated cells by macrophages

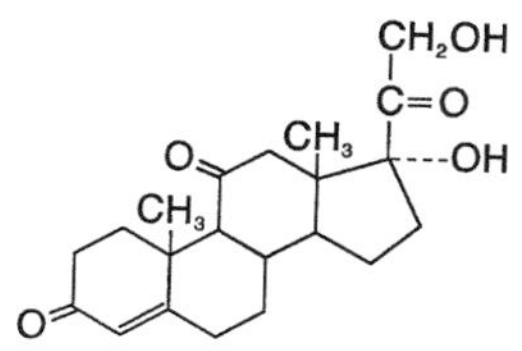

Figure 1.   Structure of cortisone.

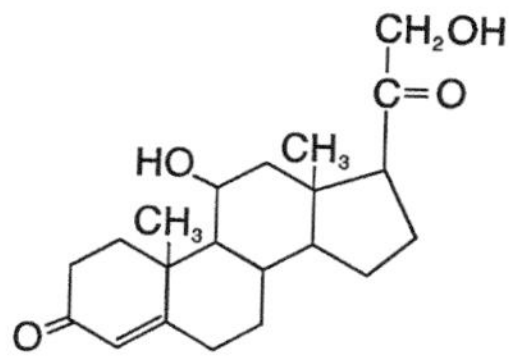

Figure 2.   Structure of corticosterone.

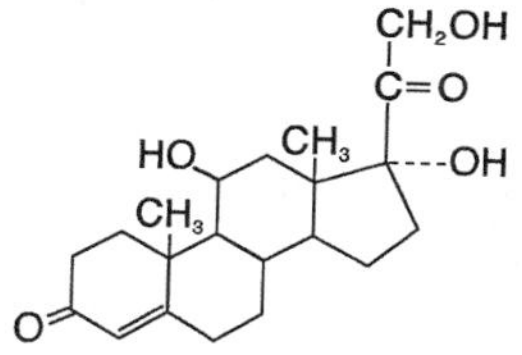

Figure 3.   Structure of cortisol.

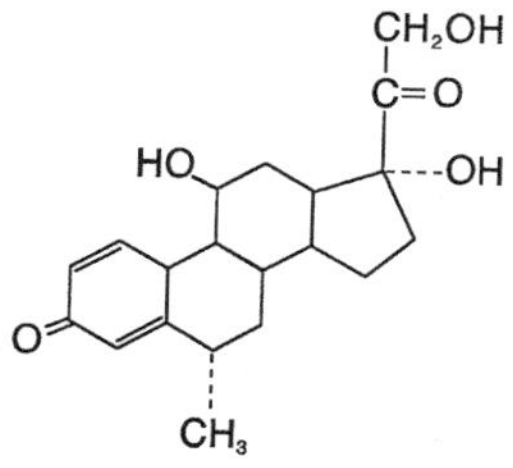

Figure 4.   Structure of 6α-methylprednisolone.

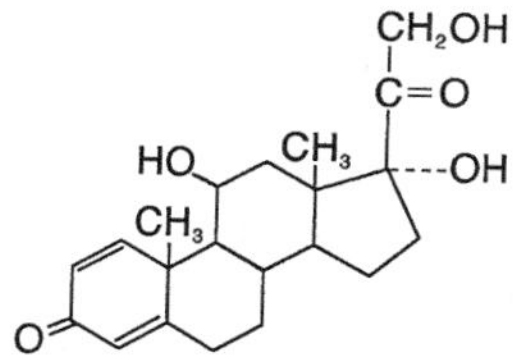

Figure 5.   Structure of prednisolone.

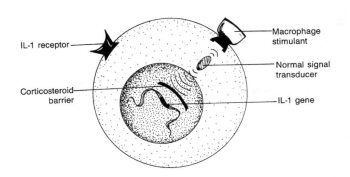

Figure 6. Mechanism of action of corticosteroids.

(Figure 6). Glucocorticoids have been widely administered for their immunosuppressive properties in autoimmune diseases such as autoimmune hemolytic anemia, systemic lupus erythematosus, Hashimoto's thyroiditis, idiopathic thrombocytopenic purpura and inflammatory bowel disease. They are also used in the treatment of various allergic reactions and for bronchial asthma. They have been widely used in organ transplantation, especially prior to the introduction of cyclosporine and related drugs. Management of rejection crises without producing bone marrow toxicity has also been achieved with these drugs. Long term usage has adverse effects that include adrenal suppression.

6-mercaptopurine (6-MP) is a powerful immunosuppressive drug used prior to the introduction of cyclosporine in organ transplantation (Figure 7). It is also an effective chemotherapeutic agent for the treatment of acute leukemia of childhood as well as other neoplastic conditions. 6-MP is a purine analog in which a thiol group replaces the 6-hydroxyl group. Hypoxanthine-guanine phosphoribosyl-transferase (HGPRT) transforms 6-MP to 6-thioinosine-5′-phosphate. This reaction product blocks various critical purine metabolic reactions. 6-MP is also incorporated into DNA as thioguanine.

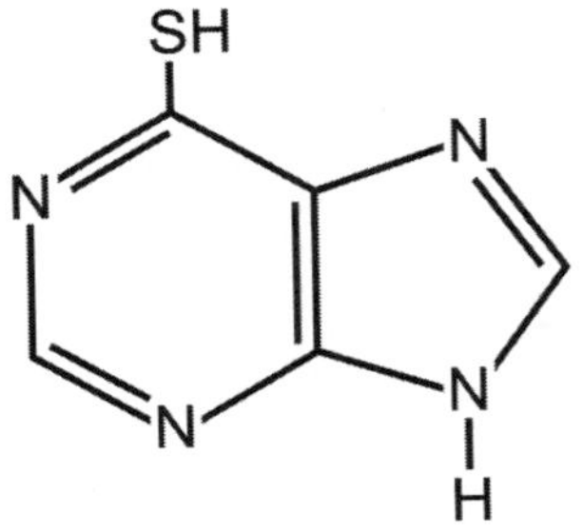

Figure 7. Structure of 6-mercaptopurine (6-MP).

Azathioprine (Figure 8) is a nitroimidazole derivative of 6-mercaptopurine, a purine antagonist. Following administration, it is converted to 6-mercaptopurine *in vivo*. Its principal action is to interfere with DNA synthesis. Of less significance is its ability to impair RNA synthesis. Azathi-

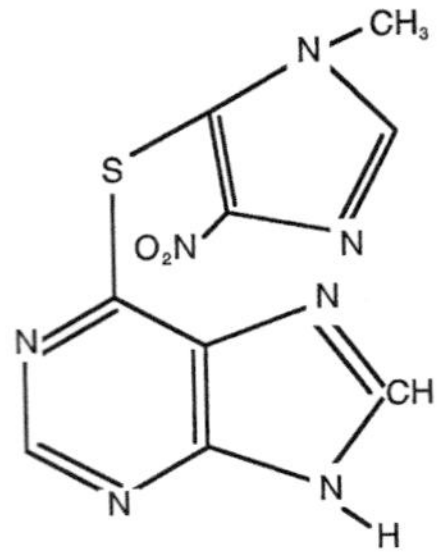

(6-[(1-methyl-4-nitro-1H-imidazol-5-yl)thio]-1H-purine)

Figure 8. Structure of azathioprine.

oprine has a greater inhibitory effect on T cell than on B cell responses, even though it suppresses both cell-mediated and humoral immunity. It diminishes circulating NK and killer cell numbers. It has been used to treat various autoimmune disorders including rheumatoid arthritis, other connective tissue diseases, autoimmune blood diseases and immunologically mediated neurological disorders. It is active chiefly against reproducing cells. The drug has little effect on immunoglobulin levels or antibody titers, but it does diminish neutrophil and monocyte numbers in the circulation.

Cyclophosphamide (N,N-bis[2-choroethyl]-tetrahydro-2H-1,3,2-oxazaphosphorine-2-amine-2-oxide) is a powerful immunosuppressive drug that is more toxic for B than for T lymphocytes (Figure 9). Therefore, it is a more effective suppressor of humoral antibody synthesis than of cell-mediated immune reactions. It is administered orally or intravenously and mediates its cytotoxic activity by cross-linking DNA strands. This alkylating action mediates target cell death. It produces dose-related lymphopenia and inhibits lymphocyte proliferation *in vitro*. The greater effect on B than on T cells is apparently related to B cells' lower rate of recovery. Cyclosphosphamide is beneficial for therapy of various immune disorders including rheumatoid arthritis, systemic lupus erythematosus-associated renal disease, Wegener's granulomatosis and other vasculitides, autoimmune hematologic disorders including idiopathic thrombocytopenic purpura, pure red cell aplasia, and autoimmune hemolytic anemia. It is used also to treat Goodpasture's syndrome and various glomerulonephritises. Its beneficial use as an immunosuppressive agent is tempered by the finding of its significant toxicity, such as its association with hemorrhagic cystitis, suppression of hematopoiesis, gastrointestinal symptoms, etc. It also may

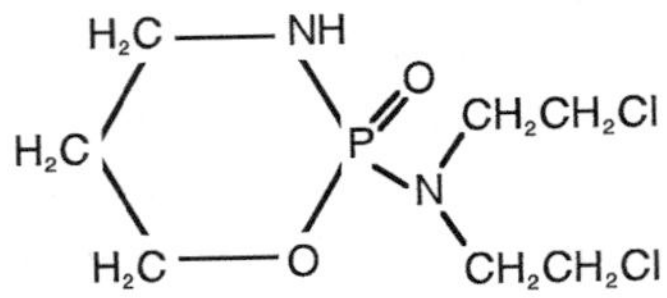

Figure 9. Structure of cyclosphosphamide.

increase the chance of opportunistic infections and be associated with an increased incidence of malignancies such as nonHodgkin's lymphoma, bladder carcinoma and acute myelogenous leukemia.

Chlorambucil (Figure 10) is an alkylating and cytotoxic drug. It is not as toxic as is cyclosphosphamide and has served as an effective therapy for selected immunological diseases such as rheumatoid arthritis, SLE, Wegener's granulomatosis, essential cryoglobulinemia, and cold agglutinin hemolytic anemia. Although chorambucil produces bone marrow suppression, it has not produced hemorrhagic cystitis and is less irritating to the GI tract than is cyclophosphamide. Chlorambucil increases the likelihood of opportunistic infections and the incidence of some tumors.

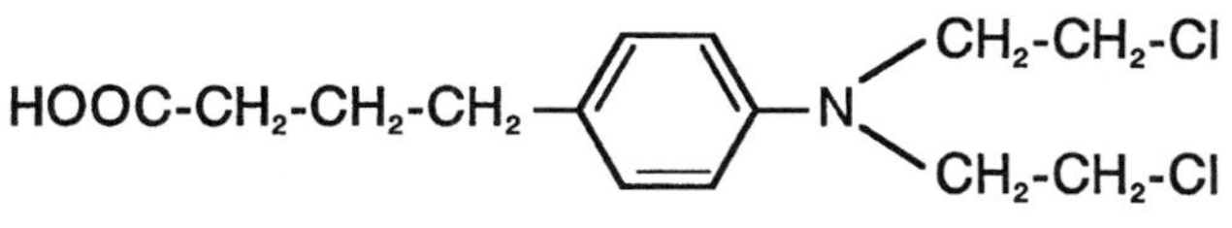

Figure 10. Structure of chlorambucil (4-[bis(2-chloroethyl)amino-phenylbutyric acid).

Busulfan (1,4-butanediol dimethanesulfonate) is an alkylating drug that is toxic to bone marrow cells. It is used to condition bone marrow transplant recipients (Figure 11).

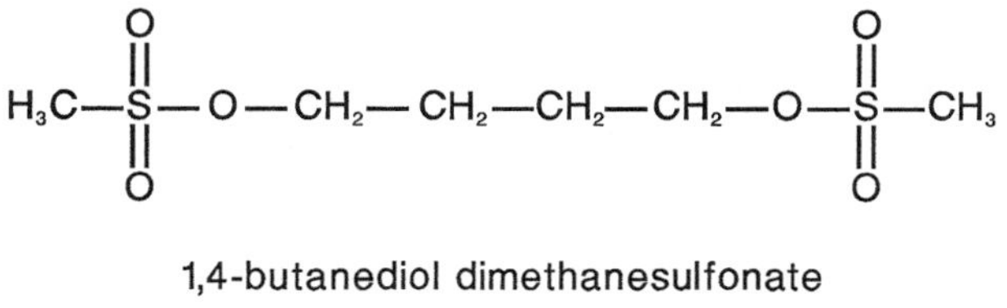

1,4-butanediol dimethanesulfonate

Figure 11. Stucture of busulfan.

Methotrexate (N-[p-[[2,4-diamino-6-pteridinyl-methyl]methylamino]benzoyl]glutamic acid) is a drug that blocks synthesis of DNA and thymidine in addition to its well known use as a chemotherapeutic agent against neoplasia (Figure 12). It blocks dihydrofolate reductase, the enzyme requisite for folic acid conversion to tetrahydrofolate. Methotrexate has been used to treat cancer, psoriasis, rheumatoid arthritis, polymyositis, Reiter's syndrome, graft-versus-host disease and steroid-dependent bronchial asthma. It inhibits both humoral and cell-mediated immune

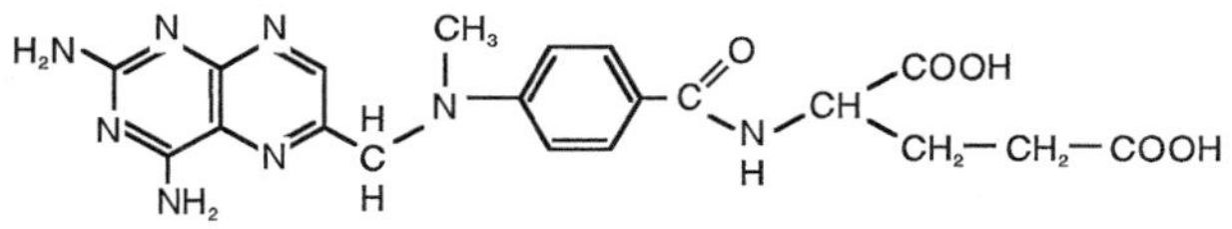

Figure 12. Structure of methotrexate.

responses. The major toxicity of methotrexate is hepatic fibrosis, which is dose related. It may also produce hypersensitivity pneumonitis and megaloblastic anemia.

Melphalan (L-phenylalanine mustard) is nitrogen mustard that is employed for therapy of multiple myeloma patients (Figure 13).

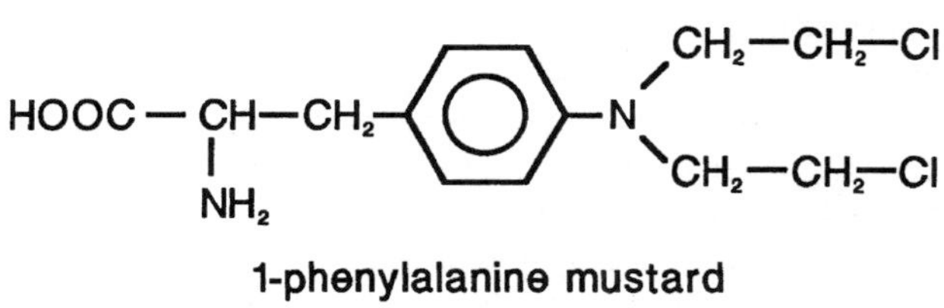

1-phenylalanine mustard

Figure 13. Structure of melphalan.

Cyclosporine (cyclosporin A) (ciclosporin) is a cyclic endecapeptide of 11 amino acid residues isolated from soil fungi which has revolutionized organ transplantation (Figure 14). Rather than acting as a cytotoxic agent, which defines the activity of a number of currently available immmunosuppressive drugs, cyclosporine (CSA) produces an immunomodulatory effect principally on the helper/inducer (CD4) lymphocytes which orchestrate the generation of an immune response. A cyclic polypeptide, CSA blocks T cell help for both humoral and cellular immunity. A primary mechanism of action is its ability to suppress interleukin-2 (IL-2) synthesis. It fails to block activation of antigen-specific suppressor T cells, and thereby assists development of antigen-specific tolerance. Side effects include nephrotoxicity and hepatotoxicity with a possible increase in B cell lymphomas. Some individuals may also develop hypertension. CSA's mechanism of action appears to include inhibition of the synthesis and release of lymphokines and alteration of expression of MHC gene products on the cell surface. CSA inhibits IL-2 mRNA formation. This does not affect IL-2 receptor expression on the cell surface. Although CSA may diminish the number of low-affinity binding sites, it does not appear to alter high-affinity binding sites on the cell surface. CSA inhibits the early

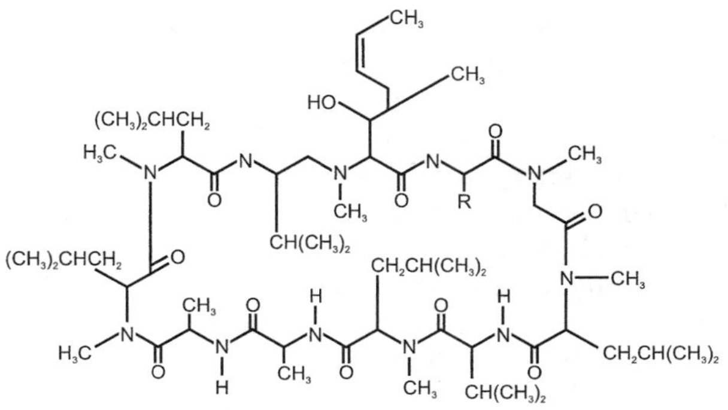

Figure 14. Structure of cyclosporine.

increase in cytosolic-free calcium which occurs in beginning activation of normal T lymphocytes. It appears to produce its effect in the cytoplasm rather than on the cell surface of a lymphocyte. This could be due to its ability to dissolve in the plasma membrane lipid bilayer. CSA's cytosolic site of action may involve calmodulin and/or cyclophilin, a protein kinase.

Although immunosuppressive action cannot be explained based upon CSA-calmodulin interaction, this association closely parallels the immunosuppressive effect. CSA produces a greater suppressive effect upon class II than upon class I antigen expression in at least some experiments. While decreasing T helper lymphocytes, the T suppressor cells appear to be spared following CSA therapy. Not only sparing but amplification of T lymphocyte suppression has been reported during CSA therapy. This is a powerful immunosuppressant that selectively affects CD4+ helper T cells without altering the activity of suppressor T cells, B cells, granulocytes and macrophages. It alters lymphocyte function but does not destroy the cells. CSA's principal immunosuppressive action is to inhibit IL-2 production and secretion. Thus, the suppression of IL-2 impairs the development of suppressor and cytotoxic T lymphocytes that are antigen-specific. It has a synergistic immunosuppressive action with corticosteroids. Corticosteroids interfere with IL-2 synthesis by inhibiting IL-1 release from monocytes and macrophages. Cyclosporine, although water insoluble, has been successfully employed as a clinical immunosuppressive agent principally in preventing rejection of organ and tissue allotransplants including kidney, heart, lung, pancreas and bone marrow. It has also been succcessful in preventing graft-vs-host reactions. The drug has some nephrotoxic properties, which may be kept to a minimum by dose reduction. As with other long term immunosuppressive agents, there may be increased risk of lymphoma development such as Epstein-Barr (EBV) and associated B cell lymphomas.

Immunophilins are high affinity receptor proteins in the cytoplasm that combine with such immunosuppressants as cyclosporin A, FK-506 and rapamycin. They prevent the activity of rotamase by blocking conversion between cis- and trans-rotamers of the peptide and protein substrate peptidyl-prolylamide bond. Immunophilins are important in transducing signals from the cell surface to the nucleus. Immunosuppressants have been postulated to prevent signal transduction mediated by T lymphocyte receptors, which blocks nuclear factor activation in activated T lymphocytes. Cyclophilin and FK506-binding proteins represent immunophilins. Drug-immunophilin complexes are implicated in the mechanism of action of the immunosuppressant drugs, cyclosporin, FK506 and rapamycin.

Cyclophilin is an 18kD protein in the cytoplasm that has peptidyl-prolyl isomerase functions. It has a unique and conserved amino acid sequence that has a broad phylogenetic distribution. It represents a protein kinase with a postulated critical role in cellular activation. It serves as a catalyst in cis-trans-rotamer interconversion. It catalyzes phosphorylation of a substrate which then serves as a cytoplasmic messenger associated with gene activation. Genes coding for the synthesis of lymphokines would be activated in helper T lymphocyte responsiveness. Cyclophilin has a high affinity for cyclosporine (CSA), which accounts for the drug's immunosuppressive action (Figure 15). Inhibition of cyclophilin-mediated activities as a consequence of CSA-cyclophilin interaction (Figure 16) could lead to inhibition of the synthesis and release of lymphokines. CSA not only inhibits primary immunization, but it may halt an ongoing immune response. This has been postulated to occur through inhibition of continued lymphokine release and by suppression of continued effector cell activation and recruitment.

FK506 (Figure 17) is a powerful immunosuppressive agent synthesized by *Streptomyces tsukubaensis*. Its principal use is for immunosuppression to prevent transplant rejection. FK506 has been used experimentally in liver transplant recipients. It interferes with the synthesis and binding of IL-2 and resembles cyclosporin, with which it may be used synergistically. Its immunosuppressive properties are 50 times greater than those of cyclosporin. It has been used in renal allotransplantation, but like cyclosporin also produces nephrotoxicity. It also has some neurotoxic effects and may have diabetogenic potential. The drug continues to be under investigation and is awaiting FDA approval.

FKBP (Figure 18) is a protein that binds FK506. It is a rotamase enzyme with an amino acid sequence that closely resembles that of protein kinase C. It serves as a receptor for both FK506 and rapamycin (Figure 19).

Rapamycin (Figure 20) is a powerful immunosuppressive drug derived from a soil fungus on Rapa Nui on Easter Island. It resembles FK506 (Figure 21) in structure, but it has a different mechanism of action. Rapamycin suppresses B and T lymphocyte proliferation, lymphokine synthesis and T cell responsiveness to IL-2. To achieve clinical immunosuppression, rapamycin is effective at concentrations one-eighth those required for FK506 and at 1% of the levels required for cyclosporin (Figure 22).

Brequinar sodium (BQR) is a recently developed antineoplastic and immunosuppressive agent (Figure 23). Its major activity is inhibition of the *de novo* biosynthesis of pyrimidine nucleosidases, resulting in inhibition of both DNA and RNA synthesis. BQR has also been shown to interfere with IgM production by IL-6 stimulated SKW6.4 cells, although in a manner independent of DNA synthesis. In transplantation studies, BQR has been shown to inhibit both the humoral and the cellular immune responses of the host, thereby significantly suppressing acute and antibody-mediated graft rejection.

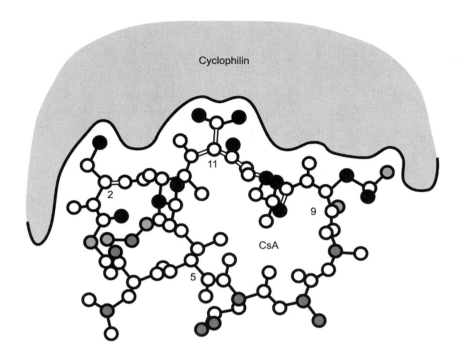

Figure 15. Cyclosporine (CSA) bound to cyclophilin.

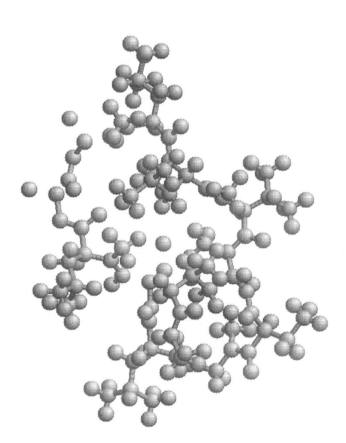

Figure 16. NMR structure of cyclosporine A as bound to cyclophilin A.

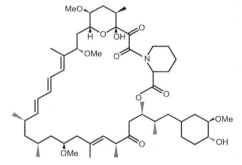

Figure 17. Structure of FK506.

Mycophenolate mofetil (Figure 24) is a new immunosuppressive drug that induces reversible antiproliferative effects specifically on lymphocytes but does not induce renal, hepatic and neurologic toxicity. Its action is based on the fact that adequate amounts of guanosine and deoxyguanosine nucleotides are requisite for lymphocytes to proliferate following antigenic stimulation. Thus, an agent that reversibly inhibits the final steps in purine synthesis, leading to a depletion of guanosine and deoxyguanosine nucleotides, could induce effective immunosuppression. Mycophenolate mofetil was found to produce these effects. It is the morpholinoethyl ester of mycophenolic acid. *In vivo*, it is hydrolyzed to the active form, mycophenolic acid, which the liver converts to mycophenolic acid goucuronide that is biologically inactive and is excreted in the urine. Mycophenolate blocks proliferation of peripheral blood mononuclear cells of humans to both B and T cell mitogens. It also blocks

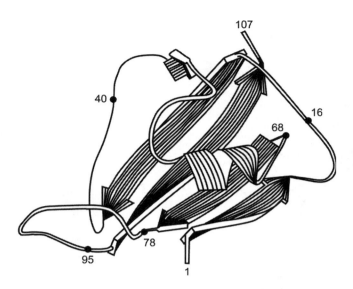

Figure 18.   Ribbon model of human FKBP.

antibody formation as evidence by inhibition of a recall response by human spleen cells challanged with tetanus toxoid. Its ability to block glycosylation of adhesion molecules that facilitate leukocyte attachment to endothelial cells and target cells probably diminishes recruitment of lymphocytes and monocytes to sites of rejection or chronic inflammation. It does not affect neutrophil chemotaxis, microbicidal activity or supraoxide production. *In vivo*, mycophenolate prevents cytotoxic T cell generation and rejection of allergeneic cells. It inhibits antibody formation in a dose-dependent manner and effectively prevents allograft rejection in animal models, especially when used in conjunction with cyclosporine. Current data suggest that the use of mycophenolate together with cyclosporine and prednisone leads to less allograft rejection than is achieved with combinations of these drugs without mycophenolate.

Anti-lymphocyte serum (or **anti-lymphocyte globulin**) is an antiserum prepared by immunizing one species, such as a rabbit or horse with lymphocytes or thymocytes from a different species, such as human (Figure 25). Antibodies present in this antiserum combine with T cells and other lymphocytes in the circulation to induce immunosuppression. ALS is used in organ transplant recipients to suppress graft rejection. The globulin fraction known as anti-lymphocyte globulin (ALG) rather than whole antiserum produces the same immunosuppressive effect.

OKT®3 (Orthoclone OKT®3) is a commercial mouse monoclonal antibody against the T cell surface marker CD3 (Figures 26 and 27). It may be used therapeutically to diminish T cell reactivity in organ allotransplant recipients experiencing a rejection episode; OKT3 may act in concert with the complement system to induce T cell lysis, or it may act as an opsonin, rendering T cells susceptible to phagocytosis. Rarely, recirculating T lymphocytes are removed in patients

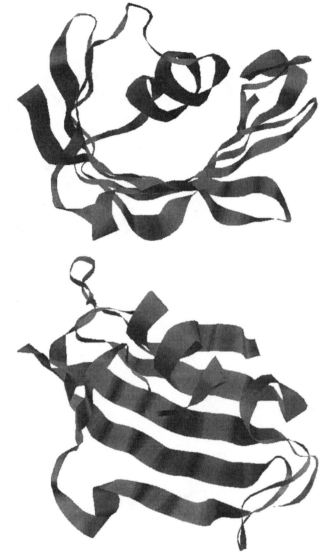

Figure 19.   Atomic structure of FKBP12-rapamycin, an immunophilin-immunosuppressant complex.

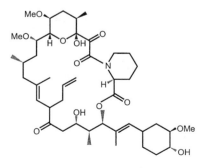

Figure 20.   Structure of rapamycin.

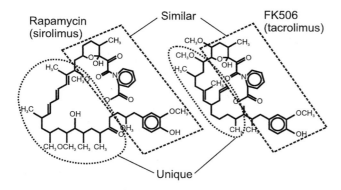

Figure 21. Uniqueness and similarities of FK506 and rapamycin.

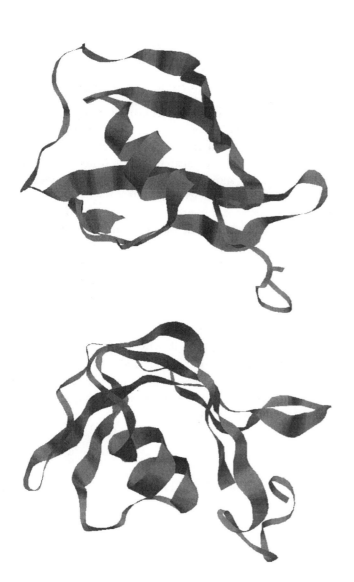

Figure 22. Human recombinant form of FK506 and rapamycin-binding protein expresseed in *E. coli*.

Figure 23. Structure of brequinar sodium (BQR.

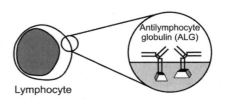

Figure 24. Structure of mycophenolate mofetil.

Figure 25. Anti-lymphocyte globulin.

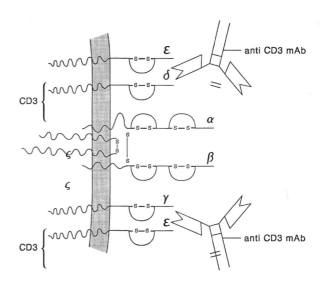

Figure 26. Anti CD3 mAb interaction with CD3 at T cell surface.

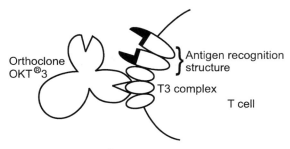

Specifically reacts with the T3-Antigen recognition structure of human T cells

Orthoclone OKT®3 blocks T cell effector function involved in renal allograft rejection

Figure 27.   OKT3 bound to the T3 complex of a T cell.

experiencing rejection crisis by thoracic duct drainage or extracorporeal irradiation of the blood.

Plasma exchange is useful for the temporary reduction in circulating antibody levels in selective diseases, such as hemolytic disease of the newborn, myasthenia gravis or Goodpasture's syndrome.

Immunosuppressive drugs act on all stages of the T and B cell maturation processes (Figure 28).

SPECIFIC IMMUNOSUPPRESSION

Anti-B and T cell receptor idiotype antibodies interact with antigenic determinants (idiotopes) at the variable N terminus of the heavy and light chains comprising the paratope region of an antibody molecule where the antigen-binding site is located. The idiotope antigenic determinants may be situated either within the cleft of the antigen-binding region or located on the periphery or outer edge of the variable region of heavy and light chain components. Anti-idiotypic antibodies also block T cell receptors for antigen for which they are specific.

Anti-target antigen antibodies may be used to block MHC class II molecules to prolong allograft survival or to remove Rh(D) positive cells to prevent sensitization of Rh(D) negative mothers.

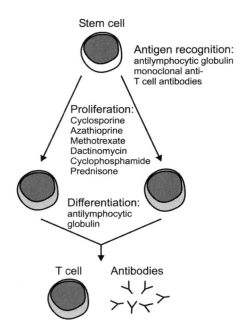

Figure 28.   Summary of the actions of immunosuppressive drugs.

Clonal deletion (negative selection) refers to the elimination of self-reactive T lymphocytes in the thymus during the development of natural self-tolerance. T cells recognize self antigens only in the context of major histocompatibility complex (MHC) molecules. Autoreactive thymocytes are eliminated following contact with self antigens expressed in the thymus before maturation is completed. The majority of CD4+ T lymphocytes in the blood circulation that survived clonal deletion in the thymus failed to respond to any stimulus. This reveals that clonal anergy participates in suppression of autoimmunity. Clonal deletion represents a critical mechanism to rid the body of autoreactive T lymphocytes. This is brought about by minor lymphocyte stimulation (mls) antigens that interact with the T cell receptor's V beta region of the T lymphocyte receptor thereby mimicking the action of bacterial super antigen. Intrathymic and peripheral tolerance in T lymphocytes can be accounted for by clonal deletion and functional inactivation of T cells reactive against self.

20

Transplantation Immunology

Transplantation is the replacement of an organ or other tissue, such as bone marrow, with organs or tissues derived ordinarily from a non-self source such as an allogeneic donor. Organs include kidney, liver, heart, lung, pancreas (including pancreatic islets), intestine or skin. In addition, bone matrix and cardiac valves have been transplanted. Bone marrow transplants are given for nonmalignant conditions such as aplastic anemia as well as to treat certain leukemias and other malignant diseases.

Transplantation immunology is the study of immunologic reactivity of a recipient to transplanted organs or tissues from a histoincompatible donor. Effector mechanisms of transplantation rejection or transplantation immunity consist of cell-mediated immunity and/or humoral antibody immunity, depending upon the category of rejection. For example, hyperacute rejection of an organ such as a renal allograft is mediated by preformed antibodies and takes place soon after the vascular anastomosis is completed in transplantation. By contrast, acute allograft rejection is mediated principally by T lymphocytes and occurs during the first week after transplantation. There are instances of humoral vascular rejection mediated by antibodies as a part of the acute rejection in response. Chronic rejection is mediated by a cellular response.

Histocompatibility is tissue compatibility as in the transplantation of tissues or organs from one member to another of the same species, an allograft, or from one species to another, a xenograft. The genes that encode antigens which should match if a tissue or organ graft is to survive in the recipient are located in the major histocompatibility complex (MHC) region. In the human this is located on the short arm of chromosome 6 (Figure 1) and in the mouse of chromosome 17. Class I and class II MHC antigens are important in tissue transplantation. The greater the match between donor and recipient, the more likely the transplant is to survive. For example, a six antigen match implies sharing of two HLA-A antigens, two HLA-B antigens, and two HLA-DR antigens between donor and recipient. Even though antigenically dissimilar grafts may survive when a powerful immunosuppressive drug such as cyclosporine is used, the longevity of the graft is still improved by having as many antigens to match as possible.

Histocompatibility antigen is one of a group of genetically encoded antigens present on tissue cells of an animal that

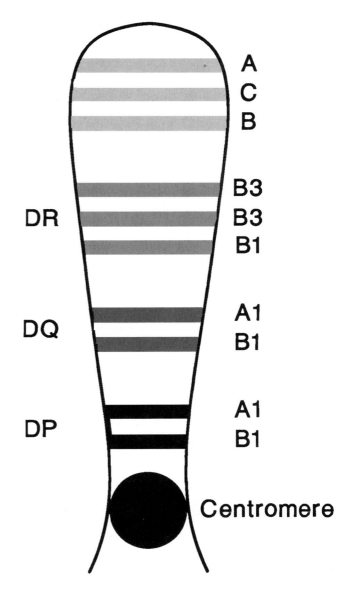

Figure 1. Human chromosome 6.

provoke a rejection response if the tissue containing them is transplanted to a genetically dissimilar recipient. These antigens are detected by typing lymphocytes on which they are expressed. In humans, these antigens are encoded by genes

353

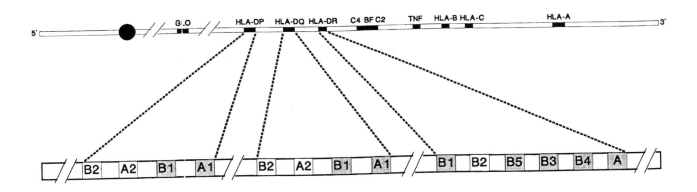

Figure 2.   Short arm of chromosome 6.

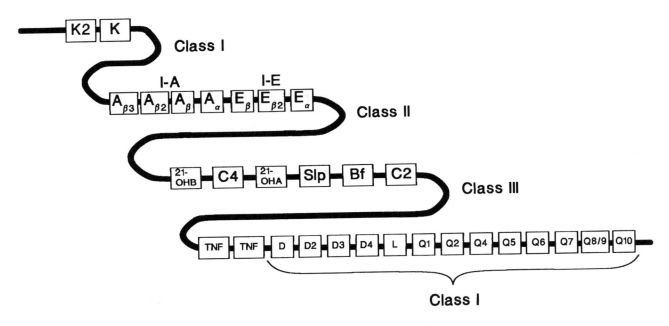

Figure 3.   H-2 complex on chromosome 17 of a mouse.

at the HLA locus on the short arm of chromosome 6 (Figure 2). In the mouse, they are encoded by genes at the H-2 locus on chromosome 17 (Figure 3).

Transplantation antigens are histocompatibility antigens which stimulate an immune response in the recipient that may lead to rejection.

A **histocompatibility locus** is a specific site on a chromosome where the histocompatibility genes that encode histocompatibility antigens are located. There are major histocompatibility loci such as HLA in the human and H-2 in the mouse across which incompatible grafts are rejected within 1 to 2 weeks. There are also several minor histocompatibility

loci, with more subtle antigenic differences, across which only slow, low level graft rejection reactions occur.

Histocompatibility testing is a determination of the MHC-class I and class II tissue type of both donor and recipient prior to organ or tissue transplantation. In the human HLA-A, HLA-B, and HLA-DR types are determined followed by crossmatching donor lymphocytes with recipient serum prior to transplantation. A mixed lymphocyte culture (MLC) is necessary in bone marrow transplantation in conjunction with molecular DNA typing. The MLC may also be requested in living related organ transplants. Organ recipients, as in renal allotransplantation, have their serum samples tested for percent reactive antibodies which reveals whether or not they have been presensitized against HLA antigens of an organ for which they may be the recipient.

HLA is an abbreviation for human leukocyte antigen. The HLA histocompatibility system in humans represents a complex of MHC class I molecules distributed on essentially all nucleated cells of the body and MHC class II molecules that are distributed on B lymphocytes, macrophages and a few other cell types. These are encoded by genes at the major histocompatibility complex. In humans the HLA locus is found on the short arm of chromosome 6. This has now been well defined and in addition to encoding surface isoantigens, genes at the HLA locus also encode immune response (*Ir*) genes. The class I region consists of HLA-A, HLA-B, and HLA-C loci and the class II region consists of the D region which is subdivided into HLA-DP, HLA-DQ, and HLA-DR subregions. Class II molecules play an important role in the induction of an immune response since antigen presenting cells must complex an antigen with class II molecules to present it in the presence of interleukin-1 to CD4+ T lymphocytes. Class I molecules are important in presentation of intracellular antigen to CD8+ T lymphocytes as well as an effector functions of target cells. Class III molecules encoded by genes located between those that encode class I and class II molecules include C2, BF, C4a, and C4b. Class I and class II molecules play an important role in the transplantation of organs and tissues. The microlymphocytotoxicity assay is used for HLA-A, -B, -C, -DR, and -DQ typing. The primed lymphocyte test is used for DP typing.

HLA-A is a class I histocompatibility antigen (Figure 4) in humans which is expressed on nucleated cells of the body. Tissue typing to identify an individual's HLA-A antigens employs lymphocytes.

HLA-B is a class I histocompatibility antigen (Figure 5) in humans which is expressed on nucleated cells of the body. Tissue typing to define an individual's HLA-B antigens employs lymphocytes.

HLA-C is a class I histocompatibility antigen in humans which is expressed on nucleated cells of the body. Lymphocytes are employed for tissue typing to determine HLA-C antigens. HLA-C antigens play little or no role in graft rejection.

The human MHC class II region is the **HLA-D region** which is comprised of three subregions designated DR, DQ and DP. Multiple genetic loci are present in each of these. DN (previously DZ) and DO subregions are each comprised of one genetic locus. Each class II HLA molecule is comprised of one α and one β chain that constitute a heterodimer. Genes within each subregion encode a particular class II molecule's α and β chains. Class II genes that encode α chains are designated A whereas class II genes that encode β chains are designated B. A number is used following A or B if a particular subregion contains two or more A or B genes.

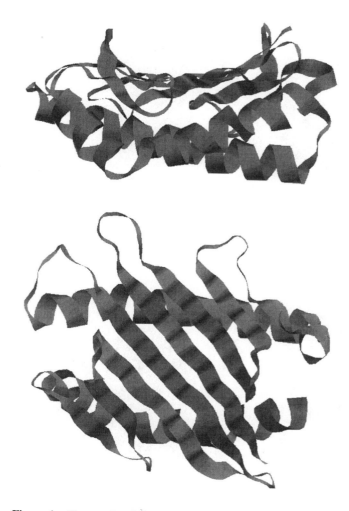

Figure 4. Human class I histocompatibility antigen (HLA-A 0201) complexed with a decameric peptide from calreticulin HLA-A 0201. Human recombinant extracellular fragment expressed in *E. coli*; peptide synthetic based on sequence of human calreticulin.

The **HLA-DP subregion** is the site of two sets of genes designated HLA-DPA1 and HLA-DPB1 and the pseudogenes HLA-DPA2 and HLA-DPB2. DPα and DPβ chains encoded by the corresponding genes DPA1 and DPB1 unite to produce the DPαβ molecule. DP antigen or type is determined principally by the very polymorphic DPβ chain in contrast to the much less polymorphic DPα chain. DP molecules carry DPw1-DPw6 antigens.

The **HLA-DQ subregion** consists of two sets of genes designated DQA1 and DQB1 and DQA2 and DQB2. DQA2 and DRB2 are pseudogenes. DQα and DQβ chains, encoded by DQA1 and DQB1 genes, unite to produce the DQαβ molecule. Although both DQα and DQβ chains are polymorphic, the DQβ chain is the principal factor in determining the DQ antigen or type. DQαβ molecules carry DQw1-DQw9 specificities.

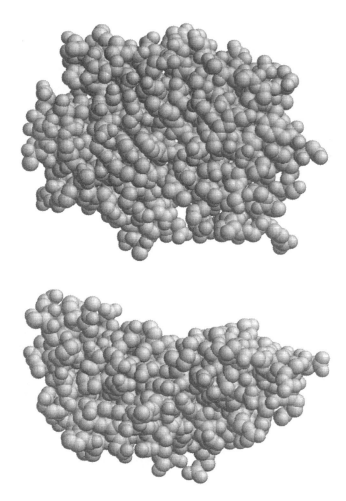

Figure 5. Class I histocompatibility antigen HLA-B*2705 complexed with nonapeptide arg-arg-ile-lys-ala-ile-thr-leu-lys (theoretical model).

The **HLA-DR subregion** is the site of one HLA-DRA gene (Figure 6). Although DRB gene number varies with DR type, there are usually three DRB genes, termed DRB1, DRB2, and DRB3 (or DR4). The DRB2 pseudogene is not expressed. The DR I chain, encoded by the DRA gene, can unite with products of DRB1 and DRB3 (or DRB4) genes which are the DR J-1 and DR J-3 (or DR J-4) chains. This yields two separate DR molecules, DR αβ-1 and DR αβ-3 (or DR αβ-4). The DR J chain determines the DR antigen (DR type) since it is very polymorphic, whereas the DR α chain is not. DR αβ-1 molecules carry DR specificities DR1-DRw18. Yet, DR αβ-3 molecules carry the DRw52 and the DR αβ-4 molecules carry the DRw53 specificity.

HLA-DR antigenic specificities are epitopes on DR gene products. Selected specificities have been mapped to defined loci. HLA serologic typing requires the identification of a prescribed antigenic determinant on a particular HLA molecular product. One typing specificity can be present on many different molecules. Different alleles at the same locus

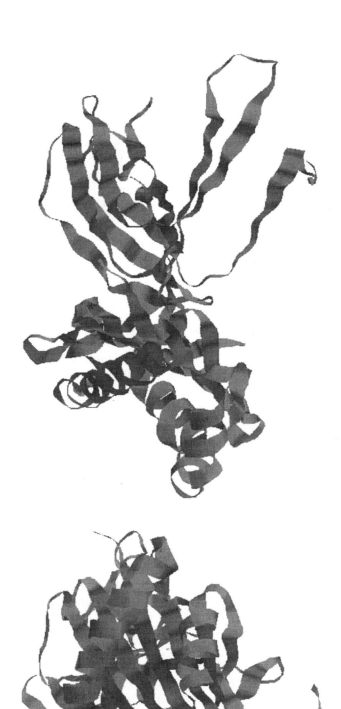

Figure 6. HLA-DR1 histocompatibility antigen.

may encode these various HLA molecules. Monoclonal antibodies are now used to recognize certain antigenic determinants shared by various molecules bearing the same HLA typing specificity. Monoclonal antibodies have been employed to recognize specific class II alleles with disease associations.

HLA-E is an HLA class I nonclassical molecule.

HLA-F is an HLA class I nonclassical molecule.

HLA-G is a polymorphic class I HLA antigen with extensive variability in the α-2 domain. It is found on trophoblasts, i.e., placenta cells and trophoblastic neoplasms. HLA-G is expressed only on cells such as placental extravillous cytotorphoblasts and choriocarcinoma that fail to express HLA-A, -B, and -C antigens. HLA-G expression is most pronounced during the first rimester of pregnancy. Trophoblast cells expressing HLA-G at the maternal-fetal junction may protect the semiallogeneic fetus from "rejection." Prominent HLA-G expression suggests maternal immune tolerance.

HLA-H is a pseudogene found in the MHC class I region that is structurally similar to HLA-A but is nonfunctional due to the absence of a cysteine residue at position 164 in its protein product and the deletion of the codon 227 nucleotide.

HLA nonclassical class I genes are located within the MHC class I region that encode products that can associate with β-2 microglobulin. However, their function and tissue distribution are different from those of HLA-A, -B, and -C molecules. Examples include HLA-E, -F, and -G. Of these onlly HLA-G is expressed on the cell surface. It is uncertain whether or not these HLA molecules are involved in peptide binding and presentation like classical class I molecules.

An **extended haplotype** consists of linked alleles in positive linkage disequilibrium situated between and including HLA-DR and LHA-B of the major histocompatibility complex of man. Examples of extended haplotypes include the association of B8/DR3/SCO1/GLO2 with membranoproliferative glomerulonephritis and of A25/B18/DR2 with complement C2 deficiency. Extended haplotypes may be a consequence of crossover oppression through environmental influences together with selected HLA types, leading to autoimmune conditions. The B27 relationship to *Klebsiella* is an example.

Linkage disequilibrium refers to the appearance of HLA genes on the same chromosome with greater frequency than would be expected by chance. This has been demonstrated by detailed studies in both populations and families, employing outbred groups where numerous different haplotypes are present. With respect to the HLA-A, -B, -C loci, a possible explanation for linkage disequilibrium is that there has not been sufficient time for the genes to reach equilibrium. However, this possibility is remote for HLA-A, -B, -D linkage disequilibrium. Natural selection has been suggested to maintain linkage disequilibrium that is advantageous. If products of two histocompatibility loci play a role in the immune response and appear on the same chromosome, they might reinforce one another and represent an advantageous association. An example of linkage disequilibrium in the HLA system of man is the occurrence on the same chromosome of HLA-A3 and HLA-B7 in the caucasian American population.

HLA disease associations are certain HLA alleles occurring in a higher frequency in individuals with particular diseases than in the general population. This type of data permits estimation of the "relative risk" of developing a disease with every known HLA allele. For example, there is a strong association between ankylosing spondylitis, which is an autoimmune disorder involving the vertebral joints, and the class I MHC allele, HLA-B27. There is a strong association between products of the polymorphic class II alleles HLA-DR and -DQ and certain autoimmune diseases, since class II MHC molecules are of great importance in the selection and activation of CD4+ T lymphocytes which regulate the immune responses against protein antigens. For example, 95% of Caucasians with insulin-dependent (type I) diabetes mellitus have HLA-DR3 or HLA-DR4 or both. There is also a strong association of HLA-DR4 with rheumatoid arthritis. Numerous other examples exist and are the targets of current investigations, especially in extended studies employing DNA probes.

HLA allelic variation is a genomic analysis that has identified specific individual allelic variants to explain HLA associations with rheumatoid arthritis, type I diabetes mellitus, multiple sclerosis and celiac disease. There is a minimum of six α and eight β genes in distinct clusters, termed HLA-DR, DQ, and DP within the HLA class II genes. DO and DN class II genes are related but map outside DR, DQ, and DP regions. There are two types of dimers along the HLA cell-surface HLA-DR class II molecules. The dimers are made up of either DRα-polypeptide associated with DRβ$_1$-polypeptide or DR with DRβ$_2$-polypeptide. Structural variation in class II gene products is linked to functional features of immune recognition leading to individual variations in histocompatibility, immune recognition and susceptibility to disease. There are two types of structural variations which include variation among DP, DQ, and DR products in primary amino acid sequence by as much as 35% and individual variation attributable to different allelic forms of class II genes. The class II polypeptide chain possesses domains which are specific structural subunits containing variable sequences that distinguish among class II α genes or class II β genes. These allelic variation sites have been suggested to form epitopes which represent individual structural differences in immune recognition.

HLA oligotyping is a recently developed method using oligonucleotide probes to supplement other histocompatibility testing techniques. Whereas, serological and cellular methods identify phenotypic characteristics of HLA proteins, oligotyping defines the genotype of the DNA that encodes HLA protein structure and specificity. Thus oligotyping can identify the DNA type even when there is a failure of expression of HLA genes which render serological techniques ineffective.

HLA tissue typing (Figure 7) is the identification of major histocompatibility complex class I and class II antigens on lymphocytes by serological and cellular techniques. The principal serological assay is microlymphocytotoxicity using microtiter plates containing predispensed anitbodies against HLA specificities to which lymphocytes of unknown specificity plus rabbit complement and vital dye are added. Following incubation, the wells are scored according to the relative proportion of cells killed. This method is employed for organ transplants such as renal allotransplants. For bone marrow transplants, mixed lymphocyte reaction procedures are performed to determine the relative degree of histocompatibility or histoincompatability between donor and recipient. Serological tests are largely being replaced by DNA typing procedures employing polymerase chain reaction (PCR) methodology and DNA or oligonucleotide probes, especially for MHC class II typing.

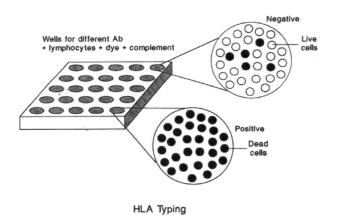

HLA Typing

Figure 7. HLA tissue typing.

Class I typing involves reactions between lymphocytes to be typed with HLA antisera of known specificity in the presence of complement. Cell lysis is detected by phase or fluorescence microscopy. This is important in parentage testing, disease association, transfusion practices, and transplantation. HLA-A, -B, and -C antigens should be defined by at least one of the following: (1) at least two different sera if both are monospecific, (2) one monospecific and two multispecific antisera, (3) at least three multispecific antisera if all multispecific are used.

Class II typing detects HLA-DR antigens using purified B cell preparations. It is based on antibody-specific, complement-

dependent disruption of the cell membrane of lymphocytes. Cell death is demonstrated by the penetration of dye into the membrane. Class II typing is more difficult than type II typing because of the variability of both B-cell isolation methods and complement toxicity. At least three antisera must be used if all are monospecific; at least five antiserum must be used for multispecific sera.

Microlymphocytotoxicity is a widely used technique for HLA tissue typing. Lymphocytes are separated from heparinized blood samples by either layering over Ficoll-hypaque (Figures 8 and 9), centrifuging and removing lymphocytes from the interface or by using beads. After appropriate washing, these purified lymphocyte preparations are counted, and aliquots are dispensed using a Hamilton syringe (Figure 10) into microtiter plate wells (Figure 11) containing predispensed quantities of antibody. When used for human histocompatibility (HLA) testing, antisera in the wells are specific for known HLA antigenic specificities. After incubation of the cells and antisera, rabbit complement is added, and the plates are again incubated. The extent of cytotoxicity induced is determined by incubating the cells with trypan blue, which enters dead cells and stains them blue, while leaving live cells unstained. The plates are read by using an inverted phase contrast microscope (Figure 12). A scoring system from 0 to 8 (where 8 implies >80% of target cells killed) is employed to indicate cytotoxicity. Most of the sera used to date are multispecific, as they are obtained from multiparous females who have been sensitized during

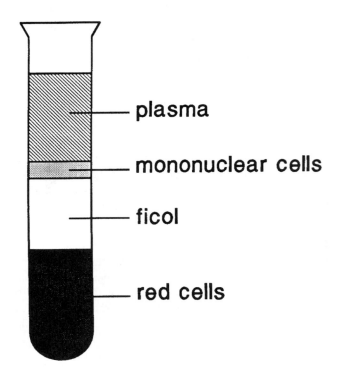

Figure 8. Cartoon of ficoll-hypaque technique of cell separation.

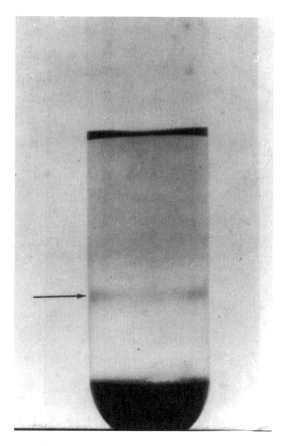

Figure 9. The separation of lymphocytes from peripheral blood by centrifugation using ficoll-hypaque.

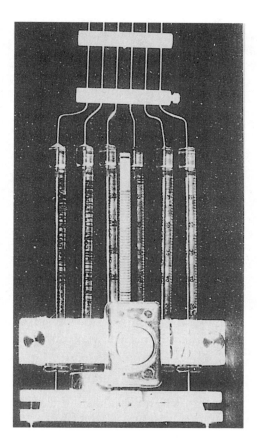

Figure 10. A Hamilton syringe that is used to dispense lymphocytes into Terasaki plates for tissue typing

pregnancy by HLA antigens determined by their spouse. Monoclonal antibodies are being used with increasing frequency in tissue typing. This technique is useful to identify HLA-A, HLA-B, and HLA-C antigens. When purified B cell preparations and specific antibodies against B cell antigens are employed, HLA-DR and HLA-DQ antigens can be identified.

A **cell tray panel** (Figure 13) is used to detect and identify HLA antibodies. Patient serum is tested against a panel of known cells. The panel (or percent) reactive antibody (PRA) is the percent of panel cells reacting with a patient's serum. It is expressed as a percentage of the total reactivity. %PRA = (# positive reactions/# cells in panel) × 100. This percentage is a useful indicator of the proportion of HLA antibodies of the patient.

Patients may have preformed antibodies against class I or II HLA antigens. If these patients receive organs that possess the corresponding antigens, they will likely experience hyperacute or delayed rejection for class I or class II incompatibilites, respectively. In order to detect such incompatibilites before transplantation, a **crossmatching procedure** is performed. The conventional crossmatching procedure (Figure 14) for organ transplants involves the combination

of donor lymphocytes with recipient serum. There are three major variables in the standard crossmatch procedure that predominantly affect the reactivity of the cell/sera sensitization. These include (1) incubation time and temperature; (2) wash steps after cell/sera sensitization; and (3) the use of additional reagents, such as antiglobulin in the test. Variations in these steps can cause wide variations in results. Lymphocytes can be separated into T and B cell categories for crossmatch procedures that are conducted at cold (4°C), room (25°C), and warm (37°C) temperatures. These permit the identification of warm anti-T cell antibodies that are almost always associated with graft rejection.

Flow cytometry can also be used to preform the crossmatching procedure. This method is highly sensitive (considerably more sensitive than the direct cytotoxicity method). Flow crossmatching is also faster, and can distinguish antibodies according to class (IgG vs. IgM) and target cell specificitity (T cells from B cells). It is a valuable procedure in organ and bone marrow transplantation and is particularly suitable to measuring antibodies against HLA class I antigens on donor T cells. False positives are rare and most errors are due to low sensitivity (lower antibody concentration). Flow crossmatching has the potential to be standardized and automated. The flow cytometry crossmatching method commonly utilizes

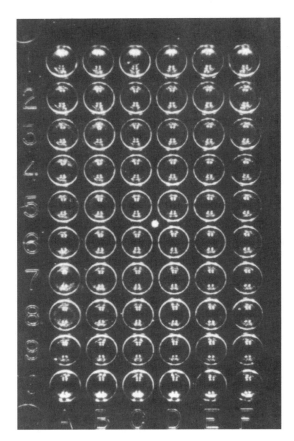

Figure 11. A Terasaki plate consisting of depressions in a plastic plate that contain predispensed antibodies to HLA antigens of various specificities and into which are placed patient lymphocytes and rabbit complement for tissue typing.

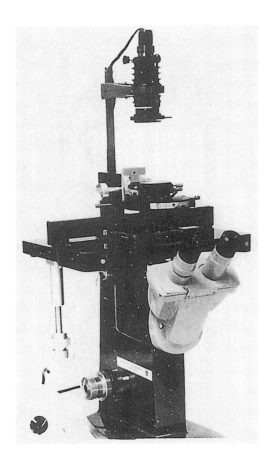

Figure 12. An inverted light microscope used to read Terasaki plates to determine tissue type.

F(ab′)$_2$ antihuman IgG conjugated to fluorescein and anti-CD3 for T cells conjugated to phycoerythrin. A two parameter display of anti-CD3 vs. IgG is generated. A positive flow crossmatch is defined as median channel shift values > 40 (Figures 15 and 16).

Splits are human leukocyte antigen (HLA) subtypes (Figure 17). For example, the base antigen HLA-B12 can be subdivided into the splits HLA-B44 and HLA-B45. The term "split" is used to designate an HLA antigen that was first believed to be a private antigen, but was later shown to be a public antigen. The former designation can be placed in parentheses following its new designation, i.e., HLA-B44(12).

A **private antigen** (Figure 18) is (1) an antigen confined to one major histocompatibility complex (MHC) molecule. (2) An antigenic specificity restricted to a few individuals. (3) A tumor antigen restricted to a specific chemically induced tumor. (4) A low-frequency epitope present on red blood cells of fewer than 0.1% of the population, i.e., Pt^a, By, Bp^a, etc. (5) HLA antigen encoded by one allele such as HLA-B27.

TRAY POS	#CNTRL	TEST	CELL ID	RACE	PANEL TYPING						
					A		B		C		BW
1A		8	10571T	H	1	2	8	35	7		6
1B		8	9891T	C	1	2	44	51	1	5 4	
1C		8	9884T	B	1	2	57	82	3	6	4 6
1D		8	9898T	B	1	23	45	49	6	7	4 6
1E		8	10356T	B	1	23	58	72	6		4 6
1F		8	10990T	O	1	24	27	37	2	6	4
2F		8	10367T	C	1	32	8	51	7		4 6
2E		8	7109T	H		13	64	6	8	4	6
2D		1	6606T	C	2	11	18	38	7		4 6
2C		1	10567T	C	2	11	37	60	3	6	4 6
2B		8	10988T	C	2	24	51	55	3		4 6
2A		1	10359T	C	2	25	57	62	5	6	4 6
3A		1	10549T	O	2	26	39	61	1	7	6
3B		1	10361T	O	2	26	54	62	1	3	6
3C		1	10570T	O	2	26	60	65	4	8	6
3D		1	9899T	B	2	30	8	58	7		4 6
3E		1	10352T	O	2	30	13	46	1	6	4 6
3F		1	10547T	C	2	31	35	47	4		4 6
4F		1	6688T	C	2	31	50	60	3	6	6
4E		1	10568T	H	2	32	41	61	2	7	6

Figure 13. Cell tray panel showing positive reactions (8s) for HLA-A1 at tray positions 1A, 1B, 1C, 1D, 1E, 1F, 2F, and 2E, and a positive reaction for HLA-A24 at position 2B.

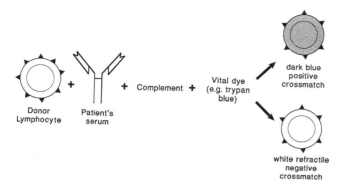

Figure 14. Crossmatching procedure.

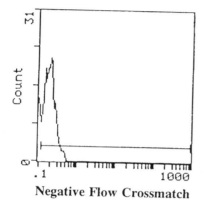

Negative Flow Crossmatch

Figure 15. Negative flow crossmatch.

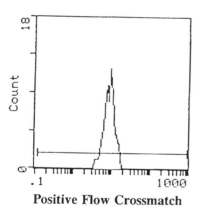

Positive Flow Crossmatch

Figure 16. Positive flow crossmatch.

Original Broad Specificities	Splits and Associated Antigens #
A2	A203#, A210 #
A9	A23, A24, A2403#
A10	A25, A26, A34, A66
A19	A29, A30, A31, A32, A33, A74
A28	A68, A69
B5	B51, B52
B7	B703#
B12	B44, B45
B14	B64, B65
B15	B62,B63, B75, B76, B77
B16	B38, B39, B3901#, B3902 #
B17	B57, B58
B21	B49, B50, B4005 #
B22	B54, B55, B56
B40	B60, B61
B70	B71, B72
Cw3	Cw9, Cw10
DR1	DR103#
DR2	DR15, DR16
DR3	DR17, DR18
DR5	DR11, DR12
DR6	DR13, DR14, DR1403 #, DR1404#
DQ1	DQ5, DQ6
DQ3	DQ7, DQ8, DQ9
Dw6	Dw18, Dw19
Dw7	Dw11, Dw17

Figure 17. Splits.

A **public antigen (supratypic antigen)** is an epitope which several distinct or private antigens have in common (Figure 18). A public antigen such as a blood group antigen is one that is present in greater than 99.9% of a population. It is detected by the indirect antiglobulin (Coombs' test). Examples include Ve, Ge, Jr, Gyª, and Okª. Antigens that occur frequently, but are not public antigens include Mns, Lewis, Duffy, P, etc. In blood banking, there is a problem finding a suitable unit of blood for a transfusion to recipients who have developed antibodies against public antigens.

Multilocus probes (Figure 19) are used to identify multiple related sequences distributed throughout each person's genome. Multilocus probes may reveal as many as 20 separate alleles. Because of this multiplicity of alleles, there is only a remote possibility that two unrelated persons would share the same pattern, i.e., about 1 in 30 billion. There is, however, a problem in deciphering the multibanded arrangement of minisatellite RFLPs, as it is difficult to ascertain which bands are allelic. Mutation rates of minisatellite HVRs remain to be demonstrated, but are recognized occasionally. This method can be used in resolving cases of disputed parentage.

Immediate spin crossmatch is a test for incompatibility between donor erythrocytes and the recipient patient's serum. This assay reveals ABO incompatibility in practically all cases, but is unable to identify IgG alloantibodies against erythrocyte antigens.

Orthotopic graft (Figure 20) is an organ or tissue transplant that is placed in the location that is usually occupied by that particular organ or tissue.

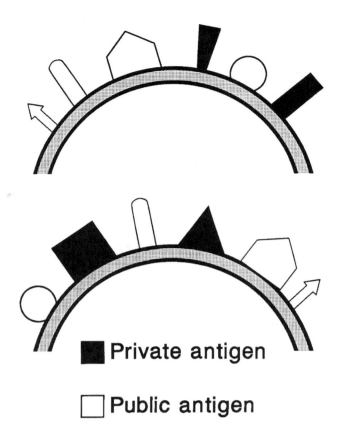

Figure 18. Public and private antigens.

Heterotopic graft is a tissue or organ transplanted to an anatomic site other than the one where it is usually found under natural conditions. For example, the anastomosis of the renal vasculature at an anatomical site that would situate the kidney in a place other than the renal fossa where it is customarily found.

A **graft** is the transplantation of a tissue or organ from one site to another within the same individual or between individuals of either the same or of a different species.

A **semisyngeneic graft** is a graft that is ordinarily accepted from an individual of one strain into an F_1 hybrid of an individual of that strain mated with an individual of a different strain (Figure 21).

Graft facilitation is a prolonged graft survival attributable to conditioning of the recipient with IgG antibody, which is believed to act as a blocking factor. It also decreases cell-mediated immunity. This phenomenon is related to immunologic enhancement of tumors by antibody and has been referred to as immunological facilitation (*facilitation immunologique*).

An **allograft** is an organ, tissue or cell transplant from one individual or strain to a genetically different individual or

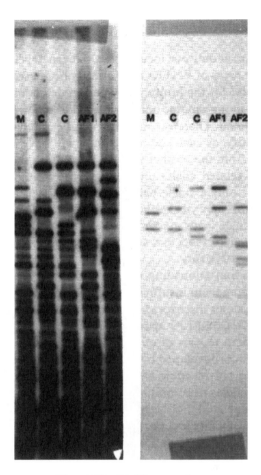

Figure 19. Multilocus probes.

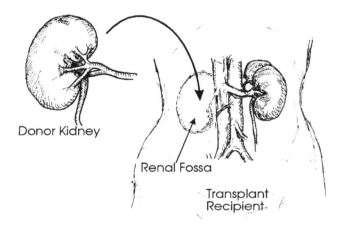

Figure 20. Orthotopic graft.

strain within the same species. Allografts are also called homografts (Figure 22).

Homograft rejection is an allograft rejection. An immune response is induced by histocompatibility antigens in the donor graft that are not present in the recipient. This is principally a cell-mediated type of immune response.

Takes

1. Autograft

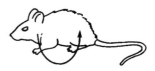

2. Isograft (Syngeneic graft)

A strain   A strain

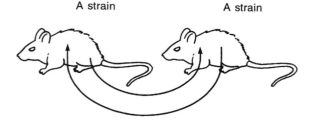

3. Semisyngeneic Graft

A strain   (AxB)F₁

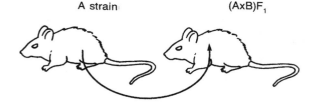

Rejects

1. Allograft

A strain   B strain

2. Semisyngeneic Graft

A strain   (AxB)F₁

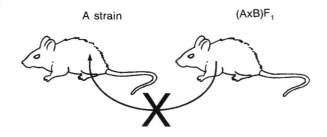

Figure 21. Semisyngeneic graft.

A **xenograft** (Figure 23) is a tissue or organ graft from a member of one species, i.e., the donor, to a member of a different species, i.e., the recipient. It is also called heterograft. Antibodies and cytotoxic T cells reject xenografts several days following transplantation.

Syngraft is a transplant from one individual to another within the same strain. Syngrafts are also called isografts.

Isograft is a tissue transplant from a donor to an isogenic recipient. Grafts exchanged between members of an inbred strain of laboratory animals such as mice are syngeneic rather than isogenic.

A **donor** is one who offers whole blood, blood products, bone marrow, or an organ to be given to another individual. Individuals who are drug addicts or test positively for certain diseases such as HIV-1 infection or hepatitis B, for example, are not suitable as donors. To be a blood donor, an individual must meet certain criteria which include blood pressure, temperature, hematocrit, pulse, and history. There are many reasons for donor rejection, including low hematocrit, skin lesions, surgery, drugs, or positive donor blood tests.

An **organ bank** is a site where selected tissues for transplantation, such as acellular bone fragments, corneas, and bone marrow, may be stored for relatively long periods until needed for transplantation. Several hospitals often share such a facility. Organs such as kidneys, liver, heart, lung, and pancreatic islets must be transplanted within 48 to 72 hours and are not suitable for storage in an organ bank.

Organ brokerage, or the selling of an organ such as a kidney from a living related donor to the transplant recipient, is practiced in certain parts of the world, but is considered unethical and is illegal in the U.S. as it is in violation of the National Organ Transplant Act (Public Law 98-507,3 USC).

Adoptive immunity (Figure 24) is the term assigned by Billingham, Brent, and Medawar (1955) to transplantation immunity induced by the passive transfer of specifically immune lymph node cells from an actively immunized animal

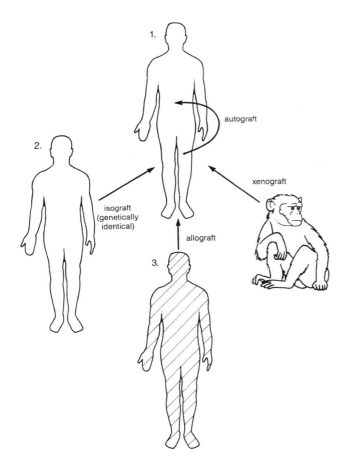

Figure 22.   Types of grafts.

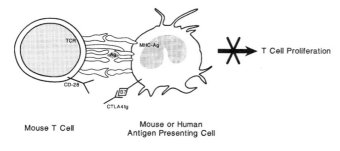

Figure 23.   Induction of tolerance to a xenogenic tissue graft.

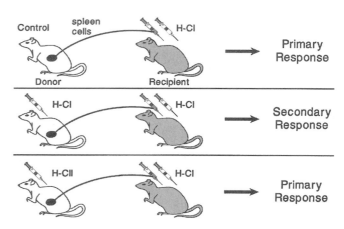

Figure 24.   Adoptive immunity.

A **skin-specific histocompatibility antigen** is a murine skin minor histocompatibility antigen termed Sk that can elicit rejection of skin, but not other tissues following transplantation from one parent into the other parent that has been irradiated and rendered a chimera by the previous injection of F1 spleen cells. The two parents are from different inbred strains of mice. The rate of rejection is relatively slow. Immunologic tolerance of F1 murine spleen cells to the skin epitope of the parent in which they are not in residence is abrogated following residence in the opposite parent.

A **split thickness graft** is a skin graft that is only 0.25 to 0.35 mm thick that consists of epidermis and a small layer of dermis. These grafts vascularize rapidly and last longer than do regular grafts. They are especially useful for skin burns, contaminated skin areas, and sites that are poorly vascularized. Thick split thickness grafts are further resistant to trauma, produce minimal contraction, and permit some amount of sensation, but graft survival is poor.

Pancreatic transplantation (Figure 25) is a treatment for diabetes. Either a whole pancreas or a large segment of it, obtained from cadavers, may be transplanted together with kidneys into the same diabetic patient. It is important for the patient to be clinically stable and for there to be as close a tissue (HLA antigen) match as possible. Graft survival is 50 to 80% at 1 year.

Islet cell transplantation is an experimental method aimed at treatment of type I diabetes mellitus. The technique has been successful in rats but less so in man. It requires sufficient functioning islets from a minimum of two cadaveric donors that have been purified, cultured and shown to produce insulin. The islet cells are administered into the portal vein. The liver serves as the host organ in the recipient who is treated with FK506 or other immunosuppressant drugs.

Bone marrow is soft tissue within bone cavities that contains hematopoietic precursor cells and hematopoietic cells

to a normal (previously nonimmune) syngeneic recipient host.

A **skin graft** uses skin from the same individual (autologous graft) or donor skin that is applied to areas of the body surface that have undergone third degree burns. A patient's keratinocytes may be cultured into confluent sheets that can be applied to the affected areas, although these may not "take" because of the absence of type IV collagen 7 S basement membrane sites for binding and fibrils to anchor the graft.

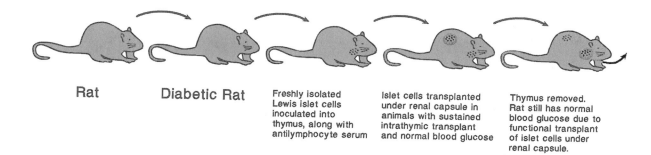

Rat   Diabetic Rat   Freshly isolated   Islet cells transplanted   Thymus removed.
                       Lewis islet cells   under renal capsule in   Rat still has normal
                       inoculated into   animals with sustained   blood glucose due to
                       thymus, along with   intrathymic transplant   functional transplant
                       antilymphocyte serum and normal blood glucose of islet cells under
                                                                      renal capsule.

Figure 25. Protocol for pancreas transplant.

that are maturing into erythrocytes, the five types of leuko-cytes, and thrombocytes. Whereas red marrow is hemopoi-etic and is present in developing bone, ribs, vertebrae, and long bones, some of the red marrow may be replaced by fat and become yellow marrow.

Bone marrow cells are stem cells from which the formed elements of the blood, including erythrocytes, leukocytes, and platelets are derived. B lymphocyte and T lymphocyte precursors are abundant. The B lymphocytes and pluripotent stem cells in bone marrow are important for reconstitution of an irradiated host. Bone marrow transplants are useful in the treatment of aplastic anemia, leukemias, and immuno-deficiencies. Patients may donate their own marrow for sub-sequent bone marrow autotransplantation if they are to receive intense doses of irradiation.

Bone marrow transplantation is a procedure used to treat both nonneoplastic and neoplastic conditions not amenable to other forms of therapy. It has been especially used in cases of aplastic anemia, acute nonlymphocytic leukemia and acute lymphocytic leukemia. 750 ml of bone marrow are removed from the iliac crest of an HLA-matched donor. Following appropriate treatment of the marrow to remove bone spicules, the cell suspension is infused intravenously into an appropriately immunosuppressed recipient who has received whole body irradiation and immunosuppressive drug therapy. Graft-versus-host episodes or acute graft-ver-sus-host disease or chronic graft-versus-host disease may follow bone marrow transplantation in selected subjects. See graft-versus-host disease. The immunosuppressed patients are highly susceptible to opportunistic infections.

Stem cells have two unique biological features that include self renewal and multilineage differentiation potential. In the past, stem cells were divided into two types that include the pluripotential stem cell and the committed stem cell. Pluri-potential stem cells were the progenitors of many different hematopoietic cells, whereas the progeny of committed stem cells were of one cell type. "Committed stem cell" is now termed "progenitor cell." Stem cells arise from yolk sac blood islands and usually are noncycling. They are not mor-phologically recognizable. Cell culture studies have yielded

much information about hematopoietic precursor cells. Hematopoietic stem cells express the progenitor cell antigen CD34, which can be detected using monoclonal antibodies and by flow cytometry.

Hematopoietic stem cell (HSC) transplants are used to reconstitute hematopoietic cell lineages and to treat neoplas-tic diseases. Twenty five percent of allogeneic marrow trans-plants in 1995 where performed using hematopoietic stem cells obtained from unrelated donors. Since only 30% of patients requiring an allogeneic marrow transplant have a sibling that is HLA-genotypically identical, it became nec-essary to identify related or unrelated potential marrow donors. It became apparent that complete HLA compatibility between donor and recipient is not absolutely necessary to reconstitute patients immunologically. Transplantation of unrelated marrow is accompanied by an increased incidence of graft-versus-host disease. Removal of mature T lympho-cytes from marrow grafts decreases the severity of GHVD but often increases the incidence of graft failure and disease relapse. HLA-phenotypically identical marrow transplants among relatives are often successful. HSC transplantation provides a method to reconstitute hematopoietic cell lin-eages with normal cells capable of continuous self-renewal.

The principal complications of HSC transplantation are graft-versus-host disease (GVHD), graft rejection, graft fail-ure, prolonged immunodeficiency, toxicity from radio-che-motherapy given pre-and post-transplantation, and GVHD prophylaxis. Methotrexate and cyclosporin A are given to help prevent acute GVHD. Chronic GVHD may also be a serious complication involving the skin, gut and liver and an associated sicca syndrome. Allogeneic HSC transplanta-tion often involves older individuals and unrelated donors. Thus, blood stem cell transplantation represents an effective method for the treatment of patients with hematologic and non-hematologic malignancies and various types of immu-nodeficiencies. The *in vitro* expansion of a small number of CD34+ cells stimulated by various combinations of cytokines appears to give hematopoietic reconstitution when reinfused after high-dose therapy. Recombinant human hematopoietic growth factors (HGF) (cytokines) may be given to counteract chemotherapy treatment-related myelotoxicity. HGF increase the number of circulating progenitor and stem cells which is important for the support of high-dose therapy in autologous as well as allogeneic HSC transplantation.

A **chimera** (Figure 26) is the presence in an individual of cells of more than one genotype. This can occur rarely under natural circumstances in dizygotic twins, as in cattle, who share a placenta in which the blood circulation has become fused, causing the blood cells of each twin to circulate in the other. More commonly, it refers to humans or other animals who have received a bone marrow transplant that provided a cell population consisting of donor and self cells. Tetraparental chimeras can be produced by experimental manipulation. The name chimera derives from a monster of Greek mythology that had the body of a goat, the head of a lion, and the tail of a serpent.

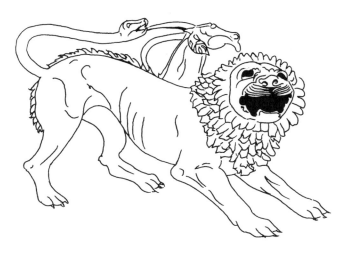

Figure 26.   Chimera.

Corneal transplants (Figure 27) are different from most other transplants in that the cornea is a "privileged site." These sites do not have lymphatic drainage. The rejection rate in corneal transplants depends on vascularization; if vascularization occurs, the cornea becomes accessible to the immune system. HLA incompatibility increases the risk of rejection if the cornea becomes vascularized. The patient can be treated with topical steroids to cause local immunosuppression.

Certain anatomical sites within the animal body provide an immunologically privileged environment which favors the prolonged survival of alien grafts. The potential for development of a blood and lymphatic vascular supply connecting graft and host may be a determining factor in the qualification of an anatomical site as an area which provides an environment favorable to the prolonged survival of a foreign graft. Immunologically privileged sites include (1) the anterior chamber of the eye, (2) the substantia propria of the cornea, (3) the meninges of the brain, (4) the testis, and (5) the cheek pouch of the Syrian hamster. Foreign grafts implanted in these sites show a diminished ability to induce

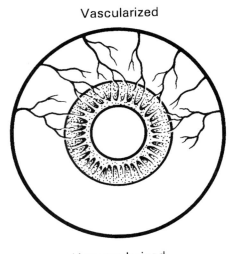

Figure 27.   Corneal transplant.

transplantation immunity in the host. These immunologically privileged sites usually fail to protect alien grafts from the immune refection mechanism in hosts previously or simultaneously sensitized with donor tissues.

The **allogeneic effect** (Figure 28) is the synthesis of antibody by B cells against a hapten in the absence of carrier-specific T cells, provided allogeneic T lymphocytes are present. Interaction of allogeneic T cells with the MHC class II molecules of B cells causes the activated T lymphocytes to produce factors that facilitate B cell differentiation into plasma cells without the requirement for helper T lymphocytes. There is allogeneic activation of T cells in the graft-versus-host reaction.

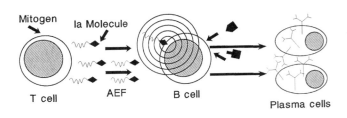

Figure 28.   Allogeneic effect factor.

Allogeneic disease includes the pathologic consequences of immune reactivity of bone marrow allotransplants in immunosuppressed recipient patients as a result of graft-versus-host reactivity in genetically dissimilar members of the same species.

Alloimmunization is defined as an immune response provoked in one member or strain of a species with an alloantigen derived from a different member or strain of the same species. Examples include the immune response in man following transplantation of a solid organ graft such as a kidney or heart from one individual to another. Alloimmunization with red blood cell antigens in humans may lead to pathologic sequelae, such as hemolytic disease of the newborn (erythroblastosis fetalis) in a third Rh(D)⁺ baby born to an Rh(D)⁻ mother.

A **take** is the successful grafting of skin that adheres to the recipient graft site three to five days following application. This is accompanied by neovascularization as indicated by a pink appearance. Thin grafts are more likely to "take" than thicker grafts, but the thin graft must contain some dermis to be successful. The term "take" also refers to an organ allotransplant that has survived hyperacute and chronic rejection.

Graft rejection (Figure 29) is an immunologic destruction of transplanted tissues or organs between two members or strains of a species differing at the major histocompatibility complex for that species (i.e., HLA in man and H-2 in the mouse). The rejection is based upon both cell-mediated and antibody-mediated immunity against cells of the graft by the histoincompatible recipient. First-set rejection usually occurs within two weeks after transplantation. The placement of a second graft with the same antigenic specificity as the first in the same host leads to rejection within one week and is termed second-set rejection. This demonstrates the presence of immunological memory learned from the first experience with the histocompatibility antigens of the graft. When the donor and recipient differ only at minor histocompatibility loci, rejection of the transplanted tissue may be delayed, depending upon the relative strength of the minor loci in which they differ. Grafts placed in a hyperimmune individual, such as those with preformed antibodies, may undergo hyperacute or accelerated rejection. Hyperacute rejection of a kidney allograft by preformed antibodies in the recipient is characterized by formation of fibrin plugs in the vasculature as a consequence of the antibodies reacting against endothelial cells lining vessels, complement fixation, polymorphonuclear neutrophil attraction and denuding of the vessel wall followed by platelet accumulation and fibrin plugging. As the blood supply to the organ is interrupted, the tissue undergoes infarction and must be removed.

White graft rejection is an accelerated rejection of a second skin graft performed within seven to 12 days after rejection of the first graft. It is characterized by lack of vascularization of the graft and its conversion to a white eschar. The characteristic changes are seen by day five after the second grafting procedure. The transplanted tissue is rendered white because of hyperacute rejection, such as a skin or kidney allograft. Preformed antibodies occlude arteries following surgical anastomosis producing infarction of the tissue graft.

Antilymphocyte serum (ALS) or **antilymphocyte globulin (ALG)** is an antiserum prepared by immunizing one species, such as a rabbit or horse, with lymphocytes or thymocytes from a different species such as a human. Antibodies present in the antiserum combine with T cells and other lymphocytes in the circulaiton to induce immunosuppression. ALS is used in organ transplant recipients to suppress graft refection (Figure 30). The globulin fraction known as ALG rather than whole antiserum produces the same immunosuppressive effect.

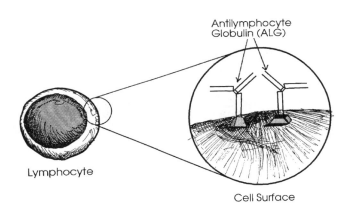

Figure 30.   Antilymphocyte globulin (ALG).

Transplantation rejection (Figure 31) is the consequence of cellular and humoral immune responses to a transplanted organ or tissue that may lead to loss of function and necessitate removal of the transplanted organ or tissue. Transplantation rejection episodes occur in many transplant recipients but are controlled by such immunosuppressive drugs as cyclosporine, rapamycin or FK506 or by monoclonal antibodies against T lymphocytes.

Hyperacute rejection (Figures 32–37) is due to preformed antibodies and is apparent within minutes following transplantation. Antibodies reacting with endothelial cells cause complement to be fixed, which attracts polymorphonuclear neutrophils, resulting in denuding of the endothelial lining of the vascular walls. This causes platelets and fibrin plugs

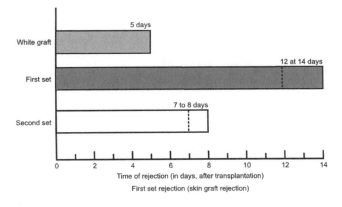

Figure 29.   Types of skin graft rejection.

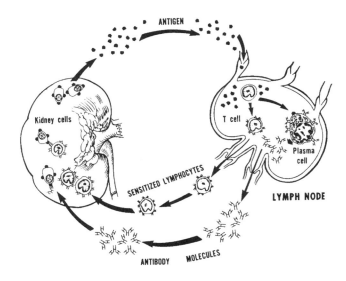

Figure 31. Rejection.

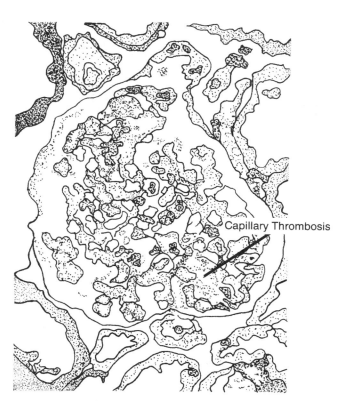

Renal Histology Showing
Hyperacute Graft Rejection

Figure 32. Cartoon of hyperacute graft rejection.

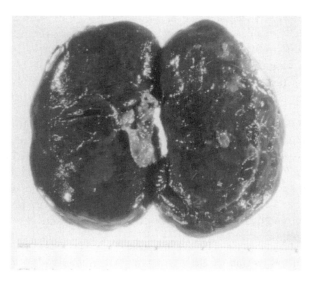

Figure 33. Hyperacute rejection of renal allotransplant showing swelling and purplish discoloration. This is a bivalved transplanted kidney. The allograft was removed within a few hours following transplantation.

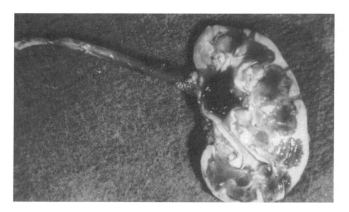

Figure 34. A bivalved transplanted kidney showing hyperacute rejection. There is extensive pale cortical necrosis. This kidney was removed five days after transplantation.

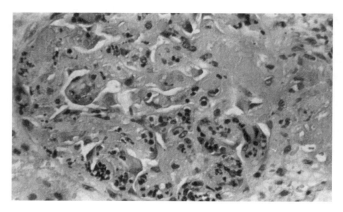

Figure 35. Microscopic view of hyperacute rejection showing a necrotic glomerulus infiltrated with numerous polymorphonuclear leukocytes. H&E stained Section 25X.

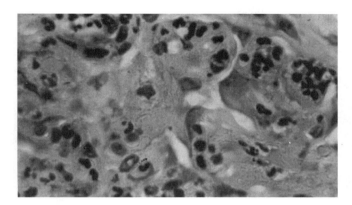

Figure 36. A high power view of the same necrotic glomerulus shown in Figure 35. There are large numbers of polymorphonuclear leukocytes present. Extensive endothelial cells destruction is apparent. H&E stained Section 50X.

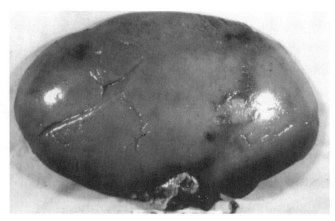

Figure 38. Acute rejection of a renal allograft in which the capsular surface shows several hemorrhagic areas. The kidney is tremendously swollen.

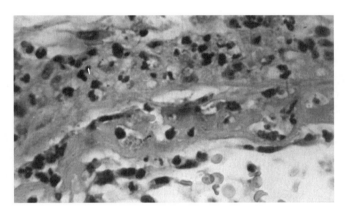

Figure 37. Microscopic view of hyperacute rejection showing necrosis of the wall of a small art arteriole.

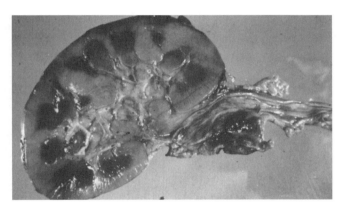

Figure 39. Acute rejection of a bivalved kidney. The cut surface buldges and is variably hemorrhagic and shows fatty degeneration of the cortex.

to block the blood flow to the transplanted organ which becomes cyanotic and must be removed. Only a few drops of bloody urine are usually produced. Segmental thrombosis, necrosis and fibrin thrombi form in the glomerular tufts. There is hemorrhage in the interstitium, mesangial cell swelling, IgG, IgM and C3 may be deposited in arteriole walls.

Acute rejection (Figures 38–44) occurs within days to weeks following transplantation and is characterized by extensive cellular infiltration of the interstitium. These cells are largely mononuclear cells and include plasma cells, lymphocytes, immunoblasts and macrophages as well as some neutrophils. Tubules become separated, and the tubular epithelium undergoes necrosis. Endothelial cells are swollen and vacuolated. There is vascular edema, bleeding with inflammation, renal tubular necrosis and sclerosed glomeruli.

Chronic rejection (Figures 45–47) occurs after more than 60 days following transplantation and may be characterized by structural changes such as interstitial fibrosis, sclerosed

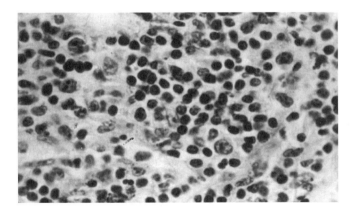

Figure 40. Microscopic view of the interstitium revealing predominantly cellular acute rejection. There is an infiltrate of variably sized lymphocytes. There is also an infiltrate of eosinophils.

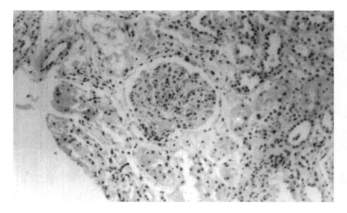

Figure 41.   Microscopic view of acute rejection showing interstitial edema. Mild lymphocytic infiltrate. In the glomerulus, there is also evidence of predominantly vast rejection with a thrombus at the vascular pole.

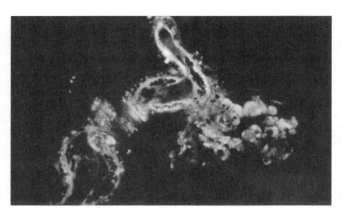

Figure 44.   Immunofluorescence preparation showing humoral rejection with high intensity fluorescence of arteriolar walls and of some glomerular capillary walls. This pattern is demonstrable in anti-immunoglobulin and anti-complement stained sections.

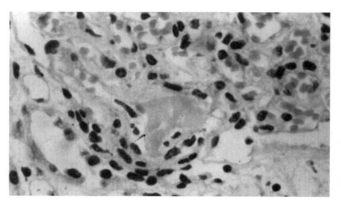

Figure 42.   A higher magnification of the thrombus at the hilus of the glomerulus.

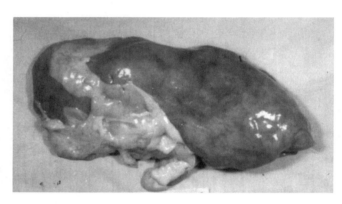

Figure 45.   Renal allotransplant showing chronic rejection. The kidney is shrunken and malformed.

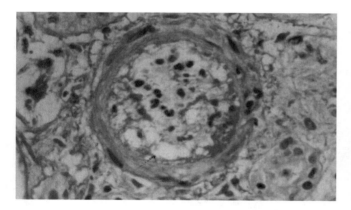

Figure 43.   A trichrome stain of a small interlobular artery showing predominantly humoral rejection. There is tremendous swelling of the intima and endothelium with some fibrin deposition and a few polymorphonuclear leukocytes.

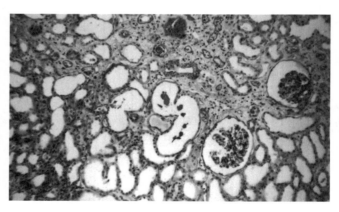

Figure 46.   Microscopic view of chronic rejection showing tubular epithelial atrophy wit interstitial fibrosis and shrinkage of glomerular capillary tufts.

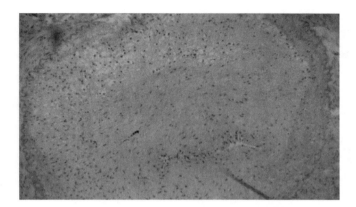

Figure 47. The wall of an artery and chronic rejection. There is obliteration of the vascular lumen with fibrous tissue. Only a slit-like lumen remains.

glomeruli, mesangial proliferative glomerulonephritis, crescent formation and various other changes.

Graft-versus-host reaction (GVHR) is the reaction of a graft containing immunocompetent cells against the genetically dissimilar tissues of an immunosuppressed recipient. Criteria requisite for a GVHR include: (1) histoincompatibility between the donor and recipient; (2) passively transferred immunologically reactive cells; (3) a recipient host who has been either naturally immunosuppressed because of immaturity or genetic defect or deliberately immunosuppressed by irradiation or drugs. The immunocompetent grafted cells are especially reactive against rapidly dividing cells. Target organs include the skin, gastrointestinal tract (including the gastric mucosa) and liver, as well as the lymphoid tissues. Patients often develop skin rashes and hepatosplenomegaly and may have aplasia of the bone marrow. GVH reaction usually develops within 7–30 days following the transplant or infusion of the lymphocytes. Prevention of the GVH reaction is an important procedural step in several forms of transplantation and may be accomplished by irradiating the transplant. The clinical course of GVH reaction may take a hyperacute, acute or chronic form as seen in graft rejection.

Graft-versus-host disease (GVHD) is a disease produced by the reaction of immunocompetent T lymphocytes of the donor graft that are histoincompatible with the tissues of the recipient into which they have been transplanted. For the disease to occur, the recipient must be either immunologically immature, immunosuppressed by irradiation or drug therapy or tolerant to the administered cells and the grafted cells must also be immunocompetent. Patients develop skin rash, fever, diarrhea, weight loss, hepatosplenomegaly and aplasia of the bone marrow. The donor lymphocytes infiltrate the skin, gastrointestinal tract and liver. The disease may be either acute or chronic. Murine GVH disease is called "runt disease," "secondary disease" or wasting disease. Both allo- and autoimmunity associated with GVHD may follow bone marrow transplantation.

20–50% of patients receiving HLA-identical bone marrow transplants still manifest GVHD with associated weight loss, skin rash, fever, diarrhea, liver disease and immunodeficiency. GVHD may be either acute, which is an alloimmune disease, or chronic, which consists of both allo- and autoimmune components. The conditions requisite for the GVH reaction include genetic differences between immunocompetent cells in the marrow graft and host tissues, immunoincompetence of the host and alloimmune differences that promote proliferation of donor cells that react with host tissues. In addition to allogenic marrow grafts, the transfusion of unirradiated blood products to an immunosuppressed patient or intrauterine transfusion from mother to fetus may lead to GVHD.

The **Simonsen phenomenon** is a graft-versus-host reaction in chick embryos that have developed splenomegaly following inoculation of immunologically competent lymphoid cells from adult chickens. Splenic lymphocytes are increased and represent a mixture of both donor and host lymphocytes.

Acute graft-versus-host reaction is the immunopathogenesis of acute GVHD consists of recognition, recruitment and effector phases. Epithelia of the skin (Figures 48–52), gastrointestinal tract (Figures 53–57), small intrahepatic biliary

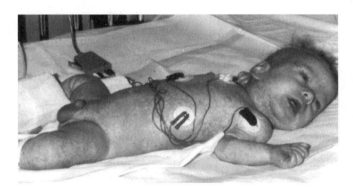

Figure 48. A diffuse erythematous to morbilliform rash in a child with acute graft vs. host disease (GVHD).

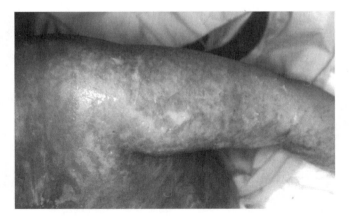

Figure 49. Diffuse erythematous skin rash in a patient with acute graft-versus-host reaction.

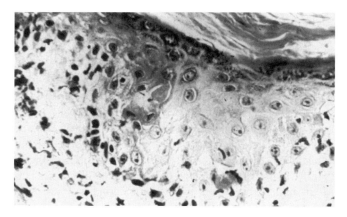

Figure 50. Histologically, there is an intense interface dermatitis with destruction of basilar cells particularly at the tips of the rete ridges, incontinence of melanin pigment and necrosis of individual epithelial cells, referred to as apoptosis.

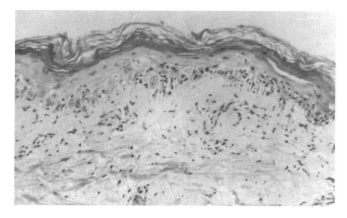

Figure 51. Histological appearance of the skin in graft-versus-host disease with disruption of the basal cell layer, hyperkeratosis and beginning sclerotic changes.

Figure 52. Papulosquamous rash in graft-versus-host disease.

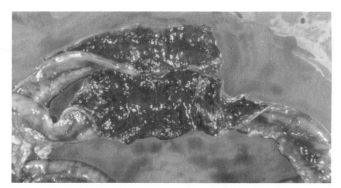

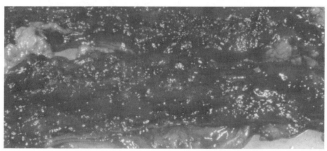

Figure 53–54. Gastrointestinal graft vs. host disease in which there is a diffuse process that usually involves the ileum and cecum most severely resulting in secretory diarrhea. Grossly there is diffuse erythema, granularity and loss of folds and when severe there is undermining and sloughing of the entire mucosa leading to fibrinopurulent clots of necrotic material. Sometimes there is frank obstruction in patients with intractable-graft-versus host disease.

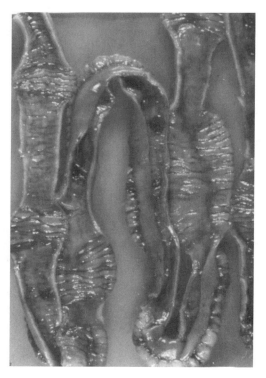

Figure 55. Stenotic and fibrotic segments alternating with more normal appearing dilated segments of gut in graft-versus-host disease.

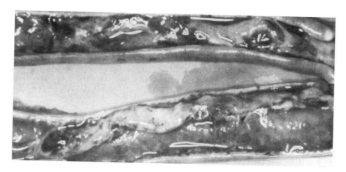

Figure 56. Sloughing of the mucosal lining of the gut in graft-versus-host disease.

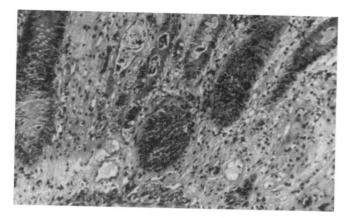

Figure 57. Histologically, graft-versus-host disease in the gut begins as a patchy destructive enteritis localized to the lower third of the crypt of Lieberkuhn.

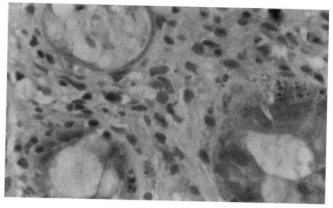

Figure 58. The earliest lesions are characterized by individual enterocyte necrosis with karyorrhectic nuclear debris, the so-called exploding crypt which progresses to a completely destroyed crypt as shown in the upper left hand corner.

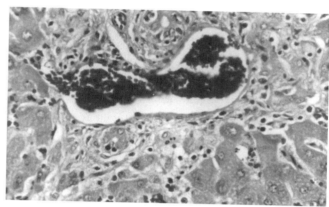

Figure 59. Hepatic graft-versus-host disease is characterized by a cholestatic hepatitis with characteristic injury and destruction of small bile ducts that resemble changes seen in rejection. In this section of early acute GVHD, there are mild portal infiltrates with striking exocytosis into bile ducts associated with individual cell necrosis and focal destruction of the bile ducts.

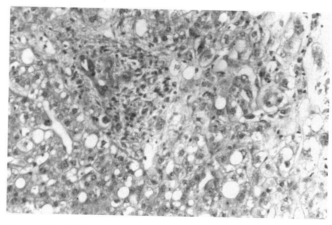

Figure 60. This liver section from a patient with GVHD demonstrates the cholestatic changes that evolve from hepatocellular ballooning to cholangiolar cholestasis with bile microliths, which signifies prolonged GVHD.

ducts and liver (Figures 58–60), and the lymphoid system constitute primary targets of acute GVHD. GVHD development may differ in severity based on relative antigenic differences between donor and host and the reactivity of donor lymphocytes against non-HLA antigens of recipient tissues. The incidence and severity of GVHD has been ascribed also to HLA-B alleles, i.e., an increased GVHD incidence associated with HLA-B8 and HLA-B35. Epithelial tissues serving as targets of GVHD include keratinocytes, erythrocytes, and bile ducts which may express Ia antigens following exposure to endogeneous interferon produced by T lymphocytes. When Ia antigens are expressed on nonlymphoid cells, they may become antigen-presenting cells for autologous antigens and aid perpetuation of autoimmunity.

Cytotoxic T lymphocytes mediate acute GVHD. Whereas most immunohistological investigations have implicated CD8+ (cytotoxic/suppressor) lymphocytes, others have identified CD4+ (T helper lymphocytes) in human GVHD. NK cells have been revealed as effectors of murine but not human GVHD. Following interaction between effector and target cells, cytotoxic granules from cytotoxic T or NK cells are distributed over the target cell membrane, leading to perforin-induced large pores across the membrane and nuclear lysis by deoxyribonuclease. Infection, rather than failure of the primary target organ (other than gastrointestinal bleeding), is the major cause of mortality in acute GVHD. Within the first few months post-transplant, all recipients demonstrate diminished immunoglobulin synthesis, decreased T helper lymphocytes and increased T suppressor cells. Acute GVHD patients manifest an impaired ability to combat viral infections. They demonstrate an increased risk of cytomegalovirus (CMV) infection, especially CMV interstitial pneumonia. GVHD may also reactivate such other viral diseases as herpes simplex.

Immunodeficiency in the form of acquired B cell lymphoproliferative disorder (BCLD) represents another serious complication of post-bone marrow transplantation. Bone marrow transplants treated with pan-T cell monoclonal antibody or those in which T lymphocytes have been depleted account for most cases of BCLD, which is associated with severe GVHD. All transformed B cells in cases of BCLD have manifested the Epstein Barr viral genome.

Chronic graft-versus-host disease (GVHD) may occur in as many as 45% of long-term bone marrow transplant recipients. Chronic GVHD (Figure 61) differs both clinically and histologically from acute GVHD and resembles autoimmune connective tissue diseases. For example, chronic GVHD patients may manifest skin lesions resembling scleroderma, sicca syndrome in the eyes and mouth, inflammation of the oral, esophageal and vaginal mucosa, bronchiolitis obliterans, occasionally myasthenia gravis, polymyositis and autoantibody synthesis. Histopathologic alterations in chronic GVHD, such as chronic inflammation and fibrotic changes in involved organs, resemble changes associated with naturally occurring autoimmune disease. The skin may reveal early inflammation with subsequent fibrotic changes.

Infiltration of lacrimal, salivary and submucosal glands by lymphoplasmacytic cells leads ultimately to fibrosis. The resulting sicca syndrome, which resembles Sjögren's syndrome, occurs in 80% of chronic GVHD patients. Drying of mucous membranes in the sicca syndrome affects the mouth, esophagus, conjunctiva, urethra and vagina. The pathogenesis of chronic GVHD involves the interaction of alloimmunity, immune dysregulation and resulting immunodeficiency and autoimmunity. The increased incidence of infection among chronic GVHD patients suggests immunodeficiency. The dermal fibrosis is associated with increased numbers of activated fibroblasts in the papillary dermis. T lymphocyte or mast cell cytokines may activate this fibroplasia that leads to dermal fibrosis in chronic GVHD.

Venoocclusive disease (VOD) is a serious liver complication after marrow transplantation (Figure 62). Histopathology of early VOD reveals concentric subendothelial widening and sublobular central venules with degeneration of surrounding pericentral hepatocytes. At this early stage, there is deposition of fibrin and Factor VIII. Late lesions of VOD show fibrous obliteration of the central venule and the sinusoids by combinations of type 3, 1 and even type 4 collagen. The clinical diagnosis of VOD is reasonably accurate based on the combination of jaundice, ascites, hepatomegaly and encephalopahty in the first two weeks posttransplant. The incidence may be higher among older patients with a diagnosis of AML or CML and with hepatitis. The mortality rate of VOD is relatively high at 32%.

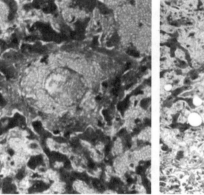
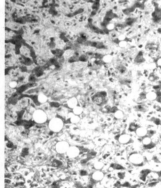

Figure 62. Venocclusive disease (VOD) accompanying graft-versus-host disease of the liver. On the left is early VOD with concentric subendothelial widening and sublobular central venules with degeneration of surrounding pericentral hepatocytes. There is deposition of fibrin and Factor VIII. On the right is a late lesion of VOD showing fibrous obliteration of the central venule and the sinusoids by combination of types 3, 1 and even type 4 collagen.

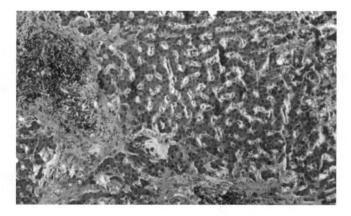

Figure 61. Chronic GVHD of the liver with pronounced inflammation and portal fibrosis with disappearance of bile ducts.

21
Tumor Immunology

Biologists have long been fascinated with possible differences between neoplastic cells (Figures 1–3) and their so-called normal counterparts or tissues of origin. This led to the search for antigens on tumors that are absent from normal tissues. The aim of finding such immunologic differences would be both for cancer testing and for cancer treatment purposes. This search has met with varying degrees of success.

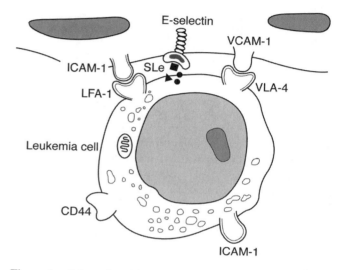

Figure 2. Schematic representation of a leukemia cell attached to an endothelial cell surface *via* adhesion molecules.

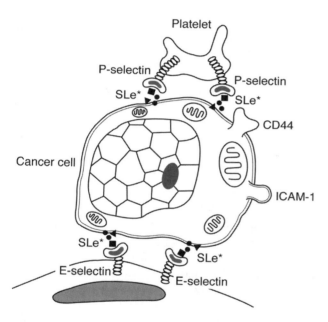

Figure 1. Schematic representation of a tumor cell attached through E-selectin molecules to an endothelial cell surface.

Modification of proteins by phosphorylation or specific proteolysis may change their covalent architecture to yield a new antigenic determinant or epitope which is called a **neoantigen**. The epitope is newly expressed on cells during development or in neoplasia. Neoantigens include tumor-associated antigens. New antigenic derterminants may also emerge when a protein changes confirmations or when a molecule is split, exposing previously unexpressed epitopes.

Tumor-associated antigens (Figure 4) are antigens designated as CA-125, CA-19-9 and CA195, among others, that may be linked to certain tumors such as lymphomas, carcinomas, sarcomas, and melanomas, but the immune response to these tumor-associated antigens is not sufficient to mount

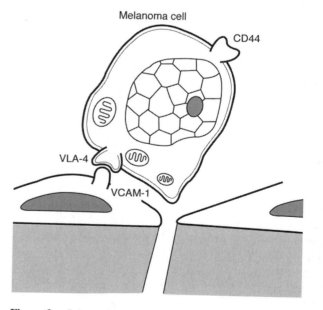

Figure 3. Schematic representation of a melanoma cell attached to an endothelial cell surface VLA-4-VCAM-1 interaction.

375

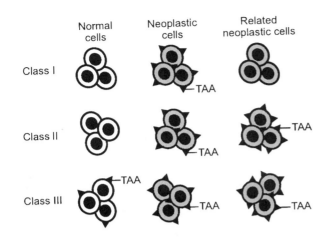

Figure 4. Schematic representation of tumor-associated antigens (TAA) among normal and neoplastic cells.

a successful cellular or humoral immune response against the neoplasm. Three classes of tumor-associated antigens have been described. Class I antigens are very specific for a certain neoplasm and are absent from normal cells. Class II antigens are found on related neoplasms from separate individuals. Class III antigens are found on malignant as well as normal cells but show increased expression in the neoplastic cells. Assays of clinical value will probably be developed for class II antigens, since they are associated with multiple neoplasms and very infrequently found in normal individuals.

Thymic-leukemia antigen (TL) is an epitope on the thymocyte membrane of TL+ mice. As the T lymphocytes mature, this antigen disappears but resurfaces if leukemia develops. TL antigens are specific and are normally present on the cell surface of thymocytes of certain mouse strains. They are encoded by a group of structural genes located at the Tla locus, in the linkage group IX, very close to the D pole of the H-2 locus on chromosome 17. There are three structural TL genes, one of which has two alleles. The TL antigens are numbered from 1 to 4 specifying four antigens: TL.1, TL.2, TL.3 and TL.4. TL.3 and TL.4 are mutually exclusive. Their expression is under the control of regulatory genes, apparently located at the same Tla locus. Normal mouse thymocytes belong to three phenotypic groups: Tl⁻, T1.2, and TL.1,2,3. Development of leukemia in the mouse induces a restructuring of the TL surface antigens of thymocytes with expression of TL.1 and TL.2 in TL⁻ cells, expression of TL.1 in TL.2 cells, and expression of TL.4 in both TL⁻ and TL.2 cells. When normal thymic cells leave the thymus, the expression of TL antigen ceases. Thus thymocytes are TL⁺ (except the TL⁻ strains) and the peripheral T cells are TL⁻. In transplantation experiments TL⁺ tumor cells undergo antigenic modulation. Tumor cells exposed to the homologous antibody, stop expressing the antigen, and

thus escape lysis when subsequently exposed to the same antibody plus complement.

CD10 (CALLA) is an antigen that has a mol wt of 100 kD. CD10 is now known to be a neutral endopetidase (enkaphalinase). It is present on many cell types, including stem cells, lymphoid progenitors of B and T cells, renal epithelium, fibroblasts, and bile canliculi.

Prostate specific antigen (PSA) is a marker in serum or tissue sections for adenocarcinoma of the prostate. PSA is a 34 kD glycoprotein found exclusively in benign and malignant epithelium of the prostate. Normal levels of PSA in males should be less than 4 ng/ml. The PSA molecule is smaller than prostatic acid phosphatase (PAP). In patients with prostate cancer, preoperative PSA serum levels are positively correlated with the disease. PSA is more stable and shows less diurnal variation than does prostatic acid phosphatase (PAP). PSA is increased in 95% of new cases of prostatic carcinoma compared with 60% for PAP. It is increased in 97% of recurrent cases compared with 66% for PAP. PSA may also be increased in selected cases of benign prostatic hypertrophy and prostatitis, but these elevations are less than those associated with adenocarcinoma of the prostate. It is inappropriate to use either PSA or PAP alone as a screen for asymptomatic males. TUR, urethral instrumentation, prostatic needle biopsy, prostatic infarct or urinary retention may also result in increased PSA values. PSA is critical for the prediction of recurrent adenocarcinoma in postsurgical patients. PSA is also a useful immunocytochemical marker for primary and metastatic adenocarcinoma of the prostate.

Oncofetal antigens (Figure 5) are markers or epitopes present in fetal tissues during development but not present, or found in minute quantities, in adult tissues. These cell-coded antigens may reappear in certain neoplasms of adults due to derepression of the gene responsible for their formation. Examples include carcinoembryonic antigen (CEA) which is found in the liver, intestine, and pancreas of the fetus but also in both malignant and benign gastrointestinal conditions. Yet it is still useful to detect recurrence of adenocarcinoma of the colon based upon demonstration of CEA in the patient's serum; α-fetoprotein (AFP) is demonstrable in approximately 70% of hepatocellular carcinomas.

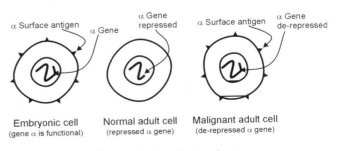

Figure 5. Oncofetal antigen.

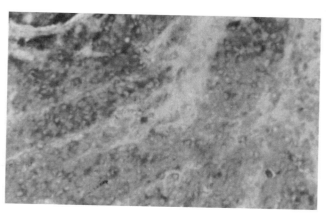

Figure 6. Carcinoembryonic antigen (CEA).

Carcinoembryonic antigen (CEA) (Figure 6) is a 200kD membrane glycoprotein epitope that is present in the fetal gastrointestinal tract in normal conditions. However, tumor cells, such as those in colon carcinoma may reexpress it. CEA was first described as a screen for identifying carcinoma by detecting nanogram quantities of the antigen in serum. It was later shown to be present in certain other conditions as well. CEA levels are elevated in almost one-third of patients with colorectal, liver, pancreatic, lung, breast, head and neck, cervical, bladder, medullarythyroid and prostatic carcinoma. However, the level may be elevated also in malignant melanoma, lymphoproliferative disease, and in smokers. Regrettably, CEA levels also increase in a variety of non-neoplastic disorders including inflammatory bowel disease, pancreatitis, and cirrhosis of the liver. Nevertheless, determination of CEA levels in the serum is valuable for monitoring the recurrence of tumors in patients whose primary neoplasm has been removed. If the patient's CEA level reveals a 35% elevation compared to the level immediately following surgery, this may signify metastases. This oncofetal antigen is comprised of one polypeptide chain with one variable region at the amino terminus and six constant region domains. CEA belongs to the immunoglobulin superfamily. It lacks specificity for cancer, thereby limiting its diagnostic usefulness.

SV-40 (simian virus 40) (Figures 7 and 8) is an oncogenic polyoma virus. It multiplies in cultures of rhesus monkey kidney and produces cytopathic alterations in African green monkey cell cultures. Inoculation into newborn hamsters leads to the development of sarcomas. SV40 has 5243 base pairs in its genome. It may follow either of two patterns of lifecycle according to the host cell. In permissive cells, such as those from African green monkeys, the virus infected cells are lysed,

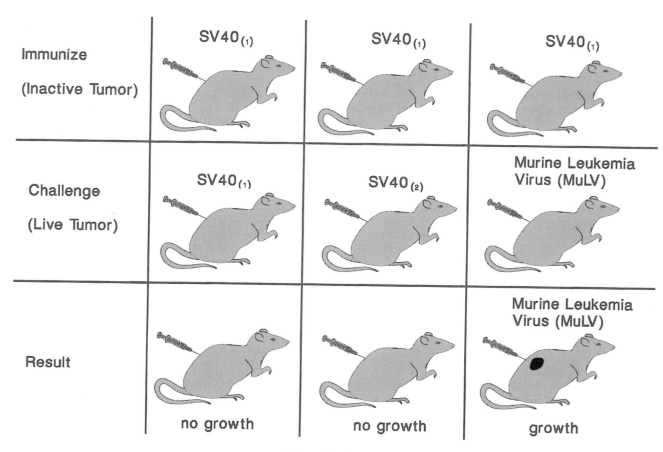

Figure 7. SV-40.

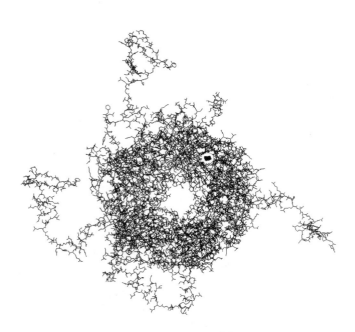

Figure 8.   SV-40. Resolution.3.1 angstroms.

causing the escape of multiple viral particles. Lysis does not occur in nonpermissive cells infected with the virus. By contrast, they may undergo oncogenic transformation in which SV40 DNA sequences become integrated into the genome of the host cell. Cells that have become transformed have characteristic morphological features and growth properties. SV40 may serve as a cloning vector. It is a diminutive icosahedral papovavirus that contains double-stranded DNA. It may induce progressive mulitfocal leukoencephalopathy. It is useful for the *in vitro* transformation of cells as a type of "permissive" infection ultimately resulting in lysis of infected host cells.

Oncogenic virus (Figure 9) is any virus, whether DNA or RNA, that can induce malignant transformation of cells. An example of a DNA virus would be human papillomavirus and an RNA virus would be retrovirus.

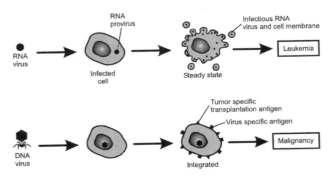

Figure 9.   Oncogenic virus.

α-Fetoprotein (Figure 10) is a principal plasma protein in the α globular fraction present in the fetus. It bears considerable homology with human serum albumin. It is produced by the embryonic yolk sac and fetal liver and consists of a 590 amino acid residue polypeptide chain structure. It may be elevated in pregnant women bearing fetuses with open neural tube defects, central nervous system defects, gastrointestinal abnormalities, immunodeficiency syndromes and various other abnormalities. After parturition, the high levels in fetal serum diminish to levels that cannot be detected. α-fetoprotein induces immunosuppression which may facilitate neonatal tolerance. Based on *in vitro* studies, it is believed to facilitate suppressor T lymphocyte function and diminish helper T lymphocyte action. Liver cancer patients reveal significantly elevated serum levels of α-fetoprotein. It is used as a marker of selected tumors such as hepatocellular carcinoma. It is detected by the ABC immunoperoxidase technique using monoclonal antibodies.

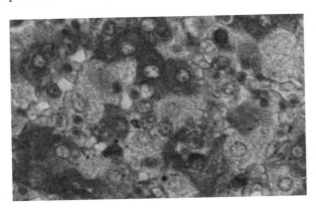

Figure 10.   α-Fetoprotein.

The **melanoma antigen-1 gene (*MAGE-1*)** in humans was derived from a malignant melanoma cell line. It encodes for an epitope that a cytotoxic T lymphocyte clone specific for melanoma recognizes. This clone was isolated from a patient bearing melanoma. MAGE-1 protein is found on one-half of all melanomas and one-fourth of all breast carcinomas, but it is not expressed on the majority of normal tissues. Even though MAGE-1 has not been shown to induce tumor rejection, cytotoxic T lymphocytes in melanoma patients manifest specific memory for MAGE-1 protein.

Tumor cells may be subject to alterations in antigenic structure. **Antigenic transformation** refers to changes in a cell's antigenic profile as a consequence of antigenic gain, deletion, reversion or other process. **Antigenic gain** refers to non-distinctive normal tissue components that are added or increased without simultaneous deletion of other normal tissue constituents. **Antigenic deletion** describes antigenic determinants that have been lost or masked in progeny of cells that usually contain them. Antigenic deletion may take place as a consequence of neoplastic transformation or mutation of parent cells resulting in disappearance or repression

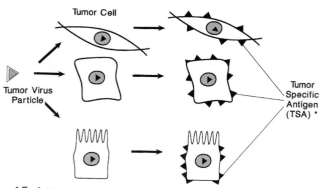

* Each tumor induced by a single virus will express the same TSA on the cell surface despite the morphology of the cell

Figure 11.   Tumor specific antigens (TSA).

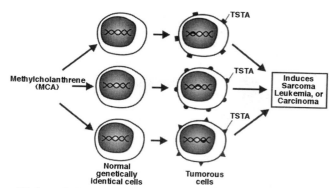

* Each genetically identical cell develops unique antigenic specificity to MCA.

Figure 12.   Tumor specific transplantation antigens (TSTA).

of the parent cell genes. **Antigenic modulation** is the loss of epitopes or antigenic determinants from a cell surface following combination with antibody. The antibodies either cause the epitope to disappear or become camouflaged by covering it. **Antigenic diversion** refers to replacement of a cell's antigenic profile by the antigens of a different normal tissue cell. Antigenic reversion is a change in antigenic profile characteristic of an adult cell to an antigenic mosaic that previously existed in the immature or fetal cell stage of the species. **Antigenic reversion** may accompany neoplastic transformation.

Tumor cells express **tumor-specific determinants** or epitopes that are identifiable also in varying quantities and forms on normal cells. **Tumor-specific antigens (TSA)**

(Figure 11) are present on tumor cells but not found on normal cells. Murine tumor-specific antigens can induce transplantation rejection in mice. **Tumor-specific transplantation antigens (TSTA)** (Figure 12) are epitopes that induce rejection of tumors transplanted among syngeneic (histocompatible) animals.

Macrophages (Figures 13 and 14) are mononuclear phagocytic cells derived from monocytes in the blood that were produced from stem cells in the bone marrow. These cells have a powerful, although nonspecific role in immune defense. These intensely phagocytic cells contain lysosomes and exert microbicidal action against microbes which they ingest. They also have effective tumoricidal activity. They may take up and degrade both protein and polysaccharide

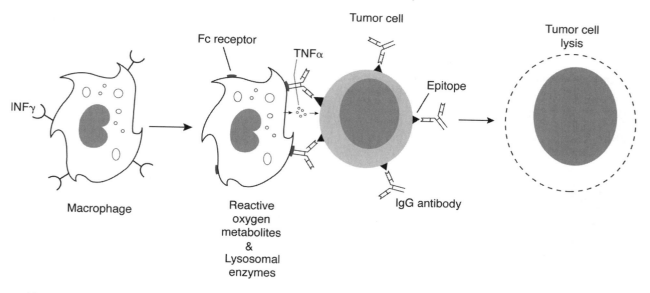

Figure 13.   Macrophage-mediated tumor cell lysis is mediated by several mechanisms. Activated macrophages express Fcγ receptors that anchor IgG molecules attached to tumor cells, but not normal cells, resulting in the release of lysosomal enzymes and reactive oxygen metabolites that lead to tumor cell lysis. Another mechanism of macrophage-mediated lysis includes the release of the cytokine tumor necrosis factor α that may unite with high affinity TNFα receptors on a tumor cell surface resulting in its lysis, or the effect of TNFα on the small blood vessels and capillaries of vascularized tumors leading to hemorrhagic necrosis producing a localized Shwartzman-like reaction.

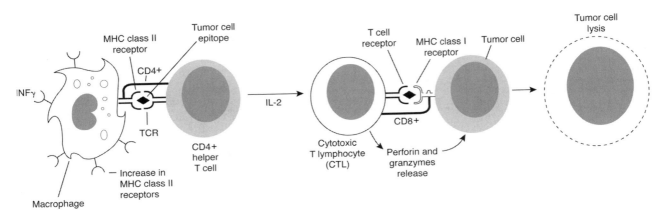

Figure 14. Macrophage-mediated tumor immunity.

antigens and present them to T lymphocytes in the context of major histocompatibility complex class II molecules. They interact with both T and B lymphocytes in immune reactions. They are freqenty found in areas of epithelium, mesothelium and blood vessels. Macrophages have been referred to as adherent cells since they readily adhere to glass and plastic and may spread on these surfaces and manifest chemotaxis. They have receptors for Fc and C3b on their surfaces, stain positively for non-specific esterase and peroxidase, and are Ia antigen positive when acting as accessory cells that present antigen to CD4+ lymphocytes in the generation of an immune response. Monocytes, which may differentiate into macrophages when they migrate into the tissues, make up 3–5% of leukocytes in the peripheral blood. Macrophages that are tissue-bound may be found in the lung alveoli, as microglial cells in the central nervous system, as Kuppfer cells in the liver, as Langerhans cells in the skin, as histiocytes in connective tissues, as well as macrophages in lymph nodes and peritoneum. Multiple substances are secreted by macrophages, including complement components C1 through C5, factors B and D, properdin, C3b inactivators and β1H. They also produce monokines such as

interleukin 1, acid hydrolase, proteases, lipases and numerous other substances.

Natural killer (NK) cells (Figures 15 and 16) attack and destroy certain virus-infected cells. They constitute an important part of the natural immune system, do not require prior contact with antigen, and are not MHC restricted by the major histocompatibility complex (MHC) antigens. NK cells are lymphoid cells of the natural immune system that express cytotoxicity against various nucleated cells including tumor cells and virus-infected cells. NK cells, killer (K) cells or antibody-dependent cell-mediated cytotoxicity (ADCC) cells induce lysis through the action of antibody. Immunologic memory is not involved as previous contact with antigen is not necessary for NK cell activity. The NK cell is approximately 15μm in diameter and has a kidney shaped nucleus with several, often three, large cytoplasmic granules. The cells are also called large granular lymphocytes (LGL). In addition to the ability to kill selected tumor cells and some virus-infected cells, they also participate in antibody-dependent cell-mediated cytotoxicity (ADCC) by anchoring antibody to the cell surface through an Fc γ receptor.

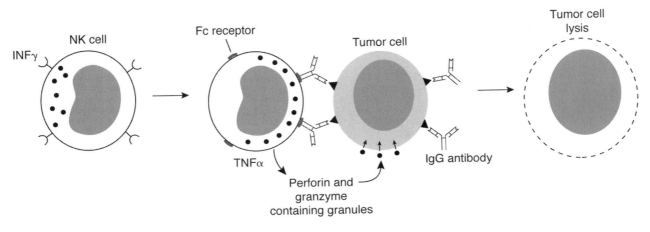

Figure 15. NK-cell mediated killing of tumor cells by antibody-dependent cell-mediated cytotoxicity.

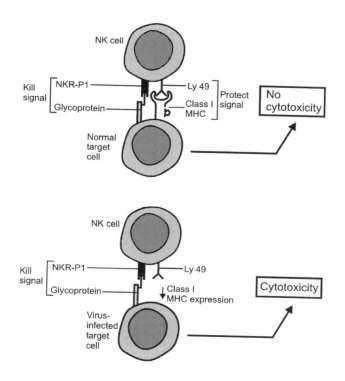

Figure 16. Proposed mechanism of NK cell cytotoxicity restricted to altered self cells. Kill signal is generated when the NK cell's NKR-PI receptor interacts with membrane glycoprotein of normal and altered self cells. The kill signal can be contermanded by interaction of the NK cells Ly49 receptor with class I MHC molecules. Thus, MHC Class I expression prevents NK cell killing of normal cells. Diminished Class I expression on altered self cells leads to their destruction.

Thus, they are able to destroy antibody coated nucleated cells. NK cells are believed to represent a significant part of the natural immune defense against spontaneously developing neoplastic cells and against infection by viruses. NK cell activity is measured by a ^{51}Cr release assay employing the K562 erythroleukemia cell line as a target.

Cytotoxic T lymphocytes (CTL) (Figure 17 and 18) are specifically sensitized T lymphocytes that are usually CD8+ and recognize antigens, through the T cell receptor, on cells of the host infected by viruses or that have become neoplastic. CD8+ cell recognition of the target is in the context of MHC class I histocompatibility molecules. Following recognition and binding, death of the target cell occurs a few hours later. CTLs secrete lymphokines that attract other lymphocytes to the area, release serine proteases and perforins that produce ion channels in the membrane of the target leading to cell lysis. Interleukin-2, produced by CD4+ T cells activates cytotoxic T cell precursors. Interferon-γ generated from CTLs activates macrophages. CTLs have a significant role in the rejection of allografts and in tumor immunity. A minor population of CD4+ lymphocytes may also be cytotoxic, but they recognize target cell antigens in the context of MHC class II molecules.

Tumor-specific IgG antibodies may act in concert with immune system cells to produce anti-tumor effects. **Antibody-dependent cell-mediated cyotoxicity (ADCC)** (Figure 19) is a reaction in which T lymphocytes, NK cells, including large granular lymphocytes, neutrophils and macrophages may lyse tumor cells, infectious agents and allogeneic cells by combining through their Fc receptors with the Fc region of IgG antibodies bound through their Fab regions to target cell surface antigens. Following linkage of Fc receptors with Fc regions, destruction of the target is accomplished through released cytokines. It represents an example of participation between antibody molecules and immune system cells to produce an effector function.

Heteroconjugate antibodies (Figure 20) are antibodies against a tumor antigen coupled covalently to an antibody specific for a natural killer cell or cytotoxic T lymphocyte surface antigen. These antibodies facilitate binding of cytotoxic effector cells or tumor target cells. Antibodies against

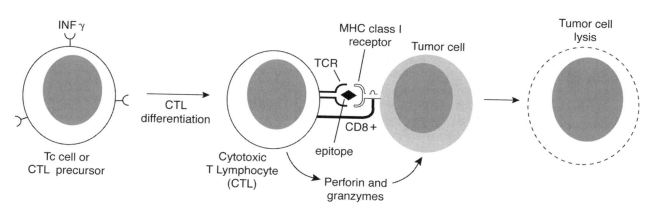

Figure 17. Cytotoxic T lymphocyte (CTL) mediated tumor lysis.

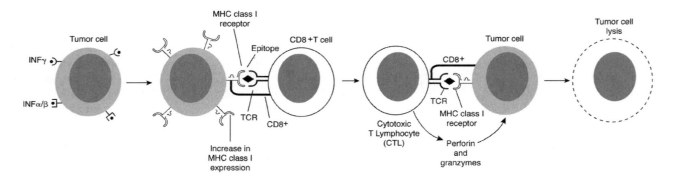

Figure 18.   CTL-mediated killing of tumor cells.

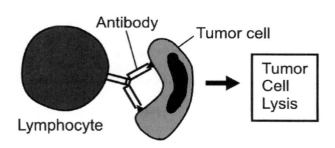

Figure 19.   ADCC.

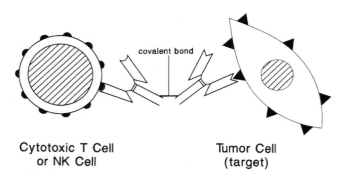

Figure 20.   Heteroconjugate antibodies.

effector cell surface markers may also be coupled covalently with hormones that bind to receptors on tumor cells.

Immunosurveillance refers to the monitoring function by cells of the immune system in recognizing, reacting against and fatally injuring aberrant cells that arise by somatic mutation and express new antigens (neoantiens) e.g., neoplastic cells. Immunosurveillance is believed to be mediated by the cellular limb of the immune response. Indirect evidence in support of the concept includes: (1) an increased incidence of tumors in aged individuals who have decreased immune competence; (2) increased tumor incidence in children with T cell immunodeficiencies; and (3) the development of neoplasms (lymphomas) in a significant number of organ or bone marrow transplant recipients who have been deliberately immunosuppressed.

Immunologic enhancement (tumor enhancement) (Figure 21) describes the prolonged survival, conversely the delayed rejection, of a tumor allograft in a host as a consequence of contact with specific antibody. Anti-tumor antibodies may have a paradoxical effect. Instead of eradicating a neoplasm, they may facilitate its survival and progressive growth in the host. Both the peripheral and central mechanisms have been postulated. Coating of tumor cells with antibody was presumed, in the past, to interfere with the ability of specifically reactive lymphocytes to destroy them, but a central effect in suppressing cell-mediated immunity, perhaps through suppressor T lymphocytes is also possible. Enhancing antibodies are blocking antibodies that favor survival of tumor or normal tissue allografts.

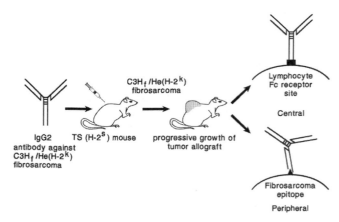

Figure 21.   Immunologic enhancement (tumor enhancement).

Immunotherapy employs immunologic mechanisms to combat disease. These include nonspecific stimulation of the immune response with BCG immunotherapy in treating certain types of cancer, and the IL-2/LAK cell adoptive immunotherapy technique for treating selected tumors.

Biological response modifiers (BRM) are a wide spectrum of molecules that alter the immune response. They include such substances as interleukins, interferons, hematopoietic colony-stimulating factors, tumor necrosis factor, B lymphocyte growth and differentiating factors, lymphotoxins, macrophage activating and chemotactic factors as well as macrophage inhibitory factor, eosinophil chemotactic factor, osteoclast activating factor, etc. BRM may modulate the immune system of the host to augment anti-tumor defense mechanisms. Some have been produced by recombinant DNA technology and are available commercially. An example is "-interferon used in the therapy of hairy cell leukemia.

Interferfon α is an immunomodulatory 189-amino acid residue glycoprotein synthesized by macrophages and B cells that are able to prevent the replication of viruses, are antiproliferative, and are pyrogenic, inducing fever. IFN-α stimulates natural killer cells and induces expression of class I MHC antigens. It also has an immunoregulatory effect through alteration of antibody responsiveness. The 14 genes that encode IFN-α are positioned on the short arm of chromosome 9 in man. Polyribonucleotides, as well as RNA or DNA viruses, may induce IFN-α secretion. Recombinant IFN-α has been prepared and used in the treatment of hairy cell leukemia, Kaposi's sarcoma, chronic myeloid leukemia, human papilloma virus-related lesions, renal cell carcinoma, chronic hepatitis, and selected other conditions. Patients may experience severe flu-like symptoms as long as the drug is administered. They also have malaise, headache, depression, and supraventricular tachycardia and may possibly develop congestive heart failure. Bone marrow suppression has been reported in some patients.

Immunoscintigraphy (Figures 22 and 23) is the formation of two-dimensional images of the distribution of radioactivity in tissues following the administration of antibodies labeled with a radionuclide that are specific for tissue antigens. A scintillation camera is used to record the images. Immunolymphoscintigraphy is a method used to determine the presence of tumor metastasis to lymph nodes. Antibody fragments or monoclonal antibodies against specific tumor antigens are radiolabeled and then detected by scintigraphy.

An **immunotoxin** (Figure 24) is produced by linking an antibody specific for target cell antigens with a cytotoxic substance, such as the toxin ricin. Upon parenteral injection, its antibody portion directs the immunotoxin to the target and its toxic portion destroys target cells on contact. An immunotoxin may also be a monoclonal antibody or one of its fractions linked to a toxic molecule such as a radioisotope, a bacterial or plant toxin or a chemotherapeutic agent. The antibody portion is intended to direct the molecule to antigens on a target cell such as those of a malignant tumor and the toxic portion of the molecule is for the purpose of destroying the target cell. Contemporary methods of recombinant DNA technology have permitted the preparation of specific hybrid molecules for use in immunotoxin therapy. Immunotoxins may have difficulty reaching the intended target tumor, may be quickly metabolized, and may stimulate

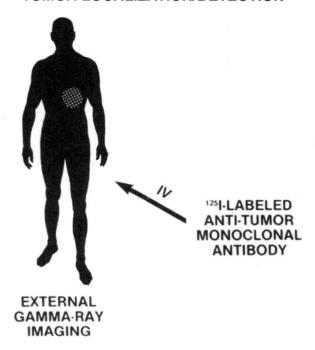

TUMOR LOCALIZATION/DETECTION

IV

^{125}I-LABELED ANTI-TUMOR MONOCLONAL ANTIBODY

EXTERNAL GAMMA-RAY IMAGING

Figure 22. Immunoscintigraphy.

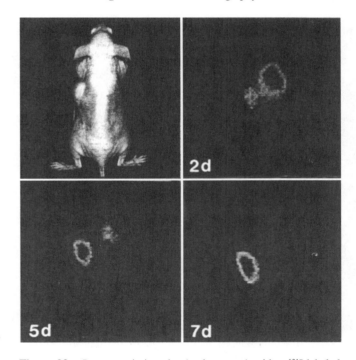

2d

5d   7d

Figure 23. Immunoscintigraphy (nude mouse) with a ^{131}I-labeled monoclonal antibody. The mouse shown bears a human colon carcinoma in its left flank. The scintigrams were recorded two, five, and seven days post injection. While the second picture shows mainly the blood pool and little of the tumor, the tumor is the major imaged spot in the body after five days; after seven days, only the tumor is recognizable.

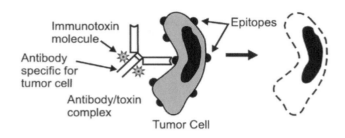

Figure 24.   Immunotoxin.

the development of anti-immunotoxin antibodies. Cross-linking proteins may likewise be unstable.

Abrin (Figure 25) and ricin are examples of immunotoxin. Abrin is a powerful toxin and lectin used in immunological research by Paul Ehrlich (circa 1900). It is extracted from the seeds of the jequirity plant and causes agglutination of erythrocytes. Ricin is a toxic protein found in seeds of *Ricinus communis* (castor bean) plants. It is a heterodimer comprised of a 30 dK α chain, which mediates cytotoxicity, and a 30 kD β chain, which interacts with cell surface galactose residues that facilitate passage of molecules into cells in endocytic vesicles. Ricin inhibits protein synthesis by linkage of a dissociated α chain in the cytosol to ribosomes. The

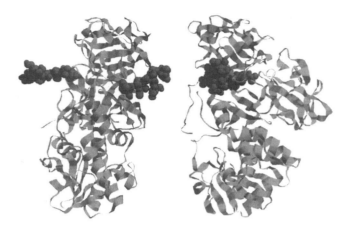

Figure 25.   Abrin — A.

ricin heterodimer or its α chain conjugated to a specific antibody serves as an immunotoxin.

Adoptive immunotherapy (Figures 26 and 27) is an experimental treatment of terminal cancer patients with metastatic tumors unresponsive to other modes of therapy by the inoculation of lymphokine-activated killer (LAK) cells or tumor-infiltrating lymphocytes (TIL) together with IL-2. This mode of therapy has shown some success in approximately one-tenth of treated individuals with melanoma or renal cell carcinoma.

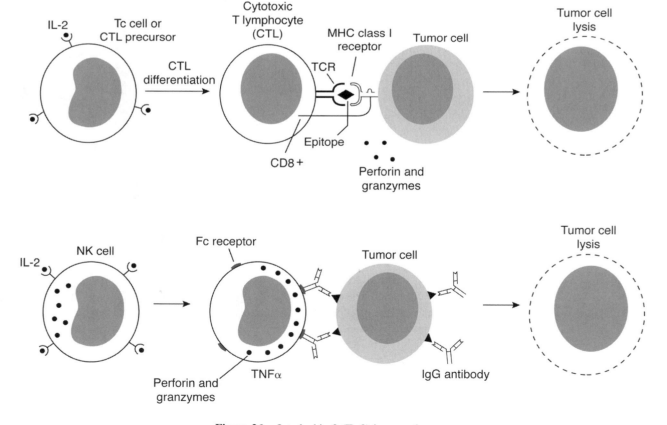

Figure 26.   Interleukin-2 (IL-2) immunotherapy.

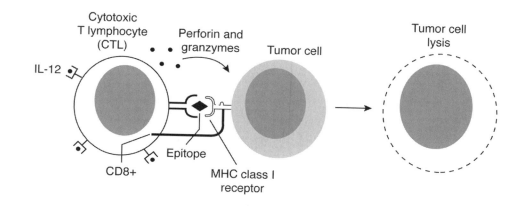

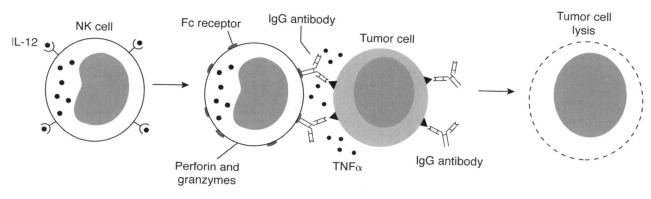

Figure 27. Interleukin-12 (IL-12) immunotherapy.

Lymphokine activated killer (LAK) cells are lymphoid cells derived from normal or tumor patients cultured in medium with recombinant IL-2 become capable of lysing NK-resistant tumor cells as revealed by ^{51}Cr-release cytotoxicity assays. These cells are also referred to as lymphokine-activated killer cells. Most LAK activity is derived from NK cells. The large granular lymphocytes (LGL) contain all LAK precursor activity and all active NK cells. In accord with the phenotype of precursor cells, LAK effector cells are also granular lymphocytes expressing markers associated with human NK cells. The asialo Gm_1+ population, known to be expressed by murine NK cells, contains most LAK precursor activity. Essentially all LAK activity resides in the LGL population in the rat. LAK cell and IL-2 immunotherapy has been employed in human cancer patients with a variety of histological tumor types when conventional therapy has been unsuccessful. Approximately one-fourth of LAK and IL-2 treated patients manifested significant responses and some individuals experienced complete remission. Serious side effects included fluid retention and pulmonary edema attributable to the administered IL-2.

Tumor infiltrating lymphocytes (TIL) are lymphocytes isolated from the tumor they are infiltrating. They are cultured with high concentrations of IL-2 leading to expansion of these activated T lymphocytes *in vitro*. TILs are very effective in destroying tumor cells and have proven much more effective than lymphokine activating killer (LAK) cells in experimental models. TILs have 50 to 100 times the antitumor activity produced by LAK cells. TILs have been isolated and grown from multiple resected human tumors including those from kidney, breast, colon and melanoma. In contrast to the non-B-non-T LAK cells, TILs nevertheless are generated from T lymphocytes and phenotypically resemble cytotoxic T lymphocytes. TILs from malignant melanoma exhibit specific cytolytic activity against cells of the tumor from which they were extracted, whereas LAK cells have a broad range of specificity. TILs appear unable to lyse cells of melanomas from patients other than those in whom the tumor originated. TILs may be tagged in order that they may be identified later.

Tumor necrosis factor α (TNFα) (Figures 28 and 29) is a cytotoxic monokine produced by macrophages stimulated with bacterial endotoxin. TNF-α participates in inflammation, wound healing, and remodeling of tissue. TNF-α, which is also called cachectin, can induce septic shock and cachexia. It is a cytokine comprised of 157 amino acid residues. It is produced by numerous types of cells including monocytes, macrophages, T lymphocytes, B lymphocytes, NK cells, and other types of cells stimulated by endotoxin or other microbial products. The genes encoding TNF-α and

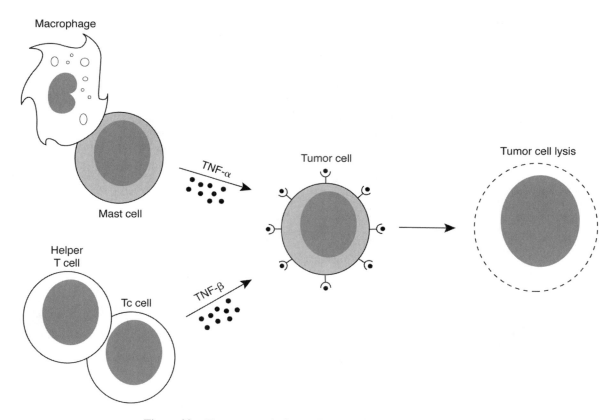

Figure 28. Tumor necrosis factor (TNF) mediated immune reaction.

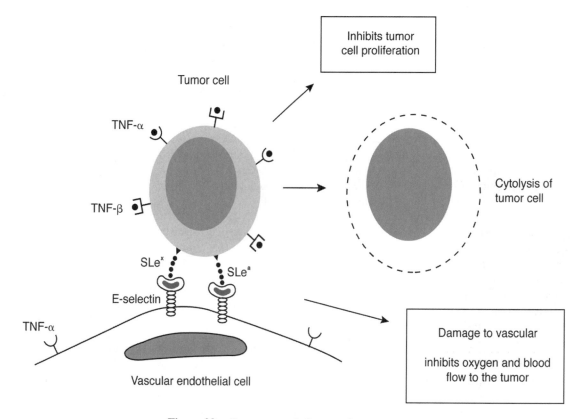

Figure 29. Tumor necrosis Immunotherapy.

TNF-β (lymphotoxin) are located on the short arm of chromosome 6 in man in the MHC region. High levels of TNF-α are detectable in the blood circulation very soon following administration of endotoxin or microorganisms. The administration of recombinant TNF-α induces shock, organ failure, hemorrhagic necrosis of tissues in experimental animals including rodents, dogs, sheep and rabbits, closely resembling the effects of lethal endotoxemia. TNF-α is produced during the first three days of wound healing. It facilitates leukocyte recruitment, induces angiogenesis and promotes fibroblast proliferation. It can combine with receptors on selected tumor cells and induce their lysis. TNF mediates the antitumor action of murine natural cytotoxic (NC) cells, which distinguishes their function from that of natural killer (NK) and cytotoxic T cells. TNF-α was termed cachectin because of its ability to induce wasting and anemia when administered on a chronic basis to experimental animals. Thus it mimics the action in cancer patients and those with chronic infection with human immunodeficiency virus or other pathogenic microorganisms. It can induce anorexia which may lead to death from malnutrition.

Tumor necrosis factor-β (TNF-β) is a 25kD protein synthesized by activated lymphocytes. It can kill tumor cells in culture, induce expression of genes, stimulate proliferation of fibroblasts and mimics most of the actions of tumor necrosis factor α (cachectin). It participates in inflammation and graft rejection and was previously termed lymphotoxin. TNF-β and TNF-α have approximately equivalent affinity for TNF receptors. Both 55kD and 80kD TNF receptors bind TNF-β. TNF-β has diverse effects that include killing of some cells and causing proliferation of others. It is the mediator whereby cytolytic T cells, natural killer cells, lymphokine-activated killer cells and "helper-killer" T cells induce fatal injury to their targets. TNF-β and TNF-α have been suggested to play a role in AIDS, possibly contributing to its pathogenesis.

Tumor necrosis factor receptor is a receptor for tumor necrosis factor that is comprised of 461 amino acid residues and possesses an extracellular domain that is rich in cysteine.

22
Immunity Against Microorganisms

NATURAL IMMUNITY

Entry of a pathogenic organism into a susceptible host is followed by invasion and colonization of tissues, circumvention of the host immune response and injury or decreased function of host tissues. Microbial immunity consists of several factors. Natural and acquired immune mechanisms facilitate the body's resistance against microorganisms. Microbes vary in the lymphocyte responsiveness and effector mechanisms they elicit. The skill with which pathogenic microorganisms resist the host's immune defense mechanisms governs their survival and pathogenicity. Paradoxically, the host response to a pathogenic microorganism, rather than the microbe itself, may induce injury to host tissues. Factors that determine the outcome of man's encounter with pathogenic microorganisms include the microbe's virulence and the size of the infecting dose on the one hand and specific defense mechanisms of the host, on the other.

Pathogenicity refers to the capacity of a microorganism to induce disease. If host defenses are decreased significantly, as in the immunocompromised host, opportunistic infections, produced by microorganisms that are not normally pathogenic for the individual, may result. There are multiple causes for diminished host resistance that include accidentally or surgically induced trauma to the mucous membranes or skin, localized lesions, leukocyte defects, complement defects, or defective B or T cell responses. Various drugs such as antibiotics may also alter the normal flora of the body. Microbes that produce opportunistic infections generally are of low virulence, i.e., their level of pathogenicity is low.

Both nonspecific constitutional factors and specific immune mechanisms provide host resistance. Nonspecific resistance mechanisms protect against body surface colonization by microorganisms with pathogenic potential, thereby blocking their penetration of underlying tissues.

Protective immunity consists of both natural, nonspecific immune mechanisms and actively acquired specific immunity that results in the defense of a host against a particular pathogenic microorganism. Protective immunity may be induced either by active immunization with a vaccine prepared from antigens of a pathogenic microorganism or by experiencing either a subclinical or clinical infection with the pathogenic microorganism.

The skin as well as mucous membranes of various anatomical regions such as the conjunctiva, nose, mouth, intestinal tract and lower genital tract have a normal commensal flora. Microbial properties, host factors and exogenous factors determine the nature of colonization. The ability of a microorganism to adhere to mucosa or epithelial cells is a significant factor. Microbes in the normal flora may compete with pathogenic microorganisms for receptors on cell surfaces. Fibronectin on epithelial cells may bind *Staphylococcus aureus* and group A hemolytic streptococci. Microbes in the commensal flora may also synthesize bacteriocins which inhibit other bacteria. They may also compete with them for nutrient substances. Thus, the normal flora serves as an effective mechanism for inducing colonization resistance. This can be interrupted by the use of broad spectrum antibiotics resulting in colonization of the surface by pathogenic microorganisms. Gram negative bacteremia may even result in an immunocompromised host. Another consequence of antibiotic therapy may be overgrowth of yeast or of *Clostridium difficile*, a toxin producing gram positive bacillus that is anaerobic and antibiotic resistant that can lead to diarrhea and colitis. Host age, hormones, nutrition and diseases such as diabetes mellitus or malignancy may influence the normal flora. For example, the vaginal flora is sparse in both prepubertal and post menopausal females but is rich in acidophilic lactobacilli during the child-bearing years of life. Lactobacilli convert glycogen to lactic acid yielding a pH of 4 to 5 which inhibits many potential pathogens that might otherwise colonize the vaginal mucosa. Microorganisms in the normal flora of various anatomical regions may induce natural antibodies that would be active against potential pathogenic microorganisms bearing cross reacting antigens.

The skin and mucous membrane serve as **mechanical barriers** to the entrance of microorganisms (Figures 1 and 2). The papilloma virus and a few other infectious agents may penetrate the skin but most microorganisms are excluded by it. Free fatty acids from sebaceous glands and lactic acid present in perspiration together with an acid pH of 5 to 6 and the dryness of the skin are unfavorable to microorganisms. *Staphylococcus aureus* may colonize hair follicles and sweat glands to produce furuncles, carbuncles, and abscesses. *Pseudomonas aeruginosa* may infect skin injured by burns. Injury to the gastric mucosa by irradiation or cytotoxic drugs may culminate in infection by the normal flora of the intestine.

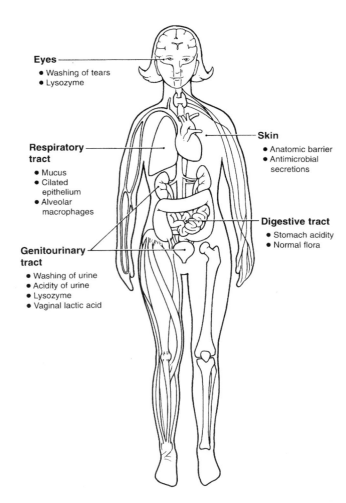

Eyes
- Washing of tears
- Lysozyme

Respiratory tract
- Mucus
- Ciliated epithelium
- Alveolar macrophages

Genitourinary tract
- Washing of urine
- Acidity of urine
- Lysozyme
- Vaginal lactic acid

Skin
- Anatomic barrier
- Antimicrobial secretions

Digestive tract
- Stomach acidity
- Normal flora

Figure 1.   External defense barriers of the human body.

Intact skin

Mucus
    Motion of cilia
    Coughing/sneezing

Cell shedding
Flushing of microbes by tears, saliva, urine, perspiration, other body fluids
Emesis and diarrhea aid microbial elimination

Figure 2.   Mechanical barriers against infection.

Lysozyme and lactoferrin are both antimicrobial substances found in **surface secretions** of the mucosa. Lysozyme induces lysis of bacterial cells through breaking the linkage connecting N-acetyl muraminic acid and N-acetylglucosamine in the walls of gram positive bacterial cells. Lactoferrin interrupts metabolism of bacterial iron.

Secretory immunoglobulin A (sIgA) can interfere with the attachment of bacteria to host cells by coating the microbes. It may also neutralize their exotoxins, inhibit their motility and agglutinate them. It is not involved in opsonization or lysis of bacteria through complement. sIgA's ability to prevent adherence of such microorganisms as *Vibrio cholerae*, *Giardia lamblia* and selected respiratory viruses to mucosal surfaces represents a significant defense mechanism. Whereas gastric acidity can destroy most microorganisms, *Mycobacterium tuberculosis* and enteroviruses are not destroyed by it. Gram negative bacteria may colonize the stomach and small intestine in subjects with achlorhydria. Unconjugated bile may prevent bacterial growth in the small gut. Intestinal peristalsis also guards against overgrowth of microorganisms in blind loops.

Inhaled microorganisms in dust or droplets greater than 5μm adhere to the mucosa lining the upper respiratory tract and are swept upward by cilia to the posterior pharynx followed by expectoration or swallowing; this is called **directional flow**. Particles less than 5μm reach the alveoli and are phagocytized by alveolar macrophages. Cigarette smoke or other pollutants, as well as bacterial or viral infection such as pertussis and influenza may diminish the sweeping action of cilia, thereby rendering the subject susceptible to secondary bacterial pneumonia. Intubation and tracheostomy may also decrease normal resistance mechanisms leading to infection. Tears and blinking actions protect the eyes causing microorganisms to be diluted and flushed out through the nasolacrimal duct into the nasopharynx. The antibacterial action of tears is attributable to lysozyme.

Even though urine can support bacterial growth in the bladder, the acid pH of urine and voiding serve as defensive mechanisms against infection. Ascending infection that is discouraged by the longer male urethra is more common in females with a shorter urethra. Urinary stasis in subjects with posterior urethral valves, prostatic hypertrophy or calculi facilitates infection.

Lysozyme can induce lysis of some gram positive bacterial cell walls but not gram negative bacteria unless antibody and complement are also present. It accentuates complement activity. Lactoferrin, a protein that binds iron, competes with microorganisms for this substance. By chelating iron, lactoferrin deprives microbes of the free iron they require for growth. Neutrophil secondary granules also contain lysozyme and lactoferrin. Beta lysin is a thrombocyte-derived antibacterial protein that is effective mainly against Gram-positive bacteria. It is released when blood platelets are disrupted, as occurs during clotting. β lysin acts as a nonantibody humoral substance that contributes to nonspecific immunity (refer to Figure 3).

An **opsonin** is a substance that adheres to the surface of a microorganism and makes it more attractive or delectable to a phagocyte. Opsonins facilitate or enhance phagocytosis of microbes which constitutes a cornerstone of constitutive defense against infection. Both nonimmune and immune substances may serve as opsonins. C3b, produced during complement activation, forms a covalent bond with the bacterial cell surface thereby rendering it susceptible to phago-

Factor	Function	Source
Lysozyme	Catalyzes hydrolysis of cell wall muco-peptide	Tears, saliva, nasal secretions, body fluids lysosomal granules
Lactoferrin, transferrin	Binds iron and competes with microorganisms for it	Specific granules of PMNs
Lactoperoxidase	May be inhibitory to many micro-organisms	Milk and saliva
Beta-lysin	Effective mainly against gram-positive bacteria	Thrombocytes, normal serum
Chemotactic factors	Induce reorientation and directed migration of PMNs, monocytes and other cells	Bacterial substances and products of cell injury and denatured proteins
Properdin	Activates complement in the absence of antibody-antigen complex	Normal plasma
Interferons	Act as immuno-modulators to increase the activities of macrophages	Leukocytes, fibroblasts, natural killer cells, T cells
Defensins	Block cell transport activities	Polymorphonuclear granules

Figure 3. Nonspecific humoral defense mechanisms.

cytosis by C3b receptor-bearing neutrophils, monocytes and macrophages. Adherence of opsonized bacteria to the phagocyte cell surface facilitates phagocytosis. Leukocyte receptors for C3b are termed CR1, CR2, CR3 and CR4. Among the pediatric population, CR3 is associated with increased susceptibility to bacterial infections, a condition termed leukocyte adhesion deficiency.

Opsonization (Figure 4) is the facilitation of the phagocytosis of microorganisms or other particles such as erythrocytes through the coating of their surfaces with either immune or nonimmune opsonins.

Fibronectin is a glycoprotein of relatively high molecular weight found on cells and in the plasma. It may serve as an opsonin and function as an adhesion molecule in cellular interactions. Fibronectin may also react with complement components. Intensive care patients often lose fibronectin from their pharynx causing alteration of the normal flora with colonization by coliforms.

Interferons contain low molecular weight glycoproteins and are characterized as α, β, and γ. Alpha and beta interferon are activated by virus infection of cells. These induce proteins with antiviral properties. By contrast, γ interferon modulates the immune response. Although interferon is not virus specific, it is cell-specific. For example, chick interferon will not protect human cells and human interferon will not protect chick cells. Interferons act at the cell surface through specific receptors. Both α and β share a common receptor whereas γ requires a separate one. Interferons activate the synthesis of antiviral substances that prevent viral mRNA translation to a greater degree than host mRNA. Interferon may activate natural killer (NK) cells and macrophages. It is produced soon after infection.

Phagocytic cells are polymorphonuclear neutrophils and eosinophils as well as macrophages (the mononuclear phagocytes) which have a critical role in defending the host against microbial infection (Figure 5). Polymorphonuclear neutrophils and occasionally eosinophils appear first in areas of acute inflammation followed later on by macrophages. Chemotactic factors, including formyl-methionyl-leucyl-phenylalanine (f-met-leu-phe) are released by actively multiplying bacteria. This is a powerful attractant for PMN's whose membrane have a specific receptor for it. Different types of infectious agents may stimulate different types of cellular response. When particles greater than 1mm become attached and engulfed by a cell, the process is known as phagocytosis. Various factors present in the serum and known as opsonins coat microorganisms or other particles and make them more delectable to phagocytic cells. These include nonspecific substances such as complement compo-

Inefficient phagocytosis

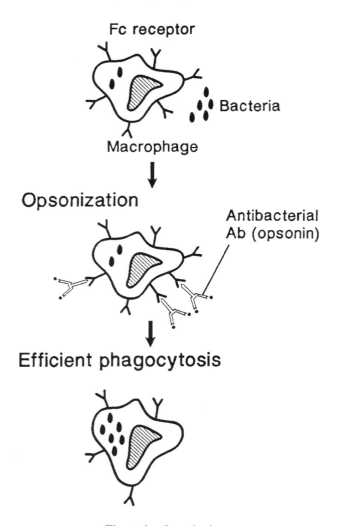

Figure 4.   Opsonization.

Microorganism	Cell Type
Extracellular bacteria	Polymorphonuclear neutrophils (PMNs)
Parasites	Eosinophils
Intracellular microorganisms (i.e., mycobacteria or fungi)	Macrophages
Viruses	Lymphocytes, NK cells

Figure 5.   Nonspecific cellular defense.

nent C3b as well as specific antibodies located in the IgG or IgG3 fractions. Capsules enable microorganisms such as pneumococci and *Hemophilus* to resist phagocytosis.

PMNs, sometimes called the soldiers of the body, are first to arrive at areas of invading and rapidly multiplying bacteria. They contain both primary or azurophilic granules and secondary or specific granules that serve as reservoirs for the digestive and hydrolytic enzymes such as lysozyme (Figure 6) before they are delivered to the phagosome. Frequently, the PMNs die after ingesting and destroying the invading microorganisms. Macrophages that serve as scavengers ingesting debris left by neutrophils killed by the microorganisms they phagocytized, are resilient and survive.

Azurophil granules (Primary granules)	Specific granules (Secondary granules)
Bacterial permeability-inducing protein (BPI)	
Cathespin G	
Cationic antimicrobial protein (CAP) 57	
Cationic antimicrobial protein (CAP) 37	
Defensins: HP1 HP2 HP3	
Elastase	
Lysozyme	
Myeloperoxidase	Bacterial chemotaxin receptors
Collagenase	
C5a receptors	
Gelatinase	
Lactoferrin	
Lysozyme	
NADPH	
Vitamin B$_{12}$-binding protein	

Figure 6.   Substances associated with neutrophils.

A **secondary granule** is a structure in the cytoplasm of polymorphonuclear leukocytes that contains vitamin B$_{12}$-binding protein, lysozyme, and lactoferrin in neutrophils. Cationic peptides are present in eosinophil secondary granules. Histamine, platelet-activating factor, and heparin are present in the secondary granules of basophils.

Mononuclear phagocytes include monocytes in the blood and macrophages in the tissues which have cell surface receptors for Fc gamma and C3b. They are also able to phagocytize microorganisms coated with opsonins and kill many but not all microorganisms during the process. Some microorganisms such as mycobacteria survive and multiply within macroph-

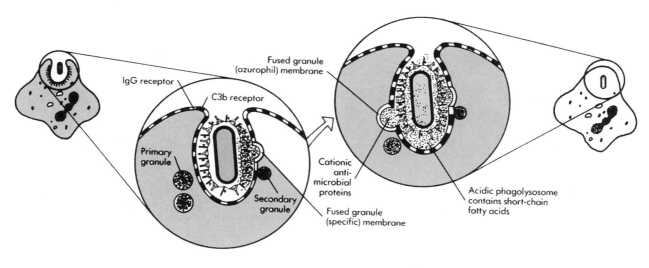

Figure 7. Steps of phagocytic endocytosis.

ages which may serve as a reservoir or transport mechanism to help them reach other areas of the body. Other intracellular microorganisms that are not killed by nonimmune macrophages include *Listeria monocytogenes, Brucella* species, *Legionella pneumophila, Cryptococcus neoformans, Toxoplasma gondii,* and *Pneumocystis carinii.* However, the development of cell-mediated immunity with the production of gamma interferon by lymphocytes is able to activate these macrophages to enable them to kill the intracellular pathogens. Activated macrophages produce interleukin-1 and tumor necrosis factor alpha which promote inflammation.

Phagocytosis (Figure 7) is an important clearance mechanism for the removal and disposition of foreign agents and particles or damaged cells. Macrophages, monocytes and polymorphonuclear leukocytes are phagocytic cells. In special circumstances other cells such as fibroblasts, may show phagocytic properties; these are called facultative phagocytes.

Phagocytosis may involve nonimmunologic or immunologic mechanisms. Nonimmunologic phagocytosis refers to the ingestion of inert particles such as latex beads or of other particles that have been modified by chemical treatment or coated with protein. Details of the recognition process of such particles are not known. Damaged cells are also phagocytized by nonimmunologic mechanisms. It is believed that in the latter case damaged cells are also coated with immunoglobulin or other proteins which facilitates their recognition.

Phagocytosis involves several steps: attachment, interiorization, and digestion (Figure 8). The initiation of ingestion is known as the "zipper mechanism". After attachment, the particle is engulfed within a fragment or plasma membrane and forms a phagocytic vacuole. This fuses with the primary lysosomes to form the phagolysosome in which the lysosomal enzymes are discharged and the enclosed material is digested. Remnants of indigestible material can be

subsequently recognized as residual bodies. The process is associated with stimulation of phagocyte metabolism.

Phagocytic dysfunction may be due to either extrinsic or intrinsic defects. The extrinsic variety encompass opsonin deficiency secondary to antibody and complement factor deficiencies; suppression of phagocytic cell numbers by immunosuppressive agents; corticosteroid-induced interference with phagocytic function; decreased neutrophils through anti-neutrophil autoantibody; and abnormal neutrophil chemotaxis as a consequence of complement deficiency or abnormal complement components. Intrinsic phagocytic dysfunction is related to enzymatic deficiencies that participate in the metabolic pathway leading to bacterial cell killing. These intrinsic disorders include chronic granulomatous disease, characterized by defects in the respiratory burst pathway, myeloperoxidase deficiency and glucose-6-phosphate dehydrogenase deficiency. Consequences of phagocytic dysfunction include increased susceptibility to bacterial infections but not viral or protozoal infections. Selected phagocytic function disorders may be associated with severe fungal infections. The severity of bacterial infections associated with phagocytic dysfunction may range from mild skin infections to fatal systemic infection.

Chemotaxis is a locomotion of cells that may be stimulated by the presence of certain substances in their environment. This locomotion may be random in direction, i.e., it is not oriented with respect to the stimulus although there is a direct cause-effect relationship between stimulus and response. In contrast, the directed locomotion implies an orientation of cell movement with respect to the inducing stimulus. The latter form of cell movement is called chemotaxis and may be positive, in which the stimulus acts as an attractant, or negative, in which the stimulus acts as a repellent.

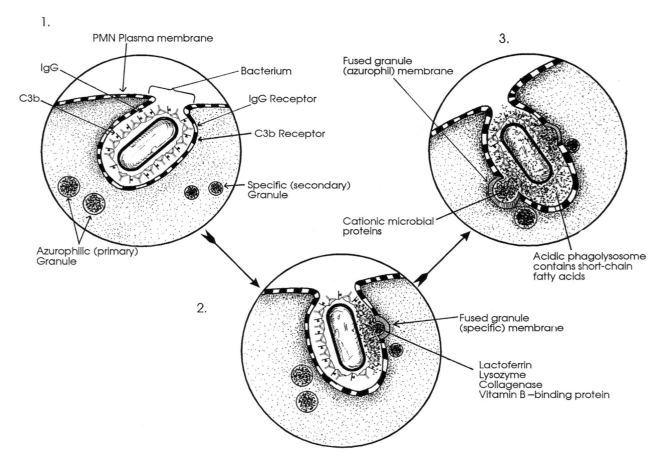

Figure 8.   Phagocytosis.

Substances which may stimulate the random cell locomotion are called cytotoxigens; those which stimulate directed migration are called cytotoxins or chemotactic factors. The main element in the effect of chemotactic factors is the presence of a concentration gradient which determines the direction of cell migration. It is said that under these circumstances a chemotactic signal is provided to the cells under consideration. In the absence of such a gradient, chemotactic factors enhance the random migration.

Phagocytes may kill microorganisms they have ingested by either of two separate mechanisms. One of these, **oxygen-dependent killing**, is activated by a powerful oxidative burst that culminates in the formation of hydrogen peroxide and other anti-microbial substances (Figure 9). In addition to this oxygen-dependent killing mechanism, phagocytized intracellular microbes may be the targets of toxic substances released from granules into the phagosome leading to microbial cell death by an oxygen-independent mechanism.

For oxygen-dependent killing of microbes, membranes of specific granules and phagosomes fuse. This permits interaction of NADPH oxidase with cytochrome b. With the aid of quinone, this combination reduces oxygen to superoxide

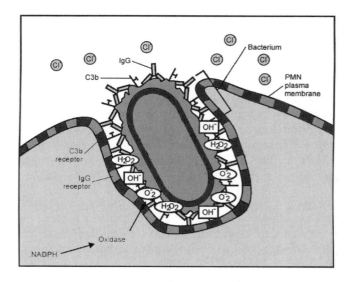

Figure 9.   Formation of Bactericide and hydrogen peroxide catalyzed by NADPH oxidase.

anion, O_2. In the presence of a catalyst superoxide dismutase, superoxidase ion is converted to hydrogen peroxide.

The clinical relevance of this process is illustrated by chronic granulomatous disease (CGD) in children who fail to form superoxide anions. They have diminished cytochrome b. Even though phagocytosis is normal, they have impaired ability to oxidize NADPH and destroy bacteria through the oxidative pathway. The oxidative mechanism kills microbes through a complex process. Hydrogen peroxide together with myeloperoxidase transforms chloride ions into hypochlorous ions that kill microorganisms. Azurophil granule fusion releases myeloperoxidase to the phagolysosome. Some microorganisms such as pneumococci may themselves form hydrogen peroxide.

Following adherence of opsonized microbes to the neutrophil plasma membrane, lysozyme and lactoferrin are discharged from specific granules into phagosomes with which they have fused. Antimicrobial cationic proteins reach phagosomes from azurophil granules. These proteins kill gram negative microbes by interrupting their cell membrane integrity. They are far less effective against gram positive microorganisms. This is **oxygen-independent killing**.

Cationic protein deficiency may be associated with chronic skin infections or abscesses. In patients with Chediak-Higashi syndrome, the neutrophil granules fuse when the cells are immature in the bone marrow. Thus, these patients' neutrophils can phagocytize bacteria but have greatly diminished ability to kill them, as their granules have already been used and are deficient in cationic proteins such as cathepsin G.

Whereas gram negative bacteria in the intestine are promptly destroyed by the oxygen-independent process, gram positive microbes such as those in the respiratory epithelium and on the skin are eliminated principally through the oxygen-dependent mechanism.

The first step in **leukocyte activation** is adhesion through surface receptors on the cell. Stimulus recognition is also mediated through membrane-bound receptors. An inducible endothelial-leukocyte adhesion molecule provides a mechanism for leukocyte-vessel wall adhesion.

Studies on H_2O_2 secretion by PMNs exposed to macrophage and lymphocyte products suggest that surface adherent leukocytes undergo a large prolonged respiratory burst. Recombinant TNF-alpha delays H_2O_2 release demonstrating that soluble factors from macrophages and lymphocytes can affect adherent PMNs with respect to cytotoxic potential. Studies on regulation of neutrophil activation by platelets reveal that platelet-derived growth factor (PDGF) does not alter the resting level of superoxide generation but inhibits the rate and extent of f-Met-Leu-Phe-induced oxidative burst. Intracellular Ca^{++} increases up-regulation of ligand-independent cell surface expression of f-Met-Leu-Phe receptors in neutrophils, whereas phorbol myristate acetate (PMA) activates down regulation of these receptors. A pertussis toxin-sensitive GTP-binding protein regulates monocyte phagocytic function.

Complement receptor 3 (CR3) facilitates the ability of phagocytes to bind and ingest opsonized particles. There is a relatively large family of homologous adhesion-promoting receptor proteins, including leukocyte proteins, that identify the sequence Arg-Gly-Asp. Molecules found to be powerful stimulators of PMN activity include recombinant IFN-gamma, granulocyte-macrophage colony-stimulating factor, TNF and lymphotoxin. Investigations of storage sites for the several protein receptors have revealed a mobile intracellular storage compartment in human neutrophils. Chemotactic stimuli, such as f-Met-Leu-Phe, may cause translocation of granules acting as storage sites to the cell surface, which could be requisite for neutrophil adhesion and chemotaxis.

Dephosphorylation pathways for inositol triphosphate isomers culminate in the elevation of intracellular Ca^{++} and protein kinase C activation. NADPH oxidase, which utilizes hexose monophosphate shunt generated NADPH, catalyzes the respiratory burst. Both Ca^{++} and protein kinase C play a key role in the activated pathway. Activated human neutrophils manifest an elevated expression of complement decay-accelerating factor, which protects erythrocytes from injury by autologous complement. Transduction of decay-accelerating factors to the cell surface following stimulation by chemoattractants may be significant in protecting PMNs from complement-mediated injury. This type of process would permit PMNs to manifest unreserved function in sites of inflammation.

Although not phagocytic, **natural killer (NK) cells** attack and destroy certain virus infected cells. They constitute a part of the natural immune system, do not require prior contact with antigen and are not MHC restricted. On contacting a virus-infected cell, NK cells produce perforin that leads to the formation of pores in the infected cell membrane leading to osmotic lysis. Interferon enhances NK cell activity. These cells appear to be large granular lymphocytes and are significant in antiviral defense and in surveillance against the development of neoplasia. NK cells lyse certain virus-infected cells without MHC restriction. Questions remain concerning the phenotype of NK cells, even though several monoclonal antibodies reactive with them are available. The natural immune system, in which the NK cells are key participants, does not involve memory. It does not require sensitization and cannot be enhanced by specific antigens. Other nonmemory cells include polymorphonuclear leukocytes and macrophages (Figure 10), which are important in early defense against infectious agents and possibly tumors. NK cells are able to lyse selected tumor target cells without prior sensitization and in the absence of antibody or complement. NK and cytotoxic T cells have been shown to share similar lytic mechanisms. Both cell types have granules

| Natural killer (NK) cells |
| Antibody-dependent cytotoxic cells |
| K cells |
| NK cells |
| Lymphokine-activated killer (LAK) cells |
| Tumor-infiltrating lymphocytes (TILS) |

Figure 10. Lymphoid cells participating in nonspecific immunity.

which contain perforin or C9-related protein which lyse target cells without antibody or complement.

NK activity is measured by a chromium release assay, employing the K562 erythroleukemia cell line as a target. Whereas NK cells mediate their effect in the absence of antibody or complement, **killer (K) cells** or **ADCC (antibody-dependent cell-mediated cytotoxicity)** cells induce lysis through the action of antibody. With the demonstration of Fc receptors on their surface, NK cells may actually be the killer (K) cells responsible for ADCC activity through attached IgG antibody. They mediate their classic effects via cell surface receptors for antigen.

Other than NK or ADCC cells, circulating monocytes or macrophages also mediate cell lysis through antibody molecules. Cytotoxic T cells (CTL) apparently recognize specific target cells through interaction with MHC antigens on the cell surface. Whereas either helper or killer T cells are directed to MHC proteins, NK cells apparently do not recognize MHC determinants. NK cell activity is located in the low density population of lymphocytes which have large granules in their cytoplasm, i.e., large granular lymphocytes (LGL). Even though NK cells are lethal to tumor cells *in vitro*, very little data exists about their *in vivo* activity. Studies in mice suggest NK cells to be important in protection against selected virus infections. NK cells are also believed to play a regulatory role in the immune system, encompassing down-regulation of antibody responses.

Humans have **innate immunity against extracellular bacteria**. Neutrophil (PMN), monocyte and tissue macrophage phagocytosis leads to rapid microbicidal action against ingested microbes from the extracellular environment. The capacity of a microorganism to resist phagocytosis and digestion in phagocytic cells is a principal feature of its virulence. Complement activation represents a significant mechanism for ridding the body of invading microorganisms. A **peptidoglycan layer** (Figure 11) in the cell walls of gram positive bacteria as well as lipopolysaccharide, or LPS (Figure 12), in the cell walls of gram negative bacteria are able to activate the alternative pathway of complement without antibody. Also associated with LPS is flagellar antigen and somatic antigen (Figure 13).

Flagellar antigens, or **H antigens**, are epitopes on flagella of enteric bacteria that are motile and Gram negative. H is

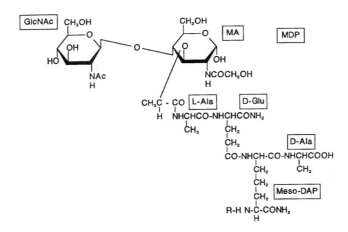

Figure 11. Peptidoglycan (murein).

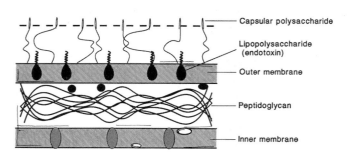

Figure 12. Cross-section of Gram negative bacterial cell wall.

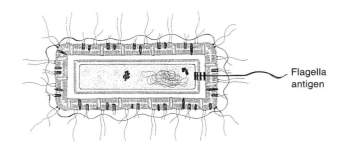

Figure 13. Bacterial cell.

from the German word "*Hauch*," which means breath, and refers to the production of a film on agar plates that resembles breathing on glass. In the Kaufmann-hite classification scheme for *Salmonella*, H antigens serve as the basis for the division of microorganisms into phase I and phase II, depending on the flagellins they contain. A single cell synthesizes only one type of flagellin. Phase variation may result in a switch to production of the other type which is genetically controlled.

A **somatic antigen**, or **O antigen**, is a lipopolysaccharide-protein antigen of enteric microorganisms which is used for their serological classification. O antigens of the *Proteus* species serve as the basis for the Weil-Felix reaction which is employed to classify *Rickettsia*. O antigens of *Shigella* permit them to be subdivided into 40 serotypes. The exterior oligosaccharide repeating unit side chain is responsible for specificity and is joined to lipid A to form lipopolysaccharide and to lipid B. The O antigen is the most variable part of the lipopolysaccharide molecule.

C3b may deposit on LPS where it is safe from the inactivating effects of factors H and I. LPS may also activate the classical complement pathway in the absence of antibody by combining with C1q. The C3b that results from activation of complement serves as an opsonin when linked to the bacterial surface making the bacterial cell more attractive to phagocytes. The membrane attack complex (MAC) induces lysis of bacterial cells. Complement reaction products play an active role in inflammation through the attraction and stimulation of leukocytes.

Lipopolysaccharides or **endotoxins** (Figure 14) induce macrophages and selected other cells such as endothelial cells of vessels to synthesize cytokines, such as interleukin-1 (IL-1), tumor necrosis factor (TNF), interleukin-6 (IL-6) and interleukin-8 (IL-8) molecules that participate in inflammation

(Figure 15). Monokines, cytokines from macrophages, activate nonspecific inflammation and facilitate lymphocyte activation by bacterial epitopes. PMNs and monocytes adhere to the endothelium of vessels in areas of infection through the action of cytokines. These inflammatory cells migrate, accumulate in local areas and become activated, enabling them to destroy the microorganisms. Local tissue injury may be an unintended consequence of these resisting processes. Fever and the formation of acute phase reactants may also be consequences of cytokine action. Some cytokines may facilitate specific immune mechanisms by stimulating both T and B cells. Excessive cytokine synthesis may lead to pathologic sequelae during infection by extracellular microorganisms. Gram negative bacterial infection can lead to disseminated intravascular coagulation (DIC) and vascular collapse known also as endotoxin shock or septic shock in which it is mediated mainly by TNF.

Endotoxin shock occurs following exposure to relatively large amounts of endotoxin produced during bacterial sepsis with *Escherichia coli*, *Pseudomonas aeruginosa*, or meningococci. It is characterized by falling blood pressure and disseminated intravascular coagulation (DIC). DIC leads to the formation of thrombi in small blood vessels, leading to such devastating consequences as bilateral cortical necrosis

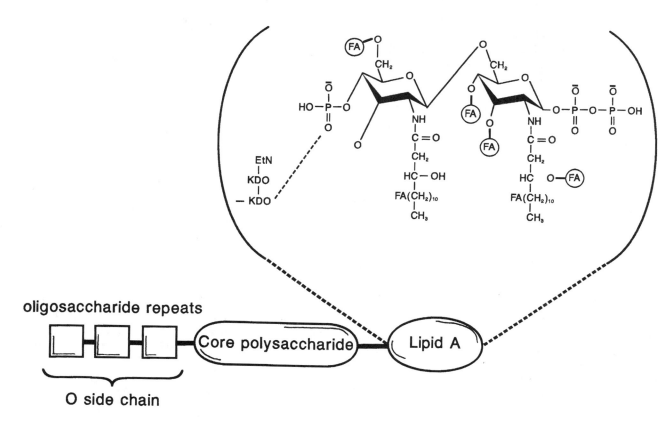

Figure 14.   Lipopolysaccharide or endotoxin.

Cell differentiation factors	Alpha interferon
CSF	Plasma proteins
Cytotoxic factors	Coagulation factors

TNFα	Oxygen metabolites
	    H_2O_2
	    Superoxide anion

Cachectin	Arachidonic acid metabolites
	    Prostaglandins
	    Thromboxanes
	    Leukotrienes

Hydrolytic enzymes
    Collagenase
    Lipase
    Phosphatase
	Complement components
	    C1 to C5
	    Properdin
	    Factors B, D, I, H

Endogenous pyrogen IL-1	

Figure 15. Secreted products of macrophages that have a protective effect on the body.

of the kidneys and blockage of the blood supply to the brain, lungs, and adrenals. When DIC affects the adrenal glands, as in certain memingococcal infections, infarction leads to adrenal insufficiency and death. This is the Waterhouse-Friderichsen syndrome.

An **enterotoxin** is a bacterial toxin that is heat stable and causes intestinal injury.

A **mitogen** is a substance. often derived from plants, that causes DNA synthesis and induces blast transformation and division by mitosis. Lectins, representing plant-derived mitogens or phytomitogens, have been widely used in both experimental and clinical immunology to evaluate T and B lymphoctye function *in vitro*. Phytohemagglutinin (PHA) is principally a human and mouse T cell mitogen, as is concanavalin A (Con A). By contrast, lipopolysaccharide (LPS) induces B lymphocyte transformation in mice, but not in humans. Staphylococcal protein A is the mitogen used to induce human B lymphocyte transformation. Poleweed mitogen (PWM) transforms B cells of both humans and mice, as well as their T cells.

Phagocytosis is the chief mechanism of **innate immunity against intracellular bacteria** whereby intracellular pathogenic microorganisms should be eliminated. However, this is frustrated by the resistance of many intracellular microbes to intracellular dissolution. Thus, the natural immune mechanism of phagocytosis is of little use in controlling infection by intracellular microorganisms. Bacteria of this category may persist in the tissues leading to chronic infection.

Natural immunity against viruses occurs when virus-infected host cells sensitize type I interferon. This blocks virus replication. Natural killer (NK) cells, which are not MHC restricted, provide early antiviral effects following infection. Type I interferon accentuates their action. Both

complement and phagocytosis play significant roles in removal of extracellular viruses.

Parasitic protozoa and helminths are adept at survival within the host through successful resistance of host **innate immune mechanisms against parasites**. Whereas parasitic stages isolated from invertebrates may be lysed through activation of the alternate complement pathway, parasites isolated from humans or other vertebrate hosts are often insusceptible to complement lysis. This could be attributable to either disappearance of surface molecules that activate complement or adherence to the surface of decay-accelerating factor (DAF) or other regulatory proteins.

Mechanisms whereby mature adult schistosomes are able to evade the immune response of the host include: low surface antigenicity; disguise; host molecule mimicry; surface antigen sequestration and shedding; reduced surface antigenicity, as well as other evasion mechanisms. Reducing surface antigenicity by host molecule masking, shedding, or sequestration of antigen represents a successful mechanism for parasites to escape the immune system. Whereas macrophages may ingest protozoa, numerous pathogenic parasites may resist intracellular killing or even replicate within the phagocyte. The outer coat of helminths helps to protect against intracellular killing by neutrophils or macrophages.

ACQUIRED IMMUNITY

Humans are confronted with a host of microorganisms with the potential to induce serious or fatal infections. Yet nature has provided appropriate molecules, cells, and receptors that can protect against these microbes. Many of these defenses are general or nonspecific and do not require previous exposure to the offending pathogen (or closely related organism). These important mechanisms constitute the **innate** or **constitutive defense system**. Another important defense system is **acquired immunity** which can develop after previous contact with the organism through infection (overt or subclinical) or by deliberate immunization with a vaccine prepared from the etiologic agent.

Naturally acquired immunity describes the protection provided by previous exposure to a pathogenic microorganism or antigenically related organism. In contrast, **artificially acquired immunity** develops as a result of immunization with vaccines — either with attenuated organisms or with killed organisms or subunit components. Toxoids provide excellent immunity against the effects of microorganisms such as *Corynebacterium diphtheriae* and *Clostridium tetani* that produce powerful exotoxins. Active immunization with appropriate booster injections leads to the development of IgG which provides immunity of long duration. Acquired immunity depends upon antibodies and T cells.

Passive immunity involves the transfer of resistance against an infectious disease agent from an immune individual to a previously susceptible recipient. **Natural passive immunity** describes the transfer of IgG antibodies across the placenta from mother to child. IgA secretory antibodies may also be passively transferred from mother to child in breast milk. **Artificially acquired passive immunity** describes the transfer of immunoglobulins from an immune individual to a nonimmune, susceptible recipient. Passive immunity of this type is more often used for prophylaxis than for therapy. It provides immediate protection of the recipient for relatively short periods (few weeks). Human sera are preferred for passive immunization to avoid serum sickness induced by foreign serum proteins. **Adoptive immunization** refers to the transfer of specifically immune lymphoid cells from one individual to another, such as occurs in bone marrow transplantation.

People can exhibit **specific immune responses to extracellular bacteria**. Antibodies are the primary agents that protect the body against extracellular bacteria (Figure 16). Microbial cell wall polysaccharides serve as thymus-independent antigens that stimulate specific IgM antibody responses. Cytokine production may even permit switching from IgM to IgG production. Protein antigens of extracellular bacteria primarily stimulate CD4+ T cells. Toxins of extracellular bacteria may activate multiple CD4+ T lymphocytes. When a bacterial toxin stimulates an entire family of T lymphocytes that express products of a certain family of V_{beta} T lymphocyte receptor genes, it is referred to as a superantigen. Immune stimulation of this type may lead to the production of abundant quantities of cytokines that lead to pathologic sequelae.

Opsonic--promote ingestion and killing by phagocytic cells (IgG)
Block attachment (IgA)
Neutralize toxins
Agglutinate bacteria--may aid in clearing
Render motile organisms nonmotile
Abs only rarely affect metabolism or growth of bacteria (Mycoplasma)
Abs, combining with antigens of the bacterial surface, activate the complement cascade, thus inducing an inflammatory response and bringing fresh phagocytes and serum Abs into the site
Abs, combining with antigens of the bacterial surface, activate the complement cascade, and through the final sequences the (MAC) membrane attack complex is formed involving C5b-C9

Figure 16. Antimicrobial actions of antibodies.

The resistance mechanisms against extracellular bacteria regrettably may include two reactions that produce tissue injury: acute inflammation and endotoxin shock. In addition, late in the course of a bacterial infection, pathogenic antibodies may appear (e.g., antibodies produced in post streptococcal glomerulonephritis and rheumatic fever). The multiple lymphocyte clones stimulated by either bacterial endotoxins or superantigens may lead to the production of autoimmunity through overriding specific T cell bypass mechanisms. Autoreactive lymphocytes may also be activated during this process.

Tetanus toxin is the exotoxin synthesized by *Clostridium tetani*. It acts on the nervous system, interrupting neuromuscular transmission and preventing synaptic inhibition in the spinal cord. It binds to a nerve cell membrane glycolipid, i.e., disialosyl ganglioside. The effects of tetanus toxin are countered by specific antitoxin.

Diphtheria toxin is a 62kD protein exotoxin synthesized and secreted by *Corynebacterium diphtheriae*. The exotoxin, which is distributed in the blood, induces neuropathy and myocarditis in humans. Tryptic enzymes nick the single chain diphtheria toxin. Thiols reduce the toxin to produce two fragments. The 40kD B fragment gains access to cells through their membranes, permitting the 21kD A fragment to enter. Whereas the B fragment is not toxic, the fragment is toxic and it inactivates elongation factor-2, thereby blocking eukaryocytic protein synthesis. Guinea pigs are especially sensitive to diphtheria toxin, which causes necrosis at injection sites, hemorrhage of the adrenals, and other pathologic consequences. Animal tests developed earlier in the century consisted of intradermal inoculation of *C. diphtheriae* suspensions into the skin of guinea pigs that were unprotected, compared to a control guinea pig that had been pretreated with passive administration of diphtheria antitoxin for protection. In later years, toxin generation was demonstrated *in vitro* by placing filter paper impregnated with antitoxin at right angles to streaks of *C. diphtheriae* microorganisms growing on media in Petri plates. Formalin treatment or storage converts the labile diphtheria toxin into toxoid.

Cholera toxin is a vibrio cholerae enterotoxin comprised of five B subunits that are cell-binding 11.6kD structures that encircle a 27kD catalase that conveys ADP-ribose to G protein, leading to continual adenyl cyclase activation. Other toxins that resemble cholera toxin in function include diphtheria toxin, exotoxin A, and pertussis toxin.

An **exotoxin** is an extracellular product of pathogenic microorganisms. Exotoxins are 3- to 500kD polypeptides produced by such microorganisms as *Cornyebacterium diphtheria*, *Clostridium tetani*, and *C. botulinum*. Vibrio cholerae produces exotoxins that elevate cAMP levels in intestinal mucosa cells and increase the flow of water and ions into the intestinal lumen, producing diarrhea. Exotoxins are polypeptides released from bacterial cells and are diffusible, thermolabile, and able to be converted to toxoids that are immunogenic, but not toxic. Bacterial exotoxins are either cytolytic, acting on cell membranes, or bipartite (A-B toxins), linking to a cell surface through the B segment of the toxin and releasing the A segment only after the molecule reaches the cytoplasm where it produces injury.

Coccidioidin is a *Coccidioides immitis* culture extract that is used in a skin test for cell-mediated immunity against the microorganism in a manner analogous to the tuberculin skin test.

Extracellular bacteria are able to evade immune mechanisms. The ability of extracellular bacteria to adhere to tissues through their surface proteins, to inhibit or inactivate complement, and to discourage phagocytosis all represent virulence mechanisms that facilitate invasion and colonization of tissues. Sialic acid-containing capsules can interfere with the alternate complement pathway. Bacterial capsules are also known to circumvent phagocytosis. Antigenic variation is another mechanism whereby bacteria may escape the development of an immune response specific for their surface antigens.

Specific immune responses can be mounted against intracellular bacteria and fungi. Some bacteria reproduce inside cells of the host. For example, mycobacteria and ***Listeria monocytogenes*** (Figure 17) are organisms of high pathogenicity that survive in phagocytic cells such as macrophages where they resist dissolution. Within the macrophage, they are not exposed to specific antibody. In addition to mycobacteria and *Listeria* species, a number of fungi are also intracellular pathogens.

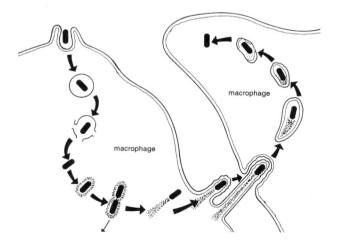

Figure 17. *Listeria.*

Cell-mediated immunity attributable to T lymphocytes is the principal mechanism whereby intracellular bacteria are eliminated by macrophages activated by gamma interferon derived from T cells. Intracellular bacterial protein antigens activate powerful T lymphocyte responsiveness and their cell wall components stimulate macrophages. CD4+ helper/inducer and CD8+ suppressor/cytotoxic t lymphocyte

subsets play significant roles in protection against intracellular bacteria. Both CD4 and CD8 T lymphocyte subsets produce gamma interferon which activates both phagocytosis and functional degradation of ingested microorganisms by macrophages.

Some intracellular microorganisms within macrophages remain resistant even in the presence of specific cell-mediated immunity. They activate macrophages which encircle the bacteria and inhibit their distribution. Infections by both mycobacteria and fungi may produce **granulomatous inflammation** (Figure 18) which leads to necrosis (death) of tissues, fibrosis, and interference with function. This represents a pathogenic immune response by the host reacting against selected intracellular bacteria.

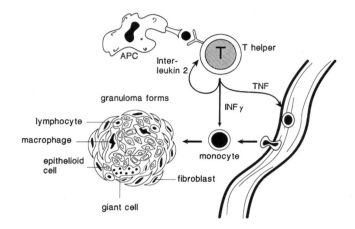

Figure 18.   Granuloma.

Caseous necrosis is tissue destruction, as occurs in tuberculosis, that has the appearance of cottage cheese (Figure 19).

Fibrinoid necrosis is tissue death in which there is a smudgy eosinophilic deposit that resembles fibrin microscopically and camouflages cellular detail. It is induced by proteases released from neutrophils that digest the tissue and cause fibrin deposition. Fibrinoid necrosis is seen in tissues in a number of connective tissue dieseases with immune mechanisms. An example is systemic lupus erythematosus. Fibrinoid necrosis is classically seen in the walls of small vessels in immune complex vasculitis such as occurs in the Arthus reaction.

Intracellular bacteria and fungi are also able to evade immune mechanisms. Intracellular bacteria's principal evasion mechanism is their ability to circumvent their killing by phagocytes. Two such microorganisms, *Mycobacterium tuberculosis* and *Legionella pneumophila* survive by preventing fusion of phagolysosomes, *Listeria monocytogenes* synthesizes a hemolysin that facilitates survival within host cells by the formation of pores within phagolysosomes permitting bacteria to escape back into the cytoplasm.

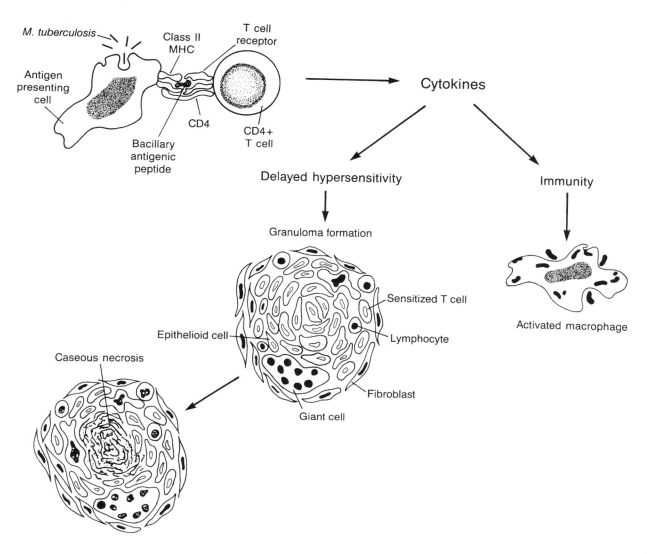

Figure 19. Caseous necrosis (tuberculosis).

Specific immune responses to viruses can occur. Viruses are obligate intracellular parasites that multiply within host cells whose nucleic acids and protein synthesis capability are subverted and appropriated for virus propogation. Viruses may injure cells they have infected by interfering with the cell's protein synthesis and normal functioning, Leading to host cell death. This constitutes a cytopathic effect. Viruses that are not cytopathic may induce a latent infection in which they remain inside host cells and induce synthesis of proteins that provoke a specific immune response. This consists of cytolytic T lymphocytes that are specific for the virus and destroy the virus infected cell. Viral proteins may induce delayed-type hypersensitivity that leads to cellular injury. Both antibodies from B cells and specifically sensitized T cells confer immunity against viruses. Before host cell invasion, specific antibodies may neutralize virions through a process known as **neutralization** (Figure 20). However, following

penetration of host cells, T-cell mediated immunity is requisite for destruction of the virus-infected host cells.

A **papovavirus** is a minute tumor virus that is icosahedral and contains double stranded DNA. Included in the group are SV40 and polyomavirus that may cause malignant and benign tumors. Permissive or nonpermissive infections occur with papovavirus; Following permisive infection of monkey cells, papovavirus replicates, leading to lysis. T antigens, which are early papovavirus proteins that occur in nonpermissive rodent cells, can lead to transformation of the cells that is not reversible if the viral genome is integrated into the host genome. It is reversible if the cell can eliminate the viral genome.

HPV (human papilloma virus) has the potential to be oncogenic and occurs most frequently in individuals with multiple sexual partners. There are 46 HPV genotypes. It can be demonstrated by *in situ* hybridization in proliferations of

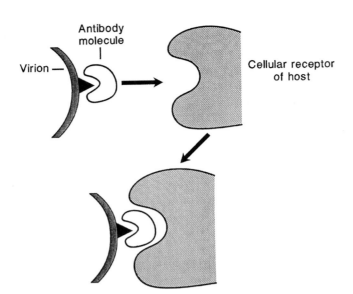

Figure 20. Neutralizing antibody molecules.

epithelial cells that are benign, such as condyloma accuminatum, or malignant, such as squamous cell carcinoma of the uterine cervix. Whereas HPV types 6 and 11 are not usually premalignant, HPV types 16, 18, 31, 33, and 35 are linked to cervical intraepithelial neoplasia (CIN), cervical dysplasia, and anogenital cancer. HPV is predicted to induce derepression as a neoplastic mechanism. HPV encodes E6, a viral protein that combines with the tumor suppressor protein p53.

Herpes virus (Figure 21) is a DNA virus family that contains a central icosahedral core of double stranded DNA. There is a lipoprotein envelope that is trilaminar and 100nm in diameter and a nucleus that is 30–43nm in diameter. Herpes viruses may persist for years in a dormant state. Six types have been described. HHV-1 (herpes simplex -1) can account for oral lesions such as fever blisters. HHV-2 (herpes simplex-2) produces lesions below the waistline and is sex-

ually transmitted. It may produce venereal disease of the vagina and vulva as well as herpetic ulcers of the penis. Both simplex-1 and simplex-2 may infect the brain (Figure 22). HHV-3 (varicella-zoster virus, VZV) occurs clinically as either an acute form known as chickenpox or chronic form termed shingles. HHV-4 (Epstein-Barr virus, EBV), HHV-5 (cytomegalovirus, CMV), HHV-6 (human B cell lymphotrophic virus) and HHV-7 are the other types of herpesvirus.

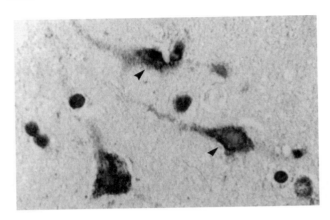

Figure 22. Herpes simplex in the brain.

Cytomegalovirus (CMV) is a herpes (DNA) virus group (Figure 23) that is distributed worldwide and is not often a problem except in individuals who are immunocompromised, such as the recipients of organ or bone marrow transplants or individuals with acquired immunodeficiency syndrome (AIDS). Histopathologically, typical inclusion bodies that resemble an owl's eye are found in multiple tissues. CMV is transmitted in the blood.

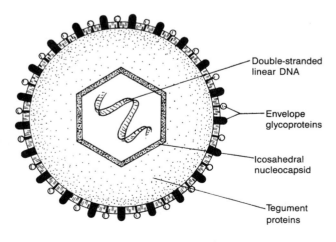

Double-stranded
linear DNA

Envelope
glycoproteins

Icosahedral
nucleocapsid

Tegument
proteins

Figure 21. Herpes virus.

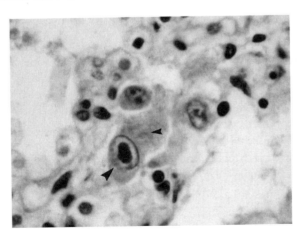

CMV inclusion bodies

▲ intranuclear and

▲ intracytoplasmic

Figure 23. Cytomegalovirus.

Owl eye appearance (Figure 24) consists of inclusions found by light microscopy in cytomegalovirus (CMV) infection. CMV-infected epithelial cells are enlarged and exhibit prominent eosinophilic intranuclear inclusions that are half the size of the nucleus and are encircled by a clear halo.

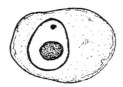

Figure 24. Owl Eye Appearance.

Chickenpox (varicella) is a human herpes virus type 3 (HHV-3) induced in acute infection that occurs usually in children less than 10 years of age. There is anorexia, malaise, low fever, and a prodromal rash following a two week incubation period. Erythematous papules appear in crops and intensify for three to four days. They are very pruritic. Complications include viral pneumonia, secondary bacterial infection, thrombocytopenia, glomerulonephritis, myocarditis, and other conditions. HHV-3 may become latent when chickenpox resolves. Its DNA may become integrated into the dorsal route ganglion cells. This may be associated with the development of Herpes zoster or shingles later in life.

Shingles (herpes zoster) is a viral infection that occurs in a band-like pattern according to distribution in the skin of involved nerves. It is usually a reactivation of the virus that causes chickenpox.

A **parvovirus** is a minute icosahedral virus comprised of single-stranded DNA that may replicate in previously uninfected host cells or in those already infected with adenovirus.

A **picornavirus** is a small RNA virus with a naked capsid structure. More than 230 viruses categorized as enteroviruses, rhinoviruses, cardioviruses, and aphthoviruses comprise this family.

Poliovirus (Figure 25) is a picornavirus of the genus enteroviridae. There are three polio serotypes. Polio and other enteroviruses are spread mainly by the fecal-oral route. Poliomyelitis occurs around the world; however, in the western hemisphere the wildtype virus has been eliminated by successful vaccines.

An **echovirus (enteric cytopathogenic human orphan virus)** is comprised of 30 types within the picornavirus family. It is cytopathic in cell culture and produces clinical manifestations in patients that include upper respiratory tract infections, diarrhea, exanthema, viremia, and sometimes poliomyelitis and viral meningitis.

A **rotavirus** (Figure 26) is a double-stranded RNA virus that is encapsulated and belongs to the reovirus family. It is 70 nm in diameter and causes epidemics of gastroenteritis,

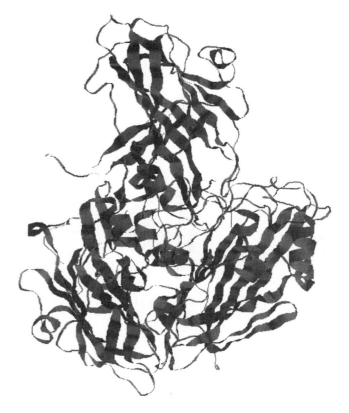

Figure 25. Type 3 Sabin strain human poliovirus.

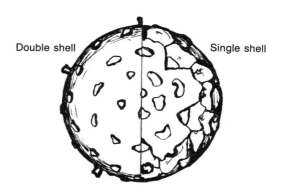

Figure 26. Rotavirus.

which are usually relatively mild but may be severe in children less than 2 years of age.

Rabies (Figure 27) is an infection produced by an RNA virus following a bite from an infected animal. The virus passes across the neuromuscular junction and infects the nerve from which it reaches the central nervous system. It also reaches salivary glands of lower animals. The virus infection leads to cerebral edema, congestion, round cell infiltration of the spinal cord and grey matter in the brain stem and profound loss of Purkinje cells. Negri bodies are found prominently in the medulla oblongata, hippocampus and cerebellum. Clinically, the fury associated with the disease is

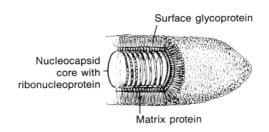

Figure 27. Rabies virus.

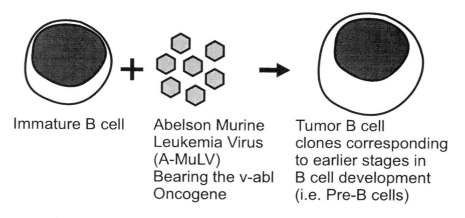

Figure 28. Abelson murine leukemia virus.

due to irritability of the central nervous system. There is fever, hyperethesia and anoxia aggression. It may be paralytic. Human rabies is rare in the United States. It is more common in other animals, with most of the cases appearing in skunks and raccoons. Fewer cases occur in bats, and only 2% each in dogs and cats. The virus is transmitted from one person to another by inhalation or by corneal transplantation, but not by human bites.

Abelson murine leukemia virus (A-MuLV) is a B cell murine leukemia inducing retrovirus that bears the v-*abl* oncogene (Figure 28). The virus has been used to immortalize immature B lymphocytes to produce pre-B cell or less differentiated B cell lines in culture. These have been useful in unraveling the nature of immunoglobulin differentiation such as H and L chain immunoglobulin gene assembly as well as class switching of immunoglobulin.

Hepatitis A (HAV) is a picornavirus which is also called enteovirus 72 (Figure 29). It is spread either person to person by the fecal-oral route or by consumption of contaminated water or food.

Hepatitis serology refers to hepatitis B antigens and antibodies against them (Figure 30). Core antigen is designated HBc. The HBc particle is comprised of double-stranded DNA and DNA polymerase. It has an association with HBe antigens. Core antigen signifies persistence of replicating hepatitis B virus. Anti-HBc antibody is a serologic indicator

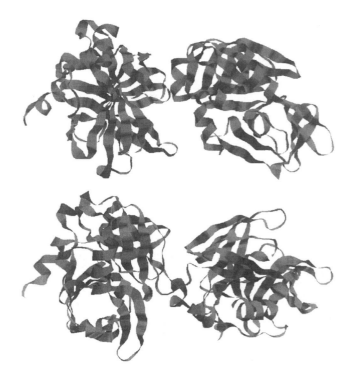

Figure 29. Hepatitis A virus 3C proteinase.

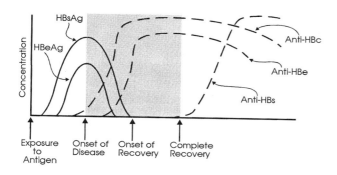

Figure 30. Hepatitis serology.

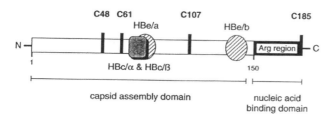

Figure 31. Schematic structure of the HBV core polypeptide. The 185 residue p21.5 polypeptide (genotype A) is shown with the amino-terminus (N) at the left and the carboxyl-terminus (C) at the right. The open region depicts the hydrophobic assimbly domain (a.a.s 1-149; open): the arg-rich nucleic acid binding region, also known as the protamine domain (a.a.s 150-185) is shown shaded. hatched ovals indicate the approximate locations of the Hbe/a and Hbe/b antigenic determinants: the shaded rectangle portrays the capsid-specific Hbc/α and Hbc/β epitopes which supposedly overlap Hbe/a. Also indicated are the four Cys esidues 48, 61, 107, and 185 (vertical bars).

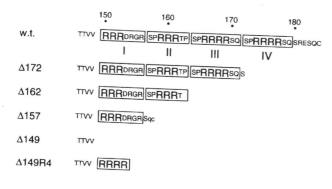

Figure 32. The protamine region of p21.5 contains four Arg-rich repeats that mediate interactions between the core protein and nucleic acid. Shown are the C-terminal amino acid sequences (residues 150-185) of wild-type (w.t.) p21.5 (top), as well as a seriew of trun-cated core proteins with defined endpoints.

of hepatitis B (Figures 31 and 32). It is an IgM antibody that increases early and is still detectable 20 years post infection. The IgM anti-HBc antibody assay is the one best antibody assay for acute hepatitis B. The HBe antigen (HBe) follows the same pattern as HBsAg antigen. When found, it

signifies a carrier state. The anti-HBe increases as HBe decreases. It appears in patients who are recovering and may last for years after the hepatitis has been resolved. The first antigen that is detectable following hepatitis B infection is surface antigen (HBs). It is detectable a few weeks before clinical disease and is highest with the first appearance of symptoms. This antigen disappears six months from infection. Antibody to HBs increases as the HBsAg levels diminish. Anti-HBs often is detectable for the lifetime of the individual.

A **hepatitis immunopathology panel** is a profile of assays that are very useful to establish the clinical and immune status of a patient believed to have hepatitis. The panel for acute hepatitis may include hepatitis B surface antigen (HBsAg), antibody to hepatitis B core antigen (anti-HBc), antihepatitis B surface antigen (anti-ABs), antihepatitis A (IgM), anti-HBe, and antihepatitis C. The panel for chronic hepatitis (carrier) includes all of these except for the antihepatitis A test.

HbsAg is the Hepatitis B virus envelope or surface antigen (Figure 33).

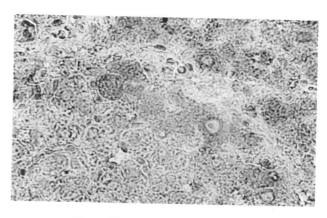

Figure 33. Hbs antigen in liver cells.

Chronic active hepatitis (autoimmune) is a disease that occurs in young females who may develop fever, arthralgias and skin rashes (Figure 34). They may be of the HLA-B8, -DR3 haplotype and suffer other autoimmune disorders. Most develop antibodies to smooth muscle, principally against actin, and autoantibodies to liver membranes. They also have other organ- and non-organ-specific autoantibodies. A polyclonal hypergammaglobulinemia may be present. Lymphocytes infiltrating portal areas destroy hepatocytes. Injury to liver cells produced by these infiltrating lymphocytes produces piecemeal necrosis. The inflammation and necrosis are followed by fibrosis and cirrhosis. The T cells infiltrating the liver are CD4+. Plasma cells are also present and immunoglobulins may be deposited on hepatocytes. The autoantibodies against liver cells do not play a pathogenetic role in liver injury. There are no sero-

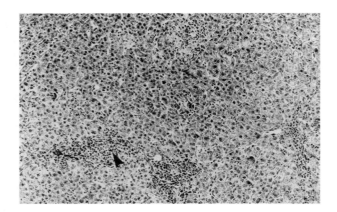

Figure 34. Chronic active hepatitis.

logic findings that are diagnostic. Corticosteroids are useful in treatment. The immunopathogenesis of autoimmune chronic active hepatitis involves antibody, K cell cytotoxicity and T cell reactivity against liver membrane antigens. Antibodies and specific T suppressor cells reactive with LSP are found in chronic active hepatitis patients, all of whom develop T cell sensitization against asialo-glycoprotein (AGR) antigen. Chronic active hepatitis has a familial predisposition.

A **DANE particle** (Figure 35) is a 42nm structure identified by electron microscopy in hepatitis B patients in the acute infective stage. The DANE particle has a 27nm-diameter icosahedral core that contains DNA polymerase.

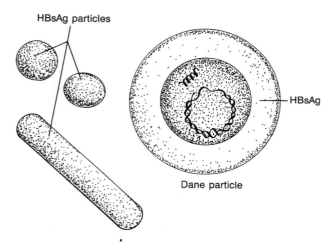

Figure 35. DANE particle.

A **prion** (Figure 36) is an infectious particle comprised of protein with appended carbohydrate. It is the most diminutive infectious agent known. The three human diseases in which prions have been implicated include kuru, Creutzfeldt-Jakob disease and Gerstmann-Straussler syndrome. They have also been implicated in the animal diseases: sheep and goat scrapie, bovine spongiform

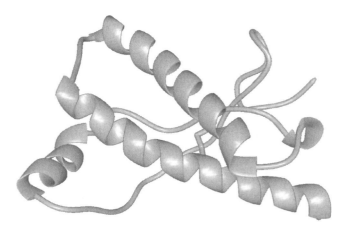

Figure 36. Prion.

encephalopathy, chronic wasting of elk and mule deer and transmissible mink encephalopathy. Prions do not induce inflammation nor do they stimulate antibody synthesis. They resist formalin, heat, ultraviolet radiation and other agents that normally inactivate viruses. They possess a 28kD hydrophobic glycoprotein particle that polymerizes forming an amyloid-like fibrillar structure.

Slow viruses are agents that induce infectious encephalitis following a lengthy latency. Slow viruses consist of conventional viruses and prions that are comprised of subverted cell proteins. Among the conventional group is measles, which induces subacute sclerosin panencephalitis, papovavirus, which induces progressive multifocal leukoencephalopathy, and rubella, which induces rare progressive rebella panencephalitis. The agents that cause kuru and Creutzfeldt-Jakob disease are among the nonconventional group of slow viruses.

Antibodies specific for viral antigenic determinants may offer early protection following viral infection. They interact with **viral capsid** (Figure 37) or envelope antigens, thereby inhibiting adherence and invasion of host cells. Antibodies may also act as opsonins that increase the attractiveness of viral particles to phagocytic cells. Secretory IgA antibody is important in neutralizing viruses on mucosal surfaces. Complement also facilitates phagocytosis and may be significant in viral lysis.

A **capsular polysaccharide** is a constituent of the protective coating around a number of bacteria such as the pneumonococus (*Streptococcus pneumoniae*) which stimulates the production of antibodies specific for its epitopes. In addition to the pneumonococcus, other microorganisms such as *Streptococci* and certain *Bacillus* species have polysaccharide capsules.

Immunization or vaccination against viruses often involves the use of an attentuated or killed virus vaccine. The anti-

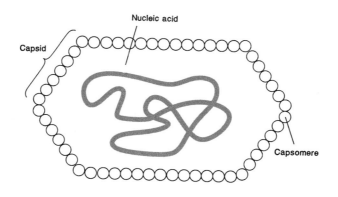

Figure 37.   Capsid.

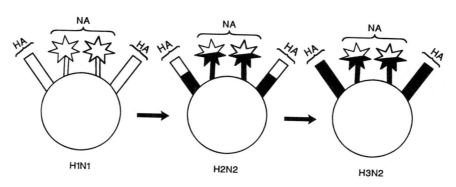

Figure 38.   Antigenic variation.

body induced is specific for the particular serologic type of the virus and protection is restricted to that serotype leaving the individual susceptible to the virus's remaining serotypes. Humoral immunity is of value only early during the course of virus infection and provides no immunity once host cells have been invaded. Antiviral immunity based upon antibody alone is insufficient to protect an individual against a viral infection. Virus neutralization does not necessarily reflect the protective action of a particular antibody.

Antiviral immunity depends primarily upon cytotoxic T cells. These cells are virus-specific CD8+ lymphocytes that can identify viral antigens presented in the context of class I MHC molecules on any virus-infected host cell with which they come into contact. The cytotoxic T lymphocytes lyse virus-infected host cells, activate intracellular enzymes that disassemble viral genomes and secrete lymphokines such as interferon.

Viruses that induce chronic infection persist for an extended period, complex with antibodies in the blood and are deposited in the vessels leading to vasculitis. Viruses may also produce disease through "molecular mimicry" in which an immune response is produced against selected amino acid sequences of the virus that are shared in common with host "self" antigens. Therefore, products of the immune reaction

(antibodies or T cells) crossreact with host tissues bearing the shared antigenic determinants, leading to injury.

Viruses are able to evade immune mechanisms. Besides the sanctuary viruses enjoy once they have entered host cells, these disease agents have additional means to escape host immune mechanisms. Viruses are especially adept at **antigenic variation** (Figure 38) whereby they may alter their surface antigenic structure once antibodies are formed against their original epitopes. This process may be repeated many times leading to the production of numerous strains of a particular virus that are antigenically and therefore serologically distinct. The **influenza** (Figures 39–41) and AIDS viruses are especially versatile in this regard.

Viruses may also induce immunosuppression in the host they infect. The AIDS virus (HIV-1) is well known to target CD4+ helper/inducer lymphocytes that are central to mounting any type of immune response. Selected viruses such as the **Epstein-Barr virus** (Figure 42) may induce immunosuppression by mechanisms that are yet to be determined but possibly attributable to genes that encode substances that dampen antiviral immune responsiveness.

Specific immune responses can be mounted against parasites. Parasites such as protozoa and helminths elicit a variety of immune responses. Helminthic infections including

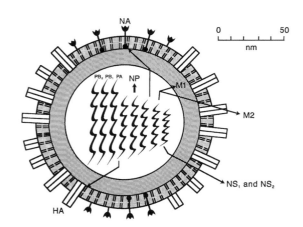

Figure 39.   Influenza virus.

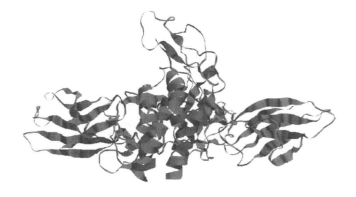

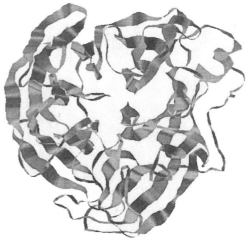

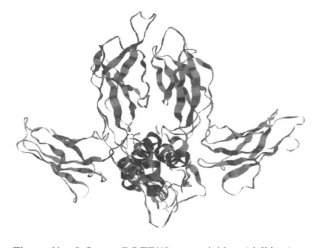

Figure 41.   Influenza B/LEE/40 neuraminidase (sialidase).

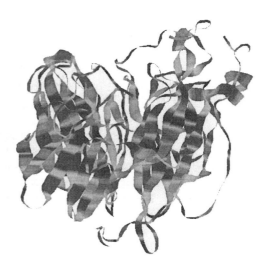

Figure 40.   Influenza A subtype N2 neuraminidase (sialidase). A/Tokyo/3/67.

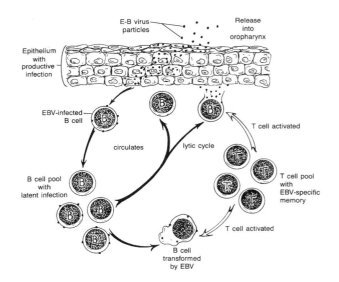

Figure 42.   Epstein-Barr virus-host interaction.

Nippostrongylus, schistosomes, and filaria evoke titers of IgE that exceed those induced by other infectious agents. Helminths specifically stimulate CD4+ helper T lymphocytes that form IL-4 and IL-5. ADCC involving eosinophils and IgE antibody is believed to be effective in immunity against helminths since the major basic protein in eosinophil granules is toxic to helminths. Coating helminths with IgE specific antibody followed by eosinophil attachment through the Fc regions leads to ADCC by eosinophils.

Ablastin is an antibody with the exclusive property of preventing reproduction of such agents as the rat parasite *Trypanosoma lewisi* (Figure 43). It does not demonstrate other antibody functions.

Parasites such as *Schistosoma mansoni* produce eggs that induce granuloma formation in such organs as the liver. Stimulated CD4+ T lymphocytes activate macrophages, which leads to granuloma formation and isolation of the eggs. The development of fibrosis interrupts the venous blood supply to the liver, leading to hypertension and cirrhosis.

Intracellular protozoa often activate specific cytotoxic T cells. They represent a critical mechanism to prevent dissemination of intracellular malarial parasites. Parasite antigen-antibody (immune) complexes may be trapped in the renal microvasculature leading to immune complex glomerulonephritis.

Parasites are capable of evading immune mechanisms. Animal parasites have developed remarkable mechanisms to

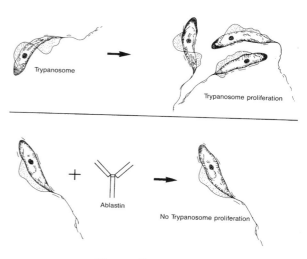

Figure 43.   Ablastin.

establish chronic infections in the vertebrate host. Natural immunity to them is weak, and the parasites have devised novel and ingenious mechanisms to circumvent specific immunity. Parasites either camouflage their own antigens or interfere with host immunity. Some parasites mask their antigens by coating themselves with host proteins, which prevents their detection by host immune mechanisms. Some develop resistance by biochemical alterations of their surface coat. They are also adept at changing their surface antigens by antigenic variation which may frustrate attempts to prophylactic immunization. Other parasites, such as *Entamoeba histolytica*, may shed their antigenic coats.

23

Immunologic Methods:
Measurement of Antigens and Antibodies

Just as the eclectic science of immunology intersects essentially all of the basic biological sciences, it makes use of many biochemical techniques such as chromatography and protein fractionation. It also employs the newer methods of molecular genetics such as gene sequencing and related techniques. Advances in technology have armed the immunologist with the powerful tools of PCR technology, immunophenotyping by flow cytometry, hybridomas and monoclonal antibodies, DNA typing, enzyme-linked immnosorbent assay (ELISA), and radiolabelling of immune system molecules. In addition, the time honored methods of precipitation, agglutination, complement fixation and related techniques long have been used by the immunologist. Since its inception, immunologic science has not only maintained a unique nomenclature but also special techniques that elucidated some of Nature's most jealously guarded secrets through scientific investigation. Inbred mice, of known genetic constitution, and more recently transgenic animals, including knockout mice, offer new avenues for elucidating

some of immunology's most perplexing conundrums. Great tomes are currently available that describe the myriad of Immunological techniques now available. A representative number of the more commonly used ones are described here (Figures 1–4).

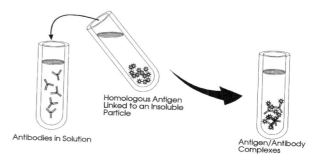

Figure 1. Absorption is the elimination of antibodies from a mixture by adding soluble antigens or the elimination of soluble antigen from a mixture by adding antibodies.

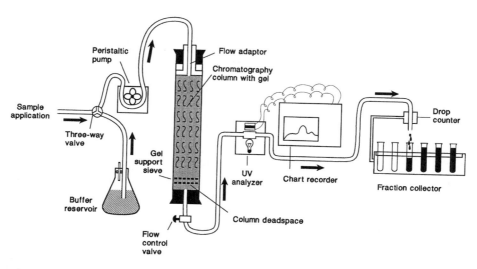

Figure 2. Column Chromatography. Arrows indicate direction of flow. Chromatography refers to a group of methods employed for the separation of proteins.

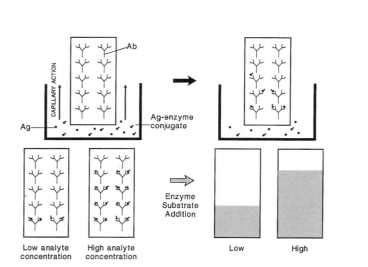

Figure 3.   Immunochromatography.

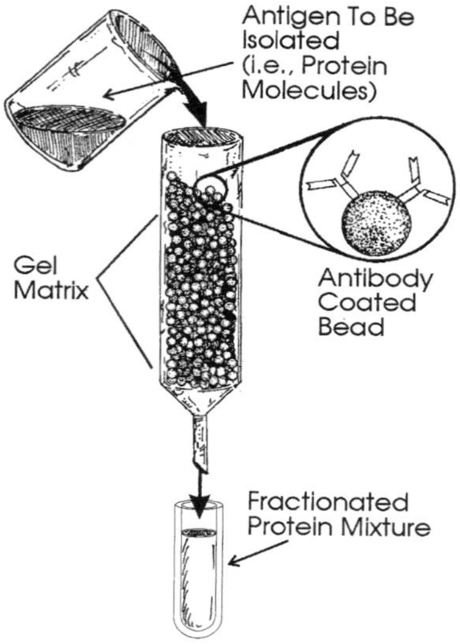

Figure 4.   Absorption chromatography is a method to separate molecules based on their absorptive characteristics. Fluid is passed over a fixed solid stationary phase.

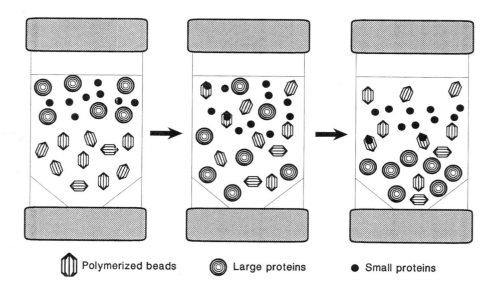

🔷 Polymerized beads   ◎ Large proteins   ● Small proteins

Figure 5.   Gel filtration chromatography.

Gel filtration chromatography (Figure 5) is a method that permits the separation of molecules on the basis of size. Porous beads are allowed to swell in buffer, water or other solutions and are packed into a column. The molecular pores of the beads will permit the entry of some molecules into them but exclude others on the basis of size. Molecules larger than the pores will pass through the column and emerge with the void volume. Since the solute molecules within the beads maintain a concentration equilibrium with solutes in the liquid phase outside the beads, molecular species of a given weight, shape, and degree of hydration move as a band. Gel chromatography using spherical agarose

gel particles is useful in the exclusion of IgM, which is present in the first peak. Of course, other molecules of similar size, such as macroglobulins are also present in this peak. IgG is present in the second peak, but the fractions of the leading side are contaminated by IgA and IgD.

Doubling dilution (Figures 6–8) is a technique used in serology to prepare serial dilutions of serum. A fixed quantity (one volume) of physiologic saline is added to each of a row of serological tubes except for the first tube in the row which receives two volumes of serum. One volume of the serum from the first tube is added to the one volume of saline

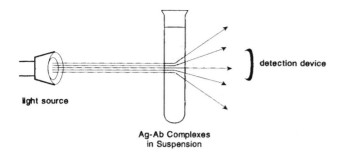

Figure 6. Turbidimetry is the quantification of a substance in suspension based on the suspension's ability to reduce forward light transmission.

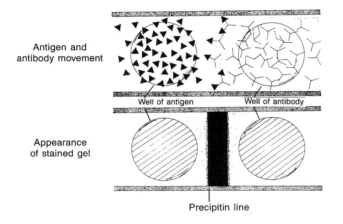

Figure 7. Gel diffusion is a method to evaluate antibodies and antigens based upon their diffusion in gels toward one another and their reaction at the point of contact in the gel.

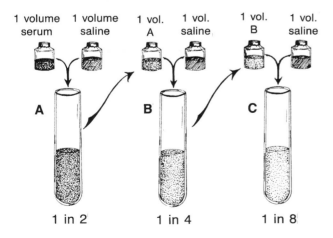

Figure 8. Doubling dilution.

in the second tube. After thoroughly mixing the contents with the transfer pipette, one volume of the second tube is transferred to the third, and the procedure is repeated down the row. This same volume is then discarded from the final tube after the contents have been thoroughly mixed. Thus, the serum dilution in each tube is double that in the preceding tube. The first tube is undiluted, the second contains a 1:2 dilution, the third a 1:4, the fourth a 1:8, etc.

Single immunodiffusion (Mancini technique) is: (1) A technique in which antibody is incorporated into agar gel and antigen is placed in a well that has been cut into the surface of the antibody-containing agar (Figure 9). Following diffusion of the antigen into the agar, a ring of precipitation forms at the point where antigen and antibody have reached equivalence. The diameter of the ring is used to quantify the antigen concentration by comparing with antigen standards. (2) The addition of antigen to a tube containing gel into which specific antibody has been incorporated. Lines of precipitation form at the site of interaction between equivalent quantities of antigen and antibody.

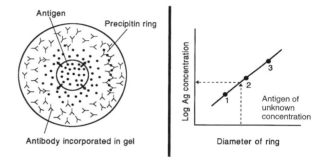

Figure 9. Single immunodiffusion (Mancini technique).

Single radial immunodiffusion (Figure 10) is a technique to quantify antigens. Plates are poured in which antibody is incorporated into agar, wells are cut and precise quantities of antigen placed in them. The antigen is permitted to diffuse into the agar containing antibody and produce a ring of precipitation upon interaction with the antibody. As diffusion proceeds, an excess of antigen develops in the area of the precipitate causing it to dissolve only to form once again at a greater distance from the site of origin. At the point where antigen and antibody have reached equivalence in the agar, a precipitation ring is produced. The precipitation ring encloses an area proportional to the concentration of antigen measured 48–72 hours following diffusion. Standard curves are employed using known antigen standards. The antigen concentration is determined from the diameter of the precipitation ring. This method can detect as little as 1–3:g/ml of antigen. Known also as the Mancini technique.

Radioimmunoassay (RIA) refers to a technique to assay either antigen or antibody which is based on radiolabeled

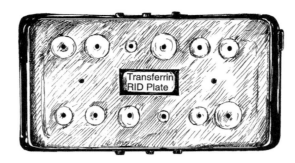

Figure 10.   Single radial immunodiffusion.

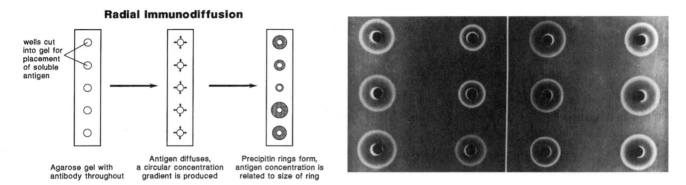

Radial Immunodiffusion

wells cut
into gel for
placement
of soluble
antigen

Agarose gel with
antibody throughout

Antigen diffuses,
a circular concentration
gradient is produced

Precipitin rings form,
antigen concentration is
related to size of ring

Figure 11.   Radial Immunodiffusion.

Figure 12.   Single Radial Immunodiffusion.

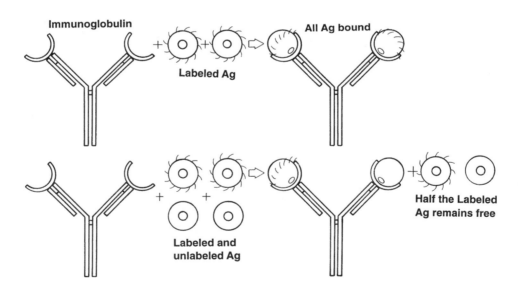

Immunoglobulin

Labeled Ag

All Ag bound

Labeled and
unlabeled Ag

Half the Labeled
Ag remains free

Figure 13.   Radioimmunoassay (RIA).

antigen competitively inhibiting the binding of antigen which is not labeled to specific antibodies (Figures 11–13). Minute quantities of enzymes, hormones or other immunogenic substances can be assayed by RIA. Enzyme immunoassays are largely replacing RIAs because of the problems associated with radioisotope regulation and disposal.

The **double diffusion test** (Figure 14) is a test in which solutions of antigen and of antibody are placed in separate wells of a gel containing electrolytes. The antigen and antibody diffuse toward one another until their molecules meet at the point of equivalence and precipitate, forming a line of precipitation in the gel. In addition to the two-dimensional

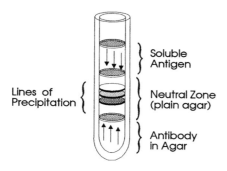

Figure 14. Double diffusion test.

technique, double immunodiffusion may be accomplished in a tube as a one dimensional technique. The Oakley-Fulthorpe test is an example of this type of reaction. This technique may be employed to detect whether antigens are similar or different or share epitopes. It may also be used to investigate antigen and antibody purity. Refer also to reaction of identity, reaction of nonidentity and reaction of partial identity.

Two-dimensional gel electrophoresis refers to a method used to characterize a protein. The protein to be analyzed is subjected to isoelectric focusing by placing the soluble protein in a pH gradient and applying an electrical charge. The protein moves to the pH where it has a neutral charge. This is followed by electrophoresis in gel at a 90° angle to separate the proteins according to size. This procedure yields a pattern known as a fingerprint that is very specific.

Immunoelectrophoresis (IEP) (Figure 15) is a method to identify antigens on the basis of their electrophoretic mobility, diffusion in gel, and formation of precipitation arcs with specific antibody. Electrophoresis in gel is combined with diffusion of a specific antibody in gel medium containing electrolyte to identify separated antigenic substances. The presence or absence of immunoglobulin molecules of various classes in a serum sample may be identified in this way. One percent agar containing electrolyte is layered onto microscope slides, allowed to gel, and patterns of appropriate troughs and wells are cut in the solidified medium. Antigen to be

identified is placed in the circular wells cut into the agar medium. This is followed by electrophoresis, which permits separation of the antigenic components according to their electrophoretic mobility, and antiserum is placed in a long trough in the center of the slide. After antibody has diffused through the agar toward each separated antigen, percipitin arcs form where the antigen and antibody interact. Abnormal amounts of immunoglobulins result in changes in the shape and position of precipitation arcs when compared with the arcs formed by antibody against normal human serum components. With monoclonal gammapathies, the arcs become broad, bulged, and displaced. The absence of immunoglobulin classes such as those found in certain immunodeficiencies can also be detected with IEP.

An **Oudin test** (Figure 16) is a type of precipitation in gel that involves single diffusion. Antiserum, incorporated into agar is placed in a narrow test tube. This is overlaid with an antigen solution which diffuses into the agar to yield precipitation rings. Also called single radial diffusion test. A band of precipitation forms at the equivalence point.

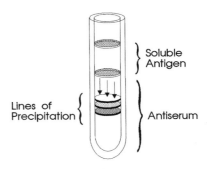

Figure 16. Oudin test.

The **Ouchterlony test** (Figure 17) is a double diffusion in gel type of precipitation test. Antigen and antibody solutions are placed in separate wells that have been cut into an agar plate prepared with electrolyte. As the antigen and antibody diffuse through the gel medium, a line of precipitation forms at the point of contact between antigen and antibody. Results are expressed as reaction of identity, reaction of partial identity or reaction of nonidentity. Refer to those entries for further details.

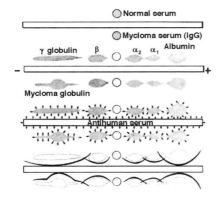

Figure 15. Immunoelectrophoresis (IEP).

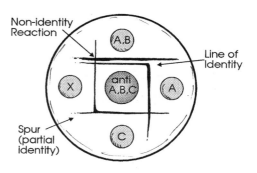

Figure 17. Ouchterlony test.

The **Oakley-Fulthorpe test** (Figure 18) is a double diffusion type of precipitation test performed by incorporating antibody into agar which is placed in the tube followed by a layer of plain agar. A solution of antigen is placed on top of the plain agar in the tube and precipitation occurs where antigen and antibody meet in the plain agar layer.

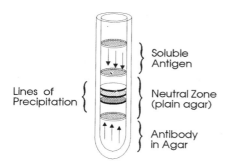

Figure 18. Oakley-Fulthorpe test.

The **Elek plate** (Figure 19) is a method to show toxin production by *Corynebacterium diphtheriae* colonies growing on an agar plate. Diphtheria antitoxin impregnated into a strip of filter paper is placed at a right angle to a streak of the microorganisms on the agar plate. Toxin formation by the growing microbes interacts with antitoxin in the filter paper to form a line of precipitation.

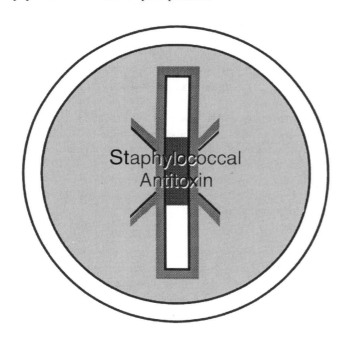

Plasma - agar plate showing
staphylocoagulase effect
inhibited by commercial antitoxin

Figure 19. Elek plate.

Rocket electrophoresis (Figure 20) describes the electrophoresis of antigen into agar-containing specific antibody. In this electro-immunodiffusion method, lines of precipitation formed in the agar by the antigen-antibody interaction assume the shape of a rocket. The antigen concentration can be quantified since the rocket-like area is proportional to the antigen concentration. This can be deduced by comparing with antigen standards. This technique has the advantage of speed since it can be completed within hours instead of longer periods required for single radial immunodiffusion. Also called Laurell rocket electrophoresis.

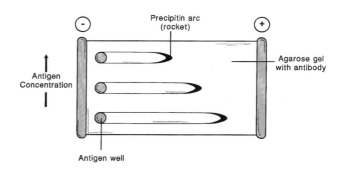

Figure 20. Rocket electrophoresis.

Electroimmunodiffusion (Figure 21) is a double diffusion in gel method in which antigen and antibody are forced toward one another in an electrical field. Precipitation occurs at the site of their interaction. Refer to Laurell rocket test and rocket immunoelectrophoresis.

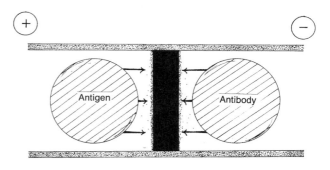

Figure 21. Electroimmunodiffusion.

The **Farr technique** (Figure 22) is an assay to measure primary binding of antibody with antigen as opposed to secondary manifestations of antibody–antigen interactions such as precipitation, agglutination, etc. It is a quantitation of an antiserum's antigen-binding properties. It is appropriate for antibodies of all immunoglobulin classzotized benzidine. A chemical substance that serves as a bivalent coupling agent that can link to protein molecules. It contains the cation. This method was used in the past to conjugate erythrocytes with antigens for use in the passive agglutination test.

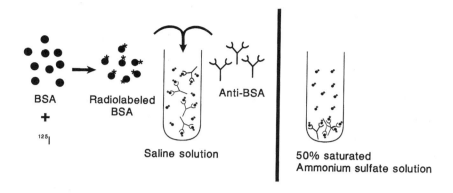

Figure 22. Farr technique.

Bis-diazotized benzidine refers to a chemical substance that serves as a bivalent coupling agent that can link to protein molecules (Figure 23). It contains the cation. This method was used in the past to conjugate erythrocytes with antigens for use in the passive agglutination test.

$$Cl^- \overset{+}{N}N - \bigotimes - \bigotimes - N\overset{+}{N} \ Cl^-$$

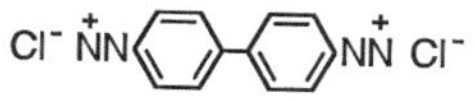

Figure 23. Bis-diazotized benzidine.

Hemagglutination (Figure 24) is the aggregation of red blood cells by antibodies, viruses, lectin, or other substances. The Hemagglutination inhibition test is an assay for antibody or antigen based on the ability to interfere with red blood cell aggregation. Certain viruses are able to agglutinate red blood cells. In the presence of antiviral antibody, the ability to agglutinate erythrocytes is inhibited. Thus, this serves as a basis to assay the antibody.

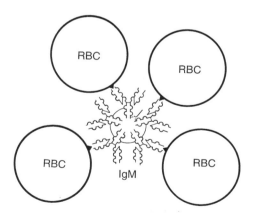

Figure 24. Hemagglutination.

The **Latex fixation test** (Figure 25) is a technique in which latex particles are used as passive carriers of soluble antigens adsorbed to their surfaces. Antibodies specific for the adsorbed antigen then cause agglutination of the coated latex particles. This has been widely used and is the basis of a rheumatoid arthritis test in which pooled human IgG molecules are coated on the surface of latex particles, which are then agglutinated by anti-immunoglobulin antibodies in the sera of rheumatoid arthritis patients.

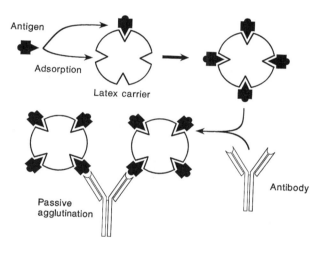

Figure 25. Latex fixation test.

Mixed agglutination (Figure 26) describes the aggregation (agglutination) produced when morphologically dissimilar cells that share a common antigen are reacted with antibody specific for this epitope. The technique is useful in demonstrating antigens on cells which by virtue of their size or irregular shape are not suitable for study by conventional agglutination tests. It is convenient to use an indicator, such as a red cell which possesses the antigen being sought. Thus, the demonstration of mixed agglutination in which the indicator cells are linked to the other cell type suspected of possessing the common antigen constitutes a positive test.

The **passive agglutination test** (Figure 27) is an assay to recognize antibodies against soluble antigens which are attached to erythrocytes, latex or other particles by either adsorption or chemical linkage. In the presence of antibodies specific for the antigen, aggregation of the passenger particles occurs. Examples of this technique include the RA latex

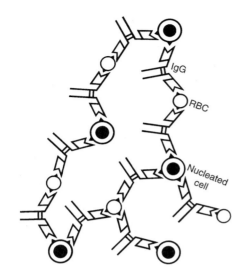

Figure 26. Mixed agglutination.

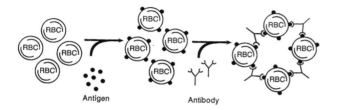

Figure 27. Passive agglutination test.

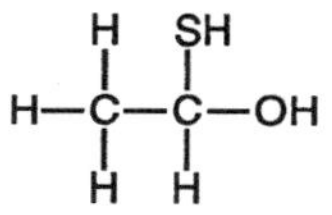

$$H-\overset{\displaystyle H}{\underset{\displaystyle H}{C}}-\overset{\displaystyle SH}{\underset{\displaystyle H}{C}}-OH$$

Figure 28. 2-mercaptoethanol agglutination test.

agglutination test, the tanned red cell technique, the bentonite flocculation test and the bis-diazotized benzidine test.

The **2-Mercaptoethanol agglutination test** (Figure 28) is a simple test to determine whether or not an agglutinating antibody is of the IgM class. If treatment of an antibody preparation, such as a serum sample, with 2-mercaptoethanol can abolish the serum's ability to produce agglutination of cells, then agglutination was due to IgM antibody. Agglutination induced by IgG antibody is unaffected by 2-mercaptoethanol treatment and just as effective after the treatment as it was before. Dithiothreitol (DTT) produces the same effect as 2-mercaptoethanol in this test.

The **Raji cell assay** (Figure 29) is an *in vitro* assay for immune complexes in serum. The technique employs Raji cells, a lymphoblastoid B lymphocyte tumor cell line that expresses receptors for complement receptor 1, complement receptor 2, FC and C1q receptors. The cell line does not express surface immunoglobulins. Following combination of Raji cells with the serum sample, the immune complex is bound and quantified using radiolabeled F(ab')$_2$ fragments of antibodies against IgG.

In the **complement fixation reaction** (Figure 30) the primary union of antigen with antibody takes place almost instantaneously and is invisible. A measured amount of complement present in the reaction mixture is taken up by complexes of antigen and antibody. The consumption or binding of complement by antigen-antibody complexes. This serves as the basis for a serologic assay in which antigen is combined with a serum specimen suspected of containing the homologous antibody. Following the addition of a measured amount of complement, which is fixed or consumed only if antibody was present in the serum and has formed a complex with the antigen, sheep red blood cells sensitized (coated) with specific antibody are added to determine whether or not complement has been fixed in the first phase of the reaction. Failure of the sensitized sheep red blood cells to lyse constitutes a positive test since no complement is available. However, sheep red blood cell lysis indicates that complement was not consumed during the first phase of the reaction, implying that homologous antibody was not present in the serum, and complement remains free to lyse the sheep red blood cells sensitized with antibody. Hemolysis constitutes a negative reaction. The sensitivity of the

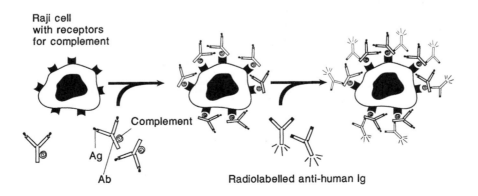

Figure 29. Raji cell assay.

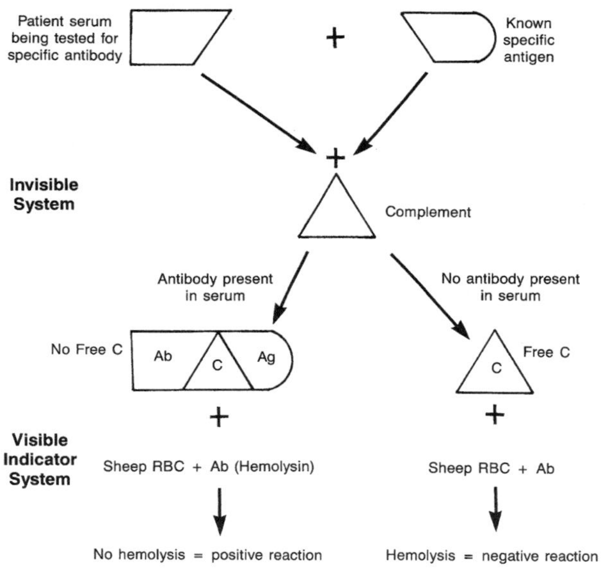

Figure 30. Complement fixation reaction.

complement fixation test falls between that of agglutination and precipitation. Complement fixation tests may be carried out in microtiter plates, which are designed for the use of relatively small volumes of reagents. The lysis of sheep red blood cells sensitized with rabbit antibody is measured either in a spectrophotometer at 413nm or by the release of ^{51}Cr from red cells that have been previously labeled with the isotope. Complement fixation can detect either soluble or insoluble antigen. Its ability to detect virus antigens in impure tissue preparations makes the test still useful in diagnosis of virus infections.

The **complement fixation assay** is a serologic test based on the fixation of complement by antigen-antibody complexes. It has been applied to many antigen-antibody systems and was widely used earlier in the century as a serologic test for syphilis.

Fluorescein (Figure 31) is a yellow dye that stains with brilliant apple green fluorescence. Its isothiocyanate derivative is widely employed to label proteins such as immunoglobulins that are useful in diagnostic medicine as well as in basic science research.

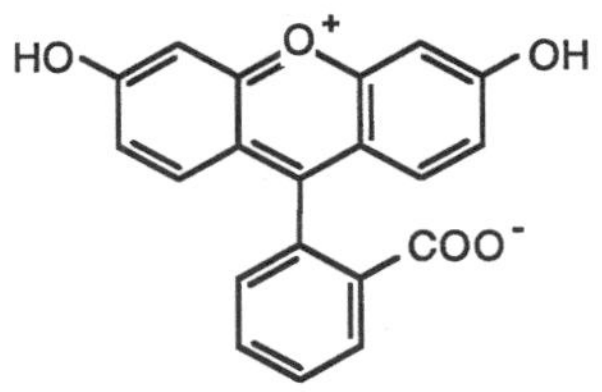

Figure 31. Flourescein.

Fluorescein isothiocyanate (Figure 32) is a widely used fluorochrome for labeling antibody molecules. It may also be used to label other proteins. Fluorescein-labeled antibodies are popular because they appear apple-green under ultraviolet irradiation, permitting easy detection of antigens of interest in tissues and cells. FITC fluoresces at 490 and 520 nm. FITC-labeled antibodies are useful for the demonstration of immune deposits in both skin and kidney biopsies.

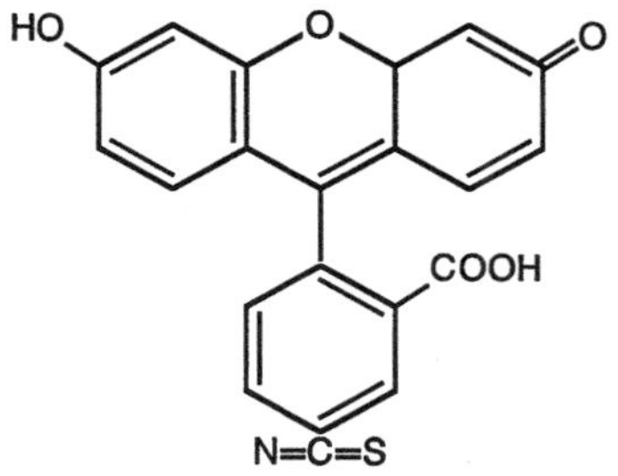

Figure 32. Fluorescein isothiocyanate (FITC).

The **fluorescent antibody technique** (Figures 33–36) is an immunofluorescence method in which antibody labeled with a fluorochrome such as fluorescein isothiocyanate (FITC) is used to identify antigen in tissues or cells when examined by ultraviolet light used in fluorescence microscopy. Besides the direct technique, antigens in tissue sections treated with unlabeled antibody can be "counterstained" with fluorescein-labeled antiimmunoglobulin to localize antigen in tissues by the indirect immunofluorescence method. The indirect fluorescence antibody technique is a method to identify antibody or antigen using a fluorochrome-labeled antibody which combines with an intermediate antibody or antigen rather than directly with the antibody or antigen being sought. The indirect test has a greater sensitivity than those of the direct fluorescence antibody technique. It is often referred to as the sandwich or double layer method.

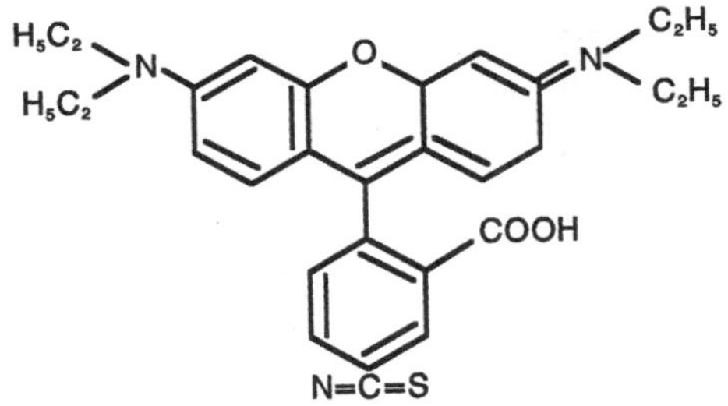

Figure 33. Rhodamine B isothiocyanate is a reddish-orange fluorochrome used to label immunoglobulins or other proteins for use in immunofluorescence studies.

The **direct fluorescence antibody method** (Figure 37) employs antibodies, either polyclonal or monoclonal, labeled with a fluorochrome such as fluorescein isothiocyanate, which yields an apple green color by immunofluorescence

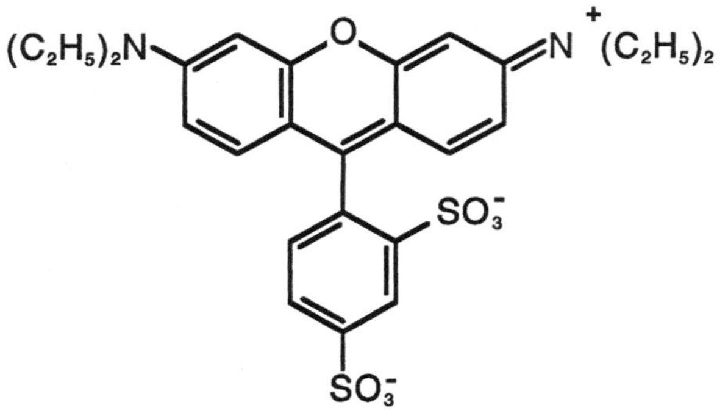

Figure 34. Rhodamine disulfonic acid is a red fluorochrome used in immunofluorescence.

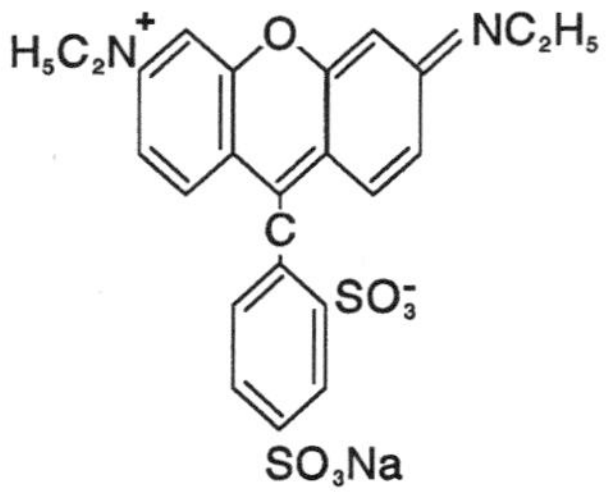

Figure 35. Lissamine rhodamine (RB200) is a fluorochrome that produces orange fluorescence. Interaction with phosphorus pentachloride yields a reactive sulphonyl chloride that is useful for labeling protein molecules to be used in immunofluorescence staining methods.

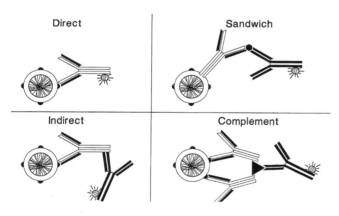

Figure 36. Flourescent antibody technique.

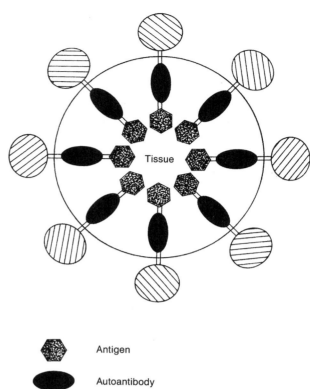

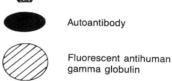

Antigen

Autoantibody

Fluorescent antihuman gamma globulin

Figure 37. Direct flourescence antibody technique.

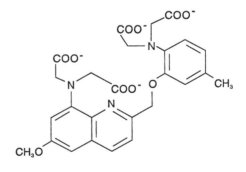

Figure 38. Quin-2.

microscopy, or rhodamine isothiocyanate, which yields a reddish-orange color, to identify a specific antigen. This technique is routinely used in immunofluorescence evaluation of renal biopsy specimens as well as skin biopsy preparations to detect immune complexes comprised of the various immunoglobulin classes or complement components.

Quin-2 (Figure 38) is a derivative of quinoline which combines with free Ca⁺⁺ to accentuate fluorescence intensity. It can be introduced into cells as an ester followed by de-esterification. When T or B lymphocytes containing Quin-2 are activated, their fluorescence intensity rises implying an elevation of free Ca⁺⁺ in the cytosol.

Ferritin labeling (Figure 39) is achieved by conjugating ferritin to antibody molecules to render them visible in histologic or cytologic specimens observed by electron microscopy. Antibodies may be labeled with ferritin by use of a cross-linking reagent such as toluene-2,4-diisocyanate. The ferritin-labeled antibody may be reacted directly with the specimen, or ferritin-labeled anti-immunoglobulin may be

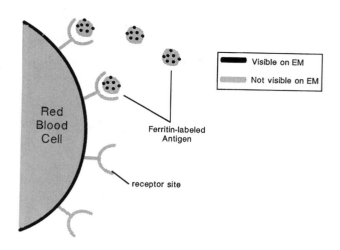

Figure 39.   Ferritin labeling.

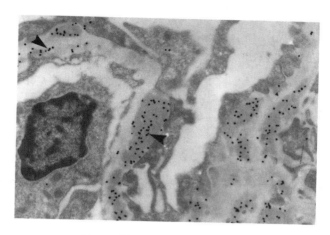

Figure 41.   Immunogold labeling.

used to react with unlabeled specific antibody attached to the target tissue antigen.

The **immunoferritin method** (Figure 40) is a technique to aid detection by electron microscopy of sites where antibody interacts with antigen of cells and tissues. Immunoglobulin may be conjugated with ferritin, an electron-dense marker, without altering its immunological reactivity. These ferritin-labeled antibodies localize molecules of antigen in subcellular areas. Electron-dense ferritin permits visualization of antibody binding to homologous antigen in cells and tissues by electron microscopy. In addition to ferritin, horseradish peroxidase-labeled antibodies may also be adapted for use in immunoelectron microscopy.

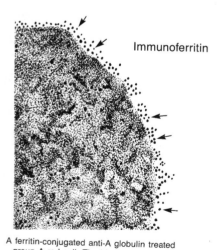

Immunoferritin

A ferritin-conjugated anti-A globulin treated group A red cell. The binding of ferritin particles to the surface of the erythrocyte denotes the site of the antigen.

Figure 40.   Immunoferritin method.

Immunogold labeling (Figure 41) is a technique to identify antigens in tissue preparations by electron microscopy. Sections are incubated with primary antibody followed by

treatment with colloidal gold-labeled anti-IgG antibody. Electron dense particles are localized at sites of antigen-antibody interactions.

The **immunoperoxidase method** (Figure 42) was introduced by Nakene and Pierce in 1966 who proposed that enzymes be used in the place of fluorochromes as labels for antibodies. Horseradish peroxidase (HRP) is the enzyme label most widely employed. The immunoperoxidase technique permits the demonstration of antigens in various types of cells and fixed tissues. This method has certain advantages that include: (1) the use of conventional light microscopy; (2) the stained preparations may be kept permanently; (3) the method may be adapted for use with electron microscopy of tissues; and (4) counterstains may be employed. The disadvantages include: (1) the demonstration of relatively minute positively staining areas is limited by the light microscope's resolution; (2) endogenous peroxidase may not have been completely eliminated from the tissue under investigation; and (3) diffusion of products resulting from the enzyme reaction away from the area where antigen is localized.

The **peroxidase-antiperoxidase (PAP)** technique employs unlabeled antibodies and a PAP reagent. This has proven highly successful for the demonstration of antigens in paraffin embedded tissues as an aid in surgical pathologic diagnosis. Tissue sections preserved in paraffin are first treated with xylene and after deparaffinization they are exposed to hydrogen peroxide solution which destroys the endogenous peroxidase activity in tissue. The sections are next incubated with normal swine serum which suppresses nonspecific binding of immunoglobulin molecules to tissues containing collagen. Thereafter, the primary rabbit antibody against the antigen to be identified is reacted with the tissue section. Primary antibody that is unbound is removed by rinsing the sections which are then covered with swine antibody against rabbit immunoglobulin. This so-called linking antibody will combine with any primary rabbit antibody in the tissue. It is added in excess which will result in one of its antigen-binding sites remaining free. After washing, the peroxidase-antiperoxidase (PAP) is

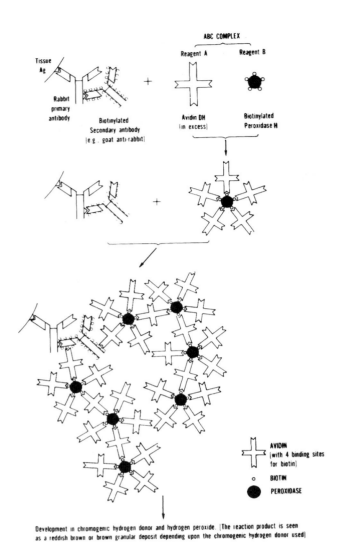

Figure 42.   Immunoperoxidase method.

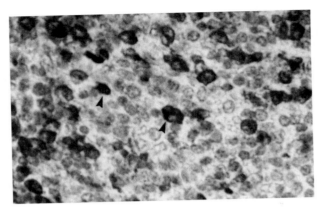

Figure 43.   Plasma cells decorated with antibody.

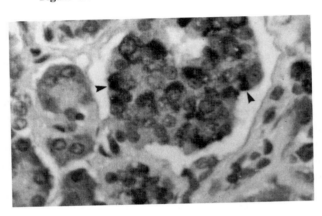

Figure 44.   Insulin in J cells.

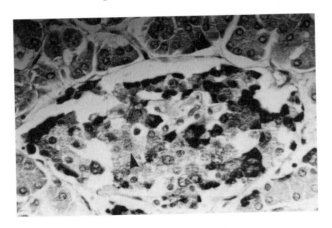

Figure 45.   Chromogranin.

placed on the section, and the antibody portion of this complex which is raised in rabbits will be bound to the free antigen-binding site of the linking antibody on the sections. The unbound PAP complex is then washed away by rinsing. To read the sections microscopically it is necessary to add a substrate of hydrogen peroxide and aminoethylcarbazole (AEC) which permits formation of a visible product that may be detected with the light microscope. The AEC is oxidized to produce a reddish brown pigment that is not water soluble. Peroxidase catalyzes the reaction. Because peroxidase occurs only at sites where the PAP is bound via linking antibody and primary antibody to antigen molecules, the antigen is identified by the reddish brown pigment. The tissue sections can then be counterstained with hematoxylin or other suitable dye, covered with mounting medium and cover slips, and read by conventional light microscopy. The PAP technique has been replaced, in part, by the avidin-biotin complex (ABC) technique.

The **PAP (peroxidase-antiperoxidase) technique** (Figures 43–47) is a method for immunoperoxidase staining of tissue to identify antigens with antibodies. This method employs unlabeled antibodies and a PAP reagent. The same PAP complex may be used for dozens of different unlabeled antibody specificities. If the primary antibody against the antigen being sought is made in the rabbit, then tissue sections treated with this reagent are exposed to sheep anti-rabbit immunoglobulin followed by the peroxidase-antiperoxidase

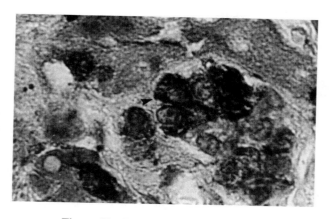

Figure 46.   Prolactin staining in pituitary.

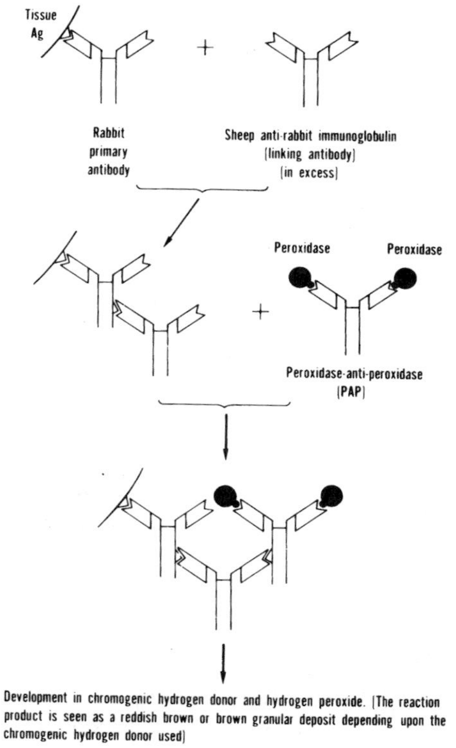

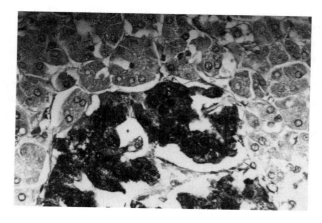

Development in chromogenic hydrogen donor and hydrogen peroxide. (The reaction product is seen as a reddish brown or brown granular deposit depending upon the chromogenic hydrogen donor used)

Figure 47.   PAP technique.

(PAP) complex. For human primary antibody, an additional step must link the human antibody into the rabbit sandwich technique. Paraffin-embedded tissue sections are first treated with xylene and after deparaffinization, they are exposed to hydrogen peroxide to destroy the endogenous peroxidase. Sections are next incubated with normal sheep serum to suppress nonspecific binding of immunoglobulin to tissue collagen. Primary rabbit antibody against the antigen to be identified is combined with the tissue section. Unbound primary antibody is removed by rinsing the sections which are then covered with sheep antibody against rabbit immunoglobulin. This linking antibody will combine with any primary

rabbit antibody in the tissue. It is added in excess which results in one of its antigen-binding sites remaining free. After washing, the peroxidase-antiperoxidase (PAP) is placed in the section, and the rabbit antibody part of this complex will be bound to the free antigen binding site of the linking antibody. The unbound PAP complex is then washed away by rinsing. A substrate of hydrogen peroxide and aminoethyl-carbazole (AEC) is placed on the tissue section leading to formation of a visible color reaction product which can be seen by light microscopy. Peroxidase is localized only at sites where the PAP is bound via linking antibody and primary antibody to antigen molecules, permitting the antigen to be identified as an area of reddish-brown pigment. Tissues may be counterstained with hematoxylin.

Neuron specific enolase (NSE) (Figure 48) is an enzyme of neurons and neuroendocrine cells as well as their derived tumors, e.g., oat cell carcinoma of lung, demonstrable by immunoperoxidase staining. NSE occurs also in some neoplasms not derived from neurons or endocrine cells.

Figure 48.   Neuron specific enolase.

The **enzyme-linked immunosorbent assay (ELISA)** (Figure 49) is an immunoassay which employs an enzyme linked to either anti-immunoglobulin or antibody specific for antigen and detects either antibody or antigen. This method is based on the sandwich or double layer technique, in which an enzyme rather than a fluorochrome is used as the label. In this method, antibody is attached to the surface of plastic tubes, wells or beads to which the antigen-containing test sample is added. If antibody is being sought in the test sample, then antigen should be attached to the plastic surface. Following antigen-antibody interaction, the enzyme-anti-immunoglobulin conjugate is added. The ELISA test is read by incubating the reactants with an appropriate substrate to yield a colored product that is measured in a spectrophotometer. Alkaline phosphatase and horseradish peroxidase are enzymes that are often employed. ELISA methods have replaced many radioimmunoassays because of their lower cost, safety, speed and simplicity in performing.

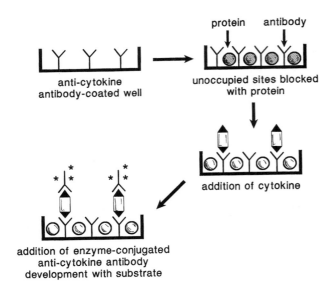

Figure 49. ELISA.

Westerm blot (immunoblot) (Figure 50) is a method to identify antibodies against proteins of precise molecular weights. It is widely used as a confirmatory test for HIV-1 antibody following the HIV-1 antibody screen test performed by the ELISA assay. Following separation of proteins by one- or two-dimensional electrophoresis, they are blotted or transferred to a nitrocellulose or nylon membrane followed by exposure to biotinylated or radioisotope-labeled antibody. The antigen under investigation is revealed by either a color reaction or autoradiography, respectively.

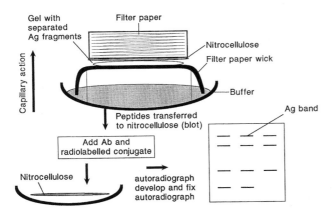

Figure 50. Western blot (immunoblot).

Southern blotting (Figure 51) is a procedure to identify DNA sequences. Following extraction of DNA from cells, it is digested with restriction endonucleases to cut DNA at precise sites into fragments. This is followed by separation of the DNA segments according to size by electrophoresis in agarose gel, denaturation with sodium hydroxide, and transfer of the single-stranded DNA to a nitrocellulose membrane by blotting. This is followed by hybridization with an

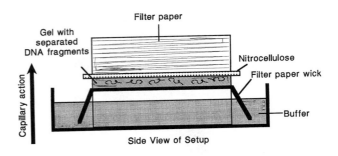

Figure 51. Southern blotting.

^{35}S- or ^{32}P-radiolabeled probe of complementary DNA. Alternatively, a biotinylated probe may be used. Autoradiography or substrate digestion identifies the location of the DNA fragments that have hybridized with the complementary DNA probe. Specific sequences in cloned and in genomic DNA can be identified by Southern blotting. Whereas DNA anaylsis is referred to as Southern blot, RNA analysis is referred to as a northern blot, and protein analysis is referred to as a western blot. A northwestern blot is one in which RNA-protein hybridizations are formed.

Northern blotting (Figure 52) is a method to identify specific mRNA molecules. Following denaturation of RNA in a particular preparation with formaldehyde to cause the molecule to unfold and become linear, the material is separated by size through gel electrophoresis and blotted onto a natural cellulose or nylon membrane. This is then exposed to a solution of labeled DNA "probe" for hybridization. This step is followed by autoradiography. Northern blotting corresponds to a similar method used for DNA fragments which is known as Southern blotting.

In situ **hybridization** (Figure 53) is a technique to identify specific DNA or RNA segments in cells or tissues or in viral plaques or colonies of microorganisms. DNA in cells or tissue fixed on glass slides must be denatured with formamide before hybridization with a radiolabeled or biotinylated DNA or RNA probe that is complementary to the tissue mRNA being sought. Proof that the probe has hybridized to its complementary strand in the tissue or cell under study must be by autoradiography or enzyme-labeled probes depending on the technique being used.

The **polymerase chain reaction (PCR)** (Figure 54) is a technique to amplify a small DNA segment beginning with as little as 1 ug. The segment of double stranded DNA is placed between two oligonucleotide primers through many cycles of amplification. Amplification takes place in a thermal cycler with one step occurring at a high temperature in the presence of DNA polymerase that is able to withstand the high temperature. Within a few hours, the original DNA segment is transformed into millions of copies. PCR methodology has been used for multiple purposes including detection of HIV-1, the prenatal diagnosis of sickle cell

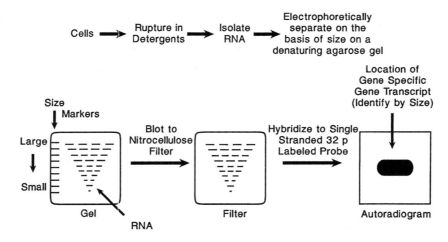

Figure 52.   Northern blotting.

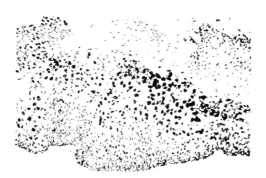

Figure 53.   *In situ* hybridization.

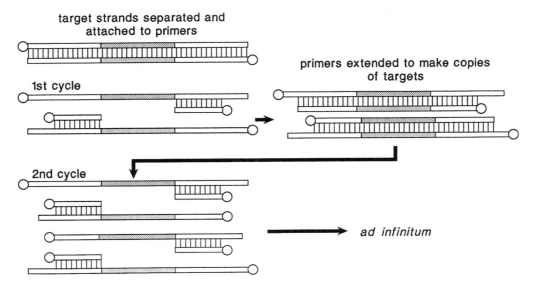

Figure 54.   Polymerase chain reaction (PCR).

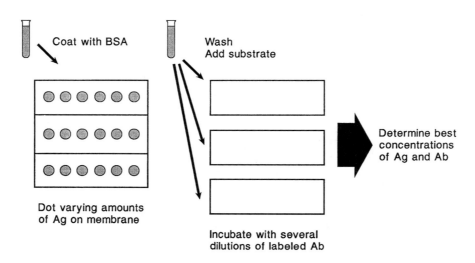

DNA Sequence

			Protein Sequence

DRI   CAG CT|T AAG TTT GAA TGT CAT TTC| TTC AAT   Glu Leu Lys Phe Glu Cys His Phe Phe Asn

1001

DR2(15 and 16)   --- |-c- --- AGG --G --- ---| --- --- ---   - Pro - Trp Val - - - - -

1002

Figure 55.   DNA Fingerprinting.

Coat with BSA

Wash
Add substrate

Dot varying amounts
of Ag on membrane

Incubate with several
dilutions of labeled Ab

Determine best
concentrations
of Ag and Ab

Figure 56.   Dot-blot.

anemia, gene rearrangements in lymphoproliferative disorders, among numerous other applications. The technique is used principally to prepare enough DNA for analysis by available DNA methods. The polymerase chain reaction has a 99.99% sensitivity. The technique is widely used in DNA diagnostic work.

DNA Fingerprinting (Figure 55) is a method to demonstrate short, tandem-repeated highly specific genomic sequences known as minisatellites. There is only a 1 in 30 billion probability that two persons would have the identical DNA fingerprint. It has greater specificity than restriction fragment length polymorphism (RFLP) analysis. Each individual has a different number of repeats. The insert-free wild-type M13 bacteriophage identifies the hypervariable minisatellites. The sequence of DNA that identifies the differences is confined to two clusters of 15 base pair repeats in the protein III gene of the bacteriophage. The specificity of this probe, known as the Jeffries probe, renders it applicable to parentage testing, human genome mapping and forensic science.

RNA may also be split into fragments by an enzymatic digestion followed by electrophoresis. A characteristic pattern for that molecule is produced and aids in identifying it.

Dot-blot (Figure 56) is a rapid hybridization method to partially quantify a specific RNA or DNA fragment found in a specimen without the need for a northern or Southern blot. After serially diluting DNA, it is "spotted" on a nylon or nitrocellulose membrane and then denatured with NaOH. It is then exposed to a heat-denatured DNA fragment probe that is believed to be complementary to the nucleic acid fragment whose identity is being sought. The probe is labeled with ^{32}P or ^{35}S. When the two strands are complementary, hybridization takes place. This is detected by autoradiography of the radiolabeled probe. Enzymatic, nonradioactive labels may also be employed.

Multilocus probes (MLPs) (Figure 57) are probes used to identify multiple related sequences distributed throughout each person's genome. Multilocus probes may reveal as many as 20 separate alleles. Because of this multiplicity of alleles, there is only a remote possibility that two unrelated persons would share the same pattern, i.e., about 1 in

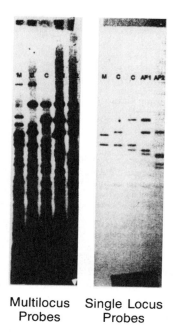

Multilocus   Single Locus
Probes   Probes

Figure 57. Multilocus probes (MLPs).

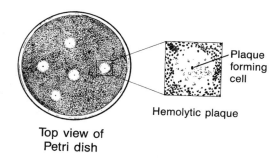

Figure 58. Plaque forming cell (PFC).

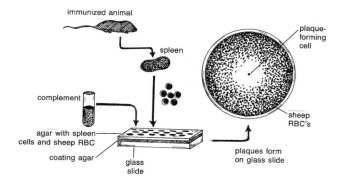

Figure 59. Jerne plaque assay.

30 billion. There is, however, a problem in desciphering the multibanded arrangement of minisatellite RFLPs as it is difficult to ascertain which bands are allelic. Mutation rates of minisatellite HVRs remain to be demonstrated, but are recognized occasionally. Used in resolving cases of disputed parentage.

The **plaque forming cell (PFC) assay** (Figure 58) is a technique for demonstrating and enumerating cells forming antibodies against a specific antigen. Mice are immunized with sheep red blood cells (SRBC). After a specified period of time, a suspension of splenic cells from the immunized mouse is mixed with antigen (SRBC), and spread on a suitable semisolid gel medium. After or during incubation at 37°C, complement is added. The erythrocytes which have anti-SRBC antibody on their surface will be lysed. Circular areas of hemolysis appear in the gel medium. If viewed under a microscope, a single antibody-forming cell can be identified in the center of the lytic area. There are several modifications of this assay since some antibodies other than IgM may fix complement less efficiently. In order to enhance the effects, an antiglobulin antibody called developing antiserum, is added to the mixture. The latter technique is called indirect PFC assay.

The **Jerne plaque assay** (Figure 59) is a technique to identify and enumerate cells synthesizing antibodies. Typically, spleen cells from a mouse immunized against sheep red blood cells are combined with melted agar or agarose in which sheep erythrocytes are suspended. After gentle mixing, the suspension is distributed into Petri plates where it gels. This is followed by incubation at 37°C, after which complement is added to the dish from a pipette. Thus, the

sheep erythrocytes surrounding cells secreting IgM antibody against them are lysed by the added complement, producing a clear zone of hemolysis resembling the effect produced by β hemolytic streptococci on blood agar. IgG antibody against sheep erythrocytes can be identified by adding anti-IgG antibody to aid lysis by complement. Whereas modifications of this method have been used to identify cells producing antibodies against a variety of antigens or haptens conjugated to the sheep red cells, it can also be used to ascertain the immunoglobulin class being secreted.

The **reverse plaque method** (Figure 60) is a method to identify antibody-secreting cells regardless of their antibody specificity. The antibody-forming cells are suspended in agarose and incubated at 37°C in petri plates with sheep red cells coated with protein A. Anti-Ig and complement are also present. Cells synthesizing and secreting immunoglobulin become encircled by Ig-anti-Ig complexes, then link to protein A on the erythrocyte surfaces. This leads to hemolytic plaques (zones of lysis). Thus, any class of immunoglobulin can be identified by this technique through the choice of the appropriate antibody.

Nylon wool (Figure 61) is a material that has been used to fractionate T and B cells from a mixture of the two based upon the tendency for B cells to adhere to the nylon wool whereas the T cells pass through. B cells are then eluted from the column. Previously, tissue typing laboratories used this technique to isolate B lymphocytes for MHC class II

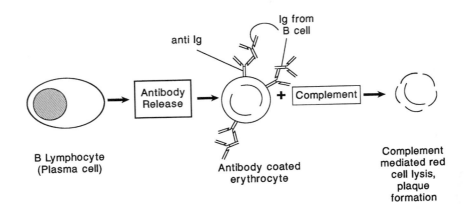

Figure 60.   Reverse plaque method.

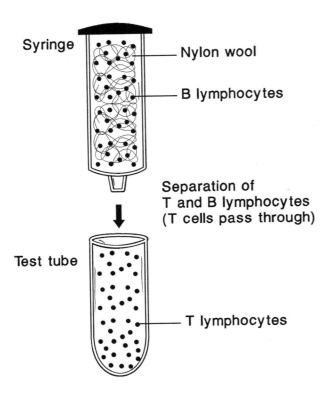

Figure 61.   Nylon wool.

(B cell) typing. Magnetic beads have replaced nylon wool for lymphocyte T and B cell separation.

Microlymphocytotoxicity (Figure 62) is a widely used technique for HLA tissue typing. Lymphocytes are separated from heparinized blood samples by either layering over Ficoll-hypaque, centrifuging and removing lymphocytes from the interface or with beads. After appropriate washing, these purified lymphocyte preparations are counted and aliquots dispensed into microtiter plate wells containing predispensed quantities of antibody. When used for human histocompatibility (HLA) testing, antisera in the wells are specific for known HLA antigenic specificities. After incu-

bation of the cells and antisera, rabbit complement is added and the plates are again incubated. The extent of cytotoxicity induced is determined by incubating the cells with trypan blue, which enters dead cells, staining them blue, but leaves live cells unstained. The plates are read by using an inverted phase contrast microscope. A scoring system from 0 to 8 (where 8 implies > 80% of target cells killed) is employed to indicate cytotoxicity. Most of the sera used to date are multispecific, as they are obtained from multiparous females who have been sensitized during pregnancy by HLA antigens determined by their spouse. Monoclonal antibodies are being used with increasing frequency in tissue typing. This technique is useful to identify HLA-A, HLA-B and HLA-C antigens. When purified B cell preparations and specific antibodies against B cell antigens are employed, HLA-DR and HLA-DQ antigens can be identified.

In the **cell-mediated lympholysis (CML)** test, responder (effector) lymphocytes are cytotoxic for donor (target) lymphocytes after the two are combined in culture (Figure 63). Target cells are labeled by incubation with ^{51}Cr at 37°C for 60 minutes. Following combination of effector and target cells in tissue culture, the release of ^{51}Cr from target cells injured by cytotoxicity represents a measure of cell-mediated lympholysis. The cell-mediated lympholysis (CML) assay gives uniform results, is relatively simple to perform, and is rather easily controlled. The effector cells can result from either *in vivo* sensitization following organ grafting or can be induced *in vitro*. Variations in effector to target cell ratios can be employed for quantification.

In the **mixed lymphocyte reaction (MLR)**, lymphocytes from potential donor and recipient are combined in tissue culture (Figure 64). Each of these lymphoid cells has the ability to respond by proliferating following stimulation by antigens of the other cell. In the one-way reaction, the donor cells are treated with mitomycin by irradiation to render them incapable of proliferation. Thus, the donor antigens stimulate the untreated responder cells. Antigenic specificities of the stimulator cells that are not present in the

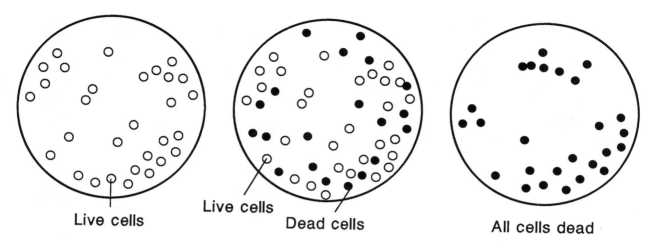

Figure 62.   Microlymphocytotoxicity.

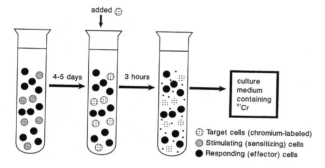

Figure 63.   Cell-mediated lympholysis (CML) test.

responder cells lead to blastogenesis of the responder lymphocytes. This leads to an increase in the synthesis of DNA and cell division. This process is followed by introduction of a measured amount of tritiated thymidine, which is incorporated into the newly synthesized DNA. The mixed lymphocyte reaction usually measures a proliferative response and not an effector cell killing response. The test is important in bone marrow and organ transplantation to evaluate the degree of histoincompatibility between donor and recipient. Also called mixed lymphocyte culture.

Lymphocyte transformation (Figure 65) is an alteration in the morphology of a lymphocyte induced by antigen, mitogen, or virus interacting with a small, resting lymphocyte. The transformed cell increases in size and in amount of cytoplasm. Nucleoli develop in the nucleus, which becomes lighter staining as the cell becomes a blast. Epstein-Barr virus transforms B cells, and the human T cell leukemia virus transforms T cells.

Macrophage/monocyte inhibitory factor (MIF) (Figure 66) is a substance synthesized by T lymphocytes in response to immunogenic challenge that inhibits the migration of macrophages. MIF is a 25kD lymphokine. Its mechanism

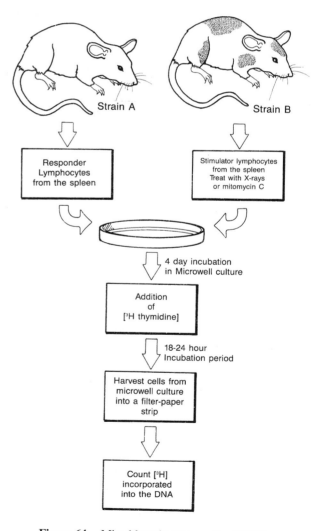

Figure 64.   Mixed lymphocyte reaction (MLR).

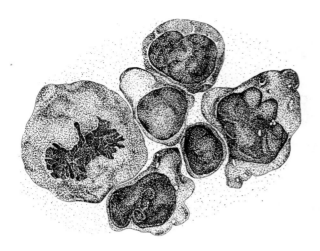

Figure 65.   Lymphocyte transformation.

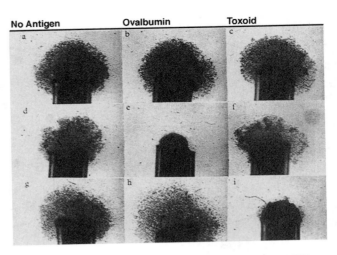

Figure 66.   Macrophage/monocyte inhibitory factor (MIF).

of action is by elevating intracellular cAMP, polymerizing microtubules and stopping macrophage migration. MIF may increase the adhesive properties of macrophages, thereby inhibiting their migration. The two types of the protein MIF include one that is 65kD with a pI of 3–4 and another that is 25kD with a pI of approximately 5.

Panning (Figure 67) is a technique to isolate lymphocyte subsets through the use of petri plates coated with monoclonal antibodies specific for lymphocyte surface markers. Thus, only lymphocytes bearing the marker being sought bind to the petri plate surface.

Immunobeads (Figure 68) are minute plastic spheres with a coating of antigen (or antibody) and may be aggregated or agglutinated in the presence of the homologous antibody. Immunobeads are used also for the isolation of specific cell subpopulations such as the separation of B cells from T cells that is useful in class II MHC typing for tissue transplantation.

The **nitroblue tetrazolium (NBT) test** (Figure 69–70) is an assay that evaluates the hexose monophosphate shunt in phagocytic cells. The soluble yellow dye, nitroblue tetrazolium, is taken up by neutrophils and monocytes during phagocytosis. In normal neutrophils, the NBT is reduced by

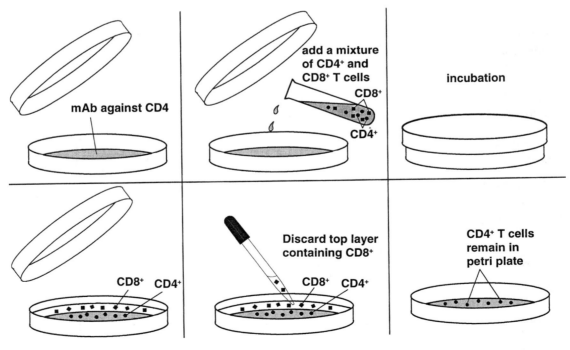

Figure 67.   Panning.

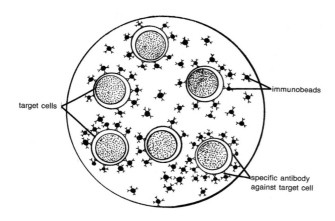

Figure 68. Immunobeads.

enzymes to insoluble, dark blue formazan crystals within the cell. Neutrophils from patients with chronic granulomatous disease are unable to reduce the nitroblue tetrazolium. The ability to reduce NBT to the insoluble deep blue formazan crystals depends on the generation of superoxide in the neutrophil being tested.

Light scatter refers to light dispersion in any direction which can be useful in the study of cells by flow cytometry (Figures 71–85). A cell passing through a laser beam both absorbs and scatters light. Fluorochrome staining of cells permits absorbed light to be remitted as fluorescence. Forward angle light scatter permits identification of a cell in flow and determination of its size. If higher angle light scatter is added, some specific cell populations may also be identified. Light scatter measured at 90° to the laser beam and flow stream yields data on cell granularity or fine structure. Light scatter depends on such factors as cell size and shape, cell orientation in flow, cellular internal structure, laser beam shape and wavelength, the angle of light collection.

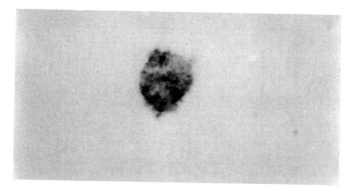

Figure 69. Nitroblue tetrazolium test (NBT).

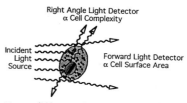

Forward Scatter—diffracted light
▾ Related to cell surface area
▾ Detected along axis of incident light in the forward direction

Side Scatter—reflected and refracted light
▾ Related to cell granularity and complexity
▾ Detected at 90° to the laser beam

Figure 71. Properties of Forward Scatter Light (FSC) and Side Scatter Light (SCC) are measured by observing how light disperses when a laser hits the cell.

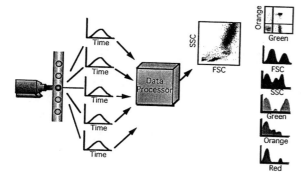

Figure 70. Flow cytometry is a fast, accurate, way to measure multiple characteristics of a single cell simultaneously. These objective measurements are made one cell at a time, at routine rates of 500 to 4000 particles per second in a moving fluid stream. A flow cytometer measures relative size (FSC), relative granularity or internal complexity (SSC) and relative florescence. Use of three color flow cytometry to analyze blood cells by size, cytoplasmic granularity and surface markers labeled with different fluorochromes

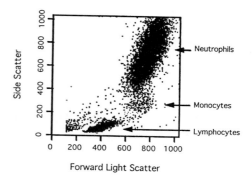

Figure 72. Each dot represents the data from one cell. The bigger the cell, the larger the FSC signal and the farther to the right the dot will appear on the x-axis. The more complex or granular the cell the larger the SCC signal and the higher it will appear on the y-axis. It is possible to discern lymphocytes, monocytes, and neutrophils in this plot.

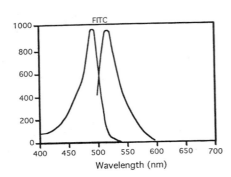

Figure 73. The absorption and emission spectra for the FITC fluorochrome are shown here. The peak absorption is around 488 nm and the peak emission is around 530 nm.

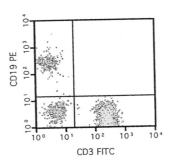

Figure 74. The FITC-positive cells fall in the lower right quadrant and PE-positive cells fall in the upper left quadrant. Cells that are positive for both FITC and PE are in the upper right quadrant.

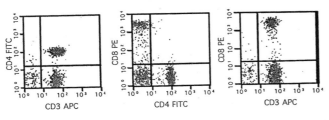

Figure 75. These are three bivariate plots displaying FITC, PE, and APC stained lymphocytes. All CD3+ cells are stained with APC, the CD4+ cells are stained with FITC, and the CD8+ cells are stained with PE.

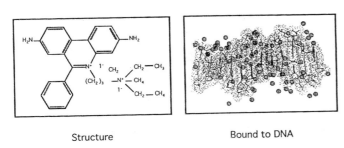

Figure 76. DNA content can be quantified by use of the fluorescent dye propidium iodide (PI). The dye intercalates between the base pairs to stain double stranded nucleic acids. The amount of DNA that PI binds is proportional to the DNA content.

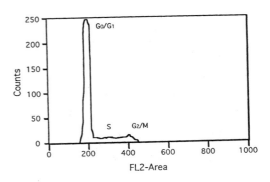

Figure 77. Staining DNA with PI and analyzing the sample by flow cytometer permits the percentage of cells in each phase of the cell cycle to be determined.

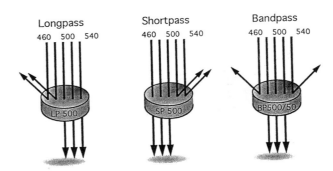

Figure 78. The specificity of an optical detector for a particular fluorescent dye is optimized by placing a filter in front of the detector which allows a narrow range of wavelengths to pass through the filter.

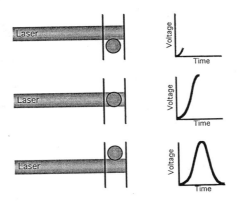

Figure 79. A pulse is created when the particle enters the laser beam and starts to scatter light. The highest point of the pulse occurs when the particle is in the center of the beam, and the maximum amount of scatter is achieved. As the particle leaves the laser, the pulse comes back down to the baseline.

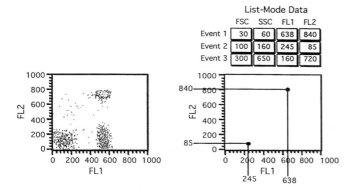

Figure 80.   Useful information can be obtained with the dot plot by determining the percentages for each population.

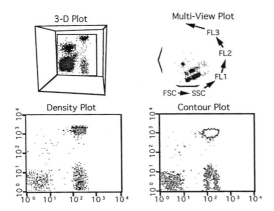

Figure 81.   The different plots can be used to clearly display and analyze populations of interest.

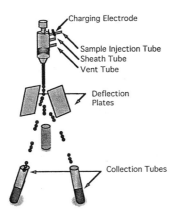

Figure 82.   Particles can be isolated after they are passed through the laser by charging the particle. Depending on the charge, the particle will either travel to the left or right sort tube, repelled or attracted toward the charged plate. All non-charged particles travel to the waste.

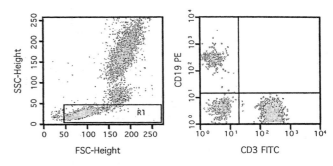

Figure 83.   The conventional method for identifying lymphocyte subsets is light-scatter gating. The lymphocytes are gated, markers are set using a two-color isotype control, then subsequent immunofluorescence analyses of the remaining files are completed.

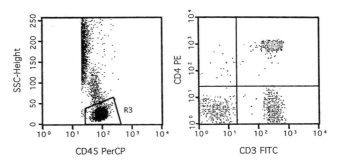

Figure 84.   Unlike traditional methods of light-scatter gating where lymphocyte gate purity and recovery are concerns, TriTEST allows the CD45-positive lymphocyte population to be gated, providing unambiguous identification.

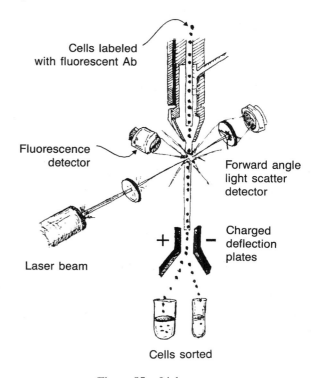

Figure 85.   Light scatter.

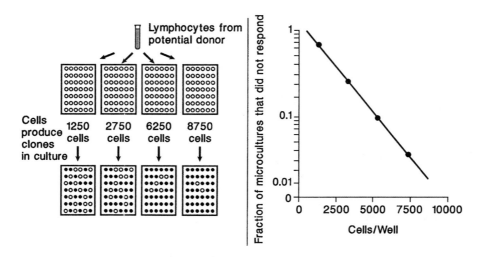

Figure 86.   Limiting dilution.

Limiting dilution (Figure 86) is a method of preparing aliquots that contain single cells through dilution to a point where each aliquot contains only one cell. The apportionment of cells by this method follows the Poissonian distribution, which yields 37% of aliquots without any cells and 63% with one or more cells. This technique can be used to estimate a certain cell's frequency in a population. For example, it may be employed to approximate the frequency of helper T lymphocytes, cytotoxic T lymphocytes or B lymphocytes in a lymphoid cell suspension or to isolate cells for cloning in the production of monoclonal antibodies.

The **prick test** (Figure 87) is an assay for immediate (IgE-mediated) hypersensitivity in humans. The epidermal surface of the skin on which drops of diluted antigen (allergen) are placed is pricked by a sterile needle passed through the allergen. The reaction produced is compared with one induced by histamine or another mast cell secretogogue. This test is convenient, simple, rapid and produces little discomfort for the patient in comparison with the intradermal test. It may even be used for infants.

The **patch test** (Figure 88) is an assay to determine the cause of skin allergy, especially contact allergic (type IV) hypersensitivity. A small square of cotton, linen or paper impregnated with the suspected allergen is applied to the skin for 24 to 48 hours. The test is read by examining the site 1 to 2 days after applying the patch. The development of redness (erythema), edema and formation of vesicles constitutes a positive test. The impregnation of tuberculin into a patch was used by Vollmer for a modified tuberculin test. There are multiple chemicals, toxins and other allergens that may induce allegic contact dermatitis in exposed members of the population.

The **Dick Test** (Figure 89) is a skin test to signify susceptibility to scarlet fever in subjects lacking protective antibody against the erythrogenic toxin of *Streptococcus pyogenes*. A

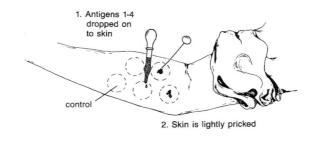

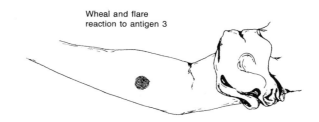

Figure 87.   Prick test.

minute quantity of diluted erythrogenic toxin is inoculated intradermally in the individual to be tested. An area of redness (erythema) occurs at the injection site 6 to 12 hours following inoculation of the diluted toxin in individuals who do not have neutralizing antibodies specific for the erythrogenic toxin and who are therefore susceptible to scarlet fever. A heat-inactivated preparation of the same diluted toxin is also injected intradermally in the same individual as a control against nonspecific hypersensitivity to other products of the preparation.

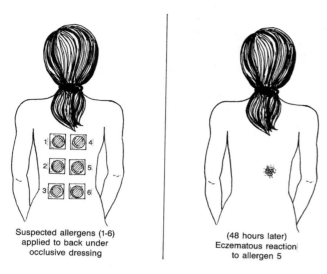

Suspected allergens (1-6) applied to back under occlusive dressing

(48 hours later) Eczematous reaction to allergen 5

Figure 88.   Patch test.

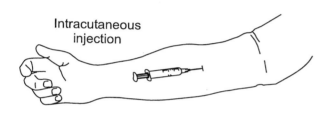

Intracutaneous injection

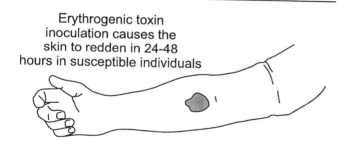

Erythrogenic toxin inoculation causes the skin to redden in 24-48 hours in susceptible individuals

Figure 89.   Dick test.

The **Rebuck skin window** (Figure 90) is a clinical method for assessing chemotaxis used *in vivo*, by making a superficial abrasion of the skin which is then covered with a glass slide. This is removed several hours later, air dried and stained for leukocyte content.

The **radioallergosorbent test (RAST)** (Figure 91) is a technique to detect specific IgE antibodies in a patient's serum. This solid phase method involves binding of the allergen-antigen complex to an insoluble support such as dextran particles or Sepharose®. The patient's serum is then passed over the allergen-support complex which permits specific IgE antibodies in the serum to bind with the allergen. After washing to remove nonreactive protein, radiolabeled anti-human IgE

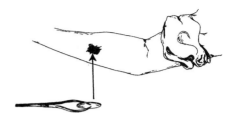

Figure 90.   Rebuck skin window.

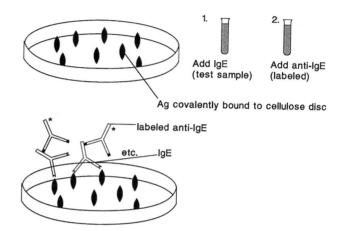

Ag covalently bound to cellulose disc

labeled anti-IgE

etc.   IgE

Figure 91.   Radioallergosorbent test (RAST).

antibody is then placed in contact with the insoluble support where it reacts with the bound IgE antibody. Both the allergen and the anti-IgE antibody must be present in excess for the test to be accurate. The amount of radioactivity on the beads is proportional to the quantity of serum antibody that is allergen-specific.

The **radioimmunosorbent test (RIST)** (Figure 92) is a solid phase radioimmunoassay to determine the serum IgE concentration. A standard quantity of radiolabeled IgE is added to the serum sample to be assayed. The mixture is then combined with Sephadex® or Dextran beads coated with antibody to human IgE. Following incubation and washing, the quantity of radiolabeled IgE bound to the beads is measured. The patient's IgE competes with the radiolabeled IgE or antibody attached to the beads. Therefore, the decrease in labeled IgE attached to the beads compared to a control in which labeled IgE combines with the beads without competition represents the patient's serum concentration of IgE. The radioallergosorbent test by comparison assays IgE levels reactive with a specific allergen.

The **paper radioimmunosorbent test (PRIST)** (Figure 93) is a technique to assay serum IgE levels. It resembles the radioimmunoabsorbent test except that filter paper discs impregnated with anti-human IgE is used in place of Sephadex discs.

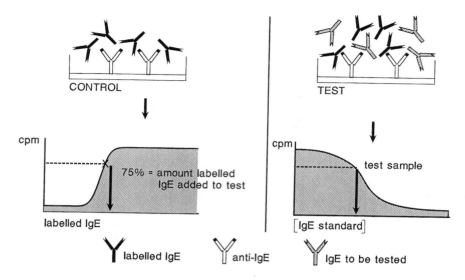

Figure 92.   Radioimmunosorbent test (RIST).

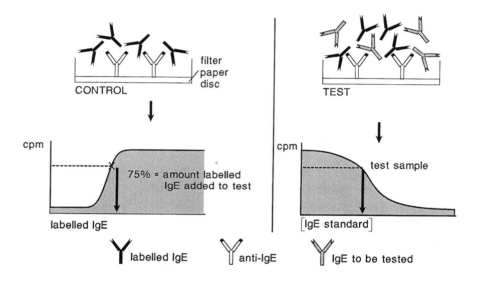

Figure 93.   Paper radioimmunosorbent test (PRIST).

The **immunoradiometric assay (IRMA)** (Figure 94) is a quantitative method to assay certain plasma proteins based on a "sandwich" technique using radiolabeled antibody, rather than radiolabeled hormone competing with hormone from a patient in the radioimmunoassay (RIA).

Immune elimination (Figure 95) refers to accelerated removal of an antigen from the blood circulation following its interaction with specific antibody and elimination of the antigen-antibody complexes through the mononuclear phagocyte system. A few days following antigen administration, antibodies appear in the circulation and eliminate the antigen at a much more rapid rate than occurs in non-immune individuals. Splenic and liver macrophages express Fc receptors that bind antigen-antibody complexes as well as complement receptors which bind those immune complexes that have already fixed complement. This is followed by removal of immune complexes through the phagocytic

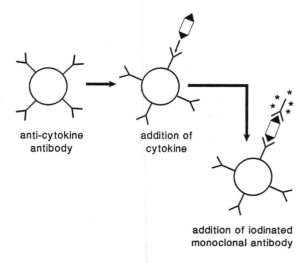

Figure 94.   Immunoradiometric assay (IRMA).

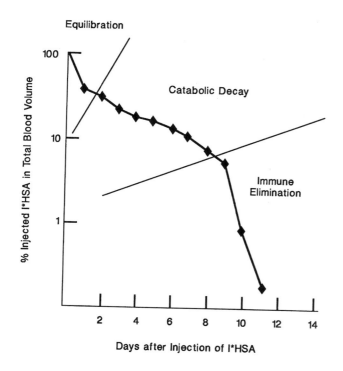

Figure 95. Immune elimination.

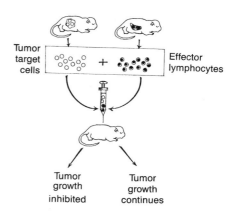

Figure 96. Winn assay.

action of mononuclear phagocytes. Immune elimination also describes an assay to evaluate the antibody response by monitoring the rate at which a radiolabeled antigen is eliminated in an animal with specific (homologous) antibodies in the circulation.

The **Winn assay** (Figure 96) is a method to determine the ability of lymphoid cells to inhibit the growth of transplantable tumors *in vivo*. Following incubation of the lymphoid cells and tumor cells *in vitro*, the mixture is injected into the skin of X-irradiated mice. Growth of the transplanted cells is followed. T lymphocytes that are specifically immune to the tumor cells will inhibit tumor growth and provide information related to tumor immunity.

Transgenic mice (Figure 97) carry a foreign gene that has been artificially and deliberately introduced into their germ line. The added genes are termed transgenes. Fertilized egg pronuclei receive microinjections of linearized DNA. These are placed in pseudopregnant female oviducts and development proceeds. About one-fourth of the mice that develop

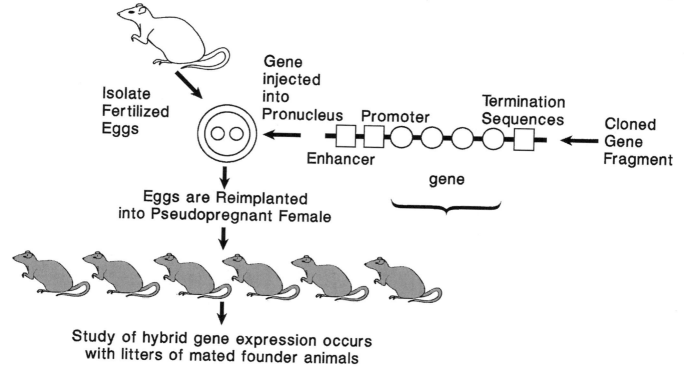

Figure 97. Transgenic mice.

following injection of several hundred gene copies into pronuclei are transgenic mice. Transgenic mice have been used to study: genes not usually expressed *in vivo*, alterations in genes that are developmentally regulated to express normal genes and cells where they are not usually expressed. Transgenic mice are also used to delete certain populations of cells with transgenes that encode toxic proteins. They are highly significant in immunologic research.

Index

I

Q

R

S